Speroff & Darney's
Clinical Guide to
Contraception

Sixth Edition

Jeffrey T. Jensen, MD, MPH
Leon Speroff Endowed Professor and Vice-Chair for Research
Department of Obstetrics and Gynecology
Oregon Health & Science University
Portland, Oregon

Mitchell D. Creinin, MD
Professor and Director of Family Planning
Department of Obstetrics and Gynecology
University of California, Davis
Sacramento, California

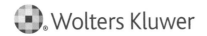
Wolters Kluwer

Philadelphia · Baltimore · New York · London
Buenos Aires · Hong Kong · Sydney · Tokyo

Acquisitions Editor: Chris Teja
Development Editor: Eric McDermott
Editorial Coordinator: Ingrid Greenlee
Marketing Manager: Phyllis Hitner
Production Project Manager: Barton Dudlick
Design Coordinator: Joseph Clark
Manufacturing Coordinator: Beth Welsh
Prepress Vendor: SPi Global

Sixth Editon

Library of Congress Cataloging-in-Publication Data
Names: Jensen, Jeffrey T., editor. | Creinin, Mitchell D., editor. | Speroff, Leon, 1935- Speroff & Darney's clinical guide to contraception.
Title: Speroff & Darney's clinical guide to contraception / [edited by] Jeffrey T. Jensen, Mitchell Creinin.
Other titles: Clinical guide to contraception
Description: Sixth edition. | Philadelphia : Wolters Kluwer, [2020] | Preceded by A clinical guide to contraception / Leon Speroff, Philip D. Darney. 5th ed. c2011. | Includes bibliographical references and index. | Summary: "This practical handbook is a current, reliable, and readable guide to today's contraceptive options. The authors provide the essential information that clinicians and patients need to choose the best contraceptive method for the patient's age and medical, social, and personal characteristics. The book concisely covers all available drugs and devices. Each contraceptive method is covered in a single chapter that includes history of the contraceptive, method of action, pharmacology (when applicable), contraindications, and use"—Provided by publisher.
Identifiers: LCCN 2019028071 | ISBN 9781975107284 (paperback)
Subjects: MESH: Contraception—methods
Classification: LCC RG136.2 | NLM WP 630 | DDC 618.1/8—dc23
LC record available at https://lccn.loc.gov/2019028071

RRS1908

CONTENTS

Contributors   vii
Foreword   ix
Preface   xi

1 Contraception, Population, and the Environment 1
Jeffrey T. Jensen, MD, MPH and Mitchell D. Creinin, MD

2 Reproduction and Hormonal Contraception ... 31
Mitchell D. Creinin, MD and Jeffrey T. Jensen, MD, MPH

3 Interpreting Evidence and Creating Clinical Guidance on Contraception 67
Kathryn M. Curtis, PhD and David Hubacher, PhD, MPH

4 Permanent Contraception 93
Aileen M. Gariepy, MD, MPH and Rebecca H. Allen, MD, MPH

5 Implantable Contraception 133
Rebecca Cohen, MD, MPH and Stephanie B. Teal, MD, MPH

6 Intrauterine Contraception 169
Jennifer E. Kaiser, MD, MSCI and David K. Turok, MD, MPH

7 Combined Hormonal Contraception 219
Carolyn L. Westhoff, MD, MSc, Surya Cooper, MD, MPH, and Ian Joseph Bishop, MD, MPH

8 Injectable Contraception 301
Laneta Dorflinger, PhD and Sharon L. Achilles, MD, PhD

9 Shorter-Acting Progestin-Only Contraception ... 329
Elizabeth Micks, MD, MPH and Sarah Prager, MD, MAS

10 Barrier Methods of Contraception 341
Jill Schwartz, MD, MPH

11 Behavioral Methods of Contraception 367
Anita L. Nelson, MD and Diana Crabtree Sokol, MD, MSc

12 Emergency Contraception 397
Nora Doty, MD, MSCR and Alison Edelman, MD, MPH

13 The History of Contraception .... ⊕
Leon Speroff, MD and Philip D. Darney, MD, MSc

Index   413

⊕ Indicates material is available online through the eBook bundled with this text. Please see the inside front cover for eBook access instructions.

CONTRIBUTORS

Sharon L. Achilles, MD, PhD
Assistant Professor
Department of Obstetrics, Gynecology
   and Reproductive Sciences Director
University of Pittsburgh
Pittsburgh, Pennsylvania

Rebecca H. Allen, MD, MPH
Associate Professor
Department of Obstetrics, Gynecology
   and Medical Science
Warren Alpert Medical School of Brown
   University
Providence, Rhode Island

Ian Joseph Bishop, MD, MPH
Assistant Professor
Chief of Family Planning
University of Miami/Jackson Memorial
   Hospital
Miami, Florida

Rebecca Cohen, MD, MPH
Assistant Professor
Department of Obstetrics and Gynecology
University of Colorado Anschutz Medical
   Campus
Aurora, Colorado

Surya Cooper, MD, MPH
Assistant Chief
Division of Family Planning
Santa Clara Valley Medical Center
San Jose, California

Mitchell D. Creinin, MD
Professor and Director of Family
   Planning
Department of Obstetrics and Gynecology
University of California, Davis
Sacramento, California

Kathryn M. Curtis, PhD
Women's Health and Fertility Branch
Division of Reproductive Health
Centers for Disease Control and
   Prevention
Atlanta, Georgia

Philip D. Darney, MD, MSc
Distinguished Research Professor
   Emeritus
Department of Obstetrics, Gynecology
   and Reproductive Sciences
University of California, San Francisco
San Francisco, California

Laneta Dorflinger, PhD
Distinguished Scientist and Director
Contraceptive Technology Innovation
FHI 360
Durham, North Carolina

Nora Doty, MD, MSCR
Assistant Professor
Department of Obstetrics and Gynecology
Hackensack Meridian Health Jersey Shore
   University Medical Center
Neptune, New Jersey

Alison Edelman, MD, MPH
Professor and Director of Family Planning
Department of Obstetrics and Gynecology
Oregon Health & Science University
Portland, Oregon

Aileen M. Gariepy, MD, MPH
Associate Professor
Section of Family Planning
Department of Obstetrics, Gynecology,
   and Reproductive Sciences
Yale School of Medicine
New Haven, Connecticut

David Hubacher, PhD, MPH
Epidemiologist
Contraceptive Technology Innovation
   Department
FHI 360
Durham, North Carolina

Jeffrey T. Jensen, MD, MPH
Leon Speroff Endowed Professor and
   Vice-Chair for Research
Department of Obstetrics and Gynecology
Oregon Health & Science University
Portland, Oregon

Jennifer E. Kaiser, MD, MSCI
Assistant Professor
Department of Obstetrics and
  Gynecology
University of Utah
Salt Lake City, Utah

Elizabeth Micks, MD, MPH
Assistant Professor
Department of Obstetrics and
  Gynecology
University of Washington
Seattle, Washington

Anita L. Nelson, MD
Professor Emeritus
Department of Obstetrics and
  Gynecology
University of California, Los Angeles
Los Angeles, California

Sarah Prager, MD, MAS
Professor and Director of Family
  Planning
Department of Obstetrics and
  Gynecology
University of Washington
Seattle, Washington

Jill Schwartz, MD, MPH
Professor
Department of Obstetrics and
  Gynecology
CONRAD/Eastern Virginia Medical
  School
Norfolk, Virginia

Diana Crabtree Sokol, MD, MSc
Assistant Professor
Department of Obstetrics, Gynecology
  and Reproductive Sciences
McGovern Medical School at The
  University of Texas Health Science
  Center at Houston
Houston, Texas

Leon Speroff, MD
Professor Emeritus
Department of Obstetrics and Gynecology
  Oregon Health & Science University
Portland, Oregon

Stephanie B. Teal, MD, MPH
Professor and Chief of Family Planning
Department of Obstetrics and Gynecology
University of Colorado Anschutz Medical
  Campus
Aurora, Colorado

David K. Turok, MD, MPH
Associate Professor and Chief of Family
  Planning Division
Department of Obstetrics and Gynecology
University of Utah
Salt Lake City, Utah

Carolyn L. Westhoff, MD, MSc
Sarah Billinghurst Solomon Professor of
  Reproductive Health and Director
Division of Family Planning & Preventive
  Services
Department of Obstetrics and Gynecology
Columbia University
New York, New York

viii

FOREWORD

I t is with a sense of pride that we write an introduction for this new edition. We are proud of the progress that has been made with the development and utilization of contraceptive methods, as documented in these pages. This impressive accomplishment reflects human initiative, creativity, and dedication. This work has made a major contribution to greater freedom, equality, and opportunity for people all around the world to lead healthier, happier lives.

This edition is written by members of the Society of Family Planning (SFP) and graduates of the Fellowship in Family Planning. SFP was founded 20 years ago by the leaders of the Fellowship to advance family planning science and education. SFP and the Fellowship have played important roles in the translation of scientific knowledge into daily living and the application of research findings into clinical practice. This book presents the work of these subspecialists, and much of the cited evidence was published by Fellowship graduates and SFP members.

We believe the "new look" of this sixth edition demonstrates scientific progress and academic maturity in a field that, when we wrote the first edition 27 years ago, attracted the interest of only a few obstetrician/gynecologists and had more investigators and publications from outside the United States than within it. This new edition attests to the immense growth of family planning science in the United States and the talent of a new generation of scholars.

The fruits of this labor are not without current challenges. Family planning is a critical element in preserving our planet's resources for future generations, and therefore, contraception is both a personal and a social responsibility. We have developed effective and safe contraceptives, but affordable access and creation of more effective and acceptable methods continue to be worldwide challenges. These are challenges that cry out for responses from governments, from medical organizations, and from each one of us individually.

The purpose of the information in these pages is to teach and guide medical and nursing clinicians at all levels (students, residents, practitioners, and academicians) in the understanding and use of modern contraception. It is this evidence-based knowledge that best equips each of us to battle the misinformation that is often used in the attempts to limit reproductive choices. We thank the editors and the authors of this book for their effort and dedication in bringing this sixth edition to publication.

Leon Speroff, MD
Professor Emeritus
Department of Obstetrics and Gynecology
Oregon Health & Science University
Portland, Oregon

Philip D. Darney, MD, MSc
Distinguished Research Professor Emeritus
Department of Obstetrics, Gynecology and Reproductive Sciences
University of California, San Francisco
San Francisco, California

PREFACE

We were honored to be asked by our mentors and friends, Leon Speroff and Philip D. Darney, to take over as editors of this classic reference. As direct and early mentees of Leon and Phil, their encouragement to serve as their successors for this book was incredibly gracious and humbling. These two important leaders provided significant research and thought to the field of family planning, creating a foundation of knowledge that has allowed the specialty to advance and flourish. As we finish this new edition, we acknowledge and thank Leon and Phil, and other giants in our field that have offered support and guidance throughout our careers. For all of their work, in collaboration with many of their peers that have also provided us with support and guidance throughout our careers, we are eternally grateful.

We took on the task of updating this classic reference with several goals. First, the field has changed rapidly since publication of the fifth edition in 2011, justifying a thorough update. Next, as the Fellowship in Family Planning has continued to grow, graduating more fellows every year it made sense to provide a comprehensive textbook for the field. As the discipline has matured, rather than simply updating the chapters ourselves, we believed that engaging more voices to tell the story would provide greater expertise. Accordingly, we invited senior experts in the field to revise chapters, and many recruited junior colleagues as coauthors. Finally, we have worked with the publisher to develop a strategy for electronic updates between future editions to ensure chapters remain up-to-date.

One of our biggest challenges in meeting these objectives has been maintaining the readability and clarity of the original book. For this, we express gratitude to Leon and Phil. They told the story of modern contraception as contemporaries relating the major events and product introduction with first-hand perspective. How could we improve on a work of the masters? Because much of the original work centered on the development of oral contraception, we could see that a simple revision of the chapters seemed inadequate. So, we decided that a complete reorganization made more sense. Chapters have undergone comprehensive revision and include the latest references.

This edition begins with an overview of the need for and current use of contraception (Chapter 1), followed by a review of reproduction and hormonal therapy (Chapter 2) and interpretation of the evidence and medical eligibility requirements (Chapter 3). We then present methods in the order of typical-use effectiveness, in keeping with best counseling practice. We intentionally do not include a chapter on abortion, as other texts cover this in detail, and abortion is not a method of contraception. Getting this terminology correct deserves emphasis. Abortion is the interruption of established pregnancy and only occurs following implantation. None of the methods described in this book have an abortifacient mechanism. Despite the rhetoric and confrontational politics, the science on this is clear. We also did not separate postabortion and postpartum contraception into separate chapters as was done with prior editions; rather, we include a section within the discussion of each contraceptive method on its use during these important times in women's lives.

To keep the text concise, we removed much of background on the history of individual methods from each chapter, summarizing this in Chapter 1 and expanding the development of synthetic steroids in Chapter 2. We could not improve on the original history written by Drs. Speroff and Darney, so have consolidated this into a supplemental chapter that is available in the eBook.

The cover reflects our deep appreciation for the beauty and complexity of reproductive biology. Consider that the amazing reproductive success of humans actually requires contraception as a solution for sustainability of our species. Women carry the bulk of the risk and burden of reproduction, so the choice of whether, when, and how often to become pregnant rests with them. Across the world, and in the United States, this basic right remains under siege. The idea of life beginning with conception presents an interesting thought experiment. Sexual reproduction in most organisms reflects continuity and not a beginning or end. The alternation of generations between haploid (one set of chromosomes) and diploid (two sets or one pair) forms exemplifies that continuity. On the cover, the queen bee possesses a diploid genome. The workers surrounding her are all haploid and incapable of reproduction. Mosses and lichens are examples of plants in which the dominant form we see is haploid, and the diploid form inconspicuous. In humans, our haploid generation exists as sperm and oocytes. Nothing ever begins or ends.

The same is true with this book. This edition is not a beginning or the end. We hope this work benefits those new to the field and becomes a valuable tool for learning. We welcome suggestions for improvement. As stated in the epilogue to the fifth edition: "And so we reach our final paragraph. We do so with optimism. This book documents, within a tick of planet Earth's time, tremendous accomplishments in contraception. These accomplishments reflect initiative, creativity, and dedication. There is reason to believe, as we do, that these human traits will persevere, and we will meet the contraceptive challenges of the future."

Let us move forward with optimism backed with facts and solid science. Our work remains a vital tool toward a sustainable, verdant, respectful, and inclusive world.

Jeffrey T. Jensen, MD, MPH
Leon Speroff Endowed Professor and Vice-Chair for Research
Department of Obstetrics and Gynecology
Oregon Health & Science University
Portland, Oregon

Mitchell D. Creinin, MD
Professor and Director of Family Planning
Department of Obstetrics and Gynecology
University of California, Davis
Sacramento, California

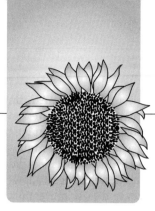

1

Contraception, Population, and the Environment

Jeffrey T. Jensen, MD, MPH and
Mitchell D. Creinin, MD

As we write this chapter, the earth's population of humans exceeds 7.7 billion. Hopefully our collective work in family planning will slow the rate of population growth over the next 80 years. If we are lucky, population will peak at just over 11 billion around 2100 before gradually stabilizing in the next millennium.[1] Achieving this goal will require us to rapidly reach a global total fertility rate (TFR) of about 2.1, a feat yet to be accomplished. We remain optimistic in pursuit of this objective as the consequences of failure are unacceptable.

Our global predicament provides evidence that Earth struggles to adequately support the current population of humans. Our ecologic footprint is not just a "catchphrase." Around 1970, the resources used daily surpassed what the Earth can maintain, meaning that Earth cannot generate resources fast enough to support our growing population.[2] Already, nations compete vigorously for the finite resources of Earth, with rising nationalism, war, famine, and migration of displaced people symptoms of massive inequality of wealth and resource distribution.[3] How will we respond to the addition of 4 billion more inhabitants by the end of the current century?

Fifty years ago, Professor Paul Ehrlich of Stanford University alerted the world to the hazards of unchecked population growth through publication of *The Population Bomb*.[4] Widely criticized as Malthusian sensationalism, his predications of exponential population growth leading to food insecurity and environmental degradation generally reflect the dilemma of our modern world.[3] In a 2014 commentary, Ehrlich urged greater activism: "All scientists should be allocating a significant amount of effort to promoting understanding and action to deal with the major drivers of environmental destruction: population growth, overconsumption by the rich, and socioeconomic inequity."[5]

Our calling of voluntary family planning represents the most humane and respectful approach to a better collective future. As health care providers, we have the privilege of delivering family planning services, and the obligation to advocate for universal access to these tools. This chapter provides a framework to view the history of contraception as a story of human innovation, dignity, and empowerment of women.

Human Population Growth

About 2 million years ago, hominoids began their ascent on the African continent and spread throughout the world.[6] By 40,000 years ago, the era of speciation of humans had ended, with only *Homo sapiens* remaining.[7] World population remained stable, and in balance with resource consumption throughout most of human history. The total human population did not reach 1 billion until about 1827.[8] Due to emerging technologies allowing exploitation of new energy resources, advances in disease prevention, and improved agricultural techniques, we reached the second billion in less than 100 years. Population growth advanced quickly to 7 billion within the next 100 years **(Table 1.1)**.[8]

It is useful to consider that the technologic achievements associated with this explosive population growth have been appreciated only recently. A 1966 report commissioned by NASA placed these gains into perspective.[9] If we consider that eight hundred human lifespans of only 60 years span roughly 50,000 years, then among the generations of those 800 people:

- 650 spent their lives in caves.
- Only the last 70 had a truly effective means of communication.
- Only the last 6 saw the printed word.
- Only the last 4 could measure time with precision.
- Only the last 2 used an electric motor.
- The majority of items that make up our current world were developed within the lifespan of the 800th person.

Correcting for one or two additional generations from 1966 does not make the comparison less remarkable today!

Peak Population

We live in the era of peak population. While we cannot change history, our collective actions today influence the future, and history should inform our

Table 1.1 Human Population Growth

Year	Population (Billions)	Years to Reach the Next Billion
1827	1	93
1920	2	37
1957	3	17
1974	4	13
1987	5	12
1999	6	12
2011	7	?

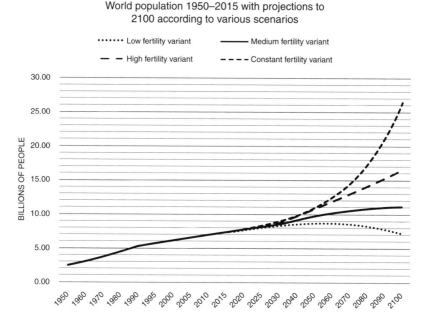

Figure 1.1 World population 1950–2015 with projections to 2100 according to various total fertility rate (TFR) scenarios. Medium fertility variant: assumes total fertility in all countries averages 1.85 children/woman; high fertility variant, 0.5 children above the medium variant; low fertility variant, 0.5 children below medium variant; constant fertility variant, assumes fertility remains at 2000–2005 estimate for each country. (Source: United Nations, Department of Economic and Social Affairs, Population Division (2017). World Population Prospects: The 2017 Revision, Volume I: Comprehensive Tables (ST/ESA/SER.A/399).)

actions and decisions. **Figure 1.1** illustrates four potential scenarios based on the United Nations Population Division's 2017 revised estimates of fertility patterns projected to 2050. The TFR provides an estimate of the number of children born per woman in a population calculated using current age-specific fertility rates. The TFR provides a better estimate of fertility and population growth than do crude birth rates, as it accounts for birth per woman over the reproductive lifespan. A TFR of 2.1 is considered replacement fertility.[1]

The United Nations Population Division's "medium" fertility estimate assumes that the TFR converges gradually to 1.85 in all nations over the next 50 years, but we can consider this more simply as reflecting replacement fertility (i.e., TFR 2.1). "High" and "low" fertility estimates assume an average of one-half a child more (or less); since women don't have half children, think of this as more women having a third child or more having only one or none. The global impact of the "third child" scenario cannot be understated. While population is expected to peak at around 11.4 billion in 2100 before stabilizing under the medium estimate, under the high fertility scenario (TFR 2.6), we reach 11 billion by 2050 and surge to over 16 billion by 2100 with no end in sight.[10] In fact, even with a rapid decline to low fertility (TFR 1.6), population would continue to grow through midcentury with a peak of around 9 billion achieved in 2050 followed by a gradual decline by the end of the century to a population similar to today. Some economists believe economic growth and wealth require an ever-expanding population and place faith that scientific and technologic advances will provide for all. We feel science is better equipped to deal with the potential challenges of transition to a smaller population where people share scarce resources more equitably.

Worldwide, fertility has declined in most developed nations, with a TFR below replacement in China, Eastern and Western Europe, Canada, Japan, Australia, and New Zealand.[1] The TFR in the United States has hovered around 2.1 for the last few years largely due to higher fertility rates among recent migrants.[11] However, since 2016, the TFR in the United States has been below 2.0, most recently 1.78.[12] Today, almost all population growth occurs in developing countries. Ten countries will account for more than half of the world's projected population over the next 30 years (ordered by their expected contribution to global growth): India, Nigeria, the Democratic Republic of Congo, Pakistan, Ethiopia, the United Republic of Tanzania, the United States, Uganda, Indonesia, and Egypt. The United Nations Population Division estimates that by 2050, 90% of the total population of earth will live in less developed nations.[1]

The consequences of this demographic transition will affect all aspects of our modern lives. A growing literature links population growth and environmental decline to war, famine, terrorism, and human migration.[13] Over the last 20 years, between 3 and 4 million people each year migrated for economic reasons from low- and middle-income nations to high-income countries.[1] Those who remained behind in the poorest nations face environmental and political challenges that threaten their daily existence.

A bulging youth population drives future population growth in less developed nations. In Africa, for example, 60% of the population is less than 25 years old.[1] Poverty and limited opportunity for a better future in poor nations provide fertile ground for civil unrest and recruitment of terrorists. The fact that the population surge occurring in the poorest nations coincides with declining fertility and overconsumption in rich nations compounds the difficulty. A lack of opportunity in poor nations fuels resentment and contributes to war, terrorism, and displaced people. The surge in migrants to rich nations and clash of cultures has given rise to xenophobic nationalist regimes in many countries, including the election of Donald Trump in the United States.

The history of our era will be the story of how the minority of earth's inhabitants living in rich nations will either share or deny earth's finite resources to the majority of inhabitants living in poor nations. The unrelenting pressure of future population growth only intensifies our challenge. Unfortunately, the politics of population growth and income inequality interfere with discussion of population policies. For this reason, many environmental and social justice advocates hesitate to prioritize family planning as a policy objective. This thinking fails to consider our fragile and inter-connected earth. Both rich and poor nations have a responsibility to limit family size and future population growth. The world can sustain neither unchecked consumption in rich nations nor high fertility in poor nations.

Population and the Environment

In a 1971 paper published in *Science*,[14] Paul Ehrlich and John Holdren pro-vided a useful formula linking environmental impact to population:

$$I = P \times A \times T$$

where:

I = environmental impact
P = population size
A = affluence (a measure of consumption)
T = technology (a measure of energy use to support the affluence)

This formula allows us to compare the relative environmental impact of different states. Rich nations like the United States, with high affluence and wasteful energy policies and a relatively large population size, have the greatest overall global environmental impact. In rich nations with stable populations, a dual strategy of embracing policies that reduce both the **T** (such as substituting renewable energy for coal) and **A** (changing the ethos to "enough" rather than "more") diminishes overall impact. While poor nations such as India with low per capita affluence and energy use have a compara-tively lower global impact, we cannot neglect the contribution of a large and growing population. Understandably, citizens of poor nations aspire to gain the wealth common in rich nations, and as income rises, so does energy use and consumption. Even small gains in **A** and **T** contribute greatly to **I** with large and growing populations. Moreover, migrants to the United States and Europe from poor regions understandably seek to consume at North American and European levels, increasing global **I** even faster.

As biologists, we see a world of finite resources under significant stress at our current population under siege by a global economic policy that assumes human ingenuity will continue to provide for any number of humans. This ingenuity hypothesis faces an enormous test in the coming decades. Without population growth, at current rates of economic growth, China is projected to outpace the United States in use of all resources by 2035, consuming roughly two thirds of the world's production of grain and meat.[15] China is not the only nation seeking a bigger piece of the global resource pie. Will we see global cooperation or conflict as nations vigor-ously compete for earth's limited resources?

The wild-card effects of global warming and degradation of ecosystem services contribute further to our concerns about overpopulation. A recent assessment of the impact of rising temperatures on global yields of major crops predicted that each degree Celsius increase in global mean temperature would, on average, reduce global yields of wheat by 6.0%, rice by 3.2%, maize by 7.4%, and soybean by 3.1%.[16] The overuse of aquifers and competition for freshwater sources also threaten agricultural productivity.[17]

The only variable that will reduce **I** under all scenarios is reduction in **P**. We cannot overemphasize the importance of voluntary contraception and global family planning policies as the most humane and practical approach to a just and peaceful future for our grandchildren. The Centers for Disease Control and Prevention (CDC) recognized the importance of these issues, citing family planning as one of the 10 great public health achievements of the 20th century.[18]

History of Contraception

Reproduction represents the most essential biologic activity. All species compete and expand populations to the limits of available resources. Natural constraints limit population growth, and the expression of fertility cycles continually throughout life for most species. Sex is a strong instinctive activity related to a natural need to repopulate the species. Since contraception violates this core hardwired behavior, it is not surprising that strong opinions follow. Unfortunately, many fundamentalist and orthodox religious scholars dismiss contraception as unnatural without painting most of the other medical conveniences that define our modern lives, such as vaccinations, antibiotics, and surgery, with the same brush.

Like all species, early humans struggled to survive. Groups prospered and populations increased during good times. Disease and famine had the opposite effect. Primitive humans lived in balance with the natural world. Births roughly matched deaths during the initial years of human evolution with well-defined gender roles and no need for contraception. The cycle of fertility controlled women's lives and limited opportunities. Pregnancy followed menarche, and prolonged lactational amenorrhea followed birth, until a woman became pregnant again. For these reasons, women in traditional societies experienced relatively few menstrual cycles.[19] Lifespan rarely surpassed the reproductive years due to death in childbirth and natural disease. Although women today may think that having a monthly menses is "natural," human women naturally experience lack of menses due to pregnancy and lactation as well as death prior to menopause.

In contrast, a modern woman will experience hundreds of menstrual cycles over her lifetime. Contemporary women also undergo earlier menarche and start having sexual intercourse at a younger age than past generations. Even though breastfeeding has increased in recent years, the duration of exclusive breastfeeding and related contraceptive lactational amenorrhea contributes minimally to fertility control in the developed world. Therefore, women today require highly effective modern contraceptive methods to limit family size.

The history of contraception is an amazing story of innovation and scientific discovery. Many excellent references, including earlier editions of this textbook, provide details beyond the scope of this chapter. To keep the length of this edition manageable, we have compiled the comprehensive details of the history of various methods from previous editions into a supplemental chapter available in the eBook. Here, we present highlights of this amazing journey.

Contraception Prior to the Modern Era

It is impossible to unlink the history of contraception from the broader history of the women's movement. One cannot overstate the importance of highly effective reversible and permanent methods of contraception as essential tools for female empowerment. We believe that when women control their own fertility, they not only improve their own lives but also improve the lives of their children and their communities. Not surprisingly, those nations that deny women access to family planning and education suffer from poverty and social instability and rank among the most desperate places on earth.[20]

The introduction of the birth control pill in 1960 ushered in the modern era of contraception. Prior to that time, the limited available approaches for fertility regulation included the male condom, the female vaginal diaphragm, and withdrawal. Although intrauterine devices (IUDs) may have an ancient origin, devices designed specifically for contraceptive purposes did not appear until the beginning of the 20th century and did not enjoy extensive use until much later.[21]

Widespread income inequality has existed in the United States for centuries. The rich enjoy access to opportunities, including contraceptive methods, unavailable to poor persons. This great disparity has motivated many activists over the last century, including Margaret Sanger. Sanger worked tirelessly and at great peril to provide information about basic sexuality and contraception options to working-class women and men. Her activities included public speaking and the publications of pamphlets promoting the concept that every woman had a right to be "absolute mistress of her own body." This included the right to practice birth control, a term coined in *The Woman Rebel*, a series published between 1914 and 1915.[22] A 1916 pamphlet *Family Limitation* provided details on techniques for menstrual regulation and the use of vaginal pessaries (diaphragm).[23] These activities put her at risk for prosecution and imprisonment under the Comstock Act of 1873.

The Comstock Act prohibited the circulation of "obscene literature and items deemed for immoral use." Over the years, courts ruled that the Act also prohibited the distribution of contraceptive information and devices. Many states also passed laws that prohibited the use of contraceptives, even among married couples. With reproductive rights still under assault today, it is important to recognize that recognition of a constitutionally protected right to privacy that allowed married couples to use contraception did not occur until the landmark Supreme Court decision of Griswold versus the State of Connecticut in 1965. Eisenstadt versus Baird extended this right to unmarried couples in 1972.[24]

Sanger survived her legal battles and founded the American Birth Control League in 1920, which in turn became the Birth Control Federation of America and eventually Planned Parenthood Federation of America in 1942. But arguably, her most important contributions involved her support for research to improve contraceptive methods through the development of oral contraception and the founding of the Population Council in 1952.

The Birth Control Pill Story and the Development of Hormonal Contraception

Few innovations in human history rival the social impact of the approval of oral contraception in 1960. Our limited space does not allow a complete presentation of this amazing story. We highly recommend *A Good Man*, the biography of Gregory Pincus written by Leon Speroff for a detailed history.[25] We borrow heavily from Speroff's book (with permission) for this summary. More detail on hormonal contraception is also presented in Chapter 2.

In 1951, Sanger introduced Gregory Pincus, a reproductive biologist at the Worcester Institute to Katharine McCormick, the first female graduate of the Massachusetts Institute of Technology and one of the richest women in the world. McCormick first met Sanger in 1917 and had long supported her efforts. Pincus, in collaboration with M.C. Chang, had demonstrated that progesterone could inhibit ovulation. McCormick provided Pincus with funding to develop a birth control pill, spending over $2 million between 1953 and 1958.

A birth control pill required the development of orally active and potent progesterone receptor agonists. The chemist Russell Marker solved the problem of supply by developing the synthetic steps to synthesize progesterone using the Mexican yam as a plant-based substrate. The importance of Marker's work to medicine cannot be overstated. The availability of large quantities of progesterone also provided the substrate for cortisol, in high demand for therapeutic use.

With a reliable source of substrate, G.D. Searle and Syntex, companies that we would call "start-ups" today, became involved in the synthesis of progesterone and cortisol. In collaboration with other chemists, notably Carl Djerassi, the scientists' and companies' cumulative efforts led to the development of novel synthetic highly potent orally active progestins. Pincus and Chang tested these compounds for effects on ovulation in animals and moved ahead with the Searle product norethynodrel.

Pincus recognized the need for a clinical collaborator and recruited Dr. John Rock, chief of gynecology and obstetrics at Harvard, for clinical trials of a birth control pill. Rock was a leading academic gynecologist with a research interest in fertility and menstrual disorders. For more than a decade, gynecologists had recommended porcine luteal extracts for the management of menstrual disorders, and Rock had also performed clinical experiments to understand the effects of newly available pure progesterone and the recently synthesized progestins.

The initial studies Rock performed on his patients demonstrated that progesterone 300 mg/d orally could inhibit ovulation in most women. A 20-day regimen beginning on cycle day 5 was picked to cover the expected time range for ovulation and to allow for normal monthly bleeding. When the progestin norethynodrel became available in 1954, the investigative team switched to this novel agent and found complete ovulation inhibition in 50 women using 10 to 40 mg/d. Interestingly, the initial progestin products were contaminated with about 1% mestranol, a synthetic estrogen known today as the prodrug for ethinyl estradiol (EE). When women subsequently received a purified progestin without mestranol, they experienced irregular bleeding. As a result, estrogen was added back in the final design of the pill to improve cycle control, establishing the principle of cyclic combined hormonal contraception.

For those of us involved in clinical trials today, the pace of progress in the oral contraception development story seems breathtaking. Collaborating with Rock and Pincus, Celso-Ramon Garcia and Edris Rice-Wray, working in Puerto Rico, performed the first contraceptive human trial in 1956. In 1957, Enovid® (mestranol 150 µg/norethynodrel 9.85 mg) was approved by the U.S. Food and Drug Administration (FDA) for the treatment of miscarriages and menstrual disorders and, on June 23, 1960, for contraception. Lower-dose estrogen formulations followed quickly with Ortho-Novum (mestranol 60 µg/norethindrone 10 mg) approved in 1962 and Ovral (EE 50 µg/norgestrel 500 µg) in 1968.

By the late 1960s, concerns regarding an association between use of oral contraceptives and venous thromboembolism (VTE) led to government commissions investigating safety. In 1968, Vessey and Doll[26] reported a ninefold increase in the risk of VTE in users of oral contraceptives compared to nonusers. A follow-up publication by Inman in 1970 documented a clear relationship between estrogen dose and VTE.[27]

In 1969, concerns came to a head with the publication of *The Doctor's Case Against the Pill*. In this controversial book, medical journalist Barbara Seaman combined the testimony of physicians, medical researchers, and women who had used oral contraceptives to build a case against the safety of the Pill and to indict the medical-pharmaceutical establishment that had marketed it. Shortly after publication, U.S. Senator Gaylord Nelson read Seaman's book while he was conducting hearings on the pharmaceutical industry regarding alleged abuses in the use of antibiotics, barbiturates, and tranquilizers. After finishing Seaman's book, he decided to take on the birth control pill as well. The high profile and highly publicized Senate hearings in 1970 attacked the safety of the pill. More than 85% of reproductive age women followed the dramatic hearings.

One needs to put this timing in perspective. The sexual revolution that commenced during the tumultuous 60s was in full swing with new positive and permissive attitudes toward female sexuality and premarital sex, leading to a greater interest in contraception. Over the next few decades, the pharmaceutical industry introduced a number of different formulations of combined pills with novel progestins and lower doses of estrogen with the goal of improving safety and tolerability while maintaining efficacy. More recently, we have seen the introduction of nonoral combined contraceptives (vaginal rings, transdermal patches, and injectables) that provide alternatives to daily administration. We discuss the key details of the pharmacology of combined hormonal contraception in Chapter 2 and management of combined hormonal contraceptive patients in Chapter 7.

Although the 1970 Senate hearings did not ultimately affect oral contraception availability, almost 20% of current users quit taking the pill in response to the reporting. These concerns led many women to turn to the vaginal diaphragm, the method of their mother's generation. For others, the solution was an IUD.

A Brief History of the Intrauterine Device

The modern history of IUD development begins with ring devices developed by Gräfenberg in Germany and Ota in Japan prior to World War II.[21] A resurgence in interest in intrauterine contraception followed the introduction of the pill, with multiple devices introduced in the 1960s and 1970s. In 1962, the Population Council sponsored the first international conference on IUDs in New York City. The most widely used devices in the sixties included the Lippes Loop, invented in 1962, and the Saf-T-Coil introduced in 1968. Both of these plastic frame devices came in multiple sizes and can be classified as inert or nonmedicated IUDs.

A.H. Robbins introduced the Dalkon Shield in 1970, the same year as the Senate hearings on the safety of oral contraceptives. The manufacturer aggressively marketed the device to clinicians using claims that the unique smaller "anatomic" design was particularly suitable for nulliparous women as a first-line contraception choice. In 1970, clinicians screened for gonorrhea by inoculating a chocolate agar bacteriologic plate and incubating this in a high carbon dioxide chamber. Chlamydia was unknown, and no reliable test existed to diagnose "nongonococcal urethritis." Not surprisingly, changes in sexual behavior and a decreased reliance on condoms for pregnancy prevention during this time led to a surge in rates of sexually transmitted infections (STIs).

Within 3 years of market introduction, clinicians recognized a high incidence of pelvic infection (including septic abortion and pelvic abscess) in Dalkon Shield users.[28] Tatum quickly pointed out that a unique design feature of the shield, a removal string that consisted of a multifilament thread enclosed in a plastic sheath, contributed to infection risk as it provided a pathway for bacteria to ascend into the upper genital tract protected from the barrier of cervical mucus.[29] Even though by the midseventies more effective copper-releasing IUDs had been introduced, the fear of infections due to the Dalkon Shield experience tainted all IUDs, and enthusiasm for their use plummeted along with sales. Although subsequent well-designed epidemiologic studies confirmed that the elevated risk of pelvic infections seen with IUDs was confined to users of the Dalkon Shield,[30] other manufactures withdrew their products. By 1984, only the 1-year progesterone-releasing Progestasert® IUD remained on the U.S. market.

The pharmaceutical industry abandoned the copper IUD in the 1980s for corporate business decisions related to concerns for profit and liability, not for medical or scientific reasons. Fortunately, the Population Council continued research investigating copper and hormonal IUDs. These efforts led to the introduction of the Copper T 380A (Paragard®) to the U.S. market in 1988 and the levonorgestrel (LNG) intrauterine system in 2000.

The LARC Revolution

The first development in nondaily hormonal contraception involved the preparation of depot injections of progestins. An intramuscular formulation of medroxyprogesterone acetate was introduced in 1960 in the United States for the treatment of endometrial cancer, and subsequent studies confirmed a long-acting contraceptive effect.[31] Although the FDA did not approve Depo-Provera for the indication of contraception until 1992, clinicians used the preparation off-label for many years prior to this date as a growing literature supported safety and efficacy. A variety of other progestin-only and combined estrogen-progestin injectables have been developed, but none are currently marketed in the United States.

Long-acting reversible contraceptives (LARC methods) provide women with an extended duration of highly effective contraception lasting one year or longer with a single administration. In addition to the groundbreaking work on IUDs, the Population Council also performed the initial studies that led to the introduction of the contraceptive implant.[32] The first device, Norplant®, consisted of six sustained release silicone capsules filled with LNG that provided contraceptive efficacy for 5 years. This highly effective device received initial U.S. approval in 1990 but was withdrawn from the market in 2002. Although litigation related to difficult removals contributed to the business decision to withdraw Norplant, improved devices were already on the horizon. A two-rod LNG system known as Jadelle® (Bayer Healthcare Pharmaceuticals LLC), also developed by the Population Council, was FDA approved in 1996 but never marketed in the United States. However, this system, as well as a Chinese copy of the implant (called Sino-implant II), is widely available around the world.[33] The single-rod etonogestrel implant (Implanon®; Merck Pharmaceuticals) gained worldwide approval in the mid-2000s as a 3-year contraceptive. The single-rod implant greatly reduces the time and difficulty of placement and removal as compared to the older systems.[34] The implant was changed slightly in 2012 with the addition of barium in the capsule to make it radiopaque and introduction of a single-handed inserter. The new capsule is marketed as Nexplanon® or Implanon NXT®.

Why So Few Male Methods?

We often receive questions about the status of male contraception development. Why have no highly effective reversible male options been introduced to the market? The absence of a male method does not reflect a lack of research effort, as male hormonal methods have entered clinical trials, and several highly specific nonhormonal targets have been identified.[35,36] Lack of demand by men or trust by female partners does not explain the absence of a product.[37] Our litigious society provides the best explanation. Pharmaceutical companies have largely shuttered their female and male contraception research and development groups in recent years. While the increasing regulatory burden and high cost associated with bringing a new product to market explain some of this development, costly litigation plays a major role. For example, even though venous and arterial thromboses represent known risks of estrogen-containing contraceptives, rare adverse events have generated billion-dollar lawsuits against drospirenone-containing combined pills and the etonogestrel contraceptive vaginal ring. The fact that the risks associated with pregnancy exceed those associated with female contraceptive methods provides the main product liability defense. Since men do not directly achieve any health benefit through contraception use, a male method would need to have no risks. Due to the near impossible requirement of absolute safety, we do not expect to see a male hormonal or non-hormonal method marketed in the United States in the foreseeable future.

Efficacy of Contraception

Effective counseling of patients requires a thorough understanding of the performance characteristics of contraceptive methods during real-world use. The Merriam-Webster dictionary defines "efficacy" as the power to produce an effect; contrast this with "effectiveness," the product of the desired intended effect. Contraceptive methods differ in their efficacy and the characteristics of use affect their effectiveness. Correct and consistent use of a method leads to maximal efficacy. However, incorrect or inconsistent use of a highly effective method will result in poor effectiveness. When counseling women about contraception choice, clinicians must consider the patients values, attitudes, and beliefs. While we advocate for use of highly effective methods, better cannot be the enemy of good. Correct and consistent use of a least effective method may result in improved effectiveness compared to inconsistent use of a more effective method. Evidence from the Contraception Choice Project supports that the use of structured counseling information that classifies methods according to effectiveness influences decision-making, with more patients picking highly effective LARC methods.[38] Below we present details as to how we assess efficacy and effectiveness of contraceptive methods.

Definition and Measurements

Contraceptive efficacy is generally assessed by measuring the number of unplanned pregnancies that occur during a specified period of exposure to and use of a contraceptive method. The two methods used to measure contraceptive efficacy are the Pearl Index and life-table analysis.

The Pearl Index (PI), created by Raymond Pearl in 1933, is defined as the number of failures per 100 woman-years of exposure.[39] The denominator is the total months or cycles of exposure from the onset of a method until completion of the study, an unintended pregnancy, or discontinuation of the method. The quotient is multiplied by 1,200 if the denominator consists of months or by 1,300 if the denominator consists of 28-day cycles.

Since the failure rates of most methods of contraception decline with duration of use, the PI cannot compare methods with various durations of exposure. For example, the PI for a 6-month study would generally exceed that seen over 24 months. An increase in the PI will also occur due to events such as significant dropout due to adverse events or lost to follow-up that reduce the number of cycles counted in the denominator. This problem occurs commonly during clinical trials, when cycles of exposure are censored by regulatory authorities due to noncompliance with protocol requirements such as failure to complete diary entries, reported use of a condom, or lack of sexual activity. However, these rules do not apply to the occurrence of pregnancy in the same cycle. Thus, the numerator consists of all pregnancies that occur during a study (from initiation through 7 days following product discontinuation), while the denominator only includes compliant cycles with exposure to sexual activity and no use of condoms or other contraceptives. The standards regulatory authorities use to adjudicate cycles have become more rigorous over time, and this has resulted in a trend toward an increase in the PI of many recently approved methods.

The problem of the "creeping" Pearl contributes to the difficulty in comparing the efficacy of recently approved contraceptive methods to older products.[40] For example, a recent phase 3 clinical trial randomized women to receive either an approved EE 20 µg/LNG 100 µg oral contraceptive or an investigational EE/LNG patch. Although the PI for the patch (4.96) and the pill (4.02) were not significantly different, the patch did not receive market approval as the PI was deemed too high.[41] In contrast, the PI reported in the package insert for this same hormonal pill combination approved in 1997 is almost fourfold lower at 0.84. So what are the issues that could contribute to the "creeping" Pearl? Likely, one or more of the following is impacting all studies performed today:

- The agencies require inclusion of a broader population of women in studies today, including women who are obese and younger (<18 years old). Thus, the population characteristics between studies done today and those done decades prior are usually different.
- Studies done in the United States commonly have higher failure rates than those done in Europe or in which a significant proportion of women are from Europe. U.S. women tend to be less compliant, especially in studies using non-LARC products.
- Women who volunteer for phase 3 studies today have different motivations than those of the past. When studies were performed decades ago, contraceptive access in the United States was limited as insurance companies commonly did not pay for these products. Women who accessed studies were highly motivated by the financial reward of accessing effective contraception. Research demonstrated that the

13

financial benefit, largely related to accessing contraception for free, drove women's participation in studies of modern methods.[42] Today, broader coverage of contraceptives means women who strongly desired contraception are not the ones necessarily volunteering for these trials. As such, the motivation to be compliant and prevent pregnancy is likely different today.

To accurately compare methods at various durations of exposure, we use the method of life-table analysis.

Life-table analysis calculates a failure rate for each month of use, allowing a direct comparison of cumulative failure rate for any specific length of exposure. Women who leave a study for any reason other than unintended pregnancy are removed from the analysis, contributing their exposure only until the time of the exit. As most pregnancies occur during the first 6 months of use of a new method, life-table analysis allows a better comparison of early and ongoing risk. Since women typically become better at using any method over time and those most susceptible to failure become pregnant early or discontinue, the remaining group of experienced users contributes more cycles of exposure the longer a study continues, decreasing the overall PI. The use of life-table analysis also allows comparison of studies with variable lengths of exposure. For this reason, one must always consider the overall length of exposure for a study reporting a PI.

Contraceptive Failure

We classify contraceptive failure according to results expected with "perfect" and "typical" use. "Perfect-use" failure is a calculated unreal estimation that reflects method effectiveness under terms of optimal conditions of correct and consistent use, while "typical-use" failure reflects the effectiveness of the method under the usual circumstances that dominate the daily lives of our patients. Perfect-use failure rates are determined in clinical trials, in which the combination of highly motivated subjects and frequent support from the study personnel yields optimum results. Moreover, for the perfect-use calculations, women who did not follow all directions in the protocol are removed from the calculation. Although studies will also calculate "typical-use" rates, the study environment still does not reflect the real world. Typical-use failure rates are more accurately estimated from data on contraception use and pregnancy collected from the periodic U.S. National Survey of Family Growth (NSFG) representative samples, using data from the Guttmacher Institute's Abortion Patient Survey to correct for underreporting of induced abortion. These real-world data provide the basis for summary tables that illustrate perfect and typical-use contraceptive failure in U.S. women.[43] In **Table 1.2**, we have updated these results with newer estimates from the most recent data reported from the 2006–2010 cycle of the NSFG.[44]

The 2006–2010 NSFG analysis demonstrated that 63% of failures occur during the first 6 months of use of most methods. LARC methods provide a

Table 1.2 Perfect and Typical Failure Rate for Contraceptive Methods

Method	Percent of Women Experiencing Pregnancy in the First Year of Use	
	Lowest Expected (Perfect Use)	Typical Use
No method	85	85
Fertility awareness–based methods		15
Standard days	5	12
Two-day method	4	14
Ovulation method	3	23
Natural cycles	1	8
Symptothermal postovulation	0.4	2
Coitally related methods		
Spermicides	16	21
Male condom	2	13
Female condom	5	21
Withdrawal	4	20
Sponge (parous women)	20	27
Sponge (nulliparous women)	9	14
Diaphragm	16	7
Short-acting hormonal methods		
Combined pill	0.3	7
Patch	0.3	7
Vaginal ring/vaginal contraceptive system	0.3	7
Progestin-only pill	0.3	7
Depo-medroxyprogesterone acetate	0.2	4
Long-acting reversible methods		
Copper T380A IUD	0.6	0.8
Levonorgestrel IUS (13.5 mg)	0.3	0.4
Levonorgestrel IUS (19.5 mg)	0.2	0.2
Levonorgestrel IUS (52 mg)	0.1	0.1
Etonogestrel implant	0.1	0.1
Permanent methods		
Female occlusion, partial salpingectomy	0.5	0.5
Female bilateral salpingectomy	0*	0*
Male	0.1	0.15

*Only rare case reports exist of conception without fallopian tubes, resulting in an estimate that so closely approaches nil that a value of zero is assigned to this outcome.
Adapted from **Trussell J,** *Contraceptive Efficacy in Contraceptive Technology*, 21st ed., Ardent Media, Inc., New York, 2018, Table 26-1, pp 844–845.

notable exception, with failures evenly distributed over the duration of use. This difference demonstrates that those methods that require compliance have higher failure rates early in use, whereas those methods that eliminate compliance as a factor for effectiveness result in intermittent and low numbers of failure over time. Users of withdrawal experienced the highest probability of failure (20%) within 1 year, followed by users of the male condom (13%), the pill (7%), and depo-medroxyprogesterone acetate (4%).[43] In contrast, the 12-month probability of failure for LARC methods was 1%.[44] Overall, the risk of failure with condom use declined from 18% in 1995 to 13% in 2006–2010, and the failure risk of hormonal methods dropped from 8% to 6%. This change likely reflects a shift away from use of condoms and short-acting hormonal methods among those women at highest risk for typical-use failure.

While the overall probability of failure decreased for all demographic groups from 1995 to 2006–2010, health disparities remained. Risk factors for contraception failure include parity ≥1, black race or Hispanic ethnicity, and poverty.[44] While age was not associated with an overall risk of contraceptive failure, women ages 25 to 29 using hormonal methods and IUDs experienced higher failure rates than older or younger women. Married and never-married women were less likely to experience contraception failure than cohabiting or formerly married women.

Contraception in the United States

The NSFG provides a representative scientific sampling of contraceptive and reproductive behavior in the United States. The initial cycles of the NSFG surveys were based on personal interviews of a national sample of women 15 to 44 years of age and conducted as periodic surveys in 1973, 1976, 1982, 1988, and 1995. These surveys provided reliable national data on marriage, divorce, contraception, infertility, and the health of women and infants in the United States. The sampling included reproductive age men in the 2002 cycle. Beginning in 2006, the NSFG shifted from a periodic survey to continuous interviewing with periodic presentation of findings. The most current available datasets reflect results from data collected between 2015 and 2017.[45]

Approximately two thirds (65%) of reproductive age U.S. women use some method of contraception, with little difference seen in the overall use prevalence over the last decade. Most of the 35% of women who report nonuse are either seeking pregnancy or are not at risk for pregnancy due a variety of reasons. Notably, and of great interest to our field, over 7% of reproductive age women report both nonuse and heterosexual intercourse within 3 months of the survey date. The incidence of nonuse increased from 5.2% to 7.4% between the 1995 and 2002 sample.[46] Between the 2006–2010 and 2011–2013 samples, we observed an encouraging slight decline in nonuse in at-risk women from 7.7% to 6.9% suggesting that changes in health policy, such as no-cost contraception, might be impacting use.[47]

Unfortunately, nonuse among at-risk women rebounded back up to 7.9% in the most recent sample.[45] The presence of this persistent large group of at-risk nonusers provides strong evidence to support continued efforts to develop novel methods and research directed to better understand the circumstances associated with nonuse.

Among women at risk for unintended pregnancy, about 90% report use of a contraceptive method.[45] Of these, 28.7% reported use of female permanent contraception in 2015–2017, a 3.5% increase from 2011 to 2013. During the same time period, use of LARC methods also increased by over 3% to 10.3%. The gains in use of both LARC and permanent methods support a general increase in LARC use and not simply a shift away from permanent methods among women who have completed desired family size. A separate analysis of use trends using data through 2014 only has shown that most of the increase LARC uptake reflects IUD use; this increased 6% from 2008 to 2014, while implant use grew only 2%.[48] About a third of women using contraceptives report current use of a moderately effective short-acting hormonal method (oral contraceptives, patch, ring, and injectable); pill use dominates this category.[48] However, the overall use prevalence of the pill declined from 15.5% of all U.S. women in 2011–2013 to 12.6% in 2015–2017, a drop of almost 3%. The use of coital methods increased from 2008 to 2014 due to a 3% increase in withdrawal and 1% increase in natural family planning. More research is needed to understand the significance of these changes. **Figure 1.2** details how contraception use patterns have changed in the United States in the 2011–2014 and 2015–2017 NSFG samples.

While we welcome the shift to LARC methods, their increased availability has not decreased nonuse of contraception. The growing use of less effective method such as withdrawal suggests that many women find many available modern methods unacceptable.

Unintended Pregnancy

The proportion of pregnancies considered unintended has declined to 45% in 2011 from 51% in 2008. However, roughly equal proportions of women experiencing an unintended pregnancy will continue the pregnancy or seek abortion.[49] Although race and ethnicity influence the rate of unintended pregnancy, poverty explains the majority of the effect (**Figure 1.3**). We cannot emphasize this point more emphatically. The ratio of unintended pregnancy rates between those women below the poverty level and those 200% above the poverty level has continued to worsen over the last two decades, even with a decline in the overall unintended pregnancy rate. In 1994, the unintended pregnancy rate was 2.6 times higher among women below the poverty level; the ratios were 5.3 in 2008 and 5.6 in 2011. Without a doubt, the broad public availability and use of highly effective contraceptive methods remain our most important tool to reduce the need for abortion. We can hope that the next round of data will show not only a continued decline in unintended pregnancy rates but also a decline in the disparity between those with resources and those with fewer resources.

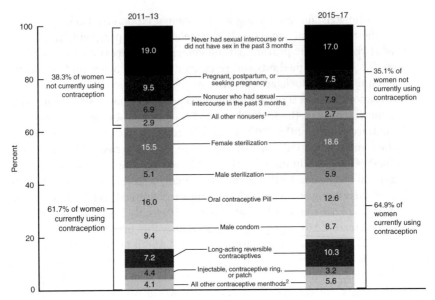

Figure 1.2 Trends in contraceptive use in the United States. Trends in contraceptive use and method mix between 2011–2013 (*left panel*) and 2015–2017 (*right panel*) among reproductive age women (ages 15 to 49 years) in the United States from the National Survey of Family Growth. (Adapted from **Daniels K, Daugherty J, Jones J,** Current contraceptive status among women aged 15–44: United States, 2011-2013, NCHS Data Brief (173):1–8, 2014; Daniels K, Abma JC, Current contraceptive status among women aged 15–49: United States, 2015–2017, NCHS Data Brief (327):1–8, 2018.)

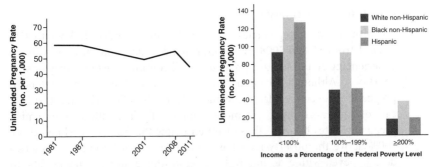

Figure 1.3 Unintended pregnancy in the United States. The rate of unintended pregnancy per 1,000 women and girls 15 to 44 years of age in the United States has declined in recent years (*left panel*), but remains disproportionately high among low-income women (*right panel*). (Adapted from **Finer LB, Zolna MR,** Declines in unintended pregnancy in the United States, 2008-2011, N Engl J Med 374:843–852, 2016.)

Teen Pregnancy

We see signs of encouragement with the most recent national health statistics. Teen pregnancy has declined dramatically over the last decade. Part of this decline may be due to a decrease in the proportion of girls 15 to 19 who report ever having had sexual intercourse from a high of 51% in 1988 to 42% in 2011–2015.[50] However, during the same time period, the proportion of teens reporting use of contraception at last sex increased from 80% to 90%.

The most recent NSFG data also show that the use of contraception at first sex increased from 75% in 2002 to 81% in 2011–2015. And, almost 6% of teens reported use of either an implant or IUD in the 2011–2015 NSFG cycle.[50]

A recent analysis evaluated trends in sexual health and contraceptive use among U.S. high school students reported in the 2013, 2015, and 2017 rounds of the nationally representative Youth Risk Behavior Survey conducted by the CDC.[51,52] This study found that the proportion of U.S. high school students who report ever having had sexual intercourse dropped slowly from 54% to 47% between 1991 and 2013 and then significantly from 47% to 41% in 2015 and reached an all-time low of 40% in 2017. Although this reduction occurred across racial, ethnic, and gender groups, the largest declines were seen among black students. Overall, a greater proportion of male (41%) than female (38%) students report ever having had intercourse. As expected, the proportion of all students reporting intercourse increases from 20% in grade 9 to 57% in grade 12.

The survey also found that contraceptive use varies by racial and ethnic background with 24% of black, 21% of Hispanic, and 12% of white sexually active female students reporting nonuse of any method at last sex in the 2017 sample. Discordantly, only 10% of black, 15% of Hispanic, and 7% of white sexually active male students reported that they or their partner had not used a method the last time they had intercourse suggesting that young men may make convenient assumptions about method use by their partners.[52] This lack of rigorous inquiry about contraceptive use by young men likely surprises no women! While the overall use of prescription contraceptive among female students has remained stable at about 35% since 2013, the prevalence of LARC method use more than doubled (2% to 5%) between 2013 and 2017.

Condom use declined among sexually active high school students from 59% in 2013 to 54% in 2017, and dual-protection use also declined. This trend is alarming, as the CDC issued a press release reporting that rates of STIs climbed during the same time period. Chlamydia infection among women 15 to 24 increased almost 8% from 715,983 cases in 2013 to 771,340 in 2017 (https://www.cdc.gov/nchhstp/newsroom/2018/press-release-2018-std-prevention-conference.html). Effective sex education and contraception counseling of teens should continue to focus on the importance of dual-protection strategies: pregnancy prevention with LARC methods and STI prevention with male or female condoms.

Public Funding of Contraception

The Contraception CHOICE Project was the first large-scale study to provide real-world evidence supporting the enhanced effectiveness of LARC methods at the population level.[53] This large prospective cohort study enrolled over 9,000 reproductive age women in St. Louis, Missouri, from 2007 to 2011 who were willing to use a contraceptive method other than the one they currently were using. Participants received structured counseling regarding various contraceptive methods that emphasized efficacy.[37] Following the counseling, the investigators allowed women to pick any method, and provided the method free of cost. During the study, women could discontinue or change methods according to their preference and with no cost constraints. CHOICE enrolled a high-risk population; 60% of the entire cohort was under 25 (15% under 20), 40% was low income, 58% identified as belonging to racial or ethnic minorities, and 63% reported a prior unintended pregnancy.[54]

The results of the CHOICE study provide useful data for clinicians and policy makers. First, women provided with structured counseling and no-cost contraception tended to pick the most effective LARC methods over moderately effective short-acting hormonal methods and least effective barriers.[53] Prior to implementation of the study, the CHOICE investigators estimated the prevalence of LARC methods at the target recruitment clinics in St. Louis as less than 5%, consistent with the NSFG data from the same period.[50] With removal of the barriers of cost, knowledge, and access, 75% of the CHOICE participants chose a LARC method at baseline enrollment; 46% picked the LNG intrauterine system, 12% a copper IUD, and 17% the etonogestrel implant.[54]

As expected, these impressive rates of LARC uptake resulted in improved outcomes. Women who selected a LARC method were more likely than users of other methods to continue use through 36 months and reported high satisfaction.[55] More importantly, this higher continuation combined with enhanced efficacy resulted in a significantly lower rate of unintended pregnancy among LARC acceptors (0.27/1,000 participant-years) than participants in CHOICE who selected a short-acting hormonal method such as the pill, vaginal ring, or patch (4.55/1,000), **a 22-fold reduction in risk!**[56]

To further illustrate the real-world benefit of removal of barriers to LARC methods, Peipert and coauthors[53] compared repeat abortion rates in the St. Louis region to Kansas City, Missouri, a community of similar size and ethnic profile subject to the same state laws. They observed a 20% decline in the number of abortions in the St. Louis area between 2008 and 2010 compared to no decline in Kansas City or the rest of Missouri and a significant decrease in the number of repeat abortions. Similar conclusions result from comparison of U.S. population data for sexually experienced teens from 2010, with significantly lower rates of teen pregnancy (159/1,000 vs. 34/1,000), birth (94/1,000 vs. 19/1,000), and abortion (42/1,000 vs. 10/1,000) seen in the CHOICE cohort.[57] Interestingly, removing the cost barriers did not remove the discrepancy in unintended pregnancy rates related to low socioeconomic status; women with low socioeconomic status experienced 3.7 unintended pregnancies/100 women-years compared to 1.94 unintended pregnancies/100 women-years among women without low socioeconomic status (adjusted HR of 1.4, 95% CI 1.1 to 1.7).[58]

Even more significant is the real-life evidence from the Colorado Family Planning Initiative (CFPI), which basically took the concept of the CHOICE project and enacted the changes in real clinics. The state of Colorado received support from a private foundation to increase the availability of LARC methods at Title X–funded clinics through provider training, counseling materials, and no-cost provision of LARC methods in 2009. The program proved wildly successful. Within 2 years, family planning caseloads had increased by 23%, and LARC use among women 15 to 24 years old grew from 5% to 19% in this high-risk population. To put these statistics in perspective, only 1 in 170 low-income women received a LARC method through Title X clinics in 2008 prior to the intervention. By 2011, this rate had increased to 1 in 15! Evaluation of key outcomes strongly supports public health benefits and cost savings. Fertility rates decreased by 29% among low-income 15 to 19 and 14% for 20- to 24-year-olds, and abortion rates fell 34% and 18%, respectively. Furthermore, in CFPI counties, the proportion of high-risk births declined by 24% between 2009 and 2011. The state of Colorado noted a 23% reduction in infant WIC program enrollment between 2010 and 2013.[59]

The availability of early results from CHOICE influenced the health care reform debate in 2009, providing key evidence for the provision of no-cost contraception as a mandatory benefit of insurance. The Affordable Care Act (ACA) became law in 2010 and mandated that all marketplace plans cover core sexual and reproductive health services including contraception and maternity care.[60] This requirement has resulted in more comprehensive coverage for everyone. Prior to the ACA, only 12% of individual private insurance plans provided comprehensive maternity coverage, and 79% provided no coverage.[61] While members of some communities have focused on the requirement for mandatory contraception coverage as a reason to oppose the ACA, clinicians understand how these comprehensive requirements support the reproductive life cycle needs of our patients. Elimination of cost sharing for LARC methods with implementation of the ACA has resulted in an increase in LARC uptake according to studies using insurance claims databases,[62] and the surge in LARC use seen in the NSFG data in recent years provides additional evidence for a relationship.

However, these benefits exist in a landscape of very expensive LARC products. A nonprofit pharmaceutical company, Medicines360, introduced a LNG 52 mg IUD at a very low public sector price with the goal of ensuring clinics could afford to stock the product and thereby increase access. Moreover, under the ACA, some states lowered the criteria for a woman to qualify for medical assistance coverage for contraception (called Medicaid expansion), but many did not. In Utah, a state that did not participate in Medicaid expansion, the availability of the lower-cost hormonal IUD to public sector clinics significantly increased uptake.[63]

According to data published by the Guttmacher Institute,[64] 6.2 million women received publicly supported contraceptive services from in the United States during 2015. Of these, 3.8 million obtained services at public Title X clinics, and 2.4 million additional women received services from private clinicians paid for by Medicaid. Almost a third of women obtaining publicly funded contraceptive services receive them through a Planned Parenthood clinic. The importance of publicly funded contraceptive services cannot be overemphasized. In 2015, Title X–funded clinics helped women avert 822,300 unintended pregnancies, preventing 387,200 unplanned births and 277,800 abortions. Without the services provided by Title X–funded clinics, the U.S. unintended pregnancy rate would increase by more than 30%, with the teen rate increasing by over 40%![64]

While equity and social justice arguments alone support the provision of no-cost contraception as a basic right for all women, the policy also makes sound fiscal sense. The investment in publicly funded contraception provides an enormous return, saving an estimated $7 for every $1 spent.[65] Expansion of public funding to include undocumented women also saves money.[66] Provision of no-cost contraception by private insurance saves money too, with estimates of $5 to $10 per member per month.[67] Evidence from the privately funded CFPI provide additional real-world evidence for the success and potential public cost savings associated with no-cost contraception coverage.[59] Despite this, and faced with overwhelming evidence of the success of the program, the Republican-led Colorado legislature voted (2015 Colorado HB 15-1194) against providing the $5 million needed to support the program in FY 2016, the year the grant support ended. We truly live in extraordinary times. Finally, the following year, the legislature did enact the needed funding.

Our lives and practices are busy, and we recognize that thorny political discussions are not everyone's cup of tea. However, we strongly believe in our obligation as clinicians and reproductive health specialists to improve both individual and public health. The acceptance of "alternative facts" degrades humanity and threatens our society. Thirty years ago, support for reproductive rights and the scientific process was overwhelmingly bipartisan. As trusted members of communities, clinicians have an opportunity and obligation to heal society by communicating facts and combating "alternative facts" when it comes to no-cost provision of all methods of contraception from public and private insurance.

While the decline in unintended pregnancy and teen pregnancy demonstrates progress, rates in the United States still exceed those of other highly developed nations. Major American problems include polarizing culture wars and antiscience rhetoric that lead to contradictory and divisive policy. Failure of many states to expand Medicaid with the ACA contributes to disparity across the United States.[68] Religious challenges to mandates for contraception coverage threaten this important social safety net.[60] The enormous diversity of people and the unequal distribution of income and opportunity in the United States only compound the problem. These factors influence the ability of our society to effectively provide education regarding sex and contraception and to effectively make contraception services available to all women.

Induced Abortion in the United States

Women require abortion to manage undesired pregnancies that result from nonuse of contraception or from contraception failure. Many women also request abortion care during otherwise desired pregnancy in the setting of serious maternal medical complications or fetal chromosomal or anatomic problems. Following the legalization of abortion in 1973 with the Roe versus Wade Supreme Court decision, the number of abortions performed in the United States reached a peak in 1981 and has subsequently declined.[69] Whereas many countries have true "national" statistics, the United States has two sources: the CDC and the Guttmacher Institute. The CDC data come from state central health agencies, the District of Columbia, and New York City with missing data from California, Maryland, and New Hampshire.[69] The Guttmacher Institute accesses primary site data with annual surveys from providers and health department data.[70] The Guttmacher data include much of the missing data from the CDC evaluations but still misses some providers due to lack of response or those that have small caseloads. The most recently published abortion statistics from the Guttmacher Institute reflect data collected in 2014. That year, an estimated 926,200 abortions were performed in the United States, 12% fewer than in 2011 with an overall abortion rate of 14.6 per 1,000 women aged 15 to 44.[70] Although many states have passed laws restricting access to abortion, overall and unintended pregnancy rates have also declined during this time interval, obscuring the impact of these legal barriers.

Between 2008 and 2014, the abortion rate for adolescents aged 15 to 19 years declined 46%, the largest of any group.[71] While abortion rates declined for all racial and ethnic groups, rates declined more for non-white women than for non-Hispanic white women. Women with incomes less than 100% of the federal poverty level continue to have the highest abortion rate of all the groups (37/1,000). These data suggest health disparities exist with respect to abortion access and family planning services.

The abortion ratio measures the proportion of pregnancies that end in abortion per 1,000 live births. As the number of unintended pregnancies declines, the proportion of desired pregnancies will increase even if the overall pregnancy rate in a population falls. Forcing women to continue an undesired pregnancy will also reduce the abortion ratio, but we would expect this to occur in the setting of an overall increase in the pregnancy rate. The fact that the abortion ratio declined from 2005 to 2014 (reaching a record low of 186/1,000)[69] in step with declines in the pregnancy rate and an increase in the use of highly effective LARC methods provides additional evidence supporting universal access to no-cost contraception. **Although the need for abortion will never go away, we can reduce the overall number of abortions by increasing access and use of contraception, the focus of this text.**

The Family Planning Health Encounter

The CHOICE project demonstrated that provision of structured information on family planning methods that emphasizes effectiveness, coupled with no-cost availability of the complete range of current options, results in high uptake of LARC methods and a reduction in unintended pregnancy and abortion rates. **Figure 1.4** provides a useful patient education tool that plainly ranks methods in terms of effectiveness and offers tips on correct and consistent use. The LARC and permanent methods are categorized as "most effective," short-acting hormonal and injectable methods as "more effective," and coital methods as "least effective." A comprehensive curriculum for contraception counseling that emphasizes LARC methods is available on the CHOICE project Web site at http://www.larcfirst.com.

While clinicians should emphasize the effectiveness of LARC methods, it is important to recognize that LARCs do not meet the needs of all women. Patient-centered counseling recognizes the priorities and concerns of individual women. While education may help a patient understand and appreciate the ease of use and benefits of LARC methods, women who regret accepting a LARC are at risk for discontinuation, in turn a risk factor for unintended pregnancy. The best method for a woman is the method that she will use consistently and correctly.[72] Noncontraceptive health benefits, such as the reduction in acne or menstrual cycle–related symptoms among users of combined pills, provide strong motivation for use.[73,74]

The family planning visit also provides an opportunity for interaction between clinician and patient to ensure good sexual health. This process includes screening and counseling strategies for the prevention of STIs. A patient visit for contraception is an excellent time for STI screening; if an infection is symptomatic, it should be diagnosed and treated during the same visit in which contraception is requested. As we move away from routine pelvic examinations, screening for chlamydia should be offered to all women under the age of 25 and for those with a recent change in partner status through collection of a self-administered vaginal swab or "dirty" (no antibacterial prep before voiding) urine. Complete and up-to-date details on recommendations for screening and treatment are available through the CDC Web site (https://www.cdc.gov/std/treatment). A positive history for STIs should trigger both screening for asymptomatic infections and counseling for safer sexual practices. Attention should be given to the contraceptive methods that have the greatest influence on the risk of STIs. The use of male condoms provides the only proven protection against STIs including human immunodeficiency virus.

Contraception and Litigation

We live in a litigious society. Clinical trials do not have the power to yield accurate data on the risk of rare adverse events. While estrogen-induced thrombosis represents the primary risk associated with hormonal

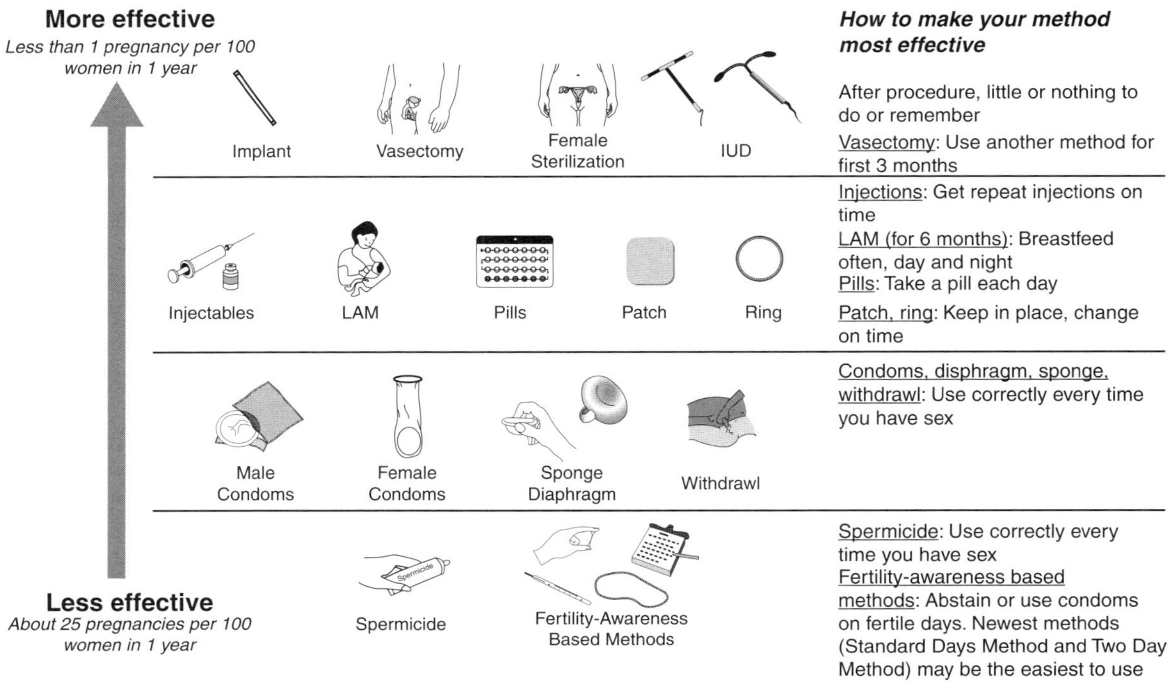

More effective
Less than 1 pregnancy per 100 women in 1 year

Less effective
About 25 pregnancies per 100 women in 1 year

Implant | Injectables

Vasectomy | Female Sterilization | IUD

LAM | Pills | Patch | Ring

Male Condoms | Female Condoms | Diaphragm | Sponge | Withdrawl

Spermicide | Fertility-Awareness Based Methods

How to make your method most effective

After procedure, little or nothing to do or remember
Vasectomy: Use another method for first 3 months

Injections: Get repeat injections on time
LAM (for 6 months): Breastfeed often, day and night
Pills: Take a pill each day
Patch, ring: Keep in place, change on time

Condoms, disphragm, sponge, withdrawl: Use correctly every time you have sex

Spermicide: Use correctly every time you have sex
Fertility-awareness based methods: Abstain or use condoms on fertile days. Newest methods (Standard Days Method and Two Day Method) may be the easiest to use

Figure 1.4 Contraceptive method education chart that ranks methods according to effectiveness. (Adapted from World Health Organization/Department of Reproductive Health and Research (WHO/RHR); Johns Hopkins Bloomberg School of Public Health (JHSPH)/Center for Communication Programs (CCP), Family planning: a global handbook for providers, CCP, Baltimore, 2007. Co-published by WHO. Available from: https://www.fphandbook.org/.)

contraception, multimillion-dollar verdicts and settlements in favor of plaintiffs who have used products as innocent as spermicides have captured national attention. Most recently, we have seen a rash of lawsuits over bizarre subjective side effects associated with microinserts used for permanent contraception with little biologic explanation of causality.[75] Considering the very widespread use of contraception, serious adverse events are extremely uncommon. The CDC has published guidelines for medical eligibility for contraception to assist clinicians as they evaluate the suitability of various methods for women with coexisting medical conditions (see Chapter 3).

Good patient communication and documentation help the clinician avoid litigation. Take a good history to fully evaluate risks and listen to the patient. Patients who sue usually claim there were contraindications or risks not conveyed by the clinician. Back up your discussion of risks, benefits, and alternatives in the medical record.

26

References

1. State of World Population 2019— Unfinished Business: The Pursuit of Rights and Choices For All, United Nations Population Fund. https://www.unfpa.org/swop-2019, 2019.

2. **WWF,** Living Planet Report 2014, In: McLellan R, Iyengar L, Jeffries B, Oerlemans N, eds. Species and Spaces, People and Places, World Wildlife Fund, Switzerland, 2014.

3. **Ehrlich PR, Ehrlich AH,** Future collapse: how optimistic should we be?, Proc Biol Sci 280:20131373, 2013.

4. **Ehrlich PR,** The Population Bomb, Ballantine Books, New York, 1968.

5. **Beattie AJ, Ehrlich PR,** Public outreach: industries depend on biodiversity too, Nature 509:563, 2014.

6. **Stringer C,** The origin and evolution of Homo sapiens, Philos Trans R Soc Lond B Biol Sci 371, 2016.

7. **Higham T, Douka K, Wood R, Ramsey CB, Brock F, Basell L, et al.,** The timing and spatiotemporal patterning of Neanderthal disappearance, Nature 512:306–309, 2014.

8. **Durand JD,** Historical estimates of world population: an evaluation, Popul Dev Rev 3:253–296, 1977.

9. **Lesher RL, Howick GJ,** Assessing Technology Transfer: Scientific and Technical Information Division, Office of Technology Utilization, National Aeronautics and Space Administration, NASA Report No. SP-50671, 1966.

10. **United Nations, Department of Economic and Social Affairs, Population Division,** World Population Prospects: The 2017 Revision, Key Findings and Advance Tables. ESA/P/WP/248. https://esa.un.org/unpd/wpp/Publications/Files/WPP2017_KeyFindings.pdf, 2017.

11. United States Census Bureau, ed, Fertility of Women in the United States: 2016, 2017.

12. **Mathews T, Hamilton BE,** Total Fertility Rates by State and Race and Hispanic Origin: United States, 2017, National Vital Statistics Reports, National Center for Health Statistics, Hyattsville, 2018.

13. **Urdal H,** A Clash of Generations? Youth Bulges and Political Violence, Int Stud Q 50:607–629, 2006.

14. **Ehrlich PR, Holdren JP,** Impact of Population Growth, Science 171:1212–1217, 1971.

15. **Brown LR,** Eco-Economy: Building an Eco-economy for the Earth, Taylor & Francis, 2013.

16. **Zhao C, Liu B, Piao S, Wang X, Lobell DB, Huang Y, et al.,** Temperature increase reduces global yields of major crops in four independent estimates, Proc Natl Acad Sci U S A 114: 9326–9331, 2017.

17. **Johansson EL, Fader M, Seaquist JW, Nicholas KA,** Green and blue water demand from large-scale land acquisitions in Africa, Proc Natl Acad Sci U S A 113:11471–11476, 2016.

18. **Centers for Disease Control and Prevention,** Achievements in public health, 1900–1999: family planning, MMWR Morb Mortal Wkly Rep 48:1073–1080, 1999.

19. **Potts M, Short R,** Ever Since Adam and Eve: The Evolution of Human Sexuality, Cambridge University Press, Cambridge, 1999.

20. **Pandey AK,** Gender Equality, Development and Women Empowerment, 1st ed. Lucknow/ New Delhi, Institute for Sustainable Development/Anmol Publications, 2003.

21. **Huber SC, Piotrow PT, Orlans FB, Kommer G,** Intrauterine devices Series B, Population Reports, 28, 1975.

22. **Sanger M,** Woman Rebel. Republished in Archives of Social History, 1976, 1914.

23. **Sanger M,** Family Limitation. https://books.google.com/ books?id=Z3AzswEACAAJ, 1916.

24. **Cushman C,** Supreme Court Decisions and Women's Rights, CQ Press. https://books.google.com/ books?id=cqnIQwAACAAJ, 2010.

25. **Speroff L,** A Good Man: Gregory Goodwin Pincus: the Man, His Story, the Birth Control Pill, Arnica Pub., 2009.

26. **Vessey MP, Doll R,** Investigation of relation between use of oral contraceptives and thromboembolic disease, Br Med J 2:199–205, 1968.

27. **Inman WH, Vessey MP, Westerholm B, Engelund A,** Thromboembolic disease and the steroidal content of oral contraceptives. A report to the Committee on Safety of Drugs, Br Med J 2:203–209, 1970.

28. **Dawood MY, Birnbaum SJ,** Unilateral tubo-ovarian abscess and intrauterine contraceptive devices, Obstet Gynecol 46:429–432, 1975.

29. **Tatum HJ, Schmidt FH, Phillips D, McCarty M, O'Leary WM,** The Dalkon Shield controversy. Structural and bacteriological studies of IUD tails, JAMA 231:711–717, 1975.

30. **Kessel E,** Pelvic inflammatory disease with intrauterine device use: a reassessment, Fertil Steril 51:1–11, 1989.

31. **Mishell DR Jr, el-Habashy MA, Good RG, Moyer DL,** Contraception with an injectable progestin. A study of its use in postpartum women, Am J Obstet Gynecol 101:1046–1053, 1968.

32. **Diaz S, Pavez M, Robertson DN, Croxatto HB,** A three-year clinical trial with levonorgestrel silastic implants, Contraception 19:557–573, 1979.

33. **Croxatto HB,** Progestin implants, Steroids 65:681–685, 2000.

34. **Ali M, Akin A, Bahamondes L, Brache V, Habib N, Landoulsi S, et al.,** Extended use up to 5 years of the etonogestrel-releasing subdermal contraceptive implant: comparison to levonorgestrel-releasing subdermal implant, Hum Reprod 31:2491–2498, 2016.

35. **Nya-Ngatchou JJ, Amory JK,** New approaches to male non-hormonal contraception, Contraception 87:296–299, 2013.

36. **Grimes DA, Lopez LM, Gallo MF, Halpern V, Nanda K, Schulz KF,** Steroid hormones for contraception in men, Cochrane Database Syst Rev (2):CD004316, 2007.

37. **Glasier AF, Anakwe R, Everington D, Martin CW, van der Spuy Z, Cheng L, et al.,** Would women trust their partners to use a male pill?, Hum Reprod 15:646–649, 2000.

38. **Madden T, Mullersman JL, Omvig KJ, Secura GM, Peipert JF,** Structured contraceptive counseling provided by the Contraceptive CHOICE Project, Contraception 88:243–249, 2013.

39. **Pearl R,** Factors in human fertility and their statistical evaluation, Lancet 222:607–611, 1933.

40. **Trussell J, Portman D,** The creeping Pearl: why has the rate of contraceptive failure increased in clinical trials of combined hormonal contraceptive pills?, Contraception 88:604–610, 2013.

41. **Kaunitz AM, Portman D, Westhoff CL, Archer DF, Mishell DR Jr Rubin A, et al.,** Low-dose levonorgestrel and ethinyl estradiol patch and pill: a randomized controlled trial, Obstet Gynecol 123:295–303, 2014.

27

42. **Hohmann H, Reid L, Creinin MD,** Women's motivation to participate in contraceptive efficacy trials, Contraception 80:270–275, 2009.

43. **Trussell J,** Contraceptive failure in the United States, Contraception 83:397–404, 2011.

44. **Sundaram A, Vaughan B, Kost K, Bankole A, Finer L, Singh S, et al.,** Contraceptive failure in the United States: estimates from the 2006-2010 National Survey of Family Growth, Perspect Sex Reprod Health 49:7–16, 2017.

45. **Daniels K, Abma JC,** Current contraceptive status among women aged 15–49: United States, 2015-2017, NCHS Data Brief (327):1–8, 2018.

46. **Mosher WD, Martinez GM, Chandra A, Abma JC, Willson SJ,** Use of contraception and use of family planning services in the United States: 1982-2002, Adv Data (350):1–36, 2004.

47. **Daniels K, Daugherty J, Jones J, Mosher W,** Current contraceptive use and variation by selected characteristics among women aged 15-44: United States, 2011-2013, NCHS Data Brief (173):1–8, 2015.

48. **Kavanaugh ML, Jerman J,** Contraceptive method use in the United States: trends and characteristics between 2008, 2012 and 2014, Contraception 97:14–21, 2018.

49. **Finer LB, Zolna MR,** Declines in unintended pregnancy in the United States, 2008–2011, N Engl J Med 374:843–852, 2016.

50. **Abma JC, Martinez GM,** Sexual activity and contraceptive use among teenagers in the United States, 2011-2015, Natl Health Stat Report (104):1–23, 2017.

51. **Ethier KA, Kann L, McManus T,** Sexual intercourse among high school students—29 States and United States Overall, 2005-2015, MMWR Morb Mortal Wkly Rep 66:1393–1397, 2018.

52. **Witwer E, Jones RK, Lindberg LD,** Sexual Behavior and Contraceptive and Condom Use Among U.S. High School Students, 2013–2017. Guttmacher Policy Report, Guttmacher Institute. https://doi.org/10.1363/2018.29941, 2018.

53. **Peipert JF, Madden T, Allsworth JE, Secura GM,** Preventing unintended pregnancies by providing no-cost contraception, Obstet Gynecol 120:1291–1297, 2012.

54. **McNicholas C, Madden T, Secura G, Peipert JF,** The contraceptive CHOICE project round up: what we did and what we learned, Clin Obstet Gynecol 57:635–643, 2014.

55. **Diedrich JT, Zhao Q, Madden T, Secura GM, Peipert JF,** Three-year continuation of reversible contraception, Am J Obstet Gynecol 213:662.e1–662.e8, 2015.

56. **Winner B, Peipert JF, Zhao Q, Buckel C, Madden T, Allsworth JE, et al.,** Effectiveness of long-acting reversible contraception, N Engl J Med 366:1998–2007, 2012.

57. **Secura GM, Madden T, McNicholas C, Mullersman J, Buckel CM, Zhao Q, et al.,** Provision of no-cost, long-acting contraception and teenage pregnancy, N Engl J Med 371:1316–1323, 2014.

58. **Iseyemi A, Zhao Q, McNicholas C, Peipert JF,** Socioeconomic status as a risk factor for unintended pregnancy in the contraceptive CHOICE Project, Obstet Gynecol 130:609–615, 2017.

59. **Ricketts S, Klingler G, Schwalberg R,** Game change in Colorado: widespread use of long-acting reversible contraceptives and rapid decline in births among young, low-income women, Perspect Sex Reprod Health 46:125–132, 2014.

60. **Tschann M, Soon R,** Contraceptive coverage and the Affordable Care Act, Obstet Gynecol Clin North Am 42:605–617, 2015.

61. **Jones RK, Sonfield A,** Health insurance coverage among women of reproductive age before and after implementation of the affordable care act, Contraception 93:386–391, 2016.

62. **Carlin CS, Fertig AR, Dowd BE,** Affordable care act's mandate eliminating contraceptive cost sharing influenced choices of women with employer coverage, Health Aff 35:1608–1615, 2016.

63. **Roth LP, Sanders JN, Simmons RG, Bullock H, Jacobson E, Turok DK,** Changes in uptake and cost of long-acting reversible contraceptive devices following the introduction of a new low-cost levonorgestrel IUD in Utah's Title X clinics: a retrospective review, Contraception 98:63–68, 2018.

64. **Frost J, Frohwirth L, Blades N, Zolna M, Douglas-Hall A, Bearak J,** Publicly Funded Contraceptive Services At U.S. Clinics, 2015. Guttmacher Policy Review, 2017.

65. **Frost JJ, Sonfield A, Zolna MR, Finer LB,** Return on investment: a fuller assessment of the benefits and cost savings of the US publicly funded family planning program, Milbank Q 92:696–749, 2014.

66. **Burlone S, Edelman AB, Caughey AB, Trussell J, Dantas S, Rodriguez MI,** Extending contraceptive coverage under the Affordable Care Act saves public funds, Contraception 87:143–148, 2013.

67. **Canestaro W, Vodicka E, Downing D, Trussell J,** Implications of employer coverage of contraception: cost-effectiveness analysis of contraception coverage under an employer mandate, Contraception 95:77–89, 2017.

68. **Johnston EM, Strahan AE, Joski P, Dunlop AL, Adams EK,** Impacts of the Affordable Care Act's medicaid expansion on women of reproductive age: differences by parental status and state policies, Womens Health Issues 28:122–129, 2018.

69. **Jatlaoui TC, Shah J, Mandel MG, Krashin JW, Suchdev DB, Jamieson DJ, et al.,** Abortion surveillance—United States, 2014, MMWR Surveill Summ 66:1–48, 2017.

70. **Jones RK, Jerman J,** Abortion incidence and service availability in the United States, 2014, Perspect Sex Reprod Health 49:17–27, 2017.

71. **Jones RK, Jerman J,** Population group abortion rates and lifetime incidence of abortion: United States, 2008-2014, Am J Public Health 107:1904–1909, 2017.

72. **Rivlin K, Isley MM,** Patient-centered contraceptive counseling and prescribing, Clin Obstet Gynecol 61:27–39, 2018.

73. **Lopez LM, Grey TW, Chen M, Denison J, Stuart G,** Behavioral interventions for improving contraceptive use among women living with HIV, Cochrane Database Syst Rev (8):CD010243, 2016.

74. **Lopez LM, Bernholc A, Chen M, Tolley EE,** School-based interventions for improving contraceptive use in adolescents, Cochrane Database Syst Rev (6):CD012249, 2016.

75. **Walter JR, Ghobadi CW, Hayman E, Xu S,** Hysteroscopic sterilization with essure: summary of the U.S. food and drug administration actions and policy implications for postmarketing surveillance, Obstet Gynecol 129:10–19, 2017.

29

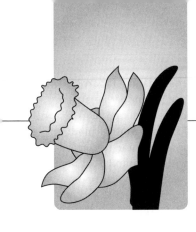

2

Reproduction and Hormonal Contraception

Mitchell D. Creinin, MD and
Jeffrey T. Jensen, MD, MPH

The discovery of the central regulatory role of hormones in reproduction led directly to the development of hormonal contraception. Beginning in 1919, Ludwig Haberlandt, a professor of physiology at the University of Innsbruck, Austria, performed a series of experiment to test the hypothesis advanced by Beard and Prenant that a product of the corpus luteum and placenta prevents ovulation.[1] Haberlandt transplanted ovarian tissue from a pregnant rabbit under the dorsal skin of an adult non-pregnant rabbit and prevented pregnancy. He later showed similar results after injecting extracts of the corpus luteum in mice, calling the approach "hormonal sterilization." The Viennese gynecologist Otfried Otto Fellner reported similar findings when administering ovarian and placental extracts to a variety of animals.[2] Haberlandt proposed injection or oral administration of an agent as a technique for fertility control and collaborated with the Hungarian pharmaceutical company Gedeon Richter in the development of an extract named Infecundin that was never tested in women. Haberlandt's early death of a heart attack in 1932, at age 47, brought an end to this effort, and Fellner disappeared after the annexation of Austria to Hitler's Germany.

Although world events contributed to the delay of these research advances, the limited availability and low potency of natural steroid hormones (SHs) from animal sources presented a more significant obstacle. This chapter tells the story of the breakthroughs leading to the wide availability of synthetic steroids and the development of hormonal contraception. To provide a framework to understand how hormonal contraception works, we first review the normal events that control the reproductive cycle.

Reproductive Endocrinology and Physiology

A complete review of reproductive endocrinology and physiology is beyond the scope of this text. In this section, we summarize the key events that regulate the natural menstrual cycle and explain how hormonal therapy affects these processes to prevent pregnancy.

Steroid Hormones

The term steroid refers to a group of lipid hormones derived from cholesterol. The lipid-like nature of SHs allows them to easily pass through cell membranes. While many tissues can synthesize steroids, the gonads (androgens, progesterone, estrogens) and adrenal glands (androgens, glucocorticoids, mineralocorticoids) are the primary SH endocrine organs. Most SHs circulate through the blood bound to specific carrier proteins. For example, estrogens and androgens circulate bound to sex hormone–binding globulin (SHBG), while glucocorticoids and progesterone bind to cortisol-binding globulin (CBG). Albumin binds all SHs with low affinity but high capacity. Only the free (unbound) hormone can exert a biologic response.[3] Route of administration, dose, metabolism, and tissue-specific receptor activity of various natural and synthetic steroid and peptide hormones also influence the biologic response.

The classical mechanism of SH action **(Figure 2.1)** requires that (1) the free SH ligand diffuses across the cell membrane; (2) the SH binds to the specific SH receptor in either the cytosol (glucocorticoids and mineralocorticoids) or cell nucleus (androgens, estrogens, progestogens); (3) the SH/receptor complex interacts with nuclear DNA to stimulate transcription of mRNA; (4) the mRNA is transported to the cytosol and ribosomes for translation; and (5) the protein synthesized causes specific cellular effects.[4] The general take-home point is that classical SH action takes time (hours to days). In other words, the clinical response following administration of a steroid requires patience. Membrane-bound SH receptors are thought to mediate nonclassical rapid responses in some tissues through direct (nonnuclear) signal transduction pathways.

In the ovary, sex steroids are produced by ovarian stromal cells. The stromal cells that border each primary germ cell differentiate into granulosa cells to form a primordial follicle. As the follicle grows and develops, each oocyte becomes surrounded by a multilayer zone of granulosa cells bordered by theca cells. Under stimulation by gonadotropins, theca cells produce androgens and the granulosa cells aromatize these androgens to estrogens.[4]

Peptide Hormones

Peptide hormones also play key roles in reproduction. The major reproductive peptide hormones that control the reproductive cycle include the hypothalamic gonadotropin-releasing hormone (GnRH) and the anterior pituitary follicle-stimulating hormone (FSH) and luteinizing hormone (LH). FSH and LH are heterodimers consisting of two peptide chains. The alpha chains are nearly identical, while the beta chains differ and provide specificity. The beta chain of human chorionic gonadotropin (hCG), a related heterodimer peptide produced by syncitiotrophoblasts, is highly similar to beta LH, differing only by an additional 24 amino acids at the carboxy-terminal end that result in a longer half-life. Thus, hCG binds to the LH receptor but circulates longer with greater bioavailability.

Other important peptide hormones include inhibin B, a product of granulosa cells; activin, produced by both the pituitary and granulosa cells; and the neuropeptides kisspeptin, dynorphin, and neurokinin B.

Peptide hormones are water soluble and cannot pass through lipid membranes. They bind to membrane receptors and influence cellular processes by acting through a second messenger **(Figure 2.2)**. Thus, unlike SHs, the

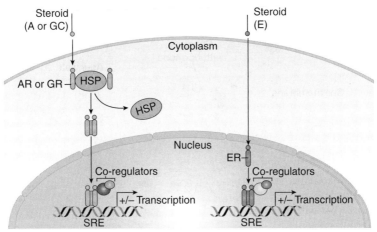

Figure 2.1 Classical Steroid Hormone Action. Steroid hormones travel in the bloodstream free or bound to binding globulins. Free hormones typically pass through the cell membrane and bind to a steroid hormone receptor in the cytosol (where binding activates the receptor and allows the complex to move to the nucleus) or directly in the nucleus. Androgen (A) and glucocorticoid (GC) receptors (AR and GR, respectively), exist primarily in the cytoplasm as monomers bound to heat shock proteins (HSPs). Binding to cytoplasmic receptors triggers release from HSPs, receptor dimerization, alterations in receptor conformation and nuclear localization. Estrogen (E) receptor (ER) and progesterone receptor are located as monomers primarily in the nucleus; steroid binding promotes dimerization and changes in receptor conformation. In both cases, nuclear dimerized receptors bind to specific steroid-response elements (SREs) and interact with several co regulators to modulate gene transcription (repression or activation). (Adapted by permission from Nature: **Levin ER, Hammes SR,** Nuclear receptors outside the nucleus: extranuclear signalling by steroid receptors. Nat Rev Mol Cell Biol 2016;17:783–797. Copyright © 2016 Springer Nature.)

effects of peptide hormones are rapid. For example, binding of GnRH to the GnRH receptor of gonadotropic cells of the anterior pituitary leads to activation of a G protein and triggers events leading to the immediate release of FSH stored in lysosomes.

Receptor Agonists and Antagonists

We use the term ligand to refer to a molecule that binds to a receptor. Ligands that bind to receptors to directly effect a physiologic response are called agonists, while those that block the response are called antagonists. The configurational changes of synthetic steroids may increase binding at the target receptor to produce a pharmacologic response as either agonists or antagonists. Some molecules also have effects on nontarget receptors. For

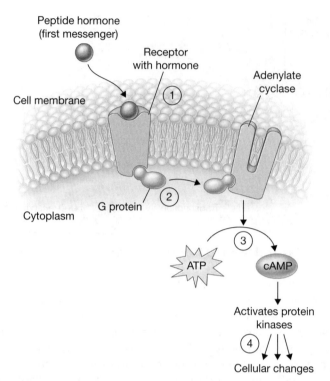

Figure 2.2 Peptide Hormone Action. Peptide hormone binds to a specific membrane-bound receptor (*1*) and induces a conformational change that in turn stimulates a G protein–coupled action (*2*) that results in the generation of a second messenger (in this case cAMP) (*3*) that initiates a series of downstream signaling events resulting in a specific cellular action (*4*).

example, levonorgestrel (LNG), a potent progestin, has weak activity at the androgen receptor.[5]

Some ligands bind to a receptor and cause an agonist or antagonist result by modulating the receptor. As a result, agonist or antagonist action from the same ligand may be tissue specific. Moieties that act on estrogen receptors are called selective estrogen receptor modulators (SERMs), and those that act on the progesterone receptor are called selective progesterone receptor modulators (SPRMs). For example, ulipristal acetate (UPA) is an SPRM that acts like progesterone at the hypothalamus to block the LH surge but opposes the action of progesterone at the level of the follicle to prevent follicle rupture.[6] While UPA also blocks progesterone receptor activity at the endometrium, this effect is less robust than another progesterone receptor modulator mifepristone.[7]

Tissue-specific reaction occurs due to the activity of cofactors that modulate the binding of the SH to its receptor. Two main distinct isoforms exist for both the estrogen (ERα and ERβ) and progesterone (PR-A and PR-B) receptors. In addition, some SH action is thought to occur through rapid signaling pathways (similar to peptide hormones) through membrane-bound receptors.[4]

The Hypothalamic-Pituitary-Ovarian Axis

Women experience regular menstrual cycles due to a highly regulated feedback loop known as the hypothalamic-pituitary-ovarian (HPO) axis **(Figure 2.3)**. The feedback control resides within centers located in the hypothalamus that respond to endocrine feedback by regulating the pulsatile release of GnRH. Several important neuropeptides participate in these pathways and affect the regulation of the reproductive cycle in a variety of ways. For example, dopamine participates in the regulation of prolactin and gonadotropin suppression important for lactational amenorrhea during breast-feeding, catecholamines modulate GnRH pulsatility and may be a factor in stress-related amenorrhea, neuropeptide Y likely participates in cycle suppression seen with poor nutrition, and opioid peptides modulate GnRH response.[4]

Many of the effects of neuropeptides are mediated through their regulation of kisspeptin neurons in the hypothalamus. These neurons respond to the low levels of ovarian steroids that are present prior to the onset of menstruation and stimulate the pulsatile release of GnRH from GnRH neurons.[8] GnRH travels thorough the hypophyseal portal vein to the anterior pituitary triggering the release of FSH. FSH stimulates granulosa cells of antral follicles to produce estradiol and inhibin B. FSH levels peak at about cycle day 4 to 6 of the follicular phase and then decline as rising levels of estradiol and inhibin B turn off the kisspeptin neurons, in turn reducing the stimulation of GnRH neurons though negative feedback. During this time, one follicle becomes dominant, likely due to paracrine signaling. The dominant follicle continues to grow and secrete estradiol and inhibin as the other follicles in the developing pool

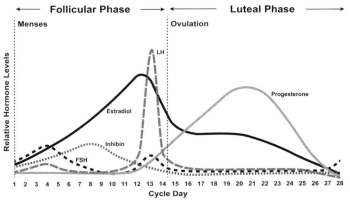

Figure 2.3 Hormonal feedback loop of the menstrual cycle showing relative relationship between changes in ovarian and pituitary hormones. FSH rises during menses in response to low levels of steroid hormones, and drops by the mid-follicular phase in response to rising levels of estradiol and inhibin. As estradiol increases, positive feedback results in the midcycle LH surge that triggers ovulation and the development of the corpus luteum, accompanied by a rise in progesterone and a decline in estradiol. The drop in progesterone initiates menstruation, and the cycle repeats. FSH, follicle stimulating hormone; LH, luteinizing hormone.

regress and undergo apoptosis. This intricate control is critical for mono-ovulation and the successful production of singleton pregnancies. The growing dominant follicle also develops LH and progesterone receptors.[4]

As the dominant follicle grows to the preovulatory stage in the late follicular phase, estradiol negative feedback switches to positive feedback as a second population of kisspeptin neurons detect the peak estradiol level and stimulate the release of GnRH with a greater pulse frequency than in the early cycle. This in turn leads to the preferential release of LH from the anterior pituitary. This LH surge develops over approximately 50 hours.

Understanding LH surge regulation is essential to hormonal contraception physiology. The kisspeptin neurons that stimulate pulsatile GnRH release causing the LH surge are regulated by the neuropeptides neurokinin B (NKB) and dynorphin (DYN), an endogenous opioid. While incompletely understood, the interaction between NKB, DYN, and kisspeptin neurons allows for the negative feedback of estradiol and inhibin B on FSH release and subsequent positive feedback that stimulates LH release.[9] Dynorphin appears responsible for the progesterone-mediated negative feedback on GnRH release that terminates the LH surge,[8] the basis for the use of progestogens to block ovulation.

Two key take-home points deserve emphasis: (1) FSH secretion stimulates follicle growth under a system of negative feedback in response to estrogen levels; and (2) progesterone receptor action can prevent or blunt the LH surge. These details explain why combined estrogen-progestogen hormonal contraception methods block follicle development and prevent ovulation, while progestogen-only methods allow follicle growth but block ovulation, resulting in estradiol production and persistent follicles in some cases.

While the above description provides details essential to the understanding of the mechanisms of hormonal contraception, we have greatly simplified the system. For example, low levels of LH secreted during the follicular phase stimulate androgen production in ovarian theca cells essential as the substrate for aromatization to estradiol in granulosa cells. A small midcycle surge of FSH increases LH receptors in the granulosa cells, transforming them into an important source for progesterone production in the luteal phase. Activin, produced by the granulosa cells, acts in an autocrine and paracrine fashion to inhibit progesterone production by the granulosa cells during the follicular phase, and reduce androgen synthesis in thecal cells, and in an endocrine fashion to augment the secretion of FSH by stimulating the synthesis of GnRH receptors in the pituitary. Progesterone and estrogen act at the level of the pituitary to increase the pituitary release of LH at midcycle. Catechol estrogens and opioid peptides also influence the regulation of menstrual cycles.[4]

Development of a Dominant Follicle

Primary germ cells cease mitotic activity early in fetal life and become arrested at prophase 1 (diplotene) of the first miotic division as primary oocytes. A single layer of granulosa cells envelops each oocyte to form a primordial follicle. While many of these follicles undergo apoptosis, growth occurs with the addition of layers of granulosa and theca cells over a process that takes about 300 days that is independent of gonadotrophins, leading to formation of primary and then secondary follicles. These follicles secrete antimüllerian hormone (AMH); the AMH level reflects the pool of healthy follicles.[10]

With continued growth, secondary follicles develop a small fluid space called the antrum over a process that takes about 65 days. At this stage, these small antral follicles become dependent on gonadotropins for further growth. Recruitment of antral follicles likely occurs in multiple waves during the cycle.[11] Under the influence of FSH, antral follicles grow and secrete estradiol and inhibin. While this process requires FSH, estradiol production results from the aromatization of androgens that are synthesized in the theca cells under the influence of low levels of LH also present during this time.[12] Selection of the dominant follicle occurs in the midfollicular phase with continued growth to form a preovulatory follicle and apoptosis of the remaining cohort.[13] Occasionally, more than one follicle will progress to the preovulatory stage and result in ovulation of more than one oocyte (and a multiple pregnancy should both fertilize). The administration of recombinant gonadotropins in controlled ovarian stimulation protocols overrides the regulation of the dominant follicle, allowing multiple follicles to progress to the preovulatory stage.

The fact that estrogen production by the ovaries requires androgen as a substrate is a point worth emphasizing. Although we think of the follicular phase as FSH dependent, small amounts of LH induce steroid synthesis in theca cells leading to the production and secretion of androstenedione, dehydroepiandrosterone, and testosterone. Under the influence of FSH, granulosa cells aromatize these androgens to estrogens. Excessive androgen production by theca cells results in symptoms of androgen excess such as acne and hirsutism. Combined hormonal contraception dramatically improves these symptoms through multiple pathways, one of which is by reducing gonadotropin stimulation, decreasing both LH and FSH. These actions provide the clinical basis for the use of combined hormonal contraceptives to treat acne and polycystic ovarian syndrome.

Ovulation and the Development of the Corpus Luteum

The LH surge initiates a series of events in the preovulatory follicle leading to a shift in SH synthesis to progesterone, resumption of meiosis by the oocyte, and the production of a variety of proteinases, collagenases, and prostaglandins needed for follicle rupture after approximately 36 hours.[4] Although serum levels of progesterone rise slowly in response to the LH surge, progesterone action within the periovulatory follicle is essential for the mediation of several pathways essential for ovulation (**Figure 2.4**).[14] For this reason, once the LH surge initiates, ovulation will often proceed even if the LH surge subsequently becomes blunted.

Understanding this mechanism provides the explanation for why UPA, a SPRM, is more effective that LNG, a progesterone receptor agonist, for emergency contraception. LNG dosing must occur prior to the start of the LH surge to prevent ovulation, while UPA remains effective if dosed prior to the LH peak. Clinically, this extends the window of effective treatment.

Following ovulation, progesterone production rises rapidly as the follicle is transformed into the corpus luteum. The corpus luteum secretes both progesterone and estradiol in response to continued episodic release of LH pulses and these steroids act centrally to suppress FSH and new follicle growth. Luteal regression begins after about 11 days in response to a variety of events. Progesterone and estradiol levels decline precipitously leading to reestablishment of conditions for a new follicular phase. Rising levels of

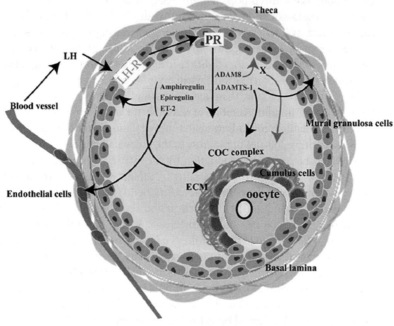

Figure 2.4 LH induces Progesterone-Mediated Action in the Preovulatory Follicle. Schematic representation of preovulatory follicle and the paracrine signaling involved in the control of progesterone receptor (PR) signaling. Luteinizing hormone (LH) acts in the granulosa cells via binding to LH receptors (LH-R). The LH surge induces PR expression in mural granulosa cells of preovulatory follicles that are otherwise devoid of PR expression. Subsequent progesterone signaling induces expression of secreted factors such as amphiregulin, epiregulin, and ET-2 that act as paracrine factors on cumulus cells that surround the oocyte to form the cumulus oocyte complex (COC) and vascular endothelial cells. In addition, progesterone induces the expression of the extracellular proteases ADAM-8 that may affect release of growth factors from the MGCs thereby further modulating intercellular cross talk, and ADAMTS-1 initiates remodeling of cumulus oocyte complex-associated extra cellular matrix as well as the follicular basement membrane. (Reprinted from **Rajaram RD, Brisken C,** Paracrine signaling by progesterone. Mol Cell Endocrinol 2012;357: 80–90. Copyright © 2011 Elsevier Ireland Ltd. With permission.)

hCG that occur with pregnancy prevent luteolysis and maintain progesterone levels to prevent decidual shedding and the onset of menses.

Menstruation

The endometrium consists of a basal layer of stem cells (basalis) and a functional layer (functionalis). During menses and the follicular phase of the ovarian cycle, rising levels of estradiol act through estrogen receptor to induce mitotic activity that begins in the basalis resulting in proliferation and the development of the functional layer.[15] Endometrial growth requires the formation of new blood vessels, and this neovascularization is also under hormonal regulation. In addition to mitotic activity, estrogen signaling induces endometrial cells to synthesize progesterone receptors.

Following ovulation, rising progesterone levels stimulate the endometrium to cease mitotic activity and undergo a secretory transformation suitable for implantation of the developing embryo. In the absence of pregnancy and rescue of the corpus luteum by hCG, progesterone levels drop within 10 to 14 days as luteolysis occurs.

Progesterone withdrawal leads to an irreversible series of events in the endometrium that result in the onset of menstruation. These actions occur within 36 hours following the drop in progesterone.[16] A key takeaway here is that normal menstruation requires estrogen-driven endometrial proliferation but occurs in response to progesterone-induced secretory transformation followed by progesterone withdrawal. Endometrial bleeding will occur following progestin withdrawal of an estrogen-primed endometrium even in the setting of continued estrogen stimulation. This explains why women using continuous estrogen therapy for postmenopausal hormone therapy experience bleeding following the sequential administration of progesterone or a progestin.

One of the important actions of progesterone signaling in the luteal phase is the down-regulation of both estrogen and progesterone receptors in the endometrial functionalis. This point deserves emphasis, as it explains why women using combined estrogen-progestogen products continuously typically develop inactive endometrium and amenorrhea following several cycles of administration. It also explains why women using combined hormonal contraception in standard cyclic regimens generally experience reduced withdrawal bleeding compared to natural cycles. In most women using standard cycles of combined methods, endometrial proliferation occurs during the hormone-free interval due to endogenous ovarian estradiol production. Upon reinitiation of the progestogen-dominant combined hormonal product, the proliferation is attenuated through progesterone receptor–mediated down-regulation. As this effect occurs through classical steroid hormone receptor action, it requires days for down-regulation to completely arrest proliferation. So, most women using combined hormonal methods experience cyclic bleeding due to endometrial proliferation that begins during the hormone-free interval.

During use of a combined hormonal contraceptive method in a traditional 21-day regimen followed by a 7-day hormone-free interval, cyclic bleeding typically occurs. During the hormone-free interval, FSH levels begin to rise and stimulate proliferation that begins in the basalis. The endometrial cells express ER and PR. Once the intake of the active hormone combination occurs, the estrogen component continues to stimulate proliferation working through the ER, while the progestin begins to down-regulate ER and PR, limiting further proliferation and initiating a secretory transformation. Menses occurs as a result of progestin withdrawal.

Women using progestin-only methods of contraception experience variable patterns of bleeding. Many women and clinicians consider amenorrhea as the optimum bleeding pattern during contraception use. Using this criterion, the LNG 52 mg intrauterine system provides the most reliable results. Users of this method have very high local levels of LNG at the endometrium, and this results in profound down-regulation of estrogen receptor and proliferation. Women using injectable depot medroxyprogesterone acetate experience high rates of amenorrhea with prolonged use, likely due to high systemic exposure leading to a profound ovarian suppression and a potent endometrial effect. However, it typically takes several months for reduced bleeding to develop. Initially, the progestogen effect results in endometrial decidualization similar to pregnancy. Over time, spotting and bleeding are common as this endometrium becomes unstable, but eventually, an inactive endometrium develops.[17] Results with contraceptive implants and progestin-only pills are less consistent, possibly due to lower endometrial levels of the progestogen and variable levels of suppression of ovarian estradiol secretion.

Some users of combined hormonal contraception experience breakthrough bleeding due to the relative dominance of the progestin component of the formulation. The management of breakthrough bleeding has led to a number of different combined hormonal regimens designed to increase endometrial proliferation (see Chapter 7). The etiology of breakthrough bleeding during the use of a progestogen-dominant contraceptive may also be abnormal blood vessel development. Successful implantation and pregnancy require substantial new blood vessel development in the endometrium. This neovascularization occurs primarily during the proliferative phase under estrogen regulation. Two types of estrogen receptor have been identified, ERα and ERβ. While most of the effects of estrogens in the reproductive tract are mediated by ERα, the endothelial cells of the endometrium express only ERβ.[18] Among the many strategies used clinically to manage breakthrough bleeding, the most successful involve increasing the dose of estrogen. Part of this effect may be mediated through stabilization of blood vessels. Recently, the use of tamoxifen, a SERM that is an antagonist for ERβ but a partial agonist for ERα, was shown to be effective for the management of breakthrough bleeding in users of contraceptive implants.[19]

The Cervix

Cervical mucus changes in response to the hormonal changes during the menstrual cycle in direct relationship to cyclic fluctuations of estrogen and progesterone. Prior to ovulation, in response to rising levels of estradiol, cervical mucus becomes fluid and penetrable by sperm. Following ovulation, in response to rising levels of progesterone, mucus thickens and becomes impenetrable. The ability of sperm to penetrate mucus is highest with ovulatory mucus and lowest during the luteal and early follicular phases. Mucus provides an important natural barrier for the upper female genital tract; by restricting penetrability to midcycle, the system reduces the opportunity for ascending infection. The dynamic nature of cervical mucus and its hormonal regulation provide an important mechanism for contraception. Since ovulation commonly occurs in users of the LNG intrauterine system, the contraceptive effect likely results from the progestin-induced thickening of cervical mucus. Progestin-only pills that allow ovulation are thought to act by inhibiting the development of favorable mucus.[20]

Mechanisms of Action of Hormonal Contraception

Combined hormonal methods contain both estrogen and progestin components. The primary mechanism of action involves blocking ovulation through the inhibition of gonadotropin secretion via an effect on both pituitary and hypothalamic centers. The progestational agent primarily suppresses LH secretion (and thus prevents ovulation), while the estrogenic agent suppresses FSH secretion (and thus prevents the emergence of a dominant follicle). Therefore, the estrogenic component contributes to the contraceptive efficacy by attenuating follicle growth. However, an estrogen-only product would not provide a practical approach even with complete follicle suppression due to unopposed endometrial proliferation.

The estrogen in the combined hormonal methods serves two other purposes. It opposes the progestin effect on the endometrium so that the two hormones balance each other to minimize irregular shedding and unwanted breakthrough bleeding, and the presence of estrogen potentiates the action of the progestational agents. The latter function of estrogen has allowed reduction of the progestin dose in CHCs over the past few decades. The mechanism for this action is probably estrogen's effect in increasing the concentration of intracellular progesterone receptors. Therefore, this minimal pharmacologic level of estrogen contributes to the efficacy of the combined methods.

Because the effect of a progestational agent will always take precedence over estrogen (unless the dose of estrogen is increased many, many fold), the endometrium, cervical mucus, and tubal function reflect progestational stimulation during continuous use. As noted above, the progestin strongly down-regulates proliferation and leads to a decidualized endometrium. Continuous use of a progestin leads to exhausted and atrophied glands, due to down-regulation of estrogen receptor. While it is tempting to conclude that these endometrial changes contribute to a contraceptive effect, we have no direct evidence for this action. For hormonal methods that work primarily by blocking ovulation, studies have not differentiated endometrial effects in cycles when a dominant follicle and ovulation occur from the effects seen in cycles when ovulation does not occur. Whether the endometrium that develops in an anovulatory cycle would be receptive is a moot point. We also know that the fertilized egg is capable of implanting ectopically. Suggesting that an effect on implantation is a mechanism of action for hormonal contraception without direct experimental evidence contributes to a narrative used by special interest groups opposed to contraception to combat public funding. Even high doses of a progestin (e.g., LNG emergency contraception) or antiprogestin SPRMs (UPA) given post ovulation do not appear to alter key implantation factors.[21,22] Most studies simply evaluate endometrial proliferation by ultrasound using stripe thickness as a surrogate for a contraceptive effect, an unproven hypothesis. In fact, data from a series of infertile women treated with clomiphene and intrauterine insemination found no difference in pregnancy rates with endometrial stripe thickness of less than 6 mm (15%), 6 to 9 mm (16%), or greater than 9 mm (19%).[23]

The cervical mucus does become thick and impervious to sperm transport with exposure to a progestin. It is possible that progestational influences on secretion and peristalsis within the fallopian tubes provide additional contraceptive effects. Even if there is some ovarian follicular activity (especially with the lowest-dose estrogen products), these progestin actions serve to ensure good contraceptive efficacy.[20]

The contraceptive effects of progestin-only products differ depending on dose, potency, and rout of administration. High systemic dose agents such as depot medroxyprogesterone acetate typically block ovulation and suppress ovarian, endometrial and cervical activity. Contraceptive implants have varying effects depending on the progestin and dose; LNG implants rely primarily over years of use on cervical mucus effects although ovulation inhibition can occur initially when hormone levels are highest. Etonogestrel implants, on the other hand, reliably block ovulation and suppress follicle growth significantly, especially during the first 2 years of use. Irregular bleeding may occur as a result of endometrial exposure to variable levels of ovarian estradiol production. Progestin-only pills are less reliable in blocking ovulation and work primarily by blocking development of fertile cervical mucus. The LNG intrauterine system infrequently blocks ovulation, but very high local levels of the progestin result in a thick nonpenetrable cervical mucus (see Chapter 6, Figure 6.2). Although the high level of local hormone also causes an inactive atrophic endometrium related to down-regulation of estrogen receptors, the reality that sperm will not penetrate the mucus means that this endometrial effect is simply a means to induce a desirable "side effect" of decreased bleeding. Cervical mucus during ovulatory cycles of the LNG-IUS during year 7 of use shows modified Insler scores similar to those observed in ovulatory women using a copper IUD; but many of these ovulations appear dysfunctional.[24] These data suggest that cervical mucus changes may not provide the only contraceptive effect of the LNG-IUS with extended use in women with ovulatory cycles. However, other mechanisms common to inert IUDs and lower levels of LNG likely prevent fertilization in most cases, making an endometrial contragestive effect the least likely mechanism.[25]

The Hormonal Contraception Story

Although early experiments demonstrated the potential of hormonal contraception, the use of products derived from animal organs resulted in tremendous variability of response. Even after the chemical structure of sex steroids was elucidated, extraction and isolation of a few milligrams required starting points measured in gallons of urine or thousands of pounds of organs. Edward Doisy, an American biochemist who first discovered SHs (estrone in 1929), reportedly processed 80,000 sow ovaries to produce 12 mg of estradiol.[26]

Marker Degradation and Progesterone

The supply problem was solved by Russell E. Marker, an American chemist known for developing the system of octane rating of gasoline. In September 1935, Marker worked at Penn State with support mainly from research grants from the Parke-Davis pharmaceutical company.

At that time, it required the ovaries from 2,500 pregnant pigs to produce 1 mg of progesterone. For several years, Marker worked on extracting hormones from the urine from pregnant animals as he pursued the goal of an abundant and inexpensive supply of progesterone. As these efforts proved futile, Marker became convinced that the solution to the problem of obtaining large quantities of SHs was in plants that contain large amounts of the plant steroid diosgenin, a sapogenin. In 1939, Marker had figured out a method, now called the Marker degradation, to convert a sapogenin molecule into a progestin, but he still needed raw materials. Marker discovered that the roots of the *Dioscorea* plant (a wild Mexican yam) provided a rich source of sapogenins. Marker was unable to obtain support from the pharmaceutical industry so he used half of his life savings to return to Mexico in October 1942 to collect yams and used these to synthesize 3 kg of progesterone, the largest lot of progesterone ever produced. United States pharmaceutical companies still refused to back Marker, and even his university refused to patent the process. Marker found a Mexican hormone laboratory headed by a Hungarian lawyer, Emeric Somlo, and a German chemist, Frederick A. Lehman; the three men agreed to form a Mexican hormone production company, named Syntex (from *synthesis* and *Mexico*). Marker left Syntex in May 1945 after he learned that he was not being paid in accordance with their agreement. He started a new company called Botanica-Mex and changed to a different species of yam (*Dioscorea barbasco*), which gave a greater yield of diosgenin, and the price of progesterone dropped significantly.[27,28]

By the 1960s, several pharmaceutical companies operated competing root-gathering operations in Mexico, closely regulated by the Mexican government that imposed annual quotas to balance harvesting with the new annual growth. Mexican yams provided the starting material for the manufacture of synthetic steroids used in oral contraceptives for about 15 years, giving way to other sources, such as soya beans, methods for total synthesis, or microbial fermentation.[29]

The Synthetic Progestational Drugs, Norethindrone and Norethynodrel

When Marker left Syntex, he took his know-how with him. Fortunately for Syntex, there still was no patent on his discoveries. George Rosenkranz left his native Hungary to study chemistry in Switzerland under the renowned steroid chemist Nobel Laureate Leopold Ruzicka.[30] Rosenkranz emigrated from Europe to Cuba to escape the Nazi regime. In 1945, he was invited for an interview with Syntex after Marker had left and was hired on the spot. Rosenkranz gave up on reconstructing Marker's process and developed his own commercial manufacture of progesterone and testosterone from Mexican yams. Soon, Syntex was making large profits providing the sex hormones as raw material to other pharmaceutical companies. Rosenkranz now had a large active laboratory and invited a young Bulgarian chemist, Carl Djerassi, to head a research group to concentrate on the synthesis of cortisone; Djerassi accepted the position and moved to Mexico City in the fall of 1949. Djerassi had also fled the Nazi regime, emigrating to the United States in 1939 when he was 16 years old.

In 2 years' time, Syntex achieved the partial synthesis of cortisone, reported in 1951.[31] The Syntex method never reached commercialization, however, because the Upjohn Company developed a more efficient process.

Djerassi and other Syntex chemists then turned their attention to the sex steroids. They discovered that the removal of the 19-carbon from yam-derived progesterone increased the progestational activity of the molecule based on similar recent work with other SHs. Chemists at Schering AG in Berlin had produced orally active versions of estradiol and testosterone in 1938, by substituting an acetylene group in the 17-position of the parent compounds. The resulting ethinyl estradiol (EE) later became the estrogen component in oral contraceptives. The product was known as ethisterone and first marketed in 1941.

On October 15, 1951, norethindrone was synthesized at Syntex by removing the 19-carbon of ethinyl testosterone.[32] The greater potency of norethindrone compared with progesterone was demonstrated in monkeys[33] and then four women at the National Institutes of Health.[34,35] Syntex supplied norethindrone to many investigators, including Gregory Pincus. Edward T. Tyler first reported its clinical use in 1955 for the treatment of menstrual disorders.[36]

Frank Colton, a chemist at G.D. Searle & Company, filed a patent for norethynodrel, a compound closely related to norethindrone, differing only in the position of the double bond, on August 31, 1953. Pincus would ultimately choose the Searle compound, norethynodrel, for clinical testing as an oral contraceptive.

The concept of oral contraception required the synthesis of highly potent, orally active progestational agents. The natural hormone progesterone has poor oral bioavailability, requires very large doses, and does not achieve a uniform response. The availability of norethindrone and norethynodrel made the development of an oral contraceptive pill feasible.

Creating a Hormonal Oral Contraceptive

Katharine Dexter McCormick (1875–1967) was a trained biologist, an early suffragist, and rich, inheriting millions from her mother and a McCormick fortune from her husband. She was the second woman to graduate from the

Massachusetts Institute of Technology, socially conscious, and a generous contributor to family planning efforts. In 1904, she married Stanley McCormick, the son of Cyrus McCormick, the founder of International Harvester. Katharine's husband suffered from schizophrenia, and she established the Neuroendocrine Research Foundation at Harvard to study schizophrenia. This brought her together with Hudson Hoagland, a neurophysiologist.

Hoagland did his graduate work at Harvard, where he studied with a reproductive biology graduate student, Gregory Pincus. Hoagland and Pincus remained in contact after completing their studies in 1927. In 1931, Hoagland, then Chair of Biology at Clark University in Worcester, Massachusetts, invited Pincus to join him. Hoagland secured funds for Pincus from philanthropists in New York City, enough for a laboratory and an assistant. This success impressed the two men, especially Hoagland, planting the idea that it would be possible to support research with private money. In 1944, Hoagland and Pincus established the Worcester Foundation for Experimental Biology. That same year, Pincus offered a fellowship to Min Chueh Chang, a Chinese Ph.D. in animal breeding. Years later, Chang would direct the testing of new progestins to effectively inhibit ovulation in animals.

Pincus developed a growing appreciation for the world's population problem. In 1951, he visited Margaret Sanger, at that time president of the Planned Parenthood Federation of America, in New York. Sanger promised a small amount of money and expressed hope that a method of contraception could be derived from the laboratory work being done by Pincus and Chang. During this meeting, Pincus formulated his thoughts derived from his mammalian research. He envisioned a progestational agent in pill form as a contraceptive, acting like progesterone in pregnancy.

When Pincus and Chang began their studies, the focus was on inhibition of ovulation, first by progesterone and then by synthetic progestins. Chang started by repeating the experiments reported by Makepeace in 1927, documenting that progesterone could inhibit ovulation.[37] The first experiment was on April 25, 1951, and Chang quickly moved to testing the newly synthesized progestins from Searle and Syntex.

Katherine McCormick learned from Hoagland of the work being done by Pincus and Chang to develop orally active progestins to inhibit ovulation. Margaret Sanger brought Pincus and Katharine McCormick together. On June 7, 1953, when 78-year-old Katharine first met with the 50-year-old Pincus at the Worcester Foundation, she wrote him a check for $20,000. A week later, Pincus and Hoagland met with McCormick and her lawyer. They signed a contract outlining the goals, the decision-making process, and the timetable. Pincus received a second check for $20,000, and McCormick agreed to fund laboratory improvements, which ended up as the completion of a new building in 1955. From 1953 to 1960, Katherine McCormick invested about $2 million in the development of an oral contraceptive.

Pincus recognized that approval of an oral contraceptive would require the involvement of a physician for human clinical trials. At a scientific conference, he met John Rock, Chief of Gynecology and Obstetrics at Harvard, and discovered their mutual interest in reproductive physiology. Ironically, Rock's interest in progestational agents stemmed from his work treating infertility.

In their first collaborative study, Pincus and Rock administered oral progesterone, 300 mg/d. Pincus suggested a 20-day regimen beginning on day 5 of the menstrual cycle.[38] He had two reasons for choosing this regimen: (1) it covered the time period during which nearly all, if not all, ovulations occurred, and (2) the withdrawal menstrual bleed at the conclusion of the treatment period would mimic the timing of a normal menstrual cycle and reassure the women that they were not pregnant.

The pace of progress was rapid. By December 1953, Pincus and Chang identified three synthetic progestins—norethindrone from Syntex and Searle's norethynodrel and norethandrolone—as the most potent and effective in inhibiting ovulation. They first administered synthetic progestins to some of Rock's patients in 1954. Of the first 50 patients to receive 10 to 40 mg of synthetic progestin (a dose extrapolated from the animal data) for 20 days each month, all failed to ovulate during treatment (causing Pincus to begin referring to the medication as "the pill"), and 7 of the 50 became pregnant after discontinuing the medication, pleasing Rock who all along was motivated to treat his infertile patients.

During this development, the scientists discovered that the initial progestin syntheses yielded products contaminated with about 1% mestranol, a synthetic estrogen. In the amounts being used, this added up to 50 to 500 μg of mestranol, a pharmacologically active dose. Mestranol undergoes demethylation in the liver to yield the potent synthetic estrogen EE. During subsequent experiments using purified progestins, women experienced breakthrough bleeding. This established the principle of the combined estrogen-progestin oral contraceptive with a progestin for ovulation inhibition and an estrogen for cycle control.

Celso-Ramon Garcia and Edris Rice-Wray, working in Puerto Rico, conducted the first clinical trial. Pincus picked Searle's norethynodrel combined with mestranol and, with great effort, convinced Searle that the commercial potential of an oral contraceptive warranted the risk of possible negative public reaction. Pincus also convinced Rock, and together they pushed the U.S. Food and Drug Administration (FDA) for acceptance of oral contraception. In 1957, Enovid (mestranol 150 μg and norethynodrel 9.85 mg) was approved for the treatment of miscarriages and menstrual disorders and, on June 23, 1960, for contraception. The pill came in a single bottle with instructions to use for 20 days and then take 5 days off. Neither Pincus nor the Worcester Foundation got rich on the pill; alas, there was no royalty agreement.

Over the ensuring few years, many companies worked feverishly to enter this new market. Syntex, a wholesale drug supplier, eventually secured licensing with the orthopedic division of Johnson & Johnson for a sales outlet for their norethindrone progestin. Ortho-Novum (mestranol and norethindrone) appeared in 1962. That same year, David Wagner, an engineer in suburban Chicago, developed a "dial-pack" dispenser after his wife experienced significant anxiety remembering how to take her pill. Syntex licensed norethindrone to Schering AG for overseas sales. Schering independently developed and patented norethindrone acetate and then introduced a contraceptive combining norethindrone acetate and EE, which rapidly became the best-selling oral contraceptive outside the United States (Anovlar). Parke-Davis marketed a combination of norethindrone acetate with EE (Norlestrin) in the United States in 1964 under cross-licensing that involved both Schering and Syntex. Wyeth Laboratories developed norgestrel, the first progestational agent completely manufactured by chemical synthesis, and introduced Ovral (norgestrel with EE) in 1968.

However, 1968 is also the year of publication of the first case-control study by Vessey and Droll detailing a ninefold increase in venous thrombosis (VT) risk and the initiation of prospective studies.[39] The competitive market for COCs had already resulted in dose reduction of estrogen to as low as 50 µg, and Inman and Vessey first reported evidence for an estrogen dose-response for VT risk in 1970.[40]

The realization that hormonal contraceptive use could result in serious adverse health outcomes led to considerable efforts to produce safer and better tolerated products and has led to the introduction of a bewildering array of different products and formulations. The solution to this clinical dilemma is relatively straightforward and the theme of the remainder of this chapter. Clinicians need to understand the pharmacologic characteristics of the various synthetic steroids and the dose-response for the physiologic effects that result in both efficacy and the potential for side effects.

Pharmacology of Steroid Contraception

Natural Estrogens and Progesterone

Estrogen is not a hormone; the term estrogen encompasses a family of natural and synthetic hormones with activity at estrogen receptors. Four estrogens exist naturally in humans: estrone (E1), estradiol (E2), estriol (E3), and estetrol (E4). These 19-carbon steroids differ by the number of hydroxy (-OH) groups present on the cyclopentanophenanthrene ring steroid backbone.

Estradiol, discovered in 1933, is the primary estrogen of the reproductive years, secreted by the ovaries from menarche through menopause. The hypothalamic-pituitary ovarian axis regulates estrogen production by stimulating ovarian follicle development. Theca cells surrounding antral follicles produce androstenedione and granulosa cells and then aromatize the androgen to estrone and estradiol. 17-beta dehydrogenase converts estrone to estradiol, the most potent natural estrogen. Conversion of estrone to estradiol occurs through 17β-hydroxysteroid dehydrogenase.

Estrone, discovered in 1929, is the primary estrogen of menopause, resulting from conversion of adrenal androstenedione by aromatase in peripheral fat. Estrone is also present during reproductive years but is much less potent than estradiol (approximately 12-fold lower).[41] However, because estrone can be converted to estradiol, peripheral production of estrone in young and old obese women can result in physiologically important levels of estradiol.

Estriol was discovered in 1930 and is primarily present during pregnancy, produced by the placenta from fetal 16-hydroxydehydroepiandosterone sulfate. The placenta also produces estrone and estradiol at quantities 10-fold lower than estriol. The rapid metabolism and low potency (80-fold less than estradiol) limit the biologic activity of estriol.[41]

Estetrol was discovered in 1965 and is primarily only present during fetal life. Estetrol is produced by the fetal liver beginning in the 9th week of pregnancy, and production ceases during the 1st week after birth. Fetal plasma levels are 12 times higher than those of the mother. Estetrol is not present in any other mammalian species except for the very last week of gestation in higher-order primates, although at a concentration 100 times lower than in humans. Estetrol is about 30- to 35-fold less potent than estradiol.[42]

When given orally, estrone, estradiol, and estriol undergo rapid hepatic metabolism through conjugation for excretion. Estradiol has a half-life of about 14 to 16 hours, with estrone and estriol even shorter. In contrast, estetrol has minimal liver metabolism with a half-life of about 28 hours.

The term progestogen refers to both natural and synthetic hormones with activity at the progesterone receptor.[5] Progesterone, a 21-carbon compound, is the only naturally occurring progestogen. Synthetic progestogens are commonly called progestins. Progesterone represents an early product of the steroid synthesis pathway and common precursor to other reproductive hormones (androgens with 19-carbons and estrogens with 18-carbons), glucocorticoids, and mineralocorticoids. The ovary is the primary source of endocrinologically active progesterone in blood, with levels increasing to nanogram concentrations in the luteal phase. To achieve these high concentrations, the corpus luteum produces milligram quantities of progesterone daily, a level of production sufficient to lower circulating levels of cholesterol in women during the luteal phase.[43]

The Estrogen Component of Combination Hormonal Contraceptives

The major obstacle to the use of sex steroids for contraception was reduced activity of the compounds when given orally due to first-pass metabolism, which also shortened the half-life of the circulating hormone. The compounding of EE in 1938 created a product with a half-life similar to oral estradiol but with much more potency when delivered orally. The discovery that progestin-only therapy resulted in breakthrough bleeding led Pincus to add back mestranol, a prodrug of EE, to the first oral contraceptive formulations. EE is the form of estrogen used in most combined hormonal contraceptives delivered orally, transdermally (patch), and vaginally (ring) today (**Figure 2.5**).

Like estradiol, EE undergoes hepatic conjugation following oral administration, but unlike estradiol, these conjugated forms remain highly potent. When delivered nonorally, EE still undergoes significant second-pass hepatic metabolism.

The metabolism of EE (particularly as reflected in blood levels) varies significantly from individual to individual and from one population to another.[44,45] There is even a range of variability at different sampling times

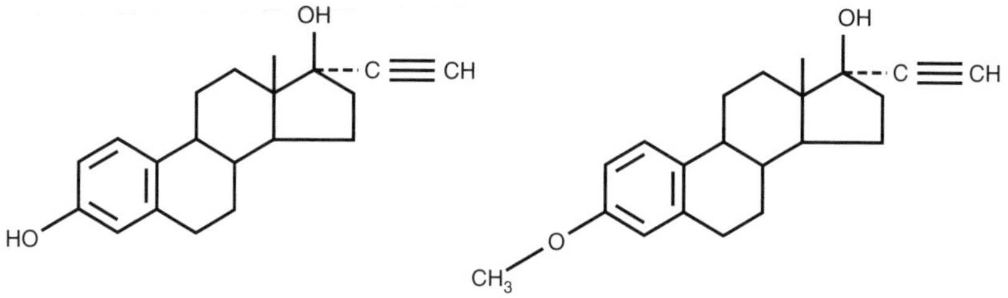

Figure 2.5 Synthetic estrogens used in combined hormonal contraception.

within the same individual. Therefore, it is not surprising that the same dose can cause side effects in one individual and not in another.

Over the past decade, oral contraceptives based on estradiol have been introduced. An estradiol-nomegestrol acetate product (Zoely®) is only available in Europe. A 5-phasic estradiol valerate-dienogest product is marketed in the United States (Natazia®) and Europe (Qlaira®). The fatty acid valeric acid ester moiety improves oral bioavailability; cleavage to 17β-estradiol and valeric acid takes place during absorption. Estradiol cypionate, another esterified estradiol, has also been used in combination with medroxyprogesterone acetate as a monthly injectable (Cyclofem,® Lunelle™). However, because the esterified estradiols are very rapidly hydrolyzed to estradiol, they are considered simply to be prodrugs for estradiol. Vaginal rings containing estradiol are currently under investigation (Clinicaltrials.gov NCT03432416).

Because EE and oral estradiol undergo extensive hepatic metabolism, these agents influence the production of hepatic globulins. The most significant clinical effects occur in relation to the hemostatic system. Thrombosis represents the most serious side effects of combined hormonal contraceptives containing EE or estradiol as the estrogen component, playing a key role in the rare major morbidity and even rarer death from cardiovascular issues. This side effect occurs in direct relationship to the degree of hepatic stimulation by the estrogen component of combined products. Although oral estradiol products exert considerable hepatic effects, they appear to have a lower impact than oral EE, as the later continue to have significant hepatic activation on second pass.[46] Nonoral estradiol administered in physiologic doses avoids first-pass effects and does not result in significant second-pass hepatic metabolism, so combined hormonal contraceptive rings with vaginal estradiol, currently under investigation, have the potential to minimize thrombosis risk.[47] Estetrol also appears to have lower impact on hemostatic factors following oral administration.[48] Confirming whether oral contraceptives currently in development using estetrol or estradiol-containing vaginal rings will have less thrombosis risk will require population-based trials.

Progestins Used in Contraceptives

In the late 1930s, chemists discovered that addition of an ethynyl group at carbon 17 of testosterone resulted in an orally active derivative, ethisterone.

In 1951, chemists at Syntex removed the 19-carbon from ethisterone, changing the major hormonal effect from that of an androgen to that of a progestogen while maintaining oral activity, creating norethindrone. Accordingly, the progestational derivatives of testosterone were designated as 19-nortestosterones (denoting the missing 19-carbon). The androgenic properties of these compounds, however, were not totally eliminated, and minimal anabolic and androgenic potential remains within the structure (**Figure 2.6**).

Progestins structurally related to progesterone were first synthesized in the 1940s, with the discovery that acetylation of the 17-hydroxy group of 17-hydroxyprogesterone produced an orally active but weak progestin. An addition at the 6-carbon position is necessary to give sufficient progestational strength for human use, probably by inhibiting metabolism.

Throughout the 1980s, the drive to develop new progestins stemmed from the belief that androgenic metabolic effects were important, especially in terms of cardiovascular disease. The new progestins developed were desogestrel, gestodene, and norgestimate.[49] Cardiovascular side effects are now known to be due to a dose-related stimulation of thrombosis by estrogen and not secondary to metabolic effects such as lipid changes.

A summary of available progestins used in contraceptives today is presented in **Table 2.1**.

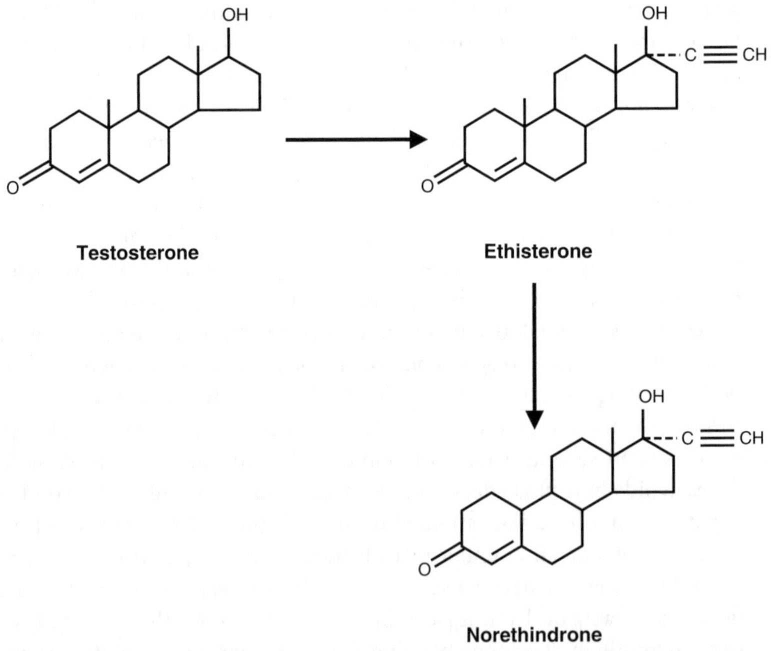

Testosterone

Ethisterone

Norethindrone

Figure 2.6 Norethindrone is a 19-Nortesterone derivative. Addition of an ethynyl group at the 17-carbon position modifies Testosterone to Ethisterone. Removal of the methyl group at the 19-carbon results in Norethisterone, also known as Norethindrone. "Nor" refers to removal of a radical, most specifically a methyl or methylene group.

Table 2.1 Progestins Used in Hormonal Contraception

Parent Hormone	Testosterone		Progesterone		Spirolactone
Derivative Hormone	19-Nortestosterone		17α-Hydroxy-progesterone	19-Norprogesterone	17α-Spironolactone
Class name	Gonanes	Estranes	Pregnanes	Norpregnanes	Spirolactone
Product name	DL-Norgestrel/levonorgestrel	Norethindrone	Medroxyprogesterone acetate	Nomegestrol acetate	Drospirenone
	Norgestimate*	Norethindrone acetate		Segesterone acetate	
	Desogestrel†	Ethynodiol diacetate			
	Gestodene¶	Norethynodrel¶			
		Lynestrenol¶			
		Dienogest‡			

*The primary metabolite, norelgestromin (levonorgestrel-3-oxime), is used in nonoral products.
†The primary metabolite, etonogestrel (3-ketodesogestrel), is used in nonoral products.
‡Dienogest is a hybrid estrane-pregnane progestin.
¶These compounds are not available in the United States.

19-Nortestosterone Agents

The 19-nortestosterone progestins consist of two families, commonly referred to as estranes and gonanes. Although all are derived from testosterone, the families primarily differ at the 13-carbon position, which has a methyl group for estranes (norethindrone, norethynodrel, norethindrone acetate, ethynodiol diacetate, and lynestrenol) and an ethyl group for gonanes (norgestrel, norgestimate, desogestrel, and gestodene). The ethyl substitution confirms more progestational and less androgenic receptor activity in vitro. Note that the term gonane refers to all molecules that contain a phenanthrene ring fused with a cyclopentane ring, the common scaffold of all SHs. Technically, the correct term for those used in reproductive health is 13-ethylgonanes.[50]

All estranes (**Figure 2.7**) are converted to the parent compound, norethindrone. Thus, the activity of norethynodrel, norethindrone acetate, ethynodiol diacetate, and lynestrenol is due to rapid conversion to norethindrone.

Norethindrone also may undergo metabolism to EE, through aromatization. While, with current doses used in CHC, this conversion is minimal, the activity can be clinically important with higher doses.[51] Norethindrone, norethynodrel, and ethynodiol diacetate also display very weak binding to the estrogen receptor.[52] Clinically, the androgenic and estrogenic activities of 19-nortestosteone derivatives are typically insignificant in the low doses used in current oral contraceptives.

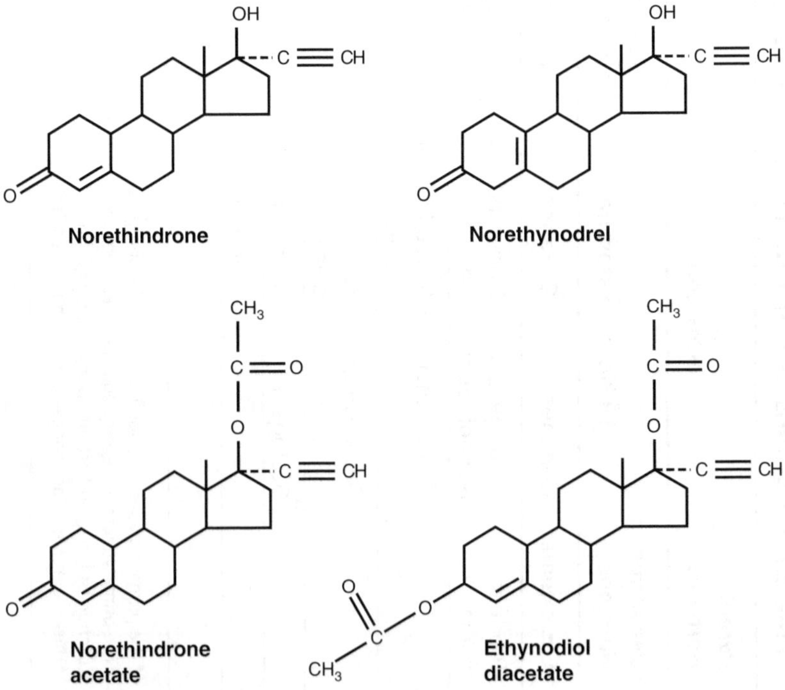

Figure 2.7 Estrane progestins.

Whereas all estranes are basically the same product (norethindrone), the gonanes are not, but can be thought of as close cousins. Norgestrel, the first gonane, is a racemic equal mixture of the dextro and levo enantiomers. The dextrorotatory form, known as D-norgestrel, is biologically inactive. L-Norgestrel (known as levonorgestrel) is the active isomer of norgestrel **(Figure 2.8)**.

Norgestimate is a prodrug with several metabolites. While each of these contribute to the activity of norgestimate, almost all of the biologic effects is attributed to levonorgestrel-3-oxime, now known as norelgestromin.[53,54] Whereas LNG and most LNG metabolites are tightly bound to SHBG, norelgestromin circulates primarily bound to albumin.[55]

Desogestrel, also a prodrug, undergoes two metabolic steps in the liver before the progestational activity is expressed in its primary active metabolite, 3-ketodesogestrel, known as etonogestrel. This metabolite differs from LNG only by a methylene group in the 11 position. Etonogestrel is not absorbed orally, but is used in both vaginal rings and implants. Although etonogestrel-containing contraceptives do not undergo first-pass metabolism, significant second-pass metabolism occurs resulting in similar biologic and metabolic effects as the parent compound.

Gestodene differs from LNG by the presence of a double bond between carbons 15 and 16. It is metabolized into many derivatives with progestational activity, but not LNG.

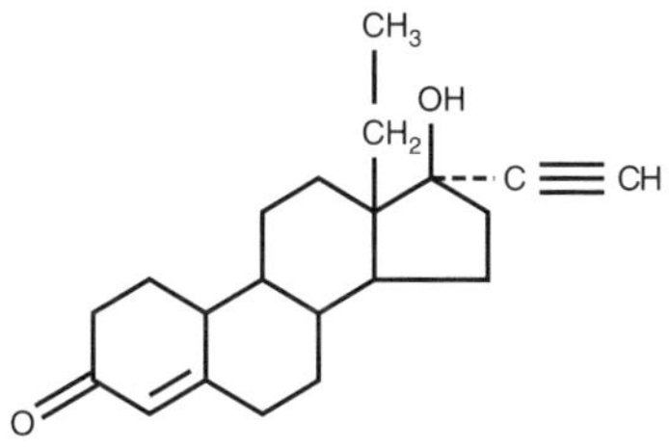

53

Levonorgestrel

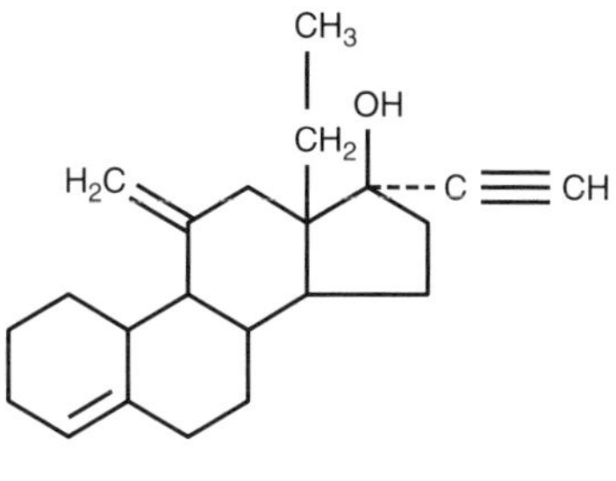

Desogestrel

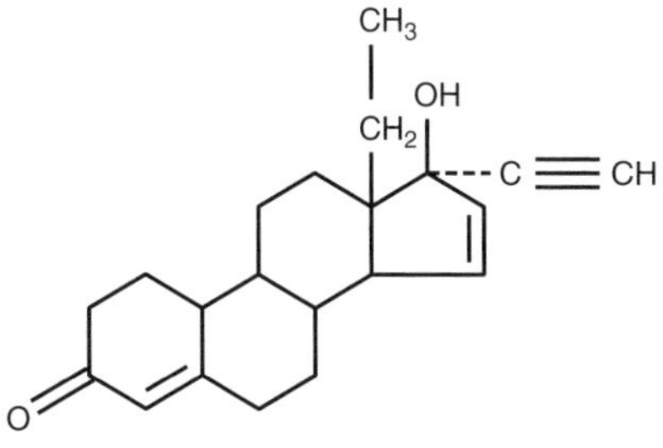

Gestodene

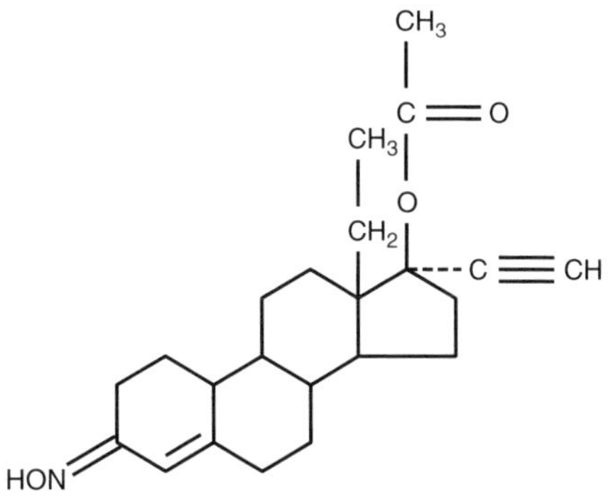

Norgestimate

Figure 2.8 Gonane progestins.

Progesterone Derivatives

Progestins derived from progesterone are classified on the basis of whether or not they possess a methyl group at the 10-carbon position (pregnanes) or lack this group (norpregnanes). Pregnanes include medroxyprogesterone acetate, megestrol acetate, chlormadinone acetate, cyproterone acetate, dydrogesterone, and medrogestone; 19-norpregnanes include nomegestrol acetate, segesterone acetate, and trimegestone. The 19-norpregnanes have strong progestational activity with no androgenic, estrogenic, or glucocorticoid activity; nomegestrol acetate also lacks mineralocorticoid activity.[56] Segesterone acetate, also known as nesterone, is not orally active and must be delivered parenterally **(Figure 2.9)**.

Dienogest is a hybrid estrane-pregnane progestin with a 19-nortestosterone base containing a cyanomethyl group instead of an ethinyl group in the 17-carbon position and an additional double bond, combining the properties of both the 19-nortestosterone family and the derivatives of progesterone[57] **(Figure 2.10)**.

Spirolactones

This class of steroids was developed in the 1950s by G.D. Searle & Company after they produced norethindrone. These steroids contain a spirane at the 17-carbon position and are technically called 17α-spirolactones. The steroids in this class all contain varying degrees of antimineralocorticoid, antiandrogenic, and progestogenic activity. The most widely known member

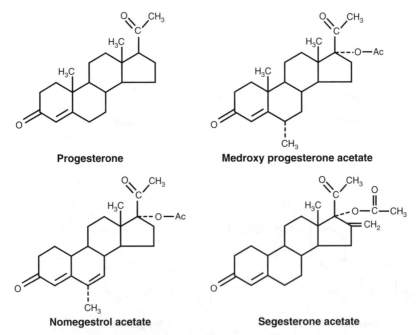

Progesterone

Medroxy progesterone acetate

Nomegestrol acetate

Segesterone acetate

Figure 2.9 Progestins derived from Progesterone.

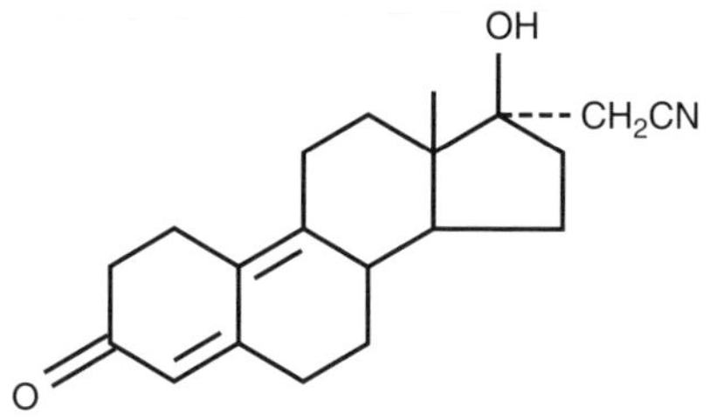

Dienogest

Figure 2.10 Dienogest is a hybrid estrane-pregnane progestin.

of this class, spironolactone, is a potassium-sparing diuretic used as an antihypertensive and, because of its antiandrogenic properties, as a treatment for hirsutism and acne. Drospirenone **(Figure 2.11)** is an analogue of spironolactone with more progestogenic activity and less antimineralocorticoid affinity than spironolactone, providing a biochemical profile very similar to progesterone.[58,59] Because drospirenone is spironolactone-like with antiandrogenic and antimineralocorticoid activity, caution is recommended in regard to serum potassium levels, avoiding its use in women with abnormal renal, adrenal, or hepatic function. However, hyperkalemia and its complications have not been a clinical problem encountered with the use of a drospirenone-containing contraceptive in the general population.[60]

Selective Progesterone Receptor Modulators

Selective progesterone receptor modulators (SPRMs) are synthetic ligands with activity as antagonists or partial agonists at the progesterone receptor. SPRMs also may have partial agonist or antagonist effects at other steroid receptors including the glucocorticoid and androgen receptor.[61] Although several SPRMs have entered clinical trials for a variety of indications, mifepristone and ulipristal acetate (UPA) have special interest in family planning **(Figure 2.12)**.

Medicinal chemists at Roussel-Uclaf in France looking for antagonists for the glucocorticoid receptor synthesized RU-486 (mifepristone) in 1980. While the compound exhibited only weak effects as a glucocorticoid receptor antagonist, the scientists discovered very potent antagonism of the progesterone

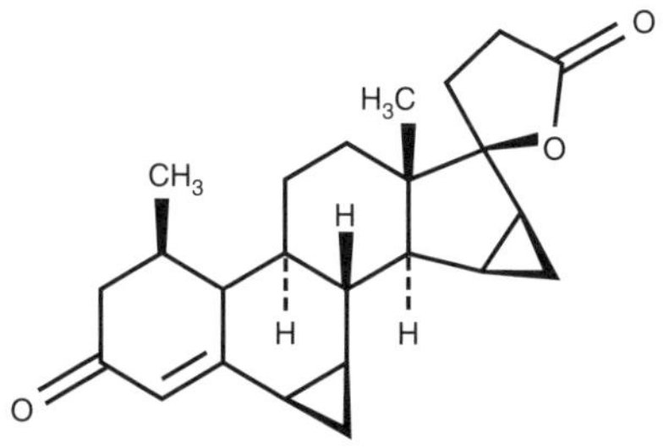

Figure 2.11 Drosperinone.

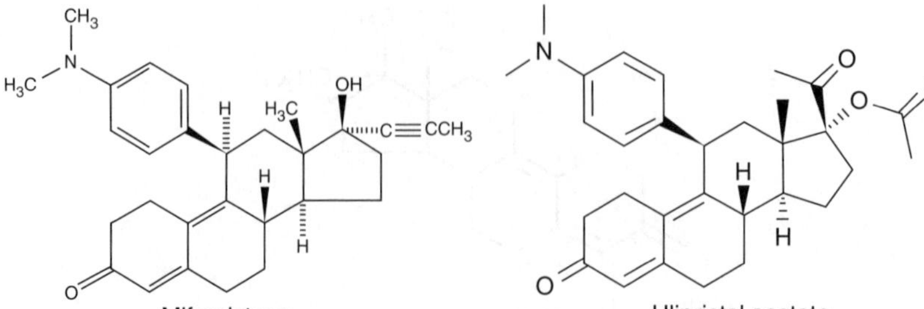

Mifepristone   Ulipristal acetate

Figure 2.12 Antiprogestins.

receptor. Subsequent studies demonstrated abortifacient properties for mifepristone during early pregnancy, and that sequential administration of a prostaglandin improved the success of expulsion. Medical abortion with the combination of mifepristone and misoprostol was first approved in France in 1988 and eventually the United States in 2000.[62]

UPA is another SPRM approved for emergency contraception and for the medical treatment of uterine fibroids in many countries.

Metabolism of Steroid Hormones

Blood Transport of Steroids

The ovaries secrete estrogens, progesterone, and androgens directly into the bloodstream. Most (approximately 70%) of the estradiol and testosterone produced by the ovaries circulate tightly bound to SHBG. About 30% circulate loosely bound to albumin. Albumin is the primary binding globulin for progesterone and the other androgens (DHEA, androstenedione, dihydrotestosterone). Another globulin CBG, also known as transcortin, binds about 18% of total progesterone.[3]

Only free hormone is available to bind to the steroid hormone receptor. Thus, increasing the amount of binding protein will decrease free hormone levels, and decreasing binding protein will increase activity. Albumin has high binding capacity due to large concentrations in the blood but has low affinity. SHBG generally has much lower capacity but high affinity. Therefore, levels of SHBG greatly influence SH activity. Most labs use indirect measurement to calculate free hormone concentration, by measuring the concentration of binding proteins to estimate the proportion free to total hormone. More recently, highly sensitive liquid chromatography–isotopic dilution tandem mass spectrometry (LC-MS/MS) methods have allowed for more precise direct measurement.[63]

Synthetic steroids also circulate bound to binding globulins. Ethinyl estradiol circulates about 90% bound to albumin.[64] All progestins bind with low affinity and high capacity to albumin. Progestins structurally related to testosterone (19-nortestosterone derivatives) bind with high affinity but low capacity to SHBG.[5] Again, contraceptive effects and off-target effects depend on free levels of the steroids.

Route of Administration, Metabolism, and Excretion

The effects of contraceptive steroid hormones differ depending on route of administration. Orally administered EE and all natural estrogens other than estetrol undergo extensive first-pass metabolism and hepatic stimulation.[65] The hepatic stimulation results in the induction of important hepatic globulins involved in coagulation and in lipid and SH transport pathways.[65] Of major interest is the induction of SHBG by estrogen. The increase in SHBG that occurs in users of EE-containing combined hormonal contraceptive methods results in a decrease in free androgen levels, an important effect that provides the basis for treatment of androgen-related symptoms such as acne and hirsutism. The degree of hepatic induction following oral estrogen administration is dose dependent.[66,67] Estetrol appears to have lesser hepatic effects than other estrogens following oral administration.[48]

Parenteral administration of estradiol at physiologic levels does not result in this same type of hepatic stimulation.[65] Estradiol undergoes isomerization to estrone, a less potent estrogen, and this is of particular importance following oral administration.[68]

Estrogens other than estetrol are eliminated from the body by metabolic conversion to inactive molecules followed by excretion in the feces and urine. The first step in this metabolism requires hydroxylation catalyzed by cytochrome P450 (CYP) enzymes in the liver.[69] Therefore, drugs that increase or decrease the activity of CYP enzymes will influence the level of circulating estrogens. CYP3A4 and CYP2C9 are the major isoforms contributing to the oxidative metabolism of EE in human liver microsomes.[70] Estetrol is primarily eliminated through the urine following minimal liver metabolism.[71]

Comparator studies evaluating the effect of ligands on the suppression of FSH and induction of hepatic globulins have demonstrated that the synthetic estrogen EE is about 100-fold more potent than estradiol.[72] Since EE passes through the liver on first pass without extensive conjugation, the liver effects of EE remain potent on recirculation. These points deserve emphasis; the enhanced effects of EE over estradiol on induction of hepatic globulins occur due to greater potency, lack of significant first-pass conjugation, and potent induction on recirculation. Furthermore, while the stimulation effects of estradiol on the liver following oral administration occur primarily as a result of first pass, EE provides potent stimulation regardless of route of administration. For this reason, hormonal contraception with transdermal or transvaginal administration of EE is associated with a risk of venous thromboembolic event (VTE) similar to that observed with oral preparations.[73] In contrast, transdermal administration of estradiol in physiologic doses for postmenopausal hormone therapy does not increase the risk of thrombosis.[74]

As noted previously, the chemical structures of progestins vary widely, and these influence their metabolism and pharmacokinetics. Many of the progestins used in oral contraceptive practice must undergo metabolism from a prodrug to an active ligand. For example, norethindrone acetate, ethynodiol diacetate, norethynodrel, and lynestrenol convert to norethindrone, desogestrel to etonogestrel, and norgestimate to levonorgestrel and norelgestromin (levonorgestrel-3-oxime). The rate of this conversion and subsequent metabolism may contribute to observed differences in efficacy and side effect profiles.[75] The major metabolic transformations that lead to progestin elimination include reduction by CYP enzymes followed by conjugation to form sulfates or glucuronides at one or more hydroxyl groups of the molecules.[76] CYP enzymes play key roles in the metabolism of progestins, with CYP3A considered the most important isoform. However, coadministration of strong CYP3A inhibitors leads to only a modest increase in exposure to EE, LNG, and norethindrone, suggesting other pathways may also be important.[76] CYP3A inhibitors do increase the half-life and area under the curve of drospirenone. More concerning is the effect of strong and moderate CYP3A inducers such as rifampin, phenytoin, and efavirenz. These enzyme inducers significantly reduce area under the curve and half-life of EE and most progestins.[76] Recent studies have documented failures of the etonogestrel contraceptive implant associated with low drug levels in women using efavirenz.[77,78]

Only the free form of a progestogen is available for pharmacologic activity. Similar to androgens, the 19-nortestosterone–derived progestins bind to SHBG. The induction of SHBG by estrogens affects the free concentration of these progestins, but at steady state is not clinically important. Obesity also affects the bioavailable level of a progestin.[79–81]

Whether progestogens have a direct effect on hepatic globulin production is controversial. Hepatocytes express estrogen and androgen receptors, but not progesterone receptors.[82] Thus, the effect of progestogens on liver function is likely mediated through the androgen receptor. This explains why at the same dose of EE, LNG pills show a smaller increase in SHBG than the antiandrogenic drospirenone.[83] While some epidemiologic research suggests that users of combined contraceptives containing androgenic progestins have a lower risk of thrombosis compared to low androgen products,[84] prospective clinical trials have not confirmed this effect.[73,85]

Practical Aspects of Route of Administration

To provide a continuous contraceptive effect, a product must deliver sufficient drug to maintain the desired pharmacodynamics effect over the entire interval between dosing. The amount of drug required is determined by the route of administration, metabolism, and mechanism of action. Since inhibition of ovulation represents the primary mechanism of action for most systemic hormonal contraceptives, an "ovulation inhibitory" concentration of a progestogen must be maintained. This level differs according to the potency of the various progestogens and route of administration. With oral and intramuscular methods, a relative "overdose" (high peak level) is delivered to ensure that the trough level (at 24 hours for oral contraceptives and 3 months for progestin-only intramuscular contraceptives) is above the ovulation inhibitory level. In contrast, implants release drug at steady state (after an initial burst) thereby resulting in lower peak and area under the curve drug levels. Injectable contraception results in the highest peak levels. Nondaily methods like implants and the ring can deliver continuous low levels systemically without

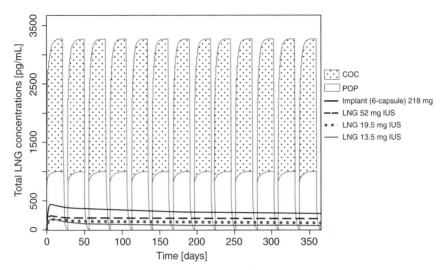

Figure 2.13 Comparison of typical levels of levonorgestrel serum levels obtained with different delivery systems. COC, combined oral contraceptives; POP, progestin-only pill; IUS, intrauterine system. Patterned areas reflect range between minimum and maximum concentrations seen with oral dosing. This narrows for COCs, as steady state is achieved during the first week of administration, and then declines to zero during the hormone-free interval. The range for POP reflects steady state with continuous dosing. (Adapted with permission from **Reinecke I, Hofmann B, Mesic E, Drenth HJ, Garmann D,** An integrated population pharmacokinetic analysis to characterize levonorgestrel pharmacokinetics after different administration routes, J Clin Pharmacol 58:1639–1654, 2018.)

a high peak. Because the hormonal IUS can be very effective with delivery of high levels of hormone locally and does not require ovulation inhibition as a mechanism of action, the amount of circulating drug is significantly lower than all other methods. **Figure 2.13** compares serum levels of LNG-containing contraceptives among women using a variety of different delivery systems.

Pharmacology Versus Marketing—Dose Versus Generation

The pharmacology of the different estrogens and progestins is already difficult enough to understand without persons or companies trying to push forward a new agenda to describe hormones. Beginning in the 1990s, pharmaceutical company marketing began to drive the way in which contraceptive products were described, to their own detriment. Prominent examples include the creation of a generation system to create the aura that newer generations of products are "better" in some way, shape, or form and renaming compounds to avoid bad press.

The nomenclature "generations" of oral contraceptive formulations did not exist in the medical world until new gonane progestins were marketed in 1992. The concepts of "high-dose" and "low-dose" oral contraceptive formulations were well known based on the estrogen content. The demarcation, with low-dose implying products with less than 50 µg of EE, was based on clinical outcomes and clear medical guidance; low-dose contraceptives had lower rates of VTEs than high-dose products.[86]

The use of the term "generation" to classify oral contraceptives lacks any scientific foundation. The marketing push in the early 1990s attempted to differentiate, on a worldwide basis, oral contraceptive formulations containing desogestrel, gestodene, and norgestimate from existing formulations, primarily those containing levonorgestrel (norgestrel) or norethindrone products. Keep in mind that all estranes are metabolized to norethindrone, so these products are basically the same.

In an instant, we had three generations of oral contraceptives:

■ First generation: EE doses of 50 µg or more, regardless of progestin
■ Second generation: EE doses less than 50 µg combined with levonorgestrel (norgestrel) or norethindrone
■ Third generation: EE doses less than 50 µg combined with desogestrel, gestodene, or norgestimate

First, why is the estrogen the deciding factor (first generation) and then it doesn't matter? This type of structure implies, based on the high-dose/low-dose concept, a lowering of VTE risk with advancing generation.

The pharmacology should hopefully be apparent: norethindrone is an estrane, while levonorgestrel, desogestrel, gestodene, and norgestimate are all gonanes. It is possible and even likely that some differences exist between progestins. But is this the right way to understand the products? Real life proved that the answer was "no."

Second, as mentioned previously, norgestimate is a prodrug. This was very confusing to the medical community. Is it a second-generation or third-generation product? As a prodrug, its primary metabolite is a LNG derivative. Pharmacologically, it makes sense that it is a second-generation product, but the pharmaceutical companies obviously would benefit from convincing providers and patients that the progestin is third generation.

Third, the second generation combines an estrane and a gonane. Are these really the same products? Should we consider the side effects the same?

Finally, the idea that the new products represented a third (newer) generation implied better everything, including safety. By the late 1990s, evidence began to accumulate that the "third-generation" pills incurred slightly higher risk of VTE than "second-generation" pills. This finding contradicts the concepts introduced by creating a first and second generation based on the high-dose/low-dose concept...how confusing. The same companies that spent a lot of money pushing that these new pills were "better" were then trying to convince everyone that they were really the same...yes, overall, they were gonanes just like LNG. In fact, we know now that the manner in which all progestins interact with EE, a potent estrogen, results in small differential effects on VTE risk.[87]

Subsequently, contraceptives containing drospirenone were introduced as "fourth-generation" products. Even though pills with dienogest and nomegestrol acetate contain estradiol and not EE, marketers also call them "fourth generation" because they are now afraid to infer a higher level of safety, even though evidence suggest equal or lower rates of VTE compared to second- and third-generation EE–containing products.[46]

Renaming compounds in a manner to avoid inference with bad outcomes, specifically, VTE, also became prominent and served to potentially confuse the clinician and scientific community. As mentioned previously, confusion over classification of norgestimate abounded and naming the progestin was part of the confusion. A company trying to differentiate a pill with norgestimate has trouble doing so when the primary metabolite is levonorgestrel-3-oxime. So, with the introduction of norgestimate-containing pills came information about the primary active metabolite, named 17-deacytlnorgestimate. Really? We are going to name a product based on what used to be there (remove something from the 17-carbon) before first-pass metabolism? Although standard organic chemistry nomenclature includes naming products based on removal of a methyl or methylene group (e.g., pregnane and norpregnane), we typically do not name a product by what is specifically removed. This is like giving directions to someone new to the area by telling them to go down a few blocks to where Johnson's Deli used to be and turn right; a stranger would not know where that business used to be and would just be confused and lost. Of course, this name served the purpose of focusing users on the new progestin (norgestimate) and not on the competitor (levonorgestrel). With the introduction of a contraceptive patch containing 17-deacytylnorgestimate (levonorgestrel-3-oxime), the name was changed to norelgestromin.

Etonogestrel is another "new" name to draw attention away from the parent compound. When desogestrel was introduced for oral contraception, the primary active metabolite was known as 3-ketodesogestrel. With the introduction of the contraceptive vaginal ring containing ethinyl estradiol and 3-ketodesogestrel, marketers were faced with a medical community concerned about the risk of VTE with ethinyl estradiol/desogestrel-containing oral contraceptives. Hence, a name change to not include "desogestrel" would avoid potential conflict.

As a community, how many generations will there be? At what point will we know if some product is really safer or better? We can better understand differences and potential benefits if we simply know what hormones are in the products we prescribe. *We recommend that clinicians understand and classify the various progestins according to the established scientific nomenclature described above and evaluate individual products according to the results of clinical trials.*

61

Generic Products

Generic products are therapeutically equivalent drugs, containing the same amount of active ingredients in the same concentration and dosage form. These products are generally less expensive versions marketed by pharmaceutical companies after patent expiration of the original drug. Generic oral contraceptives need only meet the test of bioequivalence; studies to demonstrate efficacy, side effects, and safety are not required. Meeting the test of bioequivalence requires demonstration in a small number of subjects that absorption, concentrations, and time curves are comparable to the reference drug. The generic product will be approved if the bioequivalence testing ranges from 80% to 125% of the values for the reference drug (differences no >20% lower or 25% higher). Approved, patented products must not vary more than ±10%; therefore, a generic oral contraceptive could contain only 70% of the standard dose. In the lowest-dose oral contraceptives, this could impair efficacy. However, we should hasten to point out that there has been no evidence or even anecdotal suggestions that generic oral contraceptives have reduced efficacy or cause more side effects such as breakthrough bleeding. Patients should be forewarned that generic products differ in shape, packaging, and color.

Potency

For many years, clinicians, scientists, medical writers, and even the pharmaceutical industry attempted to assign potency values to the various progestational components of hormonal contraceptives. An accurate assessment, however, has been difficult to achieve for many reasons. Progestins act on numerous target organs (e.g., the uterus, the mammary glands, and the liver), and potency varies depending on the target organ and end point being studied. In the past, animal assays, such as the Clauberg test (endometrial change in the rabbit) and the rat ventral prostate assay, were used to determine progestin potency. Although these were considered acceptable methods at the time, a better understanding of SH action and metabolism and a recognition that animal and human responses differ have led to greater reliance on data collected from human studies.

Historically, this has been a confusing issue because publications and experts used potency ranking to provide clinical advice. There is absolutely no need for confusion. Progestin potency is no longer a consideration when it comes to prescribing hormonal contraception, because the potency of the various progestins has been accounted for by appropriate adjustments of dose. For example, the biologic effect (in this case the clinical effect) of the various progestational components in current low-dose oral contraceptives is approximately the same. Our progress in lowering the doses of the steroids contained in oral contraceptives has yielded products with little serious differences. The potency of a drug does not determine its efficacy or safety, only the amount of a drug required to achieve an effect and the manner in which the hormone is delivered.

Clinical advice based on potency ranking is an artificial exercise that has not stood the test of time. There is no clinical evidence that a particular progestin is better or worse in terms of particular side effects or clinical responses. Thus, hormones should be recognized by their pharmacology, and hormonal contraceptives should be judged by their clinical characteristics: efficacy, side effects, risks, and benefits.

References

1. **Simmer HH,** On the history of hormonal contraception I. Ludwig Haberlandt (1885–1932) and his concept of "hormonal sterilization", Contraception 1:3–27, 1970.

2. **Simmer HH,** On the history of hormonal contraception II. Otfried Otto Fellner (1873–19??) and estrogens as antifertility hormones, Contraception 3:1–20, 1971.

3. **Hammond GL,** Plasma steroid-binding proteins: primary gatekeepers of steroid hormone action, J Endocrinol 230: R13–R25, 2016.

4. **Taylor HS, Pal L, Seli,** Speroff's Clinical Gynecologic Endocrinology and Infertility, 9th ed., Wolters Kluwer, Philadelphia, 2019.

5. **Stanczyk FZ, Hapgood JP, Winer S, Mishell DR,** Progestogens used in postmenopausal hormone therapy: differences in their pharmacological properties, intracellular actions, and clinical effects, Endocr Rev 34:171–208, 2013.

6. **Bouchard P, Chabbert-Buffet N, Fauser BC,** Selective progesterone receptor modulators in reproductive medicine: pharmacology, clinical efficacy and safety, Fertil Steril 96:1175–1189, 2011.

7. **Kannan A, Bhurke A, Sitruk-Ware R, Lalitkumar PG, Gemzell-Danielsson K, Williams ARW, et al.,** Characterization of molecular changes in endometrium associated with chronic use of progesterone receptor modulators: ulipristal acetate versus mifepristone, Reprod Sci 25:320–328, 2018.

8. **Clarke H, Dhillo WS, Jayasena CN,** Comprehensive review on kisspeptin and its role in reproductive disorders, Endocrinol Metab 30:124–141, 2015.

9. **Moore AM, Coolen LM, Porter DT, Goodman RL, Lehman MN,** KNDy cells revisited, Endocrinology 159:3219–3234, 2018.

10. **Seifer DB, Baker VL, Leader B,** Age-specific serum anti-Mullerian hormone values for 17,120 women presenting to fertility centers within the United States, Fertil Steril 95:747–750, 2011.

11. **Baerwald AR, Adams GP, Pierson RA,** Ovarian antral folliculogenesis during the human menstrual cycle: a review, Hum Reprod Update 18:73–91, 2012.

12. **Sanders SL, Stouffer RL,** Localization of steroidogenic enzymes in macaque luteal tissue during the menstrual cycle and simulated early pregnancy: immunohistochemical evidence supporting the two-cell model for estrogen production in the primate corpus luteum, Biol Reprod 56:1077–1087, 1997.

13. **Gougeon A,** Dynamics of follicular growth in the human: a model from preliminary results, Hum Reprod 1:81–87, 1986.

14. **Kim J, Bagchi IC, Bagchi MK,** Control of ovulation in mice by progesterone receptor-regulated gene networks, Mol Hum Reprod 15:821–828, 2009.

15. **Slayden OD, Brenner RM,** Hormonal regulation and localization of estrogen, progestin and androgen receptors in the endometrium of nonhuman primates: effects of progesterone receptor antagonists, Arch Histol Cytol 67:393–409, 2004.

16. **Slayden OD, Brenner RM,** A critical period of progesterone withdrawal precedes menstruation in macaques, Reprod Biol Endocrinol 4:S6, 2006.

17. **Maybin JA, Critchley HO,** Steroid regulation of menstrual bleeding and endometrial repair, Rev Endocr Metab Disord 13:253–263, 2012.

18. **Greaves E, Collins F, Critchley HO, Saunders PT,** ERbeta-dependent effects on uterine endothelial cells are cell specific and mediated via Sp1, Hum Reprod 28:2490–2501, 2013.

63

19. **Simmons KB, Edelman AB, Fu R, Jensen JT,** Tamoxifen for the treatment of breakthrough bleeding with the etonogestrel implant: a randomized controlled trial, Contraception 95:198–204, 2017.

20. **Han L, Taub R, Jensen JT,** Cervical mucus and contraception: what we know and what we don't, Contraception 96:310–321, 2017.

21. **Gemzell-Danielsson K, Berger C, Lalitkumar PG,** Mechanisms of action of oral emergency contraception, Gynecol Endocrinol 30:685–687, 2014.

22. **Boggavarapu NR, Berger C, von Grothusen C, Menezes J, Gemzell-Danielsson K, Lalitkumar PG,** Effects of low doses of mifepristone on human embryo implantation process in a three-dimensional human endometrial in vitro co-culture system, Contraception 94:143–151, 2016.

23. **Asante A, Coddington CC, Schenck L, Stewart EA,** Thin endometrial stripe does not affect likelihood of achieving pregnancy in clomiphene citrate/intra-uterine insemination cycles, Fertil Steril 100:1610–1614 e1, 2013.

24. **Barbosa I, Olsson SE, Odlind V, Goncalves T, Coutinho E,** Ovarian function after seven years' use of a levonorgestrel IUD, Adv Contracept 11:85–95, 1995.

25. **Ortiz ME, Croxatto HB, Bardin CW,** Mechanisms of action of intrauterine devices, Obstet Gynecol Surv 51:S42–S51, 1996.

26. **Doisy EA, Veler CD, Thayer S,** The preparation of the crystalline ovarian hormone from the urine of pregnant women, J Biol Chem 86:499–509, 1930.

27. **Marker RE,** The early production of steroid hormones, CHOC News, The Center for History of Medicine, University of Pennsylvania, 4:3, 1987.

28. **Marker RE,** Interview by Jeffrey L. Sturchio at Pennsylvania State University, Chemical Heritage Foundation, Philadelphia, Oral History: Transcript No. 0068, April 17, 1987.

29. **Djerassi C,** Problems of manufacture and distribution. The manufacture of steroidal contraceptives: technical versus political aspects, Proc R Soc B 195:175, 1976.

30. **Rosenkranz G,** The early days of Syntex, Chemical Heritage 23:10 and 12, 2004.

31. **Rosenkranz G, Pataki J, Djerassi C,** Synthesis of cortisone, J Am Chem Soc 76:4055, 1951.

32. **Djerassi C, Miramontes L, Rosenkranz G, Sondheimer F,** Synthesis of 19-nor-17alpha-ethynyltestosterone and 19-nor-17alpha-methyltestosterone, J Am Chem Soc 76:4092, 1954.

33. **Tullner WW, Hertz R,** Progestational activity of 19-norprogesterone and 19-nor-ethisterone in the Rhesus monkey, Proc Soc Exp Biol Med 94:298, 1957.

34. **Herz R, Waite JH, Thomas LB,** Progestational effectiveness of 19-nor-ethinyl-testosterone by oral route in women, Proc Soc Exp Biol Med 91:418, 1956.

35. **Tullner WW, Herz R,** High progestational activity of 19-norprogesterone, Endocrinology 52:359, 1953.

36. **Tyler ET,** Comparative evaluation of various types of administration of progesterone, J Clin Endocrinol Metab 15:881, 1955.

37. **Pincus G, Chang MC,** The effects of progesterone and related compounds on ovulation and early development in the rabbit, Acta Physiol Lat Am 3:177–183, 1953.

38. **Pincus G,** The hormonal control of ovulation and early development, Postgrad Med 24:654, 1958.

39. **Vessey MP, Doll R,** Investigation of relation between use of oral contraceptives and thromboembolic disease, Br Med J 2:199–205, 1968.

40. **Inman WH, Vessey MP, Westerholm B, Engelund A,** Thromboembolic disease and the steroidal content of oral contraceptives. A report to the Committee on Safety of Drugs, Br Med J 2:203–209, 1970.

41. **Blackburn S,** Maternal, Fetal, & Neonatal Physiology: A Clinical Perspective, 5th ed., Elsevier Health Sciences, St. Louis, MO, 2017.

42. **Coelingh Bennink HJ, Holinka CF, Diczfalusy E,** Estetrol review: profile and potential clinical applications, Climacteric 11:47–58, 2008.

43. **Jensen JT, Addis IB, Hennebold JD, Bogan RL,** Ovarian lipid metabolism modulates circulating lipids in premenopausal women, J Clin Endocrinol Metab 102:3138–3145, 2017.

44. **Goldzieher JW,** Selected aspects of the pharmacokinetics and metabolism of

ethinyl estrogens and their clinical implications, Am J Obstet Gynecol 163:318, 1990.

45. **Goldzieher J, Stanczyk FZ,** Oral contraceptives and individual variability of circulating levels of ethinyl estradiol and progestins, Contraception 78:4, 2008.

46. **Dinger J, Do Minh T, Heinemann K,** Impact of estrogen type on cardiovascular safety of combined oral contraceptives, Contraception 94:328–339, 2016.

47. **Jensen JT, Edelman AB, Chen BA, Archer DF, Barnhart KT, Thomas MA, et al.,** Continuous dosing of a novel contraceptive vaginal ring releasing Nestorone(R) and estradiol: pharmacokinetics from a dose-finding study, Contraception 97:422–427, 2018.

48. **Farris M, Bastianelli C, Rosato E, Brosens I, Benagiano G,** Pharmacodynamics of combined estrogen-progestin oral contraceptives: 2. Effects on hemostasis, Expert Rev Clin Pharmacol 10:1129–1144, 2017.

49. **Speroff L, DeCherney A,** Evaluation of a new generation of oral contraceptives, Obstet Gynecol 81:1034, 1993.

50. **Stanczyk FZ,** All progestins are not created equal, Steroids 68:879–890, 2003.

51. **Stanczyk FZ, Roy S,** Metabolism of levonorgestrel, norethindrone, and structurally related contraceptive steroids, Contraception 42:67, 1990.

52. **Edgren RA,** Progestagens, In: Givens J, ed. Clinical Uses of Steroids, Yearbook, Chicago, 1980, p 1.

53. **Kuhnz W, Blode H, Maher M,** Systemic availability of levonorgestrel after single oral administration of a noregestimate-containing combination oral contraceptive to 12 young women, Contraception 49:255, 1994.

54. **Stanczyk FZ,** Pharmacokinetics of the new progestogens and influence of gestodene and desogestrel on ethinyl-estradiol metabolism, Contraception 55:273, 1997.

55. **Hammond GL, Abrams LS, Creasy GW, Natarajan J, Allen JG, Siiteri PK,** Serum distribution of the major metabolites of noregestimate in relation to its pharmacological properties, Contraception 67:93, 2003.

56. **Sitruik-Ware RL,** New progestagens for contraceptive use, Hum Reprod Update 12:169, 2006.

57. **Foster RH, Wilde MI,** Dienogest, Drugs 56:825, 1998.

58. **Fuhrmann U, Krattenmacher R, Slater EP, Fritzemeier K-H,** The novel progestin drospirenone and its natural counterpart progesterone: biochemical profile and antiandrogenic potential, Contraception 54:243, 1996.

59. **Oelkers W, Helmerhorst FM, Wuttke W, Heithecker R,** Effect of an oral contraceptive containing drospirenone on the renin-angiotensin-aldosterone system in healthy female volunteers, Gynecol Endocrinol 14:204, 2000.

60. **Loughlin J, Seeger JD, Eng PM, Foegh M, Clifford CR, Cutone J, Walker AM,** Risk of hyperkalemia in women taking ethinylestradiol/drospirenone and other oral contraceptives, Contraception 78:377, 2008.

61. **Chabbert-Buffet N, Pintiaux A, Bouchard P,** The imminent dawn of SPRMs in obstetrics and gynecology, Mol Cell Endocrinol 358:232–243, 2012.

62. **Winikoff B, Westhoff C,** Fifteen years: looking back and looking forward, Contraception 92:177–178, 2015.

63. **Rhea JM, French D, Molinaro RJ,** Direct total and free testosterone measurement by liquid chromatography tandem mass spectrometry across two different platforms, Clin Biochem 46:656–664, 2013.

64. **Zhang H, Cui D, Wang B, Han YH, Balimane P, Yang Z, et al.,** Pharmacokinetic drug interactions involving 17alpha-ethinylestradiol: a new look at an old drug, Clin Pharmacokinet 46:133–157, 2007.

65. **Balfour JA, Heel RC,** Transdermal estradiol. A review of its pharmacodynamic and pharmacokinetic properties, and therapeutic efficacy in the treatment of menopausal complaints, Drugs 40:561–582, 1990.

66. **Ottosson UB, Carlstrom K, Johansson BG, von Schoultz B,** Estrogen induction of liver proteins and high-density lipoprotein cholesterol: comparison between estradiol valerate and ethinyl estradiol, Gynecol Obstet Invest 22:198–205, 1986.

67. **Matsui S, Yasui T, Kasai K, Keyama K, Yoshida K, Kato T, et al.,** Sex hormone-binding globulin and antithrombin III activity in women with oral ultra-low-dose estradiol, J Obstet Gynaecol 37:627–632, 2017.

65

68. **Kopper NW, Gudeman J, Thompson DJ,** Transdermal hormone therapy in postmenopausal women: a review of metabolic effects and drug delivery technologies, Drug Des Devel Ther 2:193–202, 2009.

69. **Tsuchiya Y, Nakajima M, Yokoi T,** Cytochrome P450-mediated metabolism of estrogens and its regulation in human, Cancer Lett 227:115–124, 2005.

70. **Wang B, Sanchez RI, Franklin RB, Evans DC, Huskey SE,** The involvement of CYP3A4 and CYP2C9 in the metabolism of 17 alpha-ethinylestradiol, Drug Metab Dispos 32:1209–1212, 2004.

71. **Visser M, et al.,** *In vitro* effects of estetrol on receptor binding, drug targets and human liver cell metabolism, Climacteric 11:64–68, 2008.

72. **Mashchak CA, Lobo RA, Dozono-Takano R, Eggena P, Nakamura RM, Brenner PF, et al.,** Comparison of pharmacodynamic properties of various estrogen formulations, Am J Obstet Gynecol 144:511–518, 1982.

73. **Dinger J, Mohner S, Heinemann K,** Cardiovascular risk associated with the use of an etonogestrel-containing vaginal ring, Obstet Gynecol 122:800–808, 2013.

74. **Vinogradova Y, Coupland C, Hippisley-Cox J,** Use of hormone replacement therapy and risk of venous thromboembolism: nested case-control studies using the QResearch and CPRD databases, BMJ 364:k4810, 2019.

75. **Edelman AB, Cherala G, Stanczyk FZ,** Metabolism and pharmacokinetics of contraceptive steroids in obese women: a review, Contraception 82:314–323, 2010.

76. **Zhang N, Shon J, Kim M-J, Yu C, Zhang L, Huang S-M, et al.,** Role of CYP3A in oral contraceptives clearance, Clin Transl Sci 11:251–260, 2018.

77. **Chappell CA, Lamorde M, Nakalema S, Chen BA, Mackline H, Riddler SA, et al.,** Efavirenz decreases etonogestrel exposure: a pharmacokinetic evaluation of implantable contraception with antiretroviral therapy, AIDS 31:1965–1972, 2017.

78. **Leticee N, Viard JP, Yamgnane A, Karmochkine M, Benachi A,** Contraceptive failure of etonogestrel implant in patients treated with antiretrovirals including efavirenz, Contraception 85:425–427, 2012.

79. **Edelman A, Cherala G, Lim JY, Jensen JT,** Contraceptive failures in overweight and obese combined hormonal contraceptive users, Obstet Gynecol 122:158–159, 2013.

80. **Edelman AB, Carlson NE, Cherala G, Munar MY, Stouffer RL, Cameron JL, et al.,** Impact of obesity on oral contraceptive pharmacokinetics and hypothalamic-pituitary-ovarian activity, Contraception 80:119–127, 2009.

81. **Edelman AB, Cherala G, Blue SW, Erikson DW, Jensen JT,** Impact of obesity on the pharmacokinetics of levonorgestrel-based emergency contraception: single and double dosing, Contraception 94:52–57, 2016.

82. **Shen M, Shi H,** Sex hormones and their receptors regulate liver energy homeostasis, Int J Endocrinol 2015:294278, 2015.

83. **Coelingh Bennink HJ, Zimmerman Y, Laan E, Termeer HM, Appels N, Albert A, et al.,** Maintaining physiological testosterone levels by adding dehydroepiandrosterone to combined oral contraceptives: I. Endocrine effects, Contraception 96:322–329, 2016.

84. **Lidegaard O, Nielsen LH, Skovlund CW, Skjeldestad FE, Lokkegaard E,** Risk of venous thromboembolism from use of oral contraceptives containing different progestogens and oestrogen doses: Danish cohort study, 2001–9, BMJ 343:d6423, 2011.

85. **Dinger J, Bardenheuer K, Heinemann K,** Cardiovascular and general safety of a 24-day regimen of drospirenone-containing combined oral contraceptives: final results from the International Active Surveillance Study of Women Taking Oral Contraceptives, Contraception 89:253–263, 2014.

86. **de Bastos M, Stegeman BH, Rosendaal FR, Van Hylckama Vlieg A, Helmerhorst FM, Stijnen T, Dekkers OM,** Combined oral contraceptives: venous thrombosis, Cochrane Database Syst Rev (3), Art. No.: CD010813, doi:10.1002/14651858.CD010813.pub2, 2014.

87. **Dinger J, Shapiro S,** Combined oral contraceptives, venous thromboembolism, and the problem of interpreting large but incomplete datasets, J Fam Plann Reprod Health Care 38:2–6, 2012.

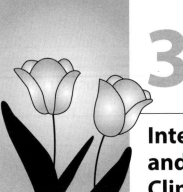

3

Interpreting Evidence and Creating Clinical Guidance on Contraception

**Kathryn M. Curtis, PhD and
David Hubacher, PhD, MPH**

C linical practice is the ultimate distillate of evidence, judgment, and experience. The safety, side effects, and benefits of treatments are established by clinical research. The clinician must determine whether results from studies are clinically relevant and useful. Incorporating research findings into clinical practice depends upon that determination. In this chapter, we provide a guide for interpreting published research and making judgments on clinical and epidemiologic studies, systematic reviews, and clinical practice guidelines.

Prior to initiating any clinical trial, regardless of design, investigators must register the study in a clinical trials database. Examples include ClinicalTrials.gov, a U.S. registry, and the EU Clinical Trials Register. These databases were created to provide information for patients, health care professionals, researchers, and the public on publicly and privately supported clinical trials. Investigators must also submit the key final results to the registry to ensure that all clinical studies, including those with negative findings, are reported. Most reputable peer-reviewed medical journals will not publish a manuscript unless trial registration was performed prior to study initiation.

The Hierarchy of Clinical Research (in Descending Order of Internal Validity)

Table 3.1 shows a general hierarchy of clinical study designs from the U.S. Preventive Services Task Force (USPSTF). **Figure 3.1** provides an algorithm to classify various study designs.

The findings and conclusions in this chapter are those of the authors and do not necessarily represent the official position of the Centers for Disease Control and Prevention.

Table 3.1 U.S. Preventive Services Task Force (USPSTF) Evidence Grading Scheme

Quality of Evidence

Level I	Properly powered and conducted RCT; well-conducted systematic review or meta-analysis of homogeneous RCTs
Level II-1	Well-designed controlled trial without randomization
Level II-2	Well-designed cohort or case-control analysis study
Level II-3	Multiple time series, with or without the intervention; results from uncontrolled studies that yield results of large magnitude
Level III	Opinions of respected authorities, based on clinical experience; descriptive studies or case reports; reports of expert committees

Strength of Recommendation

A	The USPSTF recommends the service. There is high certainty that the net benefit is substantial.
B	The USPSTF recommends the service. There is high certainty that the net benefit is moderate, or there is moderate certainty that the net benefit is moderate to substantial.
C	The USPSTF recommends selectively offering or providing this service to individual patients based on professional judgment and patient preferences. There is at least moderate certainty that the net benefit is small.
D	The USPSTF recommends against the service. There is moderate or high certainty that the service has no net benefit or that the harms outweigh the benefits.
I	The USPSTF concludes that the current evidence is insufficient to assess the balance of benefits and harms of the service. Evidence is lacking, of poor quality, or conflicting, and the balance of benefits and harms cannot be determined.

RCT, randomized controlled trial.
Source: United States Preventive Services Task Force Procedure Manual, December 2015. https://www.uspreventiveservicestaskforce.org/Page/Name/procedure-manual; accessed June 19, 2019.

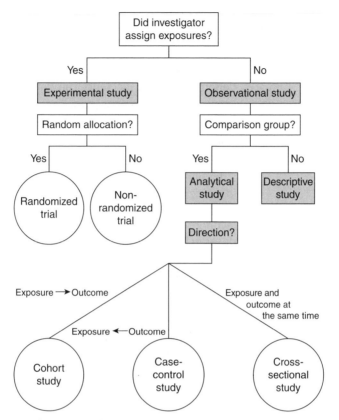

Figure 3.1 Algorithm for classification of types of clinical research. (Adapted from **Grimes DA, Schulz KF,** An overview of clinical research: the lay of the land, Lancet 359:57–61, 2002, Copyright 2002, with permission from Elsevier.)

Experimental Studies (Studies with the Exposure or Intervention Assigned by the Investigator)

Randomized Trials

A randomized trial is used to assign a treatment or intervention by chance and compare results. *Randomized controlled trials* (RCTs) are the most common type of randomized trial and involve at least two assignments: treatment(s) and control(s). Control assignments might be "standard treatment" or placebo, for example. A trial simply called a *randomized trial* is reserved for situations in which at least two experimental treatments are assigned (but no placebo or standard treatment). Participants theoretically have a random (unbiased) chance of being assigned to each group in the study, and the participant characteristics and unmeasurable influences should be nearly if not totally the same in each group. In *crossover randomized trials*, participants are randomly assigned to one treatment group and later assigned to the other group, and thus the participants serve as their own controls.

Randomized Trials

Advantages	Can provide evidence for causality. Prospective design permits person-time denominators and incidence calculations.
Disadvantages	Very expensive and time-consuming. Only a limited number of hypotheses can be evaluated in any one study.
Examples	A randomized controlled trial compared in a double-blind fashion the pregnancy rates in women using levonorgestrel 0.75 mg (*n* = 976) or ethinyl estradiol 100 mg plus levonorgestrel 0.5 mg (*n* = 979), with repeat doses in both groups 12 hours later, for emergency contraception.[1] In this study, the women receiving levonorgestrel constitute the treatment group, and the women receiving ethinyl estradiol/levonorgestrel (standard treatment), also known as the Yuzpe regimen, are the control group. Pregnancy occurred in 11 (1.1%) women in the levonorgestrel group compared with 31 (3.2%) in the Yuzpe regimen group. The crude relative risk of pregnancy for levonorgestrel compared with the Yuzpe regimen was 0.36 (95% CI, 0.18–0.70). Because the confidence interval (CI) does not include the null value of 1.0, the levonorgestrel group is superior.
	A crossover randomized trial assessed ovarian suppression during the use of combined oral contraceptives (COCs) with different durations of hormone-free interval.[2] Women were assigned to receive an ethinyl estradiol 20 µg plus norethindrone acetate 1 mg COC with either a 7-day hormone-free interval or a 4-day hormone-free interval. After 2 months, each group "crossed over" and used the other study drug for 2 months. Analysis of hormone levels in serum and cervical mucus suggested that the 4-day hormone-free interval regimen provided better ovarian suppression than the 7-day hormone-free interval regimen.

Nonrandomized Trials

In a nonrandomized trial, the intervention or exposure is still assigned by the investigator but in a nonrandom manner (e.g., by alternate assignment, odd/even subject numbers, day of the week). The essential feature of a trial involving comparisons (randomized or nonrandomized) is that participants are assigned to groups without clinical judgment or participant self-selection; many published reports labeled as trials are perhaps more accurately described as cohort studies, expanded case series, and/or prospective comparative studies. However, a trial can also be a single-arm study of a new drug or new indication for which clinical judgment is required to assess eligibility to participate. Without the benefit of randomization, nonrandomized trials may be subject to the same biases as observational studies.

Nonrandomized Trials	
Advantages	May be used when randomization is not possible for ethical or logistical reasons.
Disadvantages	Subject to selection or allocation bias (a systematic difference in how patients are assigned to the study groups) and confounding (due to the potential for baseline differences between the study groups).
Example	A nonrandomized trial evaluated a computerized contraceptive decision aid for adolescent patients.[3] Using alternate assignment (i.e., every other participant was assigned to the intervention or control groups), 456 adolescent females were assigned to the intervention group (standard education plus a contraceptive decision-making computer program), and 493 adolescent females were assigned to the control group (standard education only). The intervention group demonstrated increased short-term knowledge about oral contraceptives compared with the control group, but there were no differences in duration of oral contraceptive use over 1 year between groups.

Observational Studies (Nonexperimental Studies: Observation Without Intervention)

Observational studies that compare different groups (cohort, case-control, and cross-sectional) are higher-order studies than purely descriptive clinical reports (case series and case reports).

Cohort studies: In cohort studies, exposure information is collected from all subjects who are disease free, and subjects' experiences are recorded forward from "time zero" to determine who develops disease. Cohort studies can be prospective (starting time zero in the present and moving forward through "real time") or retrospective (starting time zero and exposures in the past and documenting subsequent disease that may have also occurred in the past).

Cohort Studies	
Advantages	Can evaluate changes over time and, if prospective, minimize recall bias. Permits person-time denominators and incidence calculations.
Disadvantages	Can be expensive, lengthy in time, and subject to selection bias and surveillance bias making the two groups being compared unequal; not well suited for studying rare outcomes; loss to follow-up can be a major source of bias.
Examples	A prospective cohort study, the International Active Surveillance Study of Women Taking Oral Contraceptives, enrolled 85,109 women who were followed prospectively for 2 to 6 years and found no increased risk of venous thromboembolism from the use of newer drospirenone-containing COCs compared with levonorgestrel-containing COCs.[4]
	A retrospective cohort study used data from the Danish national registries to identify 1,626,158 women of reproductive age and looked back over 15 years for exposure to COCs and incidence of thrombotic events. Rates of thrombotic stroke and myocardial infarction were higher among COC users compared with nonusers.[5]

Case-control studies: Case-control studies select a group of individuals with a disease or condition (cases) and compare them with a carefully selected group of individuals who do not have the disease or condition (controls). The exposure history of those with disease and those with no disease is collected and compared to determine if exposure is positively or negatively associated with being a case. The control group must be a population that would naturally produce the cases.

Case-Control Studies

Advantages	Can be relatively quick and inexpensive because investigators don't recruit participants and wait for the uncertainty of developing the disease/condition; good for rare outcomes.
Disadvantages	Subject to recall bias regarding past exposures and other errors. Usually relies on information recorded by others not with the intention of collecting data for research purposes and is, therefore, subject to missing or incomplete data. Must have sufficient (natural) levels of exposure for drawing possible associations with the disease or condition because the exposure is not controlled by the researchers; cannot estimate incidence rates, unless population-based.
Example	The World Health Organization (WHO) Collaborative Study of Cardiovascular Disease and Steroid Hormone Contraception identified 3,697 cases of stroke, myocardial infarction, or VTE among women of reproductive age, along with 9,997 controls (women without stroke, myocardial infarction, or VTE), and found no statistically significant increased risk of these thrombotic events based on an adjusted odds ratio (aOR) among oral progestin-only users (aOR 1.74; 95% CI, 0.76–3.99) or progestin-only injectable contraceptors (aOR 2.19; 95% CI, 0.66–7.26) compared with nonusers. Because the confidence interval includes the null value of 1.0, the treatment groups are not considered different than nonusers.[6]

Cross-sectional studies: Cross-sectional studies describe a group of individuals and assess exposure and disease simultaneously at one point in time.

<table>
<tr><td colspan="2">**Cross-Sectional Studies**</td></tr>
<tr><td>*Advantages*</td><td>An appropriate method to estimate prevalence; generally quick and inexpensive. Often used for exploring associations between a condition and possible causes.</td></tr>
<tr><td>*Disadvantages*</td><td>Cannot establish cause-effect relationship, cannot assess changes over time.</td></tr>
<tr><td>*Example*</td><td>The National Survey of Family Growth is a periodic cross-sectional survey conducted in the United States since the 1960s; one of the latest iterations showed that oral contraceptives were the single most prevalent form of contraception (26% among current contraception users).[7]</td></tr>
</table>

Case Reports and Case Series

Case reports: A single description or handful of descriptions of anecdotal exposures/problems/conditions. Initial reports might lead to more systematic searches for similar situations; this is often described as a *case series*.

Case series: A study in which participants are sampled if they have the outcome of interest (a particular disease or disease-related outcome); may or may not have information on exposure

Both case reports and series serve to draw attention to problems of unknown cause and often lay the groundwork for hypotheses that rule out the role of chance/coincidental occurrence. Traditionally, case reports and case series were generated from personal clinical practice, but today, the source of reports can be external, like surveying a group on a listserv for similar cases and reporting as a case series.

Case reports and case series do not have a comparison group and do not attempt to estimate the risks of disease from an exposure or estimate incidence or absolute risk; in this way, they are different from cohort studies and case-control studies.

Case Reports and Case Series

Advantages	Easy to assemble information and requires little study planning.
Disadvantages	Descriptive only: does not take a scientific approach to concluding anything about cause Does not allow for calculations of absolute risk.
Examples	A case report described migration of a transcervical female sterilization microinsert, including details of the placement procedure, detection of migration of the microinsert, and resolution of the problem, along with an accompanying literature review on the topic.[8]
	A case series of 218 pregnancies among etonogestrel implant users is described; 45 women had insufficient data to assess why pregnancy occurred, 46 were determined to have been pregnant at the time of implant insertion, 84 had unrecognized noninsertion, 30 failed for other reasons, and 13 were deemed to be product failures.[9]

Bias: Distortions Due to Study Design and Other Factors

The concerns over possible bias generally increase the more an investigation strays from standard experimental methodology. Identifying potential sources of bias and then attempting to mitigate their impact in the ascertainment of data (both exposure and disease) are essential aims of epidemiologic research. In addition, a large body of sophisticated statistical analysis and techniques have been developed to further improve the validity of research results.[10]

Detection/Surveillance/Diagnostic Bias: Systematic errors in methods of ascertainment, diagnosis, or verification of disease status. Can occur when not everyone in the study population has equal access to or utilization of medical interventions and diagnostic tests.

Publication Bias: Negative (null) studies and studies that confirm old results tend not to be published. An important source of bias in meta-analysis.

Reporting or Recall Bias: Inaccurate memory and selective recall introduce errors.

Selection Bias: Occurs when procedures for selecting study participants or influences enabling participation affect the internal and external validity of the measurements. Differences in characteristics between those selected for study and those not selected may be a result of preferential prescribing, family history, preferential referral of patients, or a healthy user effect.

For case-control studies, the source of the controls is important. Hospital-based controls are less likely to be representative of the general population than population-based controls. In cohort studies, if the selection methods for the exposed and unexposed groups lead to groups that are not representative of the target population, selection bias can result.

Information or Observer Bias: A flaw in measuring exposure or outcome that produces different results between comparison groups. Nonresponse by subjects or patients lost to follow-up can produce differences in cohort studies.

Confounding: Three characteristics are necessary, but not sufficient, for a factor to be a confounder: a risk factor for the disease, associated with the exposure of interest, and not an intermediary step in the pathway between exposure and disease. Factors such as age, body weight, and smoking are often confounders in the exposure-disease relationship. In the data analysis phase, multivariable approaches and statistical tests for examining relationships between participants' background factors and the role of such explanatory factors on disease are essential. Often, it is impossible to fully address the relationships due to errors in the measurement of confounding factors and statistical limitations (too few outcome events in relationship to the permutations of different sets of background factors). In essence, it is important to remember that statistical modeling, including multivariable analyses, cannot always make up for confounding or missing data.

The following fictitious retrospective cohort study illustrates these concepts. Returning women sophomores at unnamed state university participated in a survey to recount their freshman experiences. All women who were sexually active in their first year (n = 3,991) were included in the analysis to explore the relationship between the exposure, condom use (reported as their primary form of contraception), and the outcome, unintended pregnancy.

Crude Relative Risk Analysis

		Unintended Pregnancy?		Total	Proportion Who Experienced Unintended Pregnancy
		Yes	No		
Were condoms primary contraceptive method?	Yes	99	1,909	2,008	4.9%
	No	33	1,950	1,983	1.7%
	Total	132	3,859	3,991	

The crude relative risk is calculated as follows: 4.9%/1.7% = 3.0 (95% CI, 2.0 to 4.4). The 95% confidence interval is calculated with standard statistical analysis software. From the crude analysis, women who used condoms as their primary method of contraception were three times as likely to experience unintended pregnancy as those who did not use condoms as their primary method.

Also included in the questionnaire was the question: Did you often go to fraternity/sorority functions/parties as a freshman? As it turned out, 2,408 students did not go to such functions often, while 1,583 did. Condom use and unintended pregnancy were then re-examined separately in each stratum labeled Greek life (yes or no).

No Greek Life: Relative Risk Analysis

		Unintended Pregnancy?		Total	Proportion Who Experienced Unintended Pregnancy
		Yes	No		
Were condoms primary contraceptive method?	Yes	9	608	617	1.5%
	No	20	1,771	1,791	1.1%
	Total	29	2,379	2,408	

Relative risk: 1.5%/1.1% = 1.4 (95% CI, 0.6–2.8)

Yes Greek Life: Relative Risk Analysis

		Unintended Pregnancy?		Total	Proportion Who Experienced Unintended Pregnancy
		Yes	No		
Were condoms primary contraceptive method?	Yes	90	1,301	1,391	6.5%
	No	13	179	192	6.8%
	Total	103	1,480	1,583	

Relative risk: 6.5%/6.8% = 1.0 (95% CI, 0.5–1.7)

In each stratum (Greek life yes or no), there is no association between condom use and unintended pregnancy (the confidence intervals of both RRs include the null value of 1.0). Without consideration of Greek life as a risk factor for unintended pregnancy, one might erroneously conclude that only poor condom use was to blame. As it turned out, both condom use and unintended pregnancy were disproportionately more common among freshmen who participated in Greek life than those who did not. If the above-estimated crude relative risk of 3.0 is adjusted using the Mantel-Haenszel approach to control for the confounding role of Greek life, the risk of unintended pregnancy from condom use disappears (adjusted relative risk of 1.1; 95% CI, 0.7 to 1.7). If alcohol consumption were examined as a fourth variable, then logistic regression techniques could be used to control for Greek life and alcohol consumption simultaneously.

A Guide to Epidemiologic Terms Commonly Used
Relative Risk

The ratio of the risk of the disease or condition among those exposed and the risk among the unexposed, or the ratio of the cumulative incidence rate in the exposed and the unexposed, is also called risk ratio. In its simplest definition, relative risk compares the rate of disease in two groups, one of which has been exposed to something that is believed to either increase or decrease the risk of that disease, usually in a cohort study or randomized trial. A null value of 1.0 suggests neither an adverse effect nor a protective effect of the exposure; a value over 1.0 suggests elevated risk of the outcome, while a value under 1.0 suggests reduced risk.

Odds Ratio

The odds ratio is the measure of association calculated in case-control and cross-sectional studies. The odds ratio is a good estimate of the relative risk when the disease or condition is rare. The odds ratio does not characterize incidence or causation; it only provides an internal measure of relative risk. An important scientific mantra is "Association ≠ Causation."

Confidence Interval

By convention, we often use 95% confidence intervals. The lower and upper bounds of the interval constitute the range of error around the point estimate for that particular measurement. In practical terms, it means that if the exact study were to be done 100 times, the point estimate would fall between those values 95 times. For an odds ratio or relative risk to be statistically significant, the confidence interval must not include the null value of 1.0. When comparing confidence intervals of a rate or a measure (such as blood pressure), if the ranges overlap, the differences are not considered statistically significant.

The tighter (narrower) the range of the confidence interval, the more precise the estimate. The wider the confidence interval (CI), the more imprecise the estimate, usually because of small numbers of study subjects.

p Value

The *p* value characterizes the role (probability) that chance may play in the results. By convention, the threshold used for chance to be ruled out is a *p* value below 0.05 (significant). A *p* value of 0.05 means that there is a 5% probability that the result occurred by chance. The lower the *p* value, the more likely the result is real. (Note: a leading zero is a zero to the left of the decimal point used for clarity, but some journals do not allow them.)

Attributable Risk

Attributable risk is the difference in actual incidence of disease or condition between exposed and unexposed groups; it provides a realistic estimate of the change in incidence that is attributable to the exposure. A modest increase in relative risk will produce only a small number of cases when clinical events are rare, such as venous thromboembolism (VTE) and arterial thrombosis in young women. *If the absolute risk is very low, a statistically significant increase in relative risk may mean little or nothing in practical, real numbers.* For example, COC use is associated with a threefold increase in relative risk of VTE compared with nonuse.[11]

However, the baseline risk of VTE is relatively rare in women of reproductive age—about 5 cases per 10,000 women per year.[11] Therefore, COC users have an absolute risk of about 15 cases of VTE per 10,000 women per year, 10 of which are attributable to COC use—still a rare event.

Number Needed to Treat

The number needed to treat is the number of individuals who must be treated, usually over a 1-year time period, to produce one instance of either a positive or a negative effect.

Statistical Concepts in Hypothesis Testing

Statistical tests provide an objective methodology for evaluating whether the quantitative results obtained from an experiment or observation represent a true deviation from chance. While a full discussion of statistical tests and interpretation of results is beyond the scope of this chapter, some basic principles warrant review. First, the type of measures for endpoint analyses (e.g., means, medians, proportions, etc.) defines the statistical test used to evaluate the study hypothesis. The second major principle is that all statistical tests reflect probabilities. The degree to which we accept a result as statistically significant is somewhat arbitrary. By convention, we typically regard an outcome as statistically significant if the result has less than a 5% chance of being observed, if the null hypothesis is true.

When designing a clinical study, the investigator must consider the anticipated magnitude of the difference in the outcome between the study groups (e.g., effect size), the natural variability in the outcome in the study population (e.g., variance), and choose a level of statistical significance for evaluation of the result.

A power analysis estimates a target sample size based upon a predefined effect size and variance for the appropriate statistical test. While studies frequently report primary and secondary outcomes, the power analysis generally reflects the sample size requirement for the primary outcome only. To ensure that the study remains adequately powered to evaluate the primary outcome, investigators typically will increase the number of participants enrolled above the minimum required by the sample size calculation to account for the anticipated dropout rate.

A power analysis must consider concepts of Type 1 and Type 2 errors.

- Type 1 error (also known as α) refers to the probability of falsely concluding that a difference exists (a false-positive result). In most studies, investigators will select an α of 0.05 for evaluation of the primary outcome. In practical terms, this represents a 1 in 20 chance of a Type 1 error.
- Type 2 error (also known as β) refers to the probability of falsely accepting the null hypothesis of equality, when in fact a true difference exists (a false-negative result). Since scientists tend to be cautious, we consider the implications of a Type 2 error as less worrisome than Type 1 error. For this reason, we typically select a β of 0.2 when considering sample size. The probability of avoiding a Type 2 error is called power (power = $1 - \beta$). A study with a β of 0.2 has 80% power (e.g., 4 in 5 chance) to exclude a Type 2 error. The most common cause of a Type 2 error is a sample size being too small.

Clinicians interpreting the literature must also consider the difference between clinical significance and statistical significance. Clinical significance refers to the magnitude of difference that would reflect a clinically important result and is not influenced by sample size. In contrast, increasing sample size can result in highly statistically significant results with very small effect sizes of dubious clinical relevance. Very large database studies published in major journals frequently report highly statistically significant risk estimates of clinically unimportant effect size. Ideally, to guide clinical practice, a result should be both clinically and statistically significant.

Putting Risk into Perspective—Interpreting Findings from Epidemiologic Studies

Epidemiology is the science of detecting and understanding disease patterns in large populations. Epidemiologic studies alone do not prove causation; they identify associations between diseases and certain factors that are the first step in assessing causality.

A relative risk in the range of 1.0 to 2.0 represents an increased risk but a weak association. As explained above, confidence intervals around the relative risk help determine statistical significance of the risk. A relative risk (from a randomized trial of cohort study) of 1.5 and an odds ratio (from a case-control study) of 1.5 are mathematically equivalent and signal the same levels of risk; the hierarchy of study designs and validity attached to the estimates then differentiates the interpretation.

The clinical significance of an increase in risk is influenced by the rate of the disease in the general (unexposed) population. If the rate of the disease in the unexposed population is 10% and the relative risk is 1.4, then the risk of disease in the exposed population is 14%. If the rate of disease in the unexposed population is only 1%, then the same relative risk of 1.4 increases the actual disease risk to only 1.4%.

Criteria that strengthen the conclusion that an epidemiologic finding or association represents a true cause-and-effect relationship include the following[12]:

1. The strength of the association (the larger the relative risk, the more likely it is real).
2. Consistency, uniformity, and agreement among many studies.
3. A dose-response relationship (either with dose of a drug or an increasing effect with increasing duration of exposure).
4. Biologic plausibility of the finding (known mechanisms by which exposure could cause or influence disease).
5. An appropriate temporal relationship (the amount of time between exposure and development of disease is appropriate according to the pathogenesis of the disease).
6. Coherence of the finding with what is known about the natural history, biology, and other characteristics of the exposure and outcome relationship.

The results section of a published study objectively provides epidemiologic findings that can be used to advance science and our understanding of possible cause-and-effect relationships. Researchers typically provide outcome measures and statistical tests; together this information is used to support the conclusions of the study report. Statisticians often transform simple outcome measures such as number of incident cases, percentages, and means, to composite measures with built-in comparisons; additionally, the measures usually have a mathematical test to determine whether any differences can be considered outside the realm of chance.

Example of Interpreting Findings

A published cohort study from 2017 reported that women who currently or recently used any hormonal contraceptive had a higher risk of breast cancer than women who had never used hormonal contraceptives (relative risk, 1.20; 95% CI, 1.14 to 1.26).[13]

The relative risk of 1.20 means a 20% increased chance of developing breast cancer among women who currently or recently used any hormonal contraceptive compared with women who had never used any hormonal contraceptive. The 95% confidence interval demonstrates that if one were to conduct this exact study 100 different times, the estimated relative risk would fall between 1.14 and 1.26 in 95 of those completed studies.

The components and calculation of the relative risk are the estimated incidence rate of breast cancer among users of any hormonal contraceptive (68 cases per 100,000 per year) divided by the rate among "never users of hormonal contraception" (55 cases per 100,000 per year).

Further, the authors adjusted the relative risks by seven other factors that, if not considered, might have biased the summary measure through confounding. An important limitation for this adjustment is that a significant amount of information about important confounding factors was unavailable.

Finally, the published risk difference was estimated at 13 additional breast cancer cases per 100,000 women per year among women who currently or recently used hormonal contraception (95% range of 10–16). This converts to "number needed to treat" in the following way: to produce one instance of breast cancer, 7,690 women will need to use a hormonal contraceptive for 1 year (100,000 divided by 13 = 7,690). The estimated range of number needed to treat is 6,250 to 10,000. Therefore, while this study observed a small increase in relative risk of breast cancer associated with hormonal contraception use that is statistically significant, the absolute risk of breast cancer associated with hormonal contraceptive use is quite low (13 cases per 100,000 users per year).

Synthesizing the Evidence

While it is important for clinicians to understand how to interpret individual studies, results from a single study are generally insufficient to determine a course of clinical action or to develop an evidence-based recommendation. A systematic review synthesizes the body of evidence on a specific question and uses explicit methods to identify, critically appraise, and summarize the findings across studies, providing an overall assessment of the evidence along with a discussion of potential biases.[14,15] Systematic reviews may include meta-analysis, in which the results of individual studies are statistically combined to provide a more precise measure of effect. Looking across the totality of the evidence on a particular topic provides the clinician with a distilled review of the consistency of findings and the strength of the evidence on which to base a clinical decision. In addition to systematic reviews and meta-analyses, there are a number of other types of reviews that readers and researchers may find useful; Grant et al.[16] describe 14 review types including scoping reviews (preliminary assessment of the scope of the literature on a particular topic), rapid reviews (completeness may be determined by time constraints), and state-of-the-art reviews that address current issues.

The Cochrane Database of Systematic Reviews is a primary source for systematic reviews of the evidence in health care and contains several reviews on contraception and other reproductive health care topics (https:// fertility-regulation.cochrane.org). Reviews are developed through a standardized methodology, peer-reviewed, and updated with new evidence on a regular basis. Other sources include systematic reviews published in the literature and can be found through searching databases such as MEDLINE®, from the U.S. National Library of Medicine.

Reporting the Evidence

The final step for investigators of individual studies and systematic reviews/ meta-analyses is to clearly communicate the findings. This is most often done through publication in the peer-reviewed literature but also in the form of reports, oral presentations, and communication with scientific and lay media. It is important to "tell the story" of the research, including a precise statement of the research question, a detailed accounting of the research methods, a clear and organized summary of the results, an objective reflection on the quality of the evidence including strengths and limitations, and implications for practice and future research. Many journals encourage or require that authors follow reporting guidelines based on study type, including guidelines for randomized trials (CONSORT guidelines), observational studies (STROBE), and systematic reviews and meta-analyses (PRISMA).[17-19] These guidelines often have extensions specific to a particular type of intervention or medical condition. The EQUATOR Network (http://www.equator-network.org) provides links to many different types of reporting guidelines and extensions, as well as tips and training for publishing high-quality articles.

Translating Evidence into Clinical Guidance

Systematic reviews still need to be translated into specific recommendations for clinical action. Clinical practice guidelines are tools that provide recommendations for clinical care based on the sum and strength of the evidence, as well as other factors such as benefits and harms, patient preferences, feasibility, and cost. The Institute of Medicine (IOM) defines clinical practice guidelines as "recommendations, intended to optimize patient care, that are informed by a systematic review of evidence and an assessment of

---

Table 3.2 Trustworthy Clinical Practice Guidelines

Clinical practice guidelines are statements that include recommendations intended to optimize patient care that are informed by a systematic review of evidence and an assessment of the benefits and harms of alternative care options. Trustworthy clinical practice guidelines should:

- Be based on a systematic review of the existing evidence
- Be developed by a knowledgeable, multidisciplinary panel of experts and representatives from key affected groups
- Consider important patient subgroups and patient preferences, as appropriate
- Be based on an explicit and transparent process that minimizes distortions, biases, and conflicts of interest
- Provide a clear explanation of the logical relationships between alternative care options and health outcomes and provide ratings of both the quality of evidence and the strength of the recommendations
- Be reconsidered and revised as appropriate when important new evidence warrants modifications of recommendations

Source: Institute of Medicine, Clinical Practice Guidelines We Can Trust, The National Academies Press, Washington, DC, 2011.

---

the benefits and harms of alternative care options," and defines several characteristics of trustworthy guidelines (**Table 3.2**).[14] **Table 3.1** provides the USPSTF grading system for strength of recommendations. Clinical practice guidelines need to be implemented in the context of improving quality of care, along with development of tools and job aids for providers that may include electronic clinical decision support tools. Sources of guidelines include federal agencies, professional organizations, and other sponsoring organizations. Examples of clinical practice guidelines related to family planning and reproductive health are included in **Table 3.3**.

Medical Eligibility Criteria for Contraceptive Use and Selected Practice Recommendations for Contraceptive Use

Two key examples of clinical practice guidelines for contraception are the *Medical Eligibility Criteria for Contraceptive Use* (MEC) and the *Selected Practice Recommendations for Contraceptive Use* (SPR), produced by the World Health Organization (WHO) for a global audience.[20,21] The MEC provides recommendations for safe use of specific contraceptive methods by women with medical conditions and other characteristics, such as age and postpartum status (**Table 3.4**). Recommendations are provided using a

Table 3.3 Examples of Clinical Practice Guidelines for Family Planning and Reproductive Health

Guideline	Organization	Link
U.S. Medical Eligibility Criteria for Contraceptive Use, 2016	Centers for Disease Control and Prevention	https://www.cdc.gov/reproductivehealth/contraception/mmwr/mec/summary.html
U.S. Selected Practice Recommendations for Contraceptive Use, 2016	Centers for Disease Control and Prevention	https://www.cdc.gov/reproductivehealth/contraception/mmwr/spr/summary.html
Providing Quality Family Planning Services	Centers for Disease Control and Prevention and Office of Population Affairs	https://www.cdc.gov/reproductivehealth/contraception/qfp.htm
Clinical Guidelines on Contraception and Abortion	Society of Family Planning	https://www.societyfp.org/Resources/Clinical-guidelines.aspx
Sexually Transmitted Disease Treatment Guidelines	Centers for Disease Control and Prevention	https://www.cdc.gov/std/tg2015/default.htm
Long-Acting Reversible Contraception: Implants and Intrauterine Devices	American College of Obstetricians and Gynecologists	https://www.acog.org/Clinical-Guidance-and-Publications/Practice-Bulletins/Committee-on-Practice-Bulletins-Gynecology/Long-Acting-Reversible-Contraception-Implants-and-Intrauterine-Devices
Contraception for Adolescents	American Academy of Pediatrics	http://pediatrics.aappublications.org/content/134/4/e1257

numeric classification from 1 (safe to use) to 4 (unacceptable health risks) **(Table 3.5)**. The SPR provides recommendations for contraceptive management issues, such as when a woman can start a specific method, what exams and tests (if any) are needed and how to manage bleeding problems and other issues with contraceptive use. Use of these evidence-based guidelines can help assure that women are not exposed to inappropriate risks and are not unnecessarily denied access to contraceptive methods and services when choosing and using contraception.

Table 3.4 Summary Chart for U.S. Medical Eligibility Criteria for Contraceptive Use

Condition	Sub-Condition	Cu-IUD I	Cu-IUD C	LNG-IUD I	LNG-IUD C	Implant I	Implant C	DMPA I	DMPA C	POP I	POP C	CHC I	CHC C
Age		Menarche to <20 yrs:2; ≥20 yrs:1		Menarche to <20 yrs:2; ≥20 yrs:1		Menarche to <18 yrs:1; 18-45 yrs:1; >45 yrs:1		Menarche to <18 yrs:2; 18-45 yrs:1; >45 yrs:2		Menarche to <18 yrs:1; 18-45 yrs:1; >45 yrs:1		Menarche to <40 yrs:1; ≥40 yrs:2	
Anatomical abnormalities	a) Distorted uterine cavity	4		4									
	b) Other abnormalities	2		2									
Anemias	a) Thalassemia	2		1		1		1		1		1	
	b) Sickle cell disease‡	2		1		1		1		1		2	
	c) Iron-deficiency anemia	2		1		1		1		1		1	
Benign ovarian tumors	(including cysts)	1		1		1		1		1		1	
Breast disease	a) Undiagnosed mass	1		2		2*		2*		2*		2*	
	b) Benign breast disease	1		1		1		1		1		1	
	c) Family history of cancer	1		1		1		1		1		1	
	d) Breast cancer‡												
	i) Current	1		4		4		4		4		4	
	ii) Past and no evidence of current disease for 5 years	1		3		3		3		3		3	
Breastfeeding	a) <21 days postpartum					2*		2*		2*		4*	
	b) 21 to <30 days postpartum												
	i) With other risk factors for VTE					2*		2*		2*		3*	
	ii) Without other risk factors for VTE					2*		2*		2*		3*	
	c) 30-42 days postpartum												
	i) With other risk factors for VTE					1*		1*		1*		3*	
	ii) Without other risk factors for VTE					1*		1*		1*		2*	
	d) >42 days postpartum					1*		1*		1*		2*	
Cervical cancer	Awaiting treatment	4	2	4	2	2		2		1		2	
Cervical ectropion		1		1		1		1		1		1	
Cervical intraepithelial neoplasia		1		2		2		2		1		2	
Cirrhosis	a) Mild (compensated)	1		1		1		1		1		1	
	b) Severe‡ (decompensated)	1		3		3		3		3		4	
Cystic fibrosis‡		1*		1*		1*		2*		1*		1*	
Deep venous thrombosis (DVT)/Pulmonary embolism (PE)	a) History of DVT/PE, not receiving anticoagulant therapy												
	i) Higher risk for recurrent DVT/PE	1		2		2		2		2		4	
	ii) Lower risk for recurrent DVT/PE	1		2		2		2		2		3	
	b) Acute DVT/PE	2		2		2		2		2		4	
	c) DVT/PE and established anticoagulant therapy for at least 3 months												
	i) Higher risk for recurrent DVT/PE	2		2		2		2		2		4*	
	ii) Lower risk for recurrent DVT/PE	2		2		2		2		2		3*	
	d) Family history (first-degree relatives)	1		1		1		1		1		2	
	e) Major surgery												
	i) With prolonged immobilization	1		2		2		2		2		4	
	ii) Without prolonged immobilization	1		1		1		1		1		2	
	f) Minor surgery without immobilization	1		1		1		1		1		1	
Depressive disorders		1*		1*		1*		1*		1*		1*	

Key:

1 No restriction (method can be used)	3 Theoretical or proven risks usually outweigh the advantages
2 Advantages generally outweigh theoretical or proven risks	4 Unacceptable health risk (method not to be used)

(Continued)

86

Table 3.4 Summary Chart for U.S. Medical Eligibility Criteria for Contraceptive Use (*Continued*)

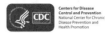

Centers for Disease Control and Prevention
National Center for Chronic Disease Prevention and Health Promotion

Condition	Sub-Condition	Cu-IUD		LNG-IUD		Implant		DMPA		POP		CHC	
		I	C	I	C	I	C	I	C	I	C	I	C
Diabetes	a) History of gestational disease	1		1		1		1		1		1	
	b) Nonvascular disease												
	i) Non-insulin dependent	1		2		2		2		2		2	
	ii) Insulin dependent	1		2		2		2		2		2	
	c) Nephropathy/retinopathy/neuropathy‡	1		2		2		3		2		3/4*	
	d) Other vascular disease or diabetes of >20 years' duration‡	1		2		2		3		2		3/4*	
Dysmenorrhea	Severe	2		1		1		1		1		1	
Endometrial cancer‡		4	2	4	2	1		1		1		1	
Endometrial hyperplasia		1		1		1		1		1		1	
Endometriosis		2		1		1		1		1		1	
Epilepsy‡	(see also Drug Interactions)	1		1		1*		1*		1*		1*	
Gallbladder disease	a) Symptomatic												
	i) Treated by cholecystectomy	1		2		2		2		2		2	
	ii) Medically treated	1		2		2		2		2		3	
	iii) Current	1		2		2		2		2		3	
	b) Asymptomatic	1		2		2		2		2		2	
Gestational trophoblastic disease‡	a) Suspected GTD (immediate postevacuation)												
	i) Uterine size first trimester	1*		1*		1*		1*		1*		1*	
	ii) Uterine size second trimester	2*		2*		1*		1*		1*		1*	
	b) Confirmed GTD												
	i) Undetectable/non-pregnant ß-hCG levels	1*	1*	1*	1*	1*		1*		1*		1*	
	ii) Decreasing ß-hCG levels	2*	1*	2*	1*	1*		1*		1*		1*	
	iii) Persistently elevated ß-hCG levels or malignant disease, with no evidence or suspicion of intrauterine disease	2*	1*	2*	1*	1*		1*		1*		1*	
	iv) Persistently elevated ß-hCG levels or malignant disease, with evidence or suspicion of intrauterine disease	4*	2*	4*	2*	1*		1*		1*		1*	
Headaches	a) Nonmigraine (mild or severe)	1		1		1		1		1		1*	
	b) Migraine												
	i) Without aura (includes menstrual migraine)	1		1		1		1		1		2*	
	ii) With aura	1		1		1		1		1		4*	
History of bariatric surgery‡	a) Restrictive procedures	1		1		1		1		1		1	
	b) Malabsorptive procedures	1		1		1		1		3		COCs: 3 P/R: 1	
History of cholestasis	a) Pregnancy related	1		1		1		1		1		2	
	b) Past COC related	1		2		2		2		2		3	
History of high blood pressure during pregnancy		1		1		1		1		1		2	
History of Pelvic surgery		1		1		1		1		1		1	
HIV	a) High risk for HIV	2	2	2	2	1		2*		1		1	
	b) HIV infection					1*		1*		1*		1*	
	i) Clinically well receiving ARV therapy	1	1	1	1	If on treatment, see Drug Interactions							
	ii) Not clinically well or not receiving ARV therapy	2	1	2	1	If on treatment, see Drug Interactions							

Abbreviations: C=continuation of contraceptive method; CHC=combined hormonal contraception (pill, patch, and ring); COC=combined oral contraceptive; Cu-IUD=copper-containing intrauterine device; DMPA = depot medroxyprogesterone acetate; I=initiation of contraceptive method; LNG-IUD=levonorgestrel-releasing intrauterine device; NA=not applicable; POP=progestin-only pill; P/R=patch/ring ‡ Condition that exposes a woman to increased risk as a result of pregnancy. *Please see the complete guidance for a clarification to this classification: www.cdc.gov/reproductivehealth/unintendedpregnancy/USMEC.htm.

87

(*Continued*)

Table 3.4 Summary Chart for U.S. Medical Eligibility Criteria for Contraceptive Use (Continued)

Condition	Sub-Condition	Cu-IUD I	Cu-IUD C	LNG-IUD I	LNG-IUD C	Implant I	Implant C	DMPA I	DMPA C	POP I	POP C	CHC I	CHC C
Hypertension	a) Adequately controlled hypertension	1*	1*	1*	1*	1*	1*	2*	2*	1*	1*	3*	3*
	b) Elevated blood pressure levels (properly taken measurements)												
	i) Systolic 140-159 or diastolic 90-99	1*	1*	1*	1*	1*	1*	2*	2*	1*	1*	3*	3*
	ii) Systolic ≥160 or diastolic ≥100‡	1*	1*	2*	2*	2*	2*	3*	3*	2*	2*	4*	4*
	c) Vascular disease	1*	1*	2*	2*	2*	2*	3*	3*	2*	2*	4*	4*
Inflammatory bowel disease	(Ulcerative colitis, Crohn's disease)	1	1	1	1	1	1	2	2	2	2	2/3*	2/3*
Ischemic heart disease‡	Current and history of	1	1	2	3	2	3	3	3	2	3	4	4
Known thrombogenic mutations‡		1*	1*	2*	2*	2*	2*	2*	2*	2*	2*	4*	4*
Liver tumors	a) Benign												
	i) Focal nodular hyperplasia	1	1	2	2	2	2	2	2	2	2	2	2
	ii) Hepatocellular adenoma‡	1	1	3	3	3	3	3	3	3	3	4	4
	b) Malignant‡ (hepatoma)	1	1	3	3	3	3	3	3	3	3	4	4
Malaria		1	1	1	1	1	1	1	1	1	1	1	1
Multiple risk factors for atherosclerotic cardiovascular disease	(e.g., older age, smoking, diabetes, hypertension, low HDL, high LDL, or high triglyceride levels)	1	1	2	2	2*	2*	3*	3*	2*	2*	3/4*	3/4*
Multiple sclerosis	a) With prolonged immobility	1	1	1	1	1	1	2	2	1	1	3	3
	b) Without prolonged immobility	1	1	1	1	1	1	2	2	1	1	1	1
Obesity	a) Body mass index (BMI) ≥30 kg/m²	1	1	1	1	1	1	1	1	1	1	2	2
	b) Menarche to <18 years and BMI ≥ 30 kg/m²	1	1	1	1	1	1	2	2	1	1	2	2
Ovarian cancer‡		1	1	1	1	1	1	1	1	1	1	1	1
Parity	a) Nulliparous	2	2	2	2	1	1	1	1	1	1	1	1
	b) Parous	1	1	1	1	1	1	1	1	1	1	1	1
Past ectopic pregnancy		1	1	1	1	1	1	1	1	2	2	1	1
Pelvic inflammatory disease	a) Past												
	i) With subsequent pregnancy	1	1	1	1	1	1	1	1	1	1	1	1
	ii) Without subsequent pregnancy	2	2	2	2	1	1	1	1	1	1	1	1
	b) Current	4	2*	4	2*	1	1	1	1	1	1	1	1
Peripartum cardiomyopathy‡	a) Normal or mildly impaired cardiac function												
	i) <6 months	2	2	2	2	1	1	1	1	1	1	4	4
	ii) ≥6 months	2	2	2	2	1	1	1	1	1	1	3	3
	b) Moderately or severely impaired cardiac function	2	2	2	2	2	2	2	2	2	2	4	4
Postabortion	a) First trimester	1*	1*	1*	1*	1*	1*	1*	1*	1*	1*	1*	1*
	b) Second trimester	2*	2*	2*	2*	1*	1*	1*	1*	1*	1*	1*	1*
	c) Immediate postseptic abortion	4	4	4	4	1*	1*	1*	1*	1*	1*	1*	1*
Postpartum (nonbreastfeeding women)	a) <21 days					1	1	1	1	1	1	4	4
	b) 21 days to 42 days												
	i) With other risk factors for VTE					1	1	1	1	1	1	3*	3*
	ii) Without other risk factors for VTE					1	1	1	1	1	1	2	2
	c) >42 days					1	1	1	1	1	1	1	1
Postpartum (in breastfeeding or non-breastfeeding women, including cesarean delivery)	a) <10 minutes after delivery of the placenta												
	i) Breastfeeding	1*	1*	2*	2*								
	ii) Nonbreastfeeding	1*	1*	1*	1*								
	b) 10 minutes after delivery of the placenta to <4 weeks	2*	2*	2*	2*								
	c) ≥4 weeks	1*	1*	1*	1*								
	d) Postpartum sepsis	4	4	4	4								

(Continued)

Table 3.4 Summary Chart for U.S. Medical Eligibility Criteria for Contraceptive Use (*Continued*)

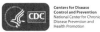

Centers for Disease Control and Prevention
National Center for Chronic Disease Prevention and Health Promotion

Condition	Sub-Condition	Cu-IUD I	Cu-IUD C	LNG-IUD I	LNG-IUD C	Implant I	Implant C	DMPA I	DMPA C	POP I	POP C	CHC I	CHC C
Pregnancy		4*	4*	4*	4*	NA*	NA*	NA*	NA*	NA*	NA*	NA*	NA*
Rheumatoid arthritis	a) On immunosuppressive therapy	2	1	2	1	1	1	2/3*	2/3*	1	1	2	2
	b) Not on immunosuppressive therapy	1	1	1	1	1	1	2	2	1	1	2	2
Schistosomiasis	a) Uncomplicated	1	1	1	1	1	1	1	1	1	1	1	1
	b) Fibrosis of the liver‡	1	1	1	1	1	1	1	1	1	1	1	1
Sexually transmitted diseases (STDs)	a) Current purulent cervicitis or chlamydial infection or gonococcal infection	4	2*	4	2*	1	1	1	1	1	1	1	1
	b) Vaginitis (*including trichomonas vaginalis and bacterial vaginosis*)	2	2	2	2	1	1	1	1	1	1	1	1
	c) Other factors relating to STDs	2*	2	2*	2	1	1	1	1	1	1	1	1
Smoking	a) Age <35	1	1	1	1	1	1	1	1	1	1	2	2
	b) Age ≥35, <15 cigarettes/day	1	1	1	1	1	1	1	1	1	1	3	3
	c) Age ≥35, ≥15 cigarettes/day	1	1	1	1	1	1	1	1	1	1	4	4
Solid organ transplantation‡	a) Complicated	3	2	3	2	2	2	2	2	2	2	4	4
	b) Uncomplicated	2	2	2	2	2	2	2	2	2	2	2*	2*
Stroke‡	History of cerebrovascular accident	1	1	2	2	2	3	3	3	2	3	4	4
Superficial venous disorders	a) Varicose veins	1	1	1	1	1	1	1	1	1	1	1	1
	b) Superficial venous thrombosis (acute or history)	1	1	1	1	1	1	1	1	1	1	3*	3*
Systemic lupus erythematosus‡	a) Positive (or unknown) antiphospholipid antibodies	1*	1*	3*	3*	3*	3*	3*	3*	3*	3*	4*	4*
	b) Severe thrombocytopenia	3*	2*	2*	2*	2*	2*	3*	2*	2*	2*	2*	2*
	c) Immunosuppressive therapy	2*	1*	2*	2*	2*	2*	2*	2*	2*	2*	2*	2*
	d) None of the above	1*	1*	2*	2*	2*	2*	2*	2*	2*	2*	2*	2*
Thyroid disorders	Simple goiter/hyperthyroid/hypothyroid	1	1	1	1	1	1	1	1	1	1	1	1
Tuberculosis‡ (see also Drug Interactions)	a) Nonpelvic	1	1	1	1	1*	1*	1*	1*	1*	1*	1*	1*
	b) Pelvic	4	3	4	3	1*	1*	1*	1*	1*	1*	1*	1*
Unexplained vaginal bleeding	(suspicious for serious condition) before evaluation	4*	2*	4*	2*	3*	3*	3*	3*	2*	2*	2*	2*
Uterine fibroids		2	2	2	2	1	1	1	1	1	1	1	1
Valvular heart disease	a) Uncomplicated	1	1	1	1	1	1	1	1	1	1	2	2
	b) Complicated‡	1	1	1	1	1	1	1	1	1	1	4	4
Vaginal bleeding patterns	a) Irregular pattern without heavy bleeding	1	1	1	1	2	2	2	2	2	2	1	1
	b) Heavy or prolonged bleeding	2*	2*	1*	2*	2*	2*	2*	2*	2*	2*	1*	1*
Viral hepatitis	a) Acute or flare	1	1	1	1	1	1	1	1	1	1	3/4*	2
	b) Carrier/Chronic	1	1	1	1	1	1	1	1	1	1	1	1
Drug Interactions													
Antiretroviral therapy All other ARV's are 1 or 2 for all methods.	Fosamprenavir (FPV)	1/2*	1*	1/2*	1*	2*	2*	2*	2*	2*	2*	3*	3*
Anticonvulsant therapy	a) Certain anticonvulsants (phenytoin, carbamazepine, barbiturates, primidone, topiramate, oxcarbazepine)	1	1	1	1	2*	2*	1*	1*	3*	3*	3*	3*
	b) Lamotrigine	1	1	1	1	1	1	1	1	1	1	3*	3*
Antimicrobial therapy	a) Broad spectrum antibiotics	1	1	1	1	1	1	1	1	1	1	1	1
	b) Antifungals	1	1	1	1	1	1	1	1	1	1	1	1
	c) Antiparasitics	1	1	1	1	1	1	1	1	1	1	1	1
	d) Rifampin or rifabutin therapy	1	1	1	1	2*	2*	1*	1*	3*	3*	3*	3*
SSRIs		1	1	1	1	1	1	1	1	1	1	1	1
St. John's wort		1	1	1	1	2	2	1	1	2	2	2	2

Updated in 2017. This summary sheet only contains a subset of the recommendations from the U.S. MEC. For complete guidance, see: http://www.cdc.gov/reproductivehealth/ unintendedpregnancy/USMEC.htm. Most contraceptive methods do not protect against sexually transmitted diseases (STDs). Consistent and correct use of the male latex condom reduces the risk of STDs and HIV.

CS266008-A

Reprinted from https://www.cdc.gov/reproductivehealth/contraception/pdf/summary-chart-us-medical-eligibility-criteria_508tagged.pdf
Use of this material does not imply an endorsement by the Centers for Disease Control and Prevention (CDC) or Health and Human Services (HHS) of any particular organization, service, or product.

The WHO encourages local adaptation at the country level, and the Centers for Disease Control and Prevention (CDC) has adapted these guidelines for use in the United States.[22,23] These guidelines are used by professional and service organizations throughout the United States, and CDC has developed provider tools and training to assist providers in their use. Together,

Table 3.5 Categories of Medical Eligibility Criteria for Contraceptive Use

Category	Definition
1	A condition for which there is no restriction for the use of the contraceptive method
2	A condition for which the advantages of using the method generally outweigh the theoretical or proven risks
3	A condition for which the theoretical or proven risks usually outweigh the advantages of using the method
4	A condition that represents an unacceptable health risk of the contraceptive method is used

Source: World Health Organization, Medical Eligibility Criteria for Contraceptive Use, World Health Organization, Geneva, 2015.

WHO and CDC work to assure that the global guidance remains up to date through continuous identification of new evidence and determination of whether changes in the recommendations are needed, based on new evidence. The guidance is updated through a comprehensive review of the recommendations about every 5 years, with release of interim guidance, as needed. Updates to the U.S. guidance follow any changes to the WHO guidance, with consideration of the need for adaptation to the U.S. context.

References

1. Randomised controlled trial of levonorgestrel versus the Yuzpe regimen of combined oral contraceptives for emergency contraception. Task Force on Postovulatory Methods of Fertility Regulation, Lancet 352:428–433, 1998.

2. **Fels H, Steward R, Melamed A, et al.,** Comparison of serum and cervical mucus hormone levels during hormone-free interval of 24/4 vs. 21/7 combined oral contraceptives, Contraception 87:732–737, 2013.

3. **Chewning B, Mosena P, Wilson D, et al.,** Evaluation of a computerized contraceptive decision aid for adolescent patients, Patient Educ Couns 38: 227–239, 1999.

4. **Dinger J, Bardenheuer K, Heinemann K,** Cardiovascular and general safety of a 24-day regimen of drospirenone-containing combined oral contraceptives: final results from the International Active Surveillance Study of Women Taking Oral Contraceptives, Contraception 89:253–263, 2014.

5. **Lidegaard O, Lokkegaard E, Jensen A, et al.,** Thrombotic stroke and myocardial infarction with hormonal contraception, N Engl J Med 366:2257–2266, 2012.

6. Cardiovascular disease and use of oral and injectable progestogen-only contraceptives and combined injectable contraceptives. Results of an international, multicenter, case-control study. World Health Organization Collaborative Study

of Cardiovascular Disease and Steroid Hormone Contraception, Contraception 57:315–324, 1998.

7. **Daniels K, Daugherty J, Jones J, et al.,** Current contraceptive use and variation by selected characteristics among women aged 15–44: United States, 2011–2013, Natl Health Stat Report 86:1–14, 2015.

8. **Ricci G, Restaino S, Di LG, et al.,** Risk of Essure microinsert abdominal migration: case report and review of literature, Ther Clin Risk Manag 10:963–968, 2014.

9. **Harrison-Woolrych M, Hill R,** Unintended pregnancies with the etonogestrel implant (Implanon): a case series from postmarketing experience in Australia, Contraception 71:306–308, 2005.

10. **Rothman KJ, Greenland S,** Precision and validity in epidemiologic studies, In: Rothman KJ, Greenland S, eds., Modern Epidemiology, 2nd ed., Lippincott-Raven Publishers, Philadelphia, 1998, pp 115–134.

11. **Bassuk SS, Manson JE,** Oral contraceptives and menopausal hormone therapy: relative and attributable risks of cardiovascular disease, cancer, and other health outcomes, Ann Epidemiol 25:193–200, 2015.

12. **Rothman KJ, Greenland S,** Causation and causal inference, In: Rothman KJ, Greenland S, eds. Modern Epidemiology, 2nd ed., Lippincott-Raven Publishers, Philadelphia, 1998, pp 7–28.

13. **Morch LS, Skovlund CW, Hannaford PC, et al.,** Contemporary hormonal contraception and the risk of breast cancer, N Engl J Med 377:2228–2239, 2017.

14. **Institute of Medicine,** Clinical Guidelines We Can Trust, The National Academies Press, Washington, DC, 2011.

15. **Liberati A, Altman DG, Tetzlaff J, et al.,** The PRISMA statement for reporting systematic reviews and meta-analyses of studies that evaluate healthcare interventions: explanation and elaboration, BMJ 339:b2700, 2009.

16. **Grant MJ, Booth A,** A typology of reviews: an analysis of 14 review types and associated methodologies, Health Info Libr J 26:91–108, 2009.

17. **Schulz KF, Altman DG, Moher D,** CONSORT 2010 statement: updated guidelines for reporting parallel group randomised trials, BMJ 340:c332, 2010.

18. **von Elm E, Altman DG, Egger M, et al.,** Strengthening the Reporting of Observational Studies in Epidemiology (STROBE) statement: guidelines for reporting observational studies, BMJ 335:806–808, 2007.

19. **Moher D, Liberati A, Tetzlaff J, et al.,** Preferred reporting items for systematic reviews and meta-analyses: the PRISMA statement, BMJ 339:b2535, 2009.

20. **World Health Organization,** Medical Eligibility Criteria for Contraceptive Use, World Health Organization, Geneva, 2015.

21. **World Health Organization,** Selected Practice Recommendations for Contraceptive Use, World Health Organization, Geneva, 2016.

22. **Curtis KM, Tepper NK, Jatlaoui TC, Berry-Bibee E, Horton LG, Zapata LB, et al.,** U.S. Medical Eligibility Criteria for Contraceptive Use, 2016, MMWR Recomm Rep 65:1–103, 2016.

23. **Curtis KM, Jatlaoui TC, Tepper NK, Zapata LB, Horton LG, Jamieson DJ, et al.,** U.S. Selected Practice Recommendations for Contraceptive Use, 2016, MMWR Recomm Rep 65:1–66, 2016.

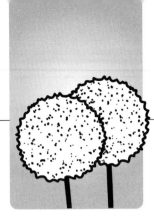

4

Permanent Contraception

Aileen M. Gariepy, MD, MPH
and Rebecca H. Allen, MD, MPH

The phrase "permanent contraception" recognizes a person's voluntary decision to complete childbearing as an active and positive decision. Although "sterilization" has been used to refer to nonreversible methods, the term can connote coercive or involuntary procedures in some settings; "permanent contraception" has been proposed as an alternative.[1] Permanent contraception is now the predominant method of contraception in the world.[2] However, the rate varies widely according to region and country (**Table 4.1**).

History

Although James Blundell proposed performing tubectomy at the time of cesarean section to avoid the need for repeat sections in women at risk of obstructed labor due to a contracted pelvis,[3] Samuel Lungren of Toledo, Ohio, published the first report of postpartum permanent contraception in 1881.[4] The method of Ralph Pomeroy, a prominent physician in Brooklyn, New York, was first described to the medical profession by his associates in 1929, 4 years after Pomeroy's death.[5] Frederick Irving of the Harvard Medical School described his technique in 1924, and the Uchida method was reported in 1946.

Few female permanent contraception procedures were performed until the 1930s when "family planning" was first suggested as an indication for surgical sterilization by Baird in Aberdeen. He required women to be older than 40 and to have had eight or more children. Mathematical formulas of this kind persisted through the 1960s. At the time, the American College of Obstetricians and Gynecologists (ACOG) recommended that voluntary permanent contraception be restricted to women or men whose age multiplied by number of children was equal to or greater than 120. In 1965, Sir Dugald Baird delivered a remarkable lecture, entitled "The Fifth Freedom," calling attention to the need to alleviate the fear of unwanted pregnancies and the important role of permanent contraception.[6] By the end of the 1960s, voluntary permanent contraception was a popular procedure but still legally restricted in some states until 1972. On the other hand, forced and coercive sterilizations were practiced in the United States during this time for both eugenic and antipoverty reasons.[7]

Table 4.1 Permanent Contraception Use in Select Regions/Countries

Region/Country	Total	Female	Male
India	40.2%	39.0%	1.2%
China	32.6%	28.2%	4.4%
United Kingdom	29.0%	8.0%	21.0%
United States	24.5%	18.6%	5.9%
Sub-Saharan Africa	1.6%	1.6%	0

Sources: United States Data: **Daniels K, Abma JC,** Current contraceptive status among women aged 15–49: United States, 2015–2017, NCHS Data Brief (327):1–8, 2018. Other World Data: **United Nations,** Trends in contraceptive use worldwide [cited June 19, 2019]. http://www.un.org/en/development/desa/population/publications/pdf/family/trendsContraceptiveUse2015Report.pdf, 2015.

Laparoscopic methods to occlude the fallopian tubes were introduced in the early 1970s. By 1982, more sterilization operations were performed for women than for men due to dramatic decreases in costs, hospital time, and pain with laparoscopy compared to laparotomy.[8] The use of laparoscopy for permanent contraception increased from only 0.6% of surgeries in 1970 to more than 35% by 1975.[9] These methods allowed women to undergo operations at times other than immediately after childbirth or during major surgery.

Hysteroscopic methods were investigated as early as 1934 when Schroeder recorded the first two attempts at hysteroscopic tubal occlusion with electrocautery initially applying electrocautery to the intramural portion of the tube.[10] As hysteroscopy advanced, this technique continued to be used but ultimately fell out favor in the 1970s due to high patency rates (20%) and risk of uterine perforation and thermal injury.[11] The neodysmium:yttrium-aluminum-garnet (Nd:YAG) laser was also trialed, but patency rates were worse than those for electrocautery (74%).[12] Research then focused on implantable devices and various plugs and screws made of nylon, silicone, ceramic, and polyethylene.[13,14] A formed-in-place silicone plug marketed under the trade name Ovabloc™ was introduced in Europe in the 1990s but was never approved in the United States. Ultimately, the Essure® coil system was approved by the European Union in 2001 and by the United States Food and Drug Administration (FDA) in 2002. Adiana®, a combination of silicone insert with thermal damage, was approved by the FDA in 2009.

Male sterilization through vasectomy began as an alternative to castration for the punishment of certain crimes and then entered the eugenics movement as means to sterilize criminals and others deemed "unimprovable."[15] As a voluntary family planning procedure, however, vasectomy first gained popularity internationally. India introduced vasectomy as a means of population control in 1952, and massive vasectomy camps were established that often used coercive techniques.[15] In the United States, vasectomy for family planning became more common in the 1960s after legal restrictions were removed on voluntary permanent contraception. Early vasectomy was performed through the inguinal canal and later moved to the scrotum. The no-scalpel vasectomy technique was developed in 1973 in China.[16]

For a complete review of the history of permanent contraception, see the online chapter available in the eBook.

Female Permanent Contraception Techniques

Interval Procedures

Procedures performed at a time unrelated to the postpartum period are classified as "interval" in timing. In the United States and most of the developed world, laparoscopy is more popular than minilaparotomy for tubal occlusion.[17] A minilaparotomy is an incision no more than a few centimeters in length. For both procedures, hospitalization is not required, and most patients are discharged within a few hours. However, in obese women, performing a true minilaparotomy can be difficult, an important consideration as obesity rates increase worldwide. Laparoscopy offers many advantages including minimal discomfort, small incision scars, and the ability to perform the procedure as an outpatient. In addition, the surgeon has an opportunity to inspect the pelvic and abdominal organs for abnormalities. The disadvantages of laparoscopic permanent contraception include the cost related to expensive equipment, the special training required, and the risks of inadvertent bowel or vessel injury. In addition, some women with a history of extensive pelvic adhesions, inability to tolerate Trendelenburg positioning, or a contraindication to general anesthesia may not be candidates for a laparoscopic procedure.

Minilaparotomy for interval procedures is an important approach if laparoscopy is not available or impossible due to adhesions. In this procedure, the surgeon makes a small suprapubic horizontal incision to access the peritoneal cavity. A uterine manipulator is used to position the fallopian tubes closer to the incision. The surgeon can place a tubal occlusion device or perform a partial or total salpingectomy. In low-resource settings, this procedure is often performed under local anesthesia alone or local anesthesia with moderate intravenous sedation.[18]

The risk of complications with interval permanent contraception procedures is low (0.9 to 1.6 per 100 procedures); risk factors for complications include obesity, prior abdominal or pelvic surgery, and diabetes.[19] The most extensive single study of female permanent contraceptive procedures comes from the landmark U.S. Collaborative Review of Sterilization (CREST), a large, multicenter, prospective study that enrolled almost 10,000 women from 1978 to 1987 and followed them at periodic intervals until 1994.[20] The CREST study compared bipolar coagulation, unipolar coagulation, silicone rubber band (Falope ring), spring clip (Hulka), interval partial salpingectomy via laparotomy, and postpartum partial salpingectomy. There were no deaths among 9,475 women who underwent laparoscopic permanent contraception in this study.[19]

Currently, laparoscopic sterilization can be achieved with any of these methods:

1. Occlusion by bipolar electrocoagulation
2. Occlusion by mechanical means (titanium clips or silicone rubber rings)
3. Removal of a portion of the fallopian tube (partial salpingectomy)
4. Removal of the entire fallopian tube (salpingectomy)

The most common laparoscopic approach for tubal occlusion or excision utilizes an umbilical port for the laparoscope and a single midline suprapubic port site for the introduction of the electrosurgical system or clip/band applying instrument. A uterine manipulator is placed transcervically to allow for better visualization of the fallopian tubes. Bilateral salpingectomy typically requires at least one additional trocar site.[21] Alternatively, "single site" laparoscopic surgery techniques allow procedures through a single umbilical port site using either a laparoscope with an operating channel (operative laparoscope) or laparoendoscopic single-site surgery (LESS) with a multichannel port.[22] All can be used with the "open" laparoscopic technique in which the laparoscopic instrument is placed into the abdominal cavity under direct visualization to decrease the risk of bowel or blood vessel puncture on blind entry.[23]

Tubal Occlusion by Electrosurgical Methods

The most common electrosurgical technique utilized in the United States is bipolar coagulation. Unipolar cautery fell out of favor due to higher rates of inadvertent thermal bowel injury.[24,25] The bipolar method of sterilization uses a specially designed forceps, typically the reusable Kleppinger bipolar forceps, to desiccate the fallopian tube at the junction of the isthmus and ampulla and destroy the tubal lumen (**Figure 4.1**). A number of single-use bipolar forceps are also available. With all of these instruments, one jaw of the forceps is the active electrode, and the other jaw is the return electrode. Current density is greatest at the point of forceps contact with tissue, and the use of a low-voltage, high-frequency current prevents the spread of electrons to nontarget tissues. As desiccation occurs at the point of high current density, tissue resistance increases, and the coagulated area eventually provides resistance to flow of the low-voltage current. Should the resistance increase beyond the voltage's capability to push electrons through the tissue, incomplete coagulation of the endosalpinx can result.[26] Although data from CREST were first reported to show that bipolar tubal electrocoagulation had a higher failure rate than other methods, a reanalysis of the data

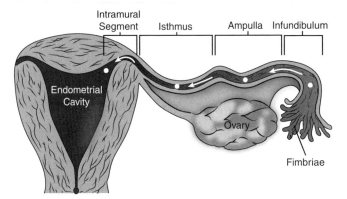

Figure 4.1 Anatomy of the Fallopian Tube. An ovum released from the ovary is swept up by the fimbria and carried through the infundibulum, ampulla, isthmus, and intramural segments of the fallopian tube aided by beating cilia and contracting smooth muscle. (Reprinted from **Patil E, Jensen JT,** Permanent contraception for women. Semin Reprod Med 34(3):139–144, 2016, with permission from Thieme. Illustration by Robin Jensen.)

focusing on procedures that ensured full fallopian tube desiccation by using electrocoagulation at three or more sites (3 cm total) indicated a comparable 5-year pregnancy rate of 3.2 pregnancies per 1,000 women.[27] The use of an ammeter will assist the surgeon in confirming complete desiccation.

Tubal Occlusion with Clips and Rings

Female sterilization by mechanical occlusion eliminates the safety concerns with electrosurgery. However, mechanical devices are subject to flaws in material, defects in manufacturing, and errors in design, all of which can alter efficacy. Two mechanical devices are in current use, the titanium Filshie clip with silicone rubber lining (**Figure 4.2**) and the Silastic (silicone elastomer) band, also known as the Falope or Yoon ring (**Figure 4.3**). The Hulka (spring) clip is no longer in use. Each of these devices requires an understanding of its mechanical function, a working knowledge of the intricate applicator necessary to apply the device, meticulous attention to maintenance of the applicators, and skillful tubal placement. These devices are less effective when used immediately postpartum on dilated tubes.[28,29] Mechanical occlusion offers a better chance for tubal reversal surgery compared to electrosurgical methods that destroy more tube; however, caution should be used with this justification for method choice since permanent, nonreversible contraception is always the goal.[30]

Filshie Clip

The Filshie clip is made of titanium lined with silicone rubber. The hinged clip is locked over the tube using a special applicator through a second incision or operating laparoscope. The clip must be applied perpendicular

The Filshie Clip

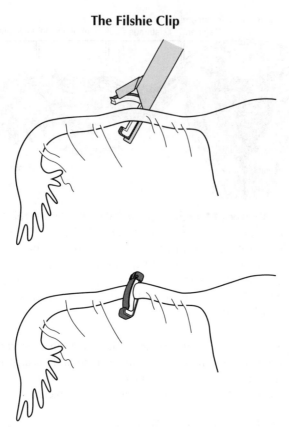

Figure 4.2 Filshie Clip.

to the isthmic portion of the tube, 1 to 2 cm from the cornua of the uterus. Care must be taken to ensure the clip completely occludes the entire tube by visualizing the tip of the applicator through the mesosalpinx. The rubber lining of the clip expands on compression to keep the tube blocked. Only 4 mm of the tube is destroyed. Clips are left permanently in place. Failure rates 1 year after the procedure approximate 1 per 1,000 women. A 15-year follow-up study in Quebec reported a cumulative failure rate of 9 per 1,000 women, whereas the 10-year failure rate in the United Kingdom was 5.6 per 1,000 women.[31,32] While the Filshie clip is also marketed for postpartum application at the time of cesarean delivery or via minilaparotomy after vaginal delivery, concerns have been raised over efficacy in this circumstance. The postpartum fallopian tubes are often hypertrophied and edematous, making correct clip application more difficult. One multicenter randomized controlled trial of 1,400 women compared the Filshie clip to partial salpingectomy.[29] At 2 years, the cumulative probability of pregnancy was 0.017 with the clip (9 pregnancies) and 0.004 with partial salpingectomy (2 pregnancies) ($p = 0.04$).

The Silastic (Falope or Yoon) Ring

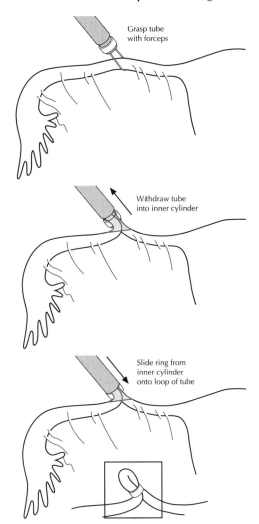

Grasp tube with forceps

Withdraw tube into inner cylinder

Slide ring from inner cylinder onto loop of tube

Figure 4.3 Falope Ring.

Silastic (Falope or Yoon) Ring

This nonreactive Silastic band has an elastic memory of 100% if stretched to no more than 6 mm for a brief time (a few minutes at most). A special applicator, 6 mm in diameter, can be placed through a second cannula or through a standard offset operating laparoscope. The applicator is designed to grasp a knuckle of tube and release the Silastic band onto a 2.5-cm loop of tube. Ten to fifteen percent of patients experience severe postoperative pelvic cramping from the tight bands (which can be reduced by the application of a local anesthetic to the tube before or after banding).[33]

The ring should be placed at the junction of the isthmic and ampullary portion each fallopian tube. Necrosis occurs promptly and a 2- to 3-cm segment of the tube is destroyed. The ring stays permanently in place. Failure rates are about 1% after 2 years, and the 10-year cumulative rate is 1.77%.[20,34] Mesosalpinx bleeding is the most common complication of Silastic ring application. It usually occurs when the forceps grab not only the tube but also a vascular fold of mesosalpinx. The mesosalpinx can also be torn on the edge of the stainless steel cylinder as the tube is drawn into the applicator. If bleeding is noted, application of the band often controls it. If the placement of additional bands or electrocoagulation fails to stop bleeding, laparotomy may be required. Silastic rings are occasionally placed on structures other than the tube. While removal of an incorrectly positioned band from the round ligament or mesosalpingeal folds typically is easily accomplished by grasping the band with the tongs of the applicator and applying gradual, increasing traction, removal is not generally necessary or recommended. Providers should be prepared to use an alternative method like electrosurgery or salpingectomy in case bands or clips cannot be applied due to adhesions or bleeding.

Total Salpingectomy

Traditionally, tubal occlusion techniques were used for laparoscopic permanent contraception as the methods were easier and thought to be associated with fewer complications than partial or total salpingectomy. Laparoscopic total salpingectomy, however, is increasingly being offered as an alternative to tubal occlusion techniques because of the potential higher efficacy and decrease in future ovarian cancer risk, so-called opportunistic salpingectomy.[35-38] In one large California health system, a one-time education campaign focusing on total salpingectomy as a means to decrease ovarian cancer risk resulted in an increase in total salpingectomy rates for interval permanent contraception from 1% in 2011 to 78% in 2016.[39] This retrospective cohort study of 9,007 tubal occlusion procedures and 1,734 total salpingectomies found that operative time increased by 3 minutes for total salpingectomy compared to tubal occlusion with no difference in estimated blood loss, readmission within 30 days, or emergency department visit within 7 days. Another retrospective cohort study compared total salpingectomy using an electrothermal bipolar tissue-sealing instrument (Ligasure) and tubal occlusive techniques.[21] The procedures included 68 tubal occlusions (19% Falope rings, 32% bipolar cautery, and 47% Filshie clips) and 81 bilateral salpingectomies. Surgical time was only 6 minutes longer for the salpingectomies, and similar rates of complications were noted.

Transcervical Approaches

Although current methods of permanent contraception are safe and effective, they require skillful surgeons and, in the case of laparoscopic and hysteroscopic operations, expensive equipment. Simpler approaches could make permanent contraception available and acceptable to more women and avoid surgery. During the 1970s and 1980s, a number of investigators developed approaches for transcervical delivery of agents to occlude the fallopian tubes.[40] While some involved the use of hysteroscopes to place occlusive devices, many techniques used sclerosing agents. Zipper developed the technique of quinacrine sterilization in which quinacrine pellets are placed to the fundus using a modified IUD inserter.[41] The pellets caused epithelial damage resulting in occlusive collagen replacement to the intramural portion of the fallopian tube.[42] Unfortunately, questions regarding potential toxicity of the approach emerged after the initiation of widespread human use in many developing nations.[43,44] Since the human use occurred in the absence of regulatory approval in the United States or Europe, these allegations led to a loss of confidence in the approach and withdrawal of support by governments and funding agencies. Although subsequently completed epidemiologic studies support the safety of quinacrine sterilization,[45,46] serious concerns regarding implementation of the program and a significantly higher (two to four times greater than surgical tubal ligation at 10 years) failure rate present significant obstacles to further research and development of the method.[47,48] The FDA placed a planned U.S. phase three clinical trial program on hold in the United States in 2006, and the sponsor withdrew support effectively ending the program.

New approaches to transcervical nonsurgical permanent contraception are under investigation. A system named FemBloc™ is being investigated in late phase clinical trials (Clinicaltrials.gov NCT03433911), but no published data exist. This system uses a proprietary catheter system to deliver a biopolymer to the intramural tube under ultrasound guidance. The transcervical administration of polidocanol foam, a sclerosing agent currently approved for the indicated for the treatment of incompetent great saphenous veins, accessory saphenous veins, and visible varicosities of the great saphenous vein system, shows potential in nonhuman primate studies.[49]

Hysteroscopic Permanent Contraception

Two hysteroscopic methods have been approved and marketed, only to be subsequently withdrawn from the market. Essure was first approved in 2002 and withdrawn in December 2018.[50] Adiana was approved in 2009[51] and withdrawn in 2012.[52] Both methods induced collagen deposition in the intramural portion of the tube over a few months. Whereas Essure delivered polyethylene terephthalate fibers to the tubal ostia, held in place by nickel-titanium (nitinol) coils, Adiana involved introduction of a silicone matrix after delivery of controlled thermal damage to the tubal lumen.

Hysteroscopic permanent contraception has several potential advantages compared to laparoscopic techniques. These advantages include no incisions or abdominal entry and the option to perform in the office setting under local anesthesia only.[53] These features make the procedure potentially beneficial for individuals at high risk for complications with abdominal surgery or general anesthesia. Two disadvantages of the previously marketed methods were the lack of immediate effectiveness and the requirement for a delayed confirmation test. These multiple steps and delay expose patients to potential pregnancy.

Both Essure and Adiana required verification of occlusion using hysterosalpingogram (HSG) or transvaginal ultrasonography. Follow-up to confirm bilateral tubal occlusion was poor, with an estimated 13% to 94% of women returning for HSG depending on the study population.[54-57] In 2015, the FDA approved transvaginal ultrasonography as an alternative to HSG in selected patients (uncomplicated placement procedure lasting ≤15 minutes and 1 to 8 trailing coils visible). One study observed an increase in follow-up rates from 77.5% for HSG to 88% (p = 0.008) for transvaginal ultrasonography.[58]

This noncompliance with HSG follow-up accounted for approximately half of all hysteroscopic tubal occlusion failures and resulting pregnancies.[53,54,59-61] In one large national comparative study, at 2 years, the pregnancy rate was 2.4% among women undergoing hysteroscopic tubal occlusion versus 2.0% among those undergoing laparoscopic procedures (HR 20, 95% CI 1.09–1.33).[54] However, among women who underwent HSG (66%), the Essure pregnancy rate fell to 1.8% and was no different than laparoscopy (HR 0.90, 95% CI 0.80–1.02). Other reasons for hysteroscopic sterilization failures include incomplete occlusion (10%), incorrect HSG interpretation (33%), and an established pregnancy before the procedure (approximately 1%).[60-63] Overall, of all women who choose hysteroscopic sterilization, at 3 months postprocedure, approximately 85% of women could rely on it for pregnancy prevention.[55,64]

Unsuccessful placement of both Essure coils occurred in 4% to 24% of procedures.[55,65-67] In one large study of 27,724 hysteroscopic tubal occlusion procedures, 4% underwent a second attempt hysteroscopically and 4% underwent a subsequent laparoscopic sterilization surgery.[54] In general, hysteroscopic tubal occlusion has a 4% to 8% rate of repeat sterilization surgery compared with less than 2% for laparoscopic procedures.[54,67,68]

Essure

Essure consists of a nickel-titanium outer coil and a stainless steel inner coil wrapped with polyethylene terephthalate fibers (**Figure 4.4**). The insert is approximately 4 cm in length and 0.8 mm in diameter, which expands to 2 mm when deployed. The hysteroscopic surgeon utilizes a specially designed, single-use, insertion catheter that uses an outer sheath to maintain the system in a wound-down state and introduce it through the tubal ostia, positioning this in the interstitial region of the tube. Withdrawal of the outer sheath allows the outer coils to expand, anchoring the system in place, spanning the uterotubal junction. The number of outer coils left trailing

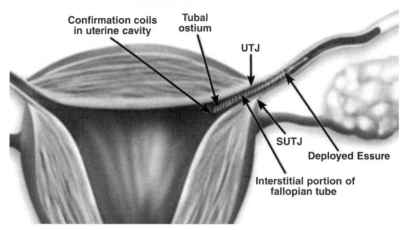

Figure 4.4 Essure Procedure. UTJ, uterotubal junction; SUTJ, serosa of uterotubal junction. (Reprinted from Essure Permanent Birth Control product information, 2018 U.S. label, with permission from Bayer Healthcare, Whippany, NJ.)

into the uterine cavity should ideally be 3 to 8, however, between 0 and 17 is acceptable. Adequate uterine distention and a thin endometrium (follicular phase or preparation with hormonal agents) are essential to be able to visualize the tubal ostia. Over several months, the polyethylene terephthalate fibers stimulate an inflammatory response that results in replacement of the tubal lumen with a fibrotic scar. Unlike laparoscopic tubal occlusion and salpingectomy procedures, this method does not provide immediate contraception. Women must use a back-up method of contraception until a confirmation of tubal occlusion by a HSG or trans-vaginal ultrasound after 3 months. If occlusion is not present at 3 months, contraception is continued and HSG is repeated 3 months later (6 months postprocedure). Contraindications include less than 6 weeks from abortion or delivery, active or recent pelvic infection, uterine or tubal pathology blocking access to tubal ostia, suspected unicornuate uterus, and known allergy to contrast media preventing ability to undergo HSG.

Serious complications with hysteroscopic tubal occlusion are rare, but there is a risk of tubal perforation and potential intra-abdominal placement of coils and bowel injury and malposition or expulsion of the coils.[69-71] Limited data exist on best practices for removal of Essure coils after insertion if needed. Case series have reported that removal may be accomplished with hysteroscopy, laparoscopy, and hysterectomy.[72-75] The most common reason cited for removal is pelvic pain.

The Essure device received expedited review from the FDA since it offered a new method of female permanent contraception that had advantages over laparoscopy.[76] While categorized as a Class III (high risk) medical device, all components of the Essure coil use materials previously approved for use in well-tolerated medical devices such as artificial joints and cardiac stents. Similarly, although a randomized clinical trial was not required, Essure developers did complete open-label safety and efficacy studies for the device. Once available, the uptake of Essure after approval was rapid, and the manufacturer estimates that more than 750,000 units were sold worldwide.[67,77-79] For example, in New York State, the use of Essure increased from 0.6% of all permanent contraception procedures in 2005 to 25.9% in 2013.[80]

Adiana

The Adiana device utilized controlled thermal damage to the lumen of the fallopian tube followed by insertion of a silicone matrix. Using hysteroscopy, a delivery catheter is inserted into the tubal ostia into the interstitial portion of the tube. The distal tip of the catheter then delivers radiofrequency energy to the lumen. The silicone matrix is then deployed in the region of thermal damage. Over the next few weeks, fibroblasts grow into the matrix, which serves as a scaffolding, and tubal occlusion occurs. HSG is performed 3 months after the procedure to confirm tubal occlusion. The company that manufactured Essure at the time, Conceptus, sued Adiana's manufacturer, Hologic, for patent infringement winning an award of $18 million. Ultimately, Hologic agreed to stop selling Adiana if Conceptus would rescind the settlement. Adiana was then removed from the market in 2012.[81]

Studies Comparing Laparoscopic and Hysteroscopic Permanent Contraception

Several retrospective cohort studies conducted in the United States and Europe have been published comparing outcomes after hysteroscopic and laparoscopic permanent contraception. The first U.S. study examined 8,048 patients undergoing hysteroscopic procedures and 44,278 undergoing laparoscopic procedures between 2005 and 2013 in New York state using a statewide claims database.[80] Women undergoing hysteroscopic procedures were more likely to be 40 years or older (25.2% vs. 20.5%, $p < 0.01$), have a history of pelvic inflammatory disease (10.3% vs. 7.2%, $p < 0.01$), major abdominal surgery (9.4% vs. 7.9%, $p < 0.01$), and cesarean section (23.3% vs. 15.4%, $p < 0.01$) compared to women undergoing laparoscopic procedures. Of women undergoing hysteroscopic permanent contraception, 50% received general anesthesia. At 1, 2, and 3 years after the procedure, the rate of pregnancy was similar, but the rate of reoperation was higher in the hysteroscopic group (1 year: OR 10.16, 95% CI 7.47–13.81; 2 years: OR 7.96, 95% CI 6.00–10.57; 3 years: OR 5.88, 95% CI 4.44–7.79). Although database studies have limited ability to infer causality due to limited control for baseline confounding, the authors of this study adjusted these odds ratio estimates for age, race, insurance status, year of procedure, major comorbidities, and history of pelvic inflammatory disease, major abdominal surgeries, and cesarean section, and the OR estimates are robust supportive of a relationship. Although pregnancy detection relied on either an emergency room visit or prenatal labs, likely underestimating overall risk of pregnancy, there is less reason to support differential bias for this outcome.

A retrospective cohort study of U.S. claims data from commercial health (i.e., private) insurance compared 42,391 women who underwent laparoscopic procedures to 27,724 women who underwent hysteroscopic tubal occlusion between 2008 and 2012.[54] Women in the hysteroscopic group had a higher rate of subsequent hysteroscopic surgeries (diagnostic hysteroscopy, endometrial ablation, myomectomy) compared to the laparoscopic group (17.5% vs. 13.4%) at 5 years, after excluding repeat hysteroscopic sterilization attempts. More women in the hysteroscopic group were diagnosed with menstrual dysfunction (26.8% vs. 22.3% at 2 years, adjusted HR 1.23, 95% CI 1.20–1.27) and had a higher rate of subsequent hysteroscopic surgeries. In contrast, they had a lower rate of subsequent intra-abdominal gynecologic surgery (15.7% vs. 17.8%) at 5 years including hysterectomy and laparoscopy. Both groups had equal rates of subsequent salpingectomy by 5 years, 1.7% versus 2.2%. There was also a lower rate of pelvic pain diagnoses in the hysteroscopic group (21% vs. 25.6%, HR 0.83, 95% CI 0.80–0.85). Women in the hysteroscopic group were more likely to become pregnant (2.4% vs. 2.0%, adjusted HR 1.20, 95% CI 1.09–1.33) in the intention-to-treat analysis, which is likely due to only 66% of women obtaining HSG to confirm occlusion. Among women who received an HSG, there was no difference in pregnancy rates compared to women undergoing laparoscopic procedures (1.8% vs. 2% at 2 years, adjusted HR 0.90, 95% CI 0.80–1.02). While statistically significant, the differences between outcomes after hysteroscopic compared to laparoscopic sterilization are very small and not clinically significant.

Another group used Medicaid claims data to compare outcomes at 24 months for 3,929 hysteroscopic tubal occlusions and 10,875 laparoscopic tubal ligations.[51] In this study, after controlling for age, race, baseline pain, and abnormal uterine bleeding diagnoses, hysteroscopic procedures were associated with a slightly lower risk of subsequent hysterectomy (OR 0.77, 95% CI 0.60–0.97) or pelvic pain diagnosis (OR 0.91, 95% CI 0.83–0.99) at 2 years postprocedure. There was no difference in abnormal uterine bleeding between groups. The inability to control for baseline confounding inherent in database studies, self-selection, and lack of information on attempted but failed hysteroscopic procedures represent major limitations of the study.

In the United Kingdom, investigators performed a comparative observational cohort study at a single hospital comparing prospectively collected data on 1,085 women who underwent hysteroscopic procedures with the retrospective data of 2,412 who had undergone laparoscopic tubal ligation with Filshie clip between 2005 and 2015.[67] Hysteroscopic tubal occlusion was successful on first attempt in 91.4% of cases, and laparoscopy was successful in 99.5% of cases (OR 18.8, 95% CI 10.2–34.4). Of the failed insertions, 6.5% resulted from device failure, 34.4% occurred due to difficulty visualizing the tubal ostia, 43% due to tubal spasm, and 16.1% due to inability of the patient to tolerate the procedure under local anesthesia. Of the failed laparoscopy procedures, 8.3% were due to mesosalpinx laceration and 91.7% due to pelvic adhesions. Most (97%) women who had successful hysteroscopic procedures returned for confirmatory testing, of whom 91% had tubal occlusion documented and could rely on Essure for contraception. In all, 902/1,085 (83.1%) of successfully performed hysteroscopic procedures with confirmatory testing were considered satisfactory, compared to 2,400/2,412 (99.5%) of laparoscopic procedures (OR 40.6, 95% CI 22.5–73.1). Women in the hysteroscopic group had six times greater odds of reoperation by 1 year postoperatively (2% vs. 0.3%, OR 6.2, 95% CI 2.8–14.0). Reoperations included removal of incorrectly placed devices, second-stage hysteroscopic procedures to achieve bilateral coil placement, and laparoscopic permanent contraception. The one-year pregnancy risk was similar, with three reported pregnancies after hysteroscopic permanent contraception and five after laparoscopic permanent contraception (OR 1.3, 95% CI 0.3–5.6). Possible limitations to external generalizability include the study population's access to universal health care, which likely facilitates radiographic confirmation testing, and lack of information on race, ethnicity, and comorbidities. Furthermore, it is unclear if pregnancy rates after hysteroscopic procedures were only measured for successful procedures, and not by intention to treat.

In Finland, investigators utilized national registries to compare pregnancy rates and repeat operations from 2009 to 2014 following 4,425 laparoscopic tubal occlusion procedures with Filshie clips, 5,631 hysteroscopic tubal occlusion procedures with Essure, and 6,216 postpartum Pomeroy partial salpingectomies.[79] There was no significant difference in pregnancy rates between the three groups, but women in the hysteroscopic group had higher rates of repeat sterilization operations (**Table 4.2**). Similar to other European studies, this analysis is limited by its external generalizability for a U.S. population due to study subjects' access to universal health care, which likely facilitates radiographic confirmation testing, and its dissimilarity to the U.S. diversity of race, ethnicity, comorbidities, and BMI, which are not reported in this study.

Finally, a large French study used national claims data to evaluate 105,357 women who underwent hysteroscopic or laparoscopic permanent contraception between 2010 and 2014.[52] Outcomes included risk of surgical complications, gynecologic outcomes (sterilization failure, second sterilization procedure, pregnancy), and medical outcomes (allergy, autoimmune disease, thyroid disorder, use of analgesics, use of migraine medication, antidepressants, benzodiazepine use, sick days, outpatient visits, suicide attempt, death) within 1 to 3 years after the procedure. Overall, 71,303 (67.7%) women underwent hysteroscopic and 34,054 (32.3%) women underwent laparoscopic permanent contraception. The risk of immediate surgical complications was lower with the hysteroscopic approach compared to the laparoscopic approach (0.13% vs. 0.78%, adjusted OR 0.18, 95% CI 0.14–0.23). There were no deaths in either group. Women in the hysteroscopic group had a higher risk of undergoing a second permanent contraception procedure at 1 year compared to the laparoscopic group (4.10% vs. 0.16%, adjusted HR 25.99, 95% CI 17.84–37.86). In addition, at one year, the

Table 4.2 Outcomes Evaluated After Hysteroscopic, Laparoscopic, and Open Permanent Contraception Procedures in Finland Between 2009 and 2014

Method	Hysteroscopic (Essure) $n = 5,631$	Laparoscopic (Filshie Clip) $n = 4,425$	Minilaparotomy (Pomeroy) $n = 6,216$
Second permanent contraception procedure*	229 (4.07%)	82 (1.85%)	53 (0.85%)
Spontaneous pregnancies[†]	38 (0.67%)	34 (0.77%)	92 (1.48%)
Spontaneous pregnancies (per 100 follow-up years)	0.20	0.25	0.26

Source: **Jokinen E, Heino A, Karipohja T, Gissler M, Hurskainen R,** Safety and effectiveness of female tubal sterilisation by hysteroscopy, laparoscopy, or laparotomy: a register based study, BJOG 124(12):1851–1857, 2017.
*$p < 0.0001$ for hysteroscopic vs. laparoscopic.
[†]$p = 0.67$ for hysteroscopic vs. laparoscopic.

hysteroscopic group had a higher risk of tubal disorder or surgery including salpingectomy (0.70% vs. 0.23%, adjusted HR 2.98, 95% CI 2.17–4.10). In contrast, women in the hysteroscopic group had a lower risk of uterine disorders (1.28% vs. 1.50%, adjusted HR 0.85, 95% CI 0.74–0.98), abnormal vaginal bleeding (0.23% vs. 0.33%, adjusted HR 0.71, 95% CI 0.52–0.96), and hysterectomy (0.43% vs. 0.81%, adjusted HR 0.54, 95% CI 0.44–0.66) compared to the laparoscopic group. At 3 years, pregnancy rates did not differ between the hysteroscopic group and the laparoscopic group (0.48% vs. 0.57%, adjusted HR 1.04, 95% CI 0.83–1.30). A composite outcome of sterilization failure (including salpingectomy, second sterilization procedure, and pregnancy) was significantly higher at 1 year in the hysteroscopic group compared to laparoscopic group (4.83% vs. 0.69%, adjusted HR 7.11, 95% CI 5.92–8.54). This difference persisted through 3 years (5.75% vs. 1.29%, adjusted HR 4.66, 95% CI 4.06–5.34). For medical complications, there was no difference between the two groups in autoimmune disease and thyroid disorders. Hysteroscopic procedures were associated with lower use of analgesics, antidepressants, benzodiazepines, outpatient visits, and sick days at 3 years compared to laparoscopic procedures. There was no real difference in the risk of suicide attempt or death in the two groups at 3 years. At 1 year, risk of allergies was slightly higher in the subgroup of women with previous allergies in those that underwent hysteroscopic versus laparoscopic permanent contraception (43.2% vs. 40.0%, adjusted HR 1.10, 95% CI 1.03–1.17), but this small difference does not seem clinically important.

Over the past decade, consumer complaints and litigation over outcomes associated with Essure hysteroscopic tubal occlusion led to increased scrutiny of the product.[68] Between 2002 and 2016, the FDA received more than 8,000 reports of complications, with most submitted after 2013.[76] The most frequently reported patient problems were pain/abdominal pain, heavier menses/menstrual irregularities, headache, fatigue, and weight fluctuations.[82] The most frequent device problems reported were categorized as patient-device incompatibility (e.g., possible nickel allergy), migration of the device, dislodged or dislocated device, breakage, device operating differently than expected, device difficult to remove, device difficult to insert, and malposition of the device. In September 2015, the FDA convened a meeting of the Obstetrics and Gynecology Devices Panel of the Medical Devices Advisory Committee to discuss the available scientific data pertaining to Essure's safety and effectiveness, hear expert scientific and clinical opinions on the risks and benefits of the device, and hear concerns and experiences of women implanted with Essure. The FDA concluded that the device could remain on the market but was concerned that some women were not receiving or understanding information regarding the risks, benefits, and alternatives of Essure. The FDA added a Black Box to the Essure prescribing information that stated that some patients implanted with the Essure system experienced perforation of the uterus and/or fallopian tubes, identification of inserts in the abdominal or pelvic cavity, persistent pain, and suspected allergic or hypersensitivity reactions.[83] Due to these concerns, relative contraindications to hysteroscopic tubal occlusion were expanded to include women with a history of any chronic pain condition, autoimmune disease, and metal allergy.[84,85] To address the lack of relevant data, the FDA also mandated the device manufacturer to conduct a new prospective comparative trial of hysteroscopic ($n = 1,400$) and laparoscopic ($n = 1,400$) permanent contraception subjects, which was planned to be completed in 2023.[86] Finally, the FDA approved a 20-page "Patient-Doctor Discussion Checklist—Acceptance of Risk and Informed Decision Acknowledgement" document developed by Bayer Healthcare, the current manufacturer of Essure, and recommended, but did not require, providers to use it. In 2017, Bayer removed Essure from all markets outside of the United States due to declining sales. In April 2018, the FDA further restricted sales and distribution of Essure to only doctors and health care facilities who actually used the FDA-approved "Patient-Doctor Discussion Checklist—Acceptance of Risk and Informed Decision Acknowledgement."[82] Bayer voluntarily removed Essure from the U.S. market in December 2018, citing declining sales. Bayer continues to stand by the safety of the product, and no recommendation exists from any regulatory body for removal of devices from asymptomatic women who have received them.

Sadly, the result of this saga is that no transcervical method of permanent contraception remains available. The story becomes a cautionary tale for contraceptive development in general. The rise and fall of Essure reflects both aggressive marketing and possibly premature and overzealous acceptance by clinicians and patients of a product that, while an excellent alterative to laparoscopy for women who could not have an abdominal procedure or lack access to a hospital-based surgery, may not have been ready to be the first-line option.

To summarize, the evidence from the various registry and comparator studies detailed above supports that Essure hysteroscopic tubal occlusion does not appear more effective than laparoscopic tubal ligation from a population perspective due to placement-related problems and failure to comply with recommended confirmation studies. These problems may also contribute to increase the short-term risk of reoperation and some gynecologic symptoms. No conclusive evidence supports additional health concerns such as allergic response to the device. Clinicians should keep these points in mind and reassure asymptomatic women who have received the device and completed a verification procedure that they can rely on Essure for contraception and expect no health issues related to the presence of the coil. Women who present with symptoms that may be attributable to Essure should be evaluated for device migration, including perforation. Evaluation should also include consideration of other treatable gynecologic or nongynecologic conditions prior to consideration of Essure coil removal or hysterectomy.

The Vaginal Approach

Prior to the availability of laparoscopy, posterior colpotomy was used to access the fallopian tubes for permanent contraception. A common technique was the Kroener fimbriectomy.[87] However, higher rates of infection and the difficulty level of the procedure, in addition to the availability of laparoscopic techniques, have caused the vast majority of clinicians to abandon this approach.[88,89] Bariatric trocars have allowed the safe and effective provision of laparoscopic tubal occlusion for obese women, so the vaginal approach offers no advantages in this circumstance. Nevertheless, the procedure is an option for the skilled vaginal surgeon.[90,91]

Male Permanent Contraception: Vasectomy

Compared to female permanent contraception, vasectomy is safer, easier, and less expensive to perform, and it is easier to verify its successful completion.[53,92,93] The operation is almost always performed under local anesthesia, usually by a urologist in an outpatient setting. Vasectomy is not immediately effective, and alternative contraception must be used until men return to confirm azoospermia by postvasectomy semen analysis (PVSA).[94] The American Urologic Association recommends PVSA testing 8 to 16 weeks after vasectomy.[92] Most men (80%) are azoospermic at

3 months and 98% to 99% at 6 months after vasectomy. Among men who return for PVSA, repeat vasectomy is necessary in ≤1% of vasectomies, when a current technique for vas deferens occlusion is used.[92] For men who have postvasectomy azoospermia or PVSA showing rare nonmotile sperm (RNMS), the risk of pregnancy after vasectomy is approximately 1 in 2,000.[95]

Surgical complications after vasectomy are rare. Symptomatic hematomas and infection occur in 1% to 2% of patients and are easily treated with heat, scrotal support, and antibiotics.[92] Rate of complications also vary by diagnostic criteria and surgeon's experience. Chronic scrotal pain after vasectomy that is associated with a negative impact on quality of life occurs in 1% to 2% of men.[95]

Most men will develop sperm antibodies following vasectomy, but no long-term sequelae have been observed, including no increased risk of coronary heart disease, stroke, hypertension, dementia, testicular or prostate cancer, or autoimmune diseases.[96-100] Adverse psychological and sexual effects have not been reported.[101] In fact, vasectomy has not been demonstrated to have any harmful effects on men's health.[92] Because the other constituents of semen are made downstream from the testes, men do not notice a decreased volume or velocity of ejaculate. Vasectomy does not change the secretion of human immunodeficiency virus (HIV) into semen, and vasectomy should not change the risk of HIV transmission.[102]

Vasectomy Methods

Since the amount of procedural discomfort and the risks of intraoperative and early postoperative complications (e.g., pain, bleeding, infection) are related mostly to vas isolation method and not to the occlusion method, the American Urological Association (AUA) recommends that isolation of the vas deferens is performed using a minimally invasive vasectomy (MIV) technique such as the no-scalpel vasectomy.[92] MIV techniques are defined as those that use a small (≤10 mm) opening of the scrotum and do not require sutures, or those that require minimal dissection of the vas and surrounding tissue, which is accomplished using special instruments. The AUA also recommends using one of four surgical techniques for occlusion of the vas deferens: (1) Mucosal cautery with fascial interposition; (2) mucosal cautery without fascial interposition; (3) open-ended vasectomy leaving the testicular end of the vas unoccluded and using mucosal cautery and fascial interposition on the abdominal end; or (4) nondivisional method of extended electrocautery. The ease of reversal is similar with all methods.

Reversibility

Fertility after vasectomy may be achieved by vasectomy reversal or by sperm retrieval by testicular aspiration with intracytoplasmic sperm injection of oocytes using techniques for assisted reproduction.[92] Approximately 2% to 6% of men undergo vasectomy reversal.[103] However, since surgical success is variable and these options may be expensive, some urologists recommend freezing a preoperative semen specimen in case of regret. A recent systematic review found that the mean postreversal pregnancy rate was 73%.[104] The prospect for pregnancy diminishes with the time elapsed from vasectomy, decreasing significantly to 30% after 10 years; the best results are achieved when reversal is performed within 3 years after vasectomy.[104,105] Another option is to collect and freeze sperm at the time of the reversal procedure for future in vitro fertilization (IVF) and intracytoplasmic sperm injection in case of reversal failure.[106] The best option is certainty that no additional children are desired.

Efficacy of Permanent Contraception

Male and female permanent contraception is highly effective at preventing pregnancy.[34] Failure rates are low but vary by method of permanent contraception and patient age. Younger women have a higher risk of failure due to their fecundity and more years of exposure to possible pregnancy before menopause occurs.[20] In addition, failures continue to accrue as each year passes, making the cumulative failure rate an important measure (**Table 4.3**). Most of the efficacy data for female permanent contraception come from the CREST study. It is worth noting that the CREST study was

Table 4.3 Permanent Contraception 1-Year and 5-Year Cumulative Failure Rates

Method	Cumulative Pregnancy Rates	
	1 Year	5 Years
Bipolar coagulation*[20,27]	0.23%	0.32%
Unipolar coagulation[20]	0.07%	0.23%
Postpartum partial salpingectomy[20]	0.06%	0.63%
Filshie clip[31,107]	0.17%	0.40%
Silastic (Falope or Yoon) ring[20]	0.59%	1.00%
Interval partial salpingectomy[20]	0.73%	1.51%
Hysteroscopic tubal occlusion for women with confirmation of bilateral occlusion[52]	0.24%	0.48%[†]
Vasectomy[108]	0.74%	1.13%
Bilateral salpingectomy[‡]	0	0

*Only with three or more sites of coagulation.
[†]Three-year cumulative failure rate.
[‡]Only rare case reports exist of conception without fallopian tubes, resulting in an estimate that so closely approaches nil that a value of zero is assigned to this outcome.

conducted during the early days of laparoscopic procedures, with earlier device versions, and different patient characteristics and comorbidities.

Since hysteroscopic permanent contraception and vasectomy require delayed confirmation and alternative contraception must be used, the risk of pregnancy should include intention-to-treat analyses. Using this approach, a 2014 study estimated that women undergoing hysteroscopic sterilization have a 10 times higher risk of pregnancy than women undergoing laparoscopic sterilization at 1 year.[109] A retrospective analysis using a commercial insurance claims database examined procedures performed from 2007 to 2013 and found that the pregnancy rate differed by whether women underwent the recommended radiologic confirmation test (one aspect of intention-to-treat analysis). The pregnancy rate was slightly higher after hysteroscopic than laparoscopic procedures (2.4% vs. 2.0%, adjusted HR 1.20, 95% CI 1.09–1.33) among all women, which is likely due to only 66% of women obtaining HSG to confirm occlusion. Among women who received an HSG, there was no difference in pregnancy rates compared to women undergoing laparoscopic procedures (1.8 vs. 2% at 2 years, adjusted HR 0.90, 95% CI 0.80–1.02).[54] The greatest risk and therefore most common cause of pregnancy after hysteroscopic sterilization is the 3- to 6-month delay between the procedure and the confirmation test, when alternative contraception is used.[54,59,109,110]

After vasectomy, men must return to confirm azoospermia by PVSA.[94] The time to achieve azoospermia is highly variable, and most PVSA studies report that 80% of men have no sperm or only RNMS by 12 weeks after vasectomy. Therefore, the American Urologic Association recommends PVSA testing 8 to 16 weeks after vasectomy.[92] Among men who return for PVSA, repeat vasectomy is necessary in ≤1% of vasectomies, when a current technique for vas deferens occlusion is used. For men who have postvasectomy azoospermia or PVSA showing RNMS, the risk of pregnancy after vasectomy is approximately 1 in 2,000.[92] The number of men who fail to return for their PVSA is unknown. Recently, an immunodiagnostic home test that detects normozoospermia and severe oligozoospermia has received FDA approval (SpermCheck Vasectomy™). A prospective, noncomparative observational study assessed the ability of SpermCheck Vasectomy to predict postvasectomy sperm counts and determined that the test was 96% accurate in predicting whether sperm counts were greater or less than a threshold of 250,000 sperm/mL, a level associated with little or no risk of pregnancy.[111]

Ectopic Pregnancy

Because procedure failure and subsequent pregnancy is a risk, all women considering a permanent contraception procedure that does not include total salpingectomy should receive counseling regarding the possibility of ectopic pregnancy.[53] Although pregnancy after female occlusive or partial salpingectomy permanent contraception is uncommon, approximately one third of such pregnancies are ectopic pregnancies.[112] Clinicians must warn women to consider the possibility of ectopic and the need for early evaluation in the event of pregnancy symptoms. In the CREST study, the 10-year cumulative probability of ectopic pregnancy after tubal occlusion by any method was 7.3 per 1,000 procedures. In general, the probability of ectopic pregnancy was greater for women under the age of 30 than for women older than age 30. In a comparator study of 817 women who became pregnant after permanent contraception, the rate of ectopic pregnancy after hysteroscopic procedures was 0.01 per 100 person-years compared to 0.07 per 100 person-years after laparoscopic procedures ($p < 0.001$).[113] Similar to the overall CREST pregnancy data, ectopic pregnancy was less common in older women. However, while permanent contraception increases the proportion of ectopic pregnancies, the overall risk of ectopic pregnancy is greatly reduced in comparison to women using no contraceptive method.

Noncontraceptive Benefits: Ovarian Cancer Risk Reduction

The lifetime incidence of ovarian cancer in average risk women is 1.3%, and ovarian cancer has the highest mortality rate of all types of gynecologic cancer.[114,115] Most ovarian serous, endometrioid, and clear cell carcinomas are derived from the fallopian tube and the endometrium and not directly from the ovary.[116-118] Evidence consistently indicates that tubal interruption is associated with a major reduction in the risk of ovarian cancer, especially endometrioid and clear cell types.[119-122] Data from the Nurses' Health Study found simple tubal occlusion procedures associated with a 67% reduced risk of ovarian cancer.[123] A recent meta-analysis showed that a previous permanent contraception procedure was associated with a 34% overall risk reduction (relative risk of 0.40 for endometrioid cancer and 0.73 for serous cancer), although no risk reduction was found for mucinous or borderline tumors.[124] Possible etiologies for the effect of permanent contraception on ovarian cancer include the creation of a mechanical barrier against ascending carcinogenic agents and prevention of endometrial and proximal Fallopian tube cell ascent into the peritoneal cavity.[125]

Rabban and colleagues[126] completed detailed histologic analysis of specimens obtained from women at high risk for hereditary breast and ovarian cancer undergoing prophylactic risk reduction salpingo-oophorectomy and demonstrated the presence of microscopic precancerous and cancerous lesions in the distal fallopian tubes of some patients. Follow-up studies have confirmed these results, leading to a new theory of a tubal etiology for serous ovarian cancer. The use of bilateral salpingectomy for permanent contraception has arisen amid calls for opportunistic prophylactic salpingectomy to prevent future ovarian cancer.[36-38,127] Opportunistic salpingectomy involves performing salpingectomy at the time of other pelvic surgeries (e.g., hysterectomy) and for permanent contraception.[35] The recommendation for salpingectomy calls for the complete removal of the tube from the fimbriated end up to the uterotubal junction; the interstitial portions of the tubes need not be removed. Interestingly, even though medical societies are recommending consideration of salpingectomy when providing permanent contraception because of increased ovarian cancer protection, a survey study found women more interested in the theoretical 100% efficacy provided by complete tubal removal than the ovarian cancer protection.[128]

Removing the entire fallopian tube including the fimbriated end appears to also reduce the risk of serous cancers, the most common and deadly type of ovarian cancer, more than simple tubal ligation.[129] In a Swedish population based study, women who underwent bilateral salpingectomy had a 65% reduction in the risk of ovarian cancer (HR 0.35, 95% CI 0.17–0.73), while women who underwent standard interruption or occlusion procedures had only a 28% reduction in risk (HR 0.72, 95% CI 0.64–0.81) compared with women who did not undergo sterilization, salpingectomy, hysterectomy, or bilateral salpingo-oophorectomy.[122] While no studies have directly compared cancer risk reduction with total salpingectomy to fimbriectomy alone, we do not recommend fimbriectomy alone (e.g., Kroener fimbriectomy) for the purpose of permanent contraception as earlier studies support an increased risk of pregnancy with this approach.[130]

Bilateral salpingectomy for permanent contraception appears safe and presumably more effective than partial salpingectomy with a lower risk for ectopic pregnancy.[37,38] The technique has been described most commonly during laparoscopic procedures but also at the time of cesarean delivery or through minilaparotomy after vaginal delivery.[38,39] Limited data suggest that opportunistic salpingectomy does not compromise ovarian function or result in premature menopause.[131–134] The practice of opportunistic salpingectomy has become widespread at the time of hysterectomy for benign indications and permanent contraception.[38,39,135,136] ACOG recommends that if laparoscopic permanent contraception is planned, then total bilateral salpingectomy should be discussed with the patient.[35] However, if salpingectomy cannot be accomplished safely, women at average risk should understand that the overall population benefit is small, and bilateral salpingectomy should not be recommended for low-risk women in the absence of a planned surgical procedure. Hopefully, the rapid acceptance of bilateral salpingectomy by clinicians will not result in future discovery of unanticipated problems such as those associated with the Essure procedure.

Counseling for Permanent Contraception

All patients undergoing surgical permanent contraception procedures should be aware of the nature of the operation, its irreversibility and alternatives, efficacy, safety, and complications. Counseling should be patient-centered and reflect the woman's goals and values.[137] Patients should not be denied permanent contraception based on age, number of previous pregnancies or children, or timing of request (e.g., at the time of abortion), and "health care providers should refrain from inserting their own biases or judgments about the appropriateness of a patient's decision to proceed with sterilization."[53,138] On the other hand, providers must be certain that the patient is not being coerced by their partner or family member into permanent contraception or by her socioeconomic constraints, for example having no access to reversible methods.[137] The history of eugenics and coerced sterilizations in the United States and worldwide must be acknowledged in current clinical practice but should also not be used to deny access to voluntary permanent contraception.

Specifically, ACOG recommends that counseling on female permanent contraception include the following points[53]:

- Permanent nature of the procedure, not intended to be reversible
- Alternative methods available, particularly long-acting reversible contraception and vasectomy, that are equally effective
- Details and risks and benefits of specific procedural approaches and anesthesia
- The possibility of failure after permanent contraception that could result in pregnancy, including ectopic pregnancy
- The need to use condoms for protection against sexually transmitted infections, including HIV
- The need to use an alternative form of contraception after hysteroscopic tubal occlusion until a confirmation test confirms appropriate placement of the coils and/or bilateral tubal occlusion
- Completion of informed consent process
- Regulations regarding interval from time of consent to procedure
- Potential effect of sterilization on future health insurance coverage (e.g., noncontraceptive uses of contraceptives, reversal or infertility treatment)

Sexuality

Permanent contraception procedures do not adversely affect sexuality.[139] Indeed, sexual life is usually positively affected as couples do not have to worry about an unwanted pregnancy. An Australian survey of 2,721 women, of whom 447 had undergone tubal ligation, reported that participants with permanent contraception were significantly less likely to lack an interest in sex, to experience vaginal dryness, and to find sex unpleasurable and more likely to experience high levels of sexual satisfaction.[140]

Menstrual Function

Patients may report menstrual changes after permanent contraception procedures. Often, this is because women discontinue hormonal contraceptives after surgery. The CREST study could find no evidence that tubal sterilization is followed by a greater incidence of menstrual changes or abnormalities.[141] The CREST study also found that the increased risk of hysterectomy after permanent contraception was concentrated in women who were treated for gynecologic disorders before tubal sterilization.[142] One retrospective cohort Medicaid claims–based study compared 3,929 women who underwent hysteroscopic tubal occlusion and 10,875 women who under-went laparoscopic tubal occlusion.[51] There was no difference between the two groups at 24 months in abnormal uterine bleeding diagnoses (defined as ≥2 diagnoses at least 2 weeks after their permanent contraception pro-cedure with at least one diagnosis occurring more than 3 months after the procedure). In contrast, an analysis of a commercial insurance claims data-base found slightly higher rates of menstrual dysfunction diagnoses after hysteroscopic compared to laparoscopic tubal occlusion (26.8% vs. 22.3% at 2 years, HR 1.23, 95% CI 1.20–1.27).[54] Investigators have not found any effect of electrocautery, rings, or clips on ovarian reserve.[143,144] Similarly, bilateral salpingectomy does not appear to be associated with any change on ovarian function.[131–134]

Since hormonal contraceptive methods generally result in improvement of menstrual bleeding disorders and cycle-related symptoms, clinicians should consider method discontinuation as a cause of new onset of these symptoms in women following a permanent contraception procedure. History taking prior to surgical contraception should include a review of menstrual cycle symptoms and hormonal treatments. Women who report a history of heavy menstrual bleeding and/or dysmenorrhea need to understand that perma-nent contraception will not manage these symptoms. In most cases, women who experience symptoms following a permanent contraception procedure will benefit from a resumption of hormonal therapy. However, many women decide to undergo a permanent contraception procedure due to intolerance of hormonal therapy. Not surprisingly, these women may be more likely to consider surgical solutions for menstrual symptoms.

Reversibility

The vast majority of women who choose permanent contraception do not regret their decision. Nevertheless, an important objective of counseling is to help women (and partners when involved) make the right choice for themselves about an irreversible decision and to minimize regret among individual women.[53,145–148] According to CREST data, the cumulative prob-ability of regret was 12.7% over 14 years of follow-up and no differences in regret were observed comparing timing after cesarean delivery, vaginal delivery, or a year later.[145] However, the risk of regret did differ by age at the time of the procedure. The probability of regret for women aged 30 years or younger was 20.3%, compared to 5.9% for women older than 30 years at the time of surgery. A more recent 2006 meta-analysis of studies of poststerilization regret concluded that women undergoing permanent contraceptive procedures at age 30 years or younger were twice as likely to report regret compared to women older than 30 years.[148] Women aged 30 years or younger at the time of their procedure were eight times more likely to undergo reversal or evaluation for IVF than older women. Similarly, men who undergo vasectomy at young ages are more likely to have the procedure reversed than those who pursue vasectomy at older ages.[53] Postabortion permanent contraception is not associated with a higher risk of regret compared to interval procedures.[145] A secondary analysis of 2002 National Survey of Family Growth data showed that 30% of black women and 27% of Hispanic women expressed desire for reversal compared with 21% of white women ($p = 0.07$).[149] After adjusting for multiple factors, however, only black women over age 30 had higher rates of regret compared to white women (adjusted OR 2.6, 95% CI 1.2–5.8). While there are trends in some studies that unmarried status and lower educational levels predict regret, these characteristics are overshadowed by age.[149]

The incidence of female permanent contraception reversal reported in most studies is between 1% and 2%.[150] The optimal method to achieve childbirth after female sterilization is unclear. Success of tubal sterilization reversal surgery ranges from 26% to 88% depending on patient age and method of sterilization.[59,151–153] There are no randomized trials that compare pregnancy outcomes or live births among women who underwent IVF compared with tubal reversal surgery. One consideration for method to achieve childbirth is cost. The American Society for Reproductive Medicine reports that reanastomosis is more cost-effective than IVF for women of all ages.[152] However, IVF is the only option for women who undergo hysteroscopic sterilization or bilateral salpingectomy. The success of IVF is not affected by previous tubal ligation.[154]

Barriers to Permanent Contraception

Barriers to accessing permanent contraception in the United States include logistical issues for postpartum procedures, federal and state consent requirements, and religiously affiliated hospitals that may prohibit the procedure.[137] For women with federally funded insurance (e.g., Medicaid), a consent form must be signed at least 30 days prior to the procedure and be accessible at the time of the procedure.[155] Additionally, regulations prohibit federal funds from being used for sterilization in women younger than 21 years of age. Women with private commercial insurance aren't subject to these federal restrictions, creating a two-tiered system of access. Nevertheless, some states have their own waiting periods and consent forms for women regardless of insurance type. These federal and state regulations were originally put in place to prevent coercion and forced sterilization among vulnerable populations. There is currently a debate about whether these regulations are still needed.[7,156,157] On the one hand, they are preventing some women from obtaining timely permanent contraception (particularly in the postpartum period) and seem patronizing; on the other hand, evidence of coerced sterilizations among incarcerated women in California has been documented as recently as 2010.[137,158] To date, there has been no move by the federal government to change these regulations. Any change would have to carefully consider the history of stratified reproduction in the United States (e.g., certain categories of people are encouraged to reproduce and parent, but others are not) and ensure that past coercive practices do not return.

Religiously affiliated hospitals may prohibit permanent contraception and other methods of contraception based on their religious doctrine. Because approximately 15% of women receive their care from a religiously affiliated hospital, they may not obtain a desired permanent contraceptive procedure.[159] Furthermore, many women are unaware of these restrictions on reproductive health care.[160] Patients should be informed of these limitations and should be offered a transfer of care if preferred.

Postabortion and Postpartum Procedures

Many women decide they wish never to become pregnant again during a desired or unintended pregnancy. Permanent contraception provides an ideal method for these women.

Postpartum

In the United States, postpartum partial salpingectomy is performed after 8% to 9% of all deliveries representing half of all permanent contraceptive procedures.[17] A U.S. study estimated postpartum permanent contraception rates from 2008 to 2013 to be 683 to 711 per 10,000 deliveries.[161] The procedure was more common in women age 35 and older and during cesarean compared to vaginal delivery. Postpartum procedures are convenient because they can be performed with a cesarean delivery or within the first 24 to 48 hours after vaginal delivery. The enlarged postpartum uterus after vaginal delivery allows access to the fallopian tubes through an infraumbilical mini-laparotomy incision. Rarely, significant abdominal adhesions may impede access to the fallopian tubes. Advantages of performing the procedure immediately after vaginal delivery include the ability to use an existing epidural anesthesia and convenience for the woman, as she need not restrict food and drink in preparation for the procedure another day.[162]

Historically, surgeons performed a partial salpingectomy technique for postpartum procedures. These techniques remove a mid-isthmic segment of fallopian tube bilaterally. Prospective studies have demonstrated that postpartum partial salpingectomy techniques have a low failure rate (0.6 per 1,000 in 1 year and 7.5 per 1,000 in 10 years).[20] The options for partial salpingectomy include the Parkland, Pomeroy (**Figure 4.5**), Uchida (**Figure 4.6**), and Irving (**Figure 4.7**) methods.

Bilateral total salpingectomy in the immediate postpartum period for permanent contraception has also been described as interest in salpingectomy increases due to its potential to decrease the risk of ovarian cancer.[35,39] In the California study mentioned above, postpartum total salpingectomy rates at cesarean delivery from 2011 to 2016 increased from 0.1% to 9.2% and at vaginal delivery from 0% to 4.5%.[39]

Several studies have compared partial and total salpingectomy at the time of cesarean delivery.[163–168] In a retrospective study, 50 women who underwent salpingectomy with LigaSure were compared to 99 women who underwent partial salpingectomy with no differences in operative time and

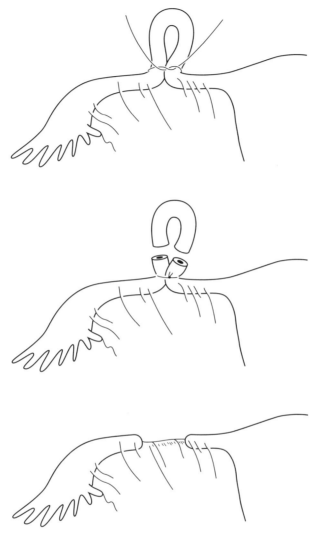

Figure 4.5 Pomeroy Method.

a similar rate of complications.[46] A randomized controlled noninferior-ity trial compared total and partial salpingectomy at the time of cesarean delivery in 37 women, also using the LigaSure device.[165] Bilateral total salpingectomy was successful in 19 out of 20 women. One procedure was converted to partial salpingectomy due to adhesions. Total operative time and estimated blood loss were not different between the groups with a mean procedure time of 5.6 minutes in the total salpingectomy group and 6.1 minutes in the partial salpingectomy group. Another small randomized trial compared total salpingectomy to partial salpingectomy in 80 women at the time of cesarean delivery, this time using traditional suture ligation

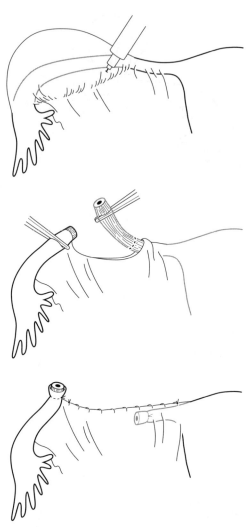

Figure 4.6 Uchida Method.

rather than Ligasure.[164] A total of 27 out of 40 (68%) of women randomized to total salpingectomy and 38 out of 40 (95%) women in the partial salpingectomy group successfully had the assigned procedure performed. Total operative time using the suture ligation technique was 15 minutes longer for the total salpingectomy group compared to partial salpingectomy. There was no difference between the groups in terms of estimated blood loss or complications. Women with higher BMIs and a longer time from skin incision to tubal operation start had an increased risk of a failed procedure. The authors did not report details as to why total salpingectomy was not able to be performed. Surgeons performed a bilateral partial salpingectomy for 8 of the 13 women who had failed total bilateral salpingectomies, performed

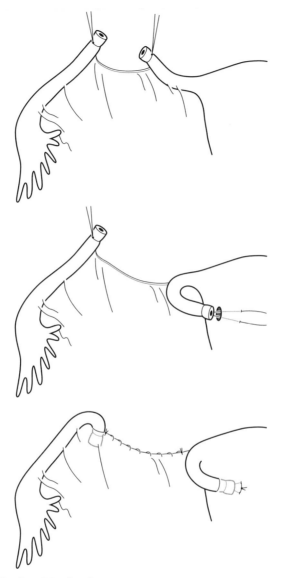

Figure 4.7 Irving Method.

a unilateral total salpingectomy or unilateral partial salpingectomy in 3 women, and were unable to perform any procedure in 2 women. A retrospective study reported more information regarding factors influencing the ability to complete a total salpingectomy.[43]

Investigators evaluated all permanent contraception procedures performed at cesarean delivery at a single institution over an 18-month period ending in April 2017. The 122 women included 32 who preferred partial salpingectomy, all of which were able to be performed. Of the 90 women who desired total salpingectomy, 17 (18.9%) could not have the procedure performed. Nine had a mixed procedure due to adhesive disease ($n = 4$), proximity to large vessels in the mesosalpinx ($n = 3$), or both ($n = 2$). Surgeons performed bilateral partial salpingectomy in 7 women due to adhesive disease ($n = 4$), engorged vasculature ($n = 10$), or unspecified reasons ($n = 2$). One woman was not able to have any procedure performed due to adhesions. The only predictive factor for not accomplishing salpingectomy was 3 or more cesarean deliveries. Surgical time for total salpingectomy averaged 9.5 to 11 minutes longer depending on whether or not the planned salpingectomy could be completed.

To perform total salpingectomy following vaginal delivery, the surgeon may need to expand or change the traditional infraumbilical minilaparotomy incision to access the full fallopian tube. Danis et al.[169] described a technique whereby a 2- to 3-cm infraumbilical vertical incision was made, and the fallopian tube was elevated outside the incision with Babcock clamps. Monopolar cautery was used to develop 2 to 3 windows in the mesosalpinx in order to suture ligate and excise the fallopian tubes. In 16 women, they found slightly longer operative time but no increase in complications compared to the 64 women who underwent partial salpingectomy.

There are often logistical issues that arise with postpartum permanent contraception after vaginal delivery in U.S. hospitals that restrict access (e.g., availability of an operating room and personnel). Unfortunately, despite the fact that ACOG considers postpartum permanent contraception to be an "urgent" not "elective" procedure given the risks of unintended pregnancy in the future,[170] many hospitals do not prioritize postpartum requests.[171] It is estimated that approximately half of women who desire postpartum permanent contraception do not obtain the procedure for logistical issues, obstetric complications, or lack of a correctly signed federal sterilization consent form dated between 30 days and 180 days prior to the procedure if they have Medicaid insurance.[171-174] Unless these women can later obtain an interval procedure, they are often left vulnerable to unintended pregnancy due to lack of insurance or logistical factors. One study of 429 Texas women desiring postpartum permanent contraception reported that of the 133 women who did not receive the requested procedure while in the hospital for cesarean or vaginal delivery, 46.7% became pregnant in the year after delivery compared to 22.3% of 1,031 patients who did not request permanent contraception.[175]

Postabortion

Many women experiencing unintended pregnancy have completed their desired family size. Given this, the request for a permanent contraception procedure at the time of surgical abortion commonly presents. Combining both procedures prevents the need for a second later surgery for women considering laparoscopic permanent contraception procedures and allows women who would prefer anesthesia for abortion to access this service. Considering the advantages, a combined procedure makes sense.

Only a few studies have evaluated the safety of combining surgical abortion with laparoscopic permanent contraception. The practice came under scrutiny due to concerns about an increased risk of complications in non-comparator studies.[176] Cheng and Rochat[177] compared data on 616 women who underwent induced abortion in the first trimester with concurrent tubal ligation with 1,805 women who had induced abortion only. They found that the complication rate with the combined procedure was slightly higher (1.8%) but within the margin seen for interval culdoscopic tubal ligation at the same institution. Investigators at the same institution followed up on these results and performed a randomized study of 406 women allocated to concurrent induced-abortion/sterilization group or sterilization 6 weeks following the abortion. They found that the abortion-attributable and sterilization-attributable complication rates for the concurrent group (3.8% and 5.2%, respectively) did not differ significantly from the interval group (6.7% and 6.9%). They also found that 4% of women who failed to return for the interval procedure experienced another unintended pregnancy.[178] Akhter and colleagues[179] used data from two United States studies: the Joint Program for the Study of Abortion and the Collaborative Review of Sterilization and found rates of complication similar to those reported by Cheng (0.9% for the abortion-only group, 1.7% for the concurrent group). Finally, a Scandinavian study reported similar complication rates with interval and combined procedures performed with laparoscopic rings.[180] All of these studies are over 30 years old. Although only one study reports results following dilation and evacuation abortions up to 18 weeks,[181] our experience with immediate postpartum procedures provides additional evidence of the safety of these combined procedures. Major advances in techniques used for laparoscopic surgery and abortion likely have reduced complication rates further.

Despite the existing safety data for combined procedures, governmental and institutional policies restrict access. Many of the same issues that create barriers for postpartum permanent contraception also affect abortion care. The most challenging provision that restricts access is the 30-day sterilization consent that women receiving Medicaid funds must sign prior to a permanent contraception procedure. Even if she is willing to wait 30 days, the Federal rules do not allow signing of these forms for procedures to be performed at the time of abortion. Additionally, inappropriate concerns that women cannot make a decision about permanent contraception while pregnant are magnified in the setting of unintended pregnancy. Despite an absence of data to support high levels of regret or interest in reversal with permanent contraception at the time of abortion, these barriers continue to exist. Clinicians should temper concerns about potential regret with the interests of the woman and the real world risk of repeat unintended pregnancy.[182]

References

1. **Jensen JT,** Permanent contraception: modern approaches justify a new name, Contraception 89:493–494, 2014.
2. **United Nations,** Trends in Contraceptive Use Worldwide, 2015 [cited April 27, 2018]. Available from: http://www.un.org/en/development/desa/population/publications/pdf/family/trendsContraceptiveUse2015Report.pdf

3. **Speert H,** Obstetric and Gynecologic Milestones Illustrated, The Parthenon Publishing Group, New York, 1996.
4. **Lungren SS,** A case of cesarean section twice successfully performed on the same patient, with remarks on the time, indications, and details of the operation, Am J Obstet Gynecol 14:78, 1881.
5. **O' Dowd MJ, Philipp EE,** The History of Obstetrics and Gynaecology, Informa Healthcare, London, 2011.
6. **Baird D,** The fifth freedom, Br Med J 234, 1966.
7. **Harris LH, Wolfe T.** Stratified reproduction, family planning care and the double edge of history. Curr Opin obstet Gynecol 26:539–544, 2014.
8. **Chandra A,** Surgical Sterilization in the United States: Prevalence and Characteristics, 1965–95, US Department of Health and Human Services, Hyattsville, 1998.
9. **Peterson HB, Greenspan JR, DeStefano F, Ory HW, Layde PM,** The impact of laparoscopy on tubal sterilization in United States hospitals, 1970 and 1975 to 1978, Am J Obstet Gynecol 140: 811–814, 1981.
10. **Quinones R, Alvarado A, Ley E,** Hysteroscopic sterilization, Int J Gynaecol Obstet 14:27–34, 1976.
11. **March CM, Israel R,** A critical appraisal of hysteroscopic tubal fulguration for sterilization, Contraception 11: 261–269, 1975.
12. **Brumsted JR, Shirk G, Soderling MJ, Reed T,** Attempted transcervical occlusion of the fallopian tube with the Nd:YAG laser, Obstet Gynecol 77:327–328, 1991.
13. **Cooper JM,** Hysteroscopic sterilization, Clin Obstet Gynecol 35:282–298, 1992.
14. **Magos A, Chapman L,** Hysteroscopic tubal sterilization, Obstet Gynecol Clin North Am 31:705–719, xii, 2004.
15. **Sheynkin YR,** History of vasectomy, Urol Clin North Am 36:285–294, 2009.
16. **Huber D,** No-scalpel vasectomy: the transfer of a refined surgical technique from China to other countries, Adv Contracept 5:217–218, 1989.
17. **Chan LM, Westhoff CL,** Tubal sterilization trends in the United States, Fertil Steril 94:1–6, 2010.
18. **World Health Organization Department of Reproductive Health and Research, Johns Hopkins Bloomberg School of Public Health/ Center for Communication Programs, Knowledge for Health Project,** Female sterilization. In: Family Planning: A Global Handbook for Providers [Internet], CCP and WHO, Baltimore and Geneva, 2018.
19. **Jamieson DJ, Hillis SD, Duerr A, Marchbanks PA, Costello C, Peterson HB,** Complications of interval laparoscopic tubal sterilization: findings from the United States Collaborative Review of Sterilization, Obstet Gynecol 96:997–1002, 2000.
20. **Peterson HB, Xia Z, Hughes JM, Wilcox LS, Tylor LR, Trussell J,** The risk of pregnancy after tubal sterilization: findings from the U.S. Collaborative Review of Sterilization, Am J Obstet Gynecol 174:1161–1168; discussion 8–70, 1996.
21. **Westberg J, Scott F, Creinin MD,** Safety outcomes of female sterilization by salpingectomy and tubal occlusion, Contraception 95:505–508, 2017.
22. **Scheib SA.** A laparoendoscopic single-site surgical approach to laparoscopic salpingectomy. J Minim Invasive Gynecol 25:326–327, 2018.
23. **Soto E, Falcone T,** Trocar placement. In: Atlas of Pelvic Anatomy and Gynecologic Surgery [Internet], 4th ed., Elsevier, Philadelphia, 2016, pp. 1235–1241.
24. **Peterson HB, Ory HW, Greenspan JR, Tyler CW Jr,** Deaths associated with laparoscopic sterilization by unipolar electrocoagulating devices, 1978 and 1979, Am J Obstet Gynecol 139:141–143, 1981.
25. **Barrett SL, Vella JM, Dellon AL,** Historical development of bipolar coagulation, Microsurgery 30:667–669, 2010.
26. **Soderstrom RM, Levy BS, Engel T,** Reducing bipolar sterilization failures, Obstet Gynecol 74:60–63, 1989.
27. **Peterson HB, Xia Z, Wilcox LS, Tylor LR, Trussell J,** Pregnancy after tubal sterilization with bipolar electrocoagulation. U.S. Collaborative Review of Sterilization Working Group, Obstet Gynecol 94:163–167, 1999.
28. **Rodriguez MI, Edelman AB, Kapp N,** Postpartum sterilization with the titanium clip: a systematic review, Obstet Gynecol 118:143–147, 2011.

124

29. **Rodriguez MI, Seuc A, Sokal DC,** Comparative efficacy of postpartum sterilisation with the titanium clip versus partial salpingectomy: a randomised controlled trial, BJOG 120:108–112, 2013.

30. **Gordts S, Campo R, Puttemans P, Gordts S,** Clinical factors determining pregnancy outcome after microsurgical tubal reanastomosis, Fertil Steril 92:1198–1202, 2009.

31. **Penfield AJ,** The Filshie clip for female sterilization: a review of world experience, Am J Obstet Gynecol 182:485–489, 2000.

32. **Trussell J, Guilbert E, Hedley A,** Sterilization failure, sterilization reversal, and pregnancy after sterilization reversal in Quebec, Obstet Gynecol 101:677–684, 2003.

33. **Harrison MS, DiNapoli MN, Westhoff CL,** Reducing postoperative pain after tubal ligation with rings or clips: a systematic review and meta-analysis. Obstet Gynecol 124:68–75, 2014.

34. **Lawrie TA, Kulier R, Nardin JM,** Techniques for the interruption of tubal patency for female sterilisation, Cochrane Database Syst Rev (8):CD003034, 2016.

35. **American College of Obstetricians and Gynecologists,** Committee opinion no. 620: Salpingectomy for ovarian cancer prevention, Obstet Gynecol 125:279–281, 2015.

36. **Ely LK, Truong M,** The role of opportunistic bilateral salpingectomy vs tubal occlusion or ligation for ovarian cancer prophylaxis, J Minim Invasive Gynecol 2017;24:371–378.

37. **Creinin MD, Zite N,** Female tubal sterilization: the time has come to routinely consider removal, Obstet Gynecol 124:596–599, 2014.

38. **McAlpine JN, Hanley GE, Woo MM, Tone AA, Rozenberg N, Swenerton KD, et al.,** Opportunistic salpingectomy: uptake, risks, and complications of a regional initiative for ovarian cancer prevention, Am J Obstet Gynecol 210: 471.e1—471.e11, 2014.

39. **Powell CB, Alabaster A, Simmons S, Garcia C, Martin M, McBride-Allen S, et al.,** Salpingectomy for sterilization: change in practice in a large integrated health care system, 2011–2016, Obstet Gynecol 130:961–967, 2017.

40. **Zatuchni GI, Shelton JD, Goldsmith A, Sciarra JJ; Program for Applied Research on Fertility Regulation,** Female Transcervical Sterilization: Proceedings of an International Workshop on Non-Surgical Methods for Female Tubal Occlusion June 22 to 24, 1982, Harper & Row, Chicago, 1983.

41. **Sokal DC, Zipper J, King T,** Transcervical quinacrine sterilization: clinical experience, Int J Gynaecol Obstet 51:S57–S69, 1995.

42. **Merchant RN, Prabhu SR, Kessel E,** Clinicopathologic study of fallopian tube closure after single transcervical insertion of quinacrine pellets, Int J Fertil Womens Med 40:47–54, 1995.

43. **Mudur G,** India to ban female sterilisation with malaria drug, BMJ 316:958, 1998.

44. **Kumar S,** Quinacrine sterilisation trials in India delayed, Lancet 345:976, 1995.

45. **Sokal DC, Hieu do T, Loan ND, Hubacher D, Nanda K, Weiner DH, et al.,** Safety of quinacrine contraceptive pellets: results from 10-year follow-up in Vietnam, Contraception 78:66–72, 2008.

46. **Sokal DC, Trujillo V, Guzman SC, Guzman-Serani R, Wheeless A, Hubacher D,** Cancer risk after sterilization with transcervical quinacrine: updated findings from a Chilean cohort, Contraception 81:75–78, 2010.

47. **Sokal DC, Hieu do T, Loan ND, Hubacher D, Nanda K, Weiner DH, et al.,** Contraceptive effectiveness of two insertions of quinacrine: results from 10-year follow-up in Vietnam, Contraception 78:61–65, 2008.

48. **Pal SK,** Quinacrine sterilization of 1997 women in Daharpur, Midnapore, West Bengal, India: a comparison of 3 protocols, Int J Gynaecol Obstet 83:S97–S100, 2003.

49. **Jensen JT, Hanna C, Yao S, Thompson E, Bauer C, Slayden OD,** Transcervical administration of polidocanol foam prevents pregnancy in female baboons, Contraception 94:527–533, 2016.

50. **Espey E, Hofler LG.** Evaluating the Long-term Safety of Hysteroscopic Sterilization. JAMA 2018;319.

125

51. **Anderson TL, Vancaillie TG.** The Adiana System for permanent contraception: safety and efficacy at 3 years. J Minim Invasive Gynecol 2011;18:612–616.

52. Conceptus(R) Announces Settlement of Patent Infringement Lawsuit with Hologic. https://globenewswire.com/news-release/2012/04/30/474765/253823/en/Conceptus-R-Announces-Settlement-of-Patent-Infringement-Lawsuit-With-Hologic.html, April 30, 2012 [cited 2018 October 7].

53. **American College of Obstetricians and Gynecologists,** ACOG Practice bulletin no. 133: benefits and risks of sterilization, Obstet Gynecol 121:392–404, 2013.

54. **Perkins RB, Morgan JR, Awosogba TP, Ramanadhan S, Paasche-Orlow MK,** Gynecologic outcomes after hysteroscopic and laparoscopic sterilization procedures, Obstet Gynecol 128: 843–852, 2016.

55. **Chudnoff SG, Nichols JE Jr, Levie M,** Hysteroscopic Essure inserts for permanent contraception: extended follow-up results of a phase III multicenter international study, J Minim Invasive Gynecol 22:951–960, 2015.

56. **Shavell VI, Abdallah ME, Diamond MP, Kmak DC, Berman JM,** Post-Essure hysterosalpingography compliance in a clinic population, J Minim Invasive Gynecol 15:431–434, 2008.

57. **Leyser-Whalen O, Berenson AB,** Adherence to hysterosalpingogram appointments following hysteroscopic sterilization among low-income women, Contraception 88:697–699, 2013.

58. **Jeirath N, Basinski CM, Hammond MA,** Hysteroscopic sterilization device follow-up rate: hysterosalpingogram versus transvaginal ultrasound, J Minim Invasive Gynecol 25:836–841, 2018.

59. **Stuart GS, Ramesh SS,** Interval female sterilization, Obstet Gynecol 131: 117–124, 2018.

60. **Munro MG, Nichols JE, Levy B, Vleugels MP, Veersema S,** Hysteroscopic sterilization: 10-year retrospective analysis of worldwide pregnancy reports, J Minim Invasive Gynecol 21:245–251, 2014.

61. **Cleary TP, Tepper NK, Cwiak C, Whiteman MK, Jamieson DJ,** Marchbanks PA, et al., Pregnancies after hysteroscopic sterilization: a systematic review, Contraception 87:539–548, 2013.

62. **Levy B, Levie MD, Childers ME,** A summary of reported pregnancies after hysteroscopic sterilization, J Minim Invasive Gynecol 14:271–274, 2007.

63. **Hitzerd E, Schreuder HW, Vleugels MP, Veersema S,** Twelve-year retrospective review of unintended pregnancies after Essure sterilization in the Netherlands, Fertil Steril 105:932–937, 2016.

64. **Gariepy AM, Creinin MD, Schwarz EB, Smith KJ,** Reliability of laparoscopic compared with hysteroscopic sterilization at 1 year: a decision analysis, Obstet Gynecol 118:273–279, 2011.

65. **Savage UK, Masters SJ, Smid MC, Hung YY, Jacobson GF,** Hysteroscopic sterilization in a large group practice: experience and effectiveness, Obstet Gynecol 114:1227–1231, 2009.

66. **Mino M, Arjona JE, Cordon J, Pelegrin B, Povedano B, Chacon E,** Success rate and patient satisfaction with the Essure sterilisation in an outpatient setting: a prospective study of 857 women, BJOG 114:763–766, 2007.

67. **Antoun L, Smith P, Gupta JK, Clark TJ,** The feasibility, safety, and effectiveness of hysteroscopic sterilization compared with laparoscopic sterilization, Am J Obstet Gynecol 217:570.e1–570.e6, 2017.

68. **Dhruva SS, Ross JS, Gariepy AM,** Revisiting Essure—Toward safe and effective sterilization, N Engl J Med 373:e17, 2015.

69. **Adelman MR, Dassel MW, Sharp HT,** Management of complications encountered with Essure hysteroscopic sterilization: a systematic review, J Minim Invasive Gynecol 21:733–743, 2014.

70. **Hurskainen R, Hovi SL, Gissler M, Grahn R, Kukkonen-Harjula K, Nord-Saari M, et al.,** Hysteroscopic tubal sterilization: a systematic review of the Essure system, Fertil Steril 94:16–19, 2010.

71. **Povedano B, Arjona JE, Velasco E, Monserrat JA, Lorente J, Castelo-Branco C,** Complications of hysteroscopic Essure((R)) sterilisation: report on 4306 procedures performed in a single centre, BJOG 119:795–799, 2012.

72. **Johal T, Kuruba N, Sule M, Mukhopadhyay S, Raje G,** Laparoscopic salpingectomy and removal of Essure hysteroscopic sterilisation device: a case series, Eur J Contracept Reprod Health Care 23:227–230, 2018.

73. **Lazorwitz A, Tocce K,** A case series of removal of nickel-titanium sterilization microinserts from the uterine cornua using laparoscopic electrocautery for salpingectomy, Contraception 96:96–98, 2017.

74. **Clark NV, Rademaker D, Mushinski AA, Ajao MO, Cohen SL, Einarsson JI,** Essure removal for the treatment of device-attributed symptoms: an expanded case series and follow-up survey, J Minim Invasive Gynecol 24:971–976, 2017.

75. **Charavil A, Agostini A, Rambeaud C, Schmitt A, Tourette C, Crochet P,** Vaginal hysterectomy with salpingectomy for Essure insert removal, J Minim Invasive Gynecol 26:695–701, 2019.

76. **Espey E, Hofler LG,** Evaluating the long-term safety of hysteroscopic sterilization, JAMA 319, 2018.

77. **Carney PI, Lin J, Xia F, Law A,** Temporal trend in the use of hysteroscopic vs laparoscopic sterilization and the characteristics of commercially insured and Medicaid-insured females in the US who have had the procedures, Int J Womens Health 8:137–144, 2016.

78. **Shavell VI, Abdallah ME, Shade GH Jr, Diamond MP, Berman JM,** Trends in sterilization since the introduction of Essure hysteroscopic sterilization, J Minim Invasive Gynecol 6:22–27, 2009.

79. **Jokinen E, Heino A, Karipohja T, Gissler M, Hurskainen R,** Safety and effectiveness of female tubal sterilisation by hysteroscopy, laparoscopy, or laparotomy: a register based study, BJOG 124:1851–1857, 2017.

80. **Mao J, Pfeifer S, Schlegel P, Sedrakyan A,** Safety and efficacy of hysteroscopic sterilization compared with laparoscopic sterilization: an observational cohort study, BMJ 351:h5162, 2015.

81. Conceptus(R) Announces Settlement of Patent Infringement Lawsuit With Hologic. April 30, 2012. [cited September 24, 2018] Available from: https://globenewswire.com/news-rel ease/2012/04/30/474765/253823/en/ Conceptus-R-Announces-Settlement-of-Patent-Infringement-Lawsuit-With-Hologic.html

82. **U.S. Food and Drug Administration,** FDA Activities: Essure. Available from: https://www.fda.gov/MedicalDevices/ ProductsandMedicalProcedures/ ImplantsandProsthetics/ EssurePermanentBirthControl/ ucm452254.htm

83. **Bayer,** Essure Label. Available from: http://labeling.bayerhealthcare.com/ html/products/pi/essure_pib_en.pdf

84. **Brito LG, Cohen SL, Goggins ER, Wang KC, Einarsson JI,** Essure surgical removal and subsequent symptom resolution: case series and follow-up survey, J Minim Invasive Gynecol 22:910–913, 2015.

85. **Yunker AC, Ritch JM, Robinson EF, Golish CT,** Incidence and risk factors for chronic pelvic pain after hysteroscopic sterilization, J Minim Invasive Gynecol 22:390–394, 2015.

86. **U.S. Food and Drug Administration,** Labeling for Permanent Hysteroscopically-Placed Tubal Implants Intended for Sterilization, 2016. Available from: https://www. fda.gov/downloads/MedicalDevices/ DeviceRegulationandGuidance/ GuidanceDocuments/UCM488020.pdf

87. **Kroener WF Jr,** Surgical sterilization by fimbriectomy, Am J Obstet Gynecol 104:247–254, 1969.

88. **Miesfeld RR, Giarratano RC, Moyers TG,** Vaginal tubal ligation—is infection a significant risk?, Am J Obstet Gynecol 137:183–188, 1980.

89. Randomized comparative study of culdoscopy and minilaparotomy for surgical contraception in women, Contraception 26:587–593, 1982.

90. **Ayhan A, Boynukalin K, Salman MC,** Tubal ligation via posterior colpotomy, Int J Gynaecol Obstet 93:254–255, 2006.

91. **Chang WH, Liu JY, Yeh YC, Wu GJ, Chiang YJ, Yu MH, et al.,** Tubal ligation via colpotomy or laparoscopy: a retrospective comparative study, Arch Gynecol Obstet 283:805–808, 2011.

92. **Sharlip ID, Belker AM, Honig S, Labrecque M, Marmar JL, Ross LS,**

127

et al., Vasectomy: AUA guideline, J Urol 188:2482–2491, 2012.

93. **Smith GL, Taylor GP, Smith KF,** Comparative risks and costs of male and female sterilization, Am J Public Health 75:370–374, 1985.

94. **Curtis KM, Jatlaoui TC, Tepper NK, Zapata LB, Horton LG, Jamieson DJ, et al.,** U.S. selected practice recommendations for contraceptive use, 2016, MMWR Recomm Rep 65:1–66, 2016.

95. **Rogers MD, Kolettis PN,** Vasectomy, Urol Clin North Am 40:559–568, 2013.

96. **Giovannucci E, Tosteson TD, Speizer FE, Vessey MP, Colditz GA,** A long-term study of mortality in men who have undergone vasectomy, N Engl J Med 326:1392–1398, 1992.

97. **Guo ZL, Xu JL, Lai RK, Wang SS,** Vasectomy and cardiovascular disease risk: A systematic review and meta-analysis, Medicine 96:e7852, 2017.

98. **Manson JE, Ridker PM, Spelsberg A, Ajani U, Lotufo PA, Hennekens CH,** Vasectomy and subsequent cardiovascular disease in US physicians, Contraception 59:181–186, 1999.

99. **Peterson HB, Huber DH, Belker AM,** Vasectomy: an appraisal for the obstetrician-gynecologist, Obstet Gynecol 76:568–572, 1990.

100. **Bernal-Delgado E, Latour-Perez J, Pradas-Arnal F, Gomez-Lopez LI,** The association between vasectomy and prostate cancer: a systematic review of the literature, Fertil Steril 70:191–200, 1998.

101. **Bertero E, Hallak J, Gromatzky C, Lucon AM, Arap S,** Assessment of sexual function in patients undergoing vasectomy using the international index of erectile function, Int Braz J Urol 31:452–458, 2005.

102. **Krieger JN, Nirapathpongporn A, Chaiyaporn M, Peterson G, Nikolaeva I, Akridge R, et al.,** Vasectomy and human immunodeficiency virus type 1 in semen, J Urol 159:820–825; discussion 5–6, 1998.

103. **Kirby EW, Hockenberry M, Lipshultz LI,** Vasectomy reversal: decision making and technical innovations, Transl Androl Urol 6:753–760, 2017.

104. **Herrel LA, Goodman M, Goldstein M, Hsiao W,** Outcomes of microsurgical vasovasostomy for vasectomy reversal: a meta-analysis and systematic review, Urology 85:819–825, 2015.

105. **Belker AM, Thomas AJ Jr, Fuchs EF, Konnak JW, Sharlip ID,** Results of 1,469 microsurgical vasectomy reversals by the Vasovasostomy Study Group, J Urol 145:505–511, 1991.

106. **Glazier DB, Marmar JL, Mayer E, Gibbs M, Corson SL,** The fate of cryopreserved sperm acquired during vasectomy reversals, J Urol 161:463–466, 1999.

107. **Sokal D, Gates D, Amatya R, Dominik R,** Two randomized controlled trials comparing the tubal ring and Filshie clip for tubal sterilization, Fertil Steril 74:525–533, 2000.

108. **Jamieson DJ, Costello C, Trussell J, Hillis SD, Marchbanks PA, Peterson HB, et al.,** The risk of pregnancy after vasectomy, Obstet Gynecol 103:848–850, 2004.

109. **Gariepy AM, Creinin MD, Smith KJ, Xu X,** Probability of pregnancy after sterilization: a comparison of hysteroscopic versus laparoscopic sterilization, Contraception 90:174–181, 2014.

110. **American College of Obstetricians and Gynecologists,** ACOG Committee Opinion No. 458: Hysterosalpingography after tubal sterilization, Obstet Gynecol 115:1343–1345, 2010.

111. **Klotz KL, Coppola MA, Labrecque M, Brugh VM III, Ramsey K, Kim KA, et al.,** Clinical and consumer trial performance of a sensitive immunodiagnostic home test that qualitatively detects low concentrations of sperm following vasectomy, J Urol 180:2569–2576, 2008.

112. **Peterson HB, Xia Z, Hughes JM, Wilcox LS, Tylor LR, Trussell J,** The risk of ectopic pregnancy after tubal sterilization. U.S. Collaborative Review of Sterilization Working Group, N Engl J Med 336:762–767, 1997.

113. **Brandi K, Morgan JR, Paasche-Orlow MK, Perkins RB, White KO,** Obstetric outcomes after failed hysteroscopic and laparoscopic sterilization procedures, Obstet Gynecol 131:253–261, 2018.

114. **National Cancer Institute Surveillance, Epidemiology, and End Results**

Program, Cancer Stat Facts: Ovarian Cancer. Available from: https://seer.cancer.gov/statfacts/html/ovary.html

115. **Siegel RL, Miller KD, Jemal A,** Cancer statistics, 2018, CA Cancer J Clin 68:7–30, 2018.

116. **Dubeau L,** The cell of origin of ovarian epithelial tumours, Lancet Oncol 9:1191–1197, 2008.

117. **Salvador S, Gilks B, Kobel M, Huntsman D, Rosen B, Miller D,** The fallopian tube: primary site of most pelvic high-grade serous carcinomas, Int J Gynecol Cancer. 19:58–64, 2009.

118. **Walker JL, Powell CB, Chen LM, Carter J, Bae Jump VL, Parker LP, et al.,** Society of Gynecologic Oncology recommendations for the prevention of ovarian cancer, Cancer 121:2108–2120, 2015.

119. **Irwin KL, Weiss NS, Lee NC, Peterson HB,** Tubal sterilization, hysterectomy, and the subsequent occurrence of epithelial ovarian cancer, Am J Epidemiol 134:362–369, 1991.

120. **Whittemore AS, Harris R, Itnyre J,** Characteristics relating to ovarian cancer risk: collaborative analysis of 12 US case–control studies. II. Invasive epithelial ovarian cancers in white women. Collaborative Ovarian Cancer Group, Am J Epidemiol 136:1184–1203, 1992.

121. **Hankinson SE, Hunter DJ, Colditz GA, Willett WC, Stampfer MJ, Rosner B, et al.,** Tubal ligation, hysterectomy, and risk of ovarian cancer. A prospective study, JAMA 270:2813–2818, 1993.

122. **Falconer H, Yin L, Gronberg H, Altman D,** Ovarian cancer risk after salpingectomy: a nationwide population-based study, J Natl Cancer Inst 107, 2015.

123. **Miracle-McMahill HL, Calle EE, Kosinski AS, Rodriguez C, Wingo PA, Thun MJ, et al.,** Tubal ligation and fatal ovarian cancer in a large prospective cohort study, Am J Epidemiol 145: 349–357, 1997.

124. **Cibula D, Widschwendter M, Majek O, Dusek L,** Tubal ligation and the risk of ovarian cancer: review and meta-analysis, Hum Reprod Update 17:55–67, 2011.

125. **Cibula D, Widschwendter M, Zikan M, Dusek L,** Underlying mechanisms of ovarian cancer risk reduction after tubal ligation, Acta Obstet Gynecol Scand 90:559–563, 2011.

126. **Rabban JT, Garg K, Crawford B, Chen LM, Zaloudek CJ,** Early detection of high-grade tubal serous carcinoma in women at low risk for hereditary breast and ovarian cancer syndrome by systematic examination of fallopian tubes incidentally removed during benign surgery, Am J Surg Pathol 38:729–742, 2014.

127. **Backes FJ,** Salpingectomy, why not?, Am J Obstet Gynecol 210:385–386, 2014.

128. **Piazza A, Schwirian K, Scott F, Wilson MD, Zite NB, Creinin MD.** Women's preferences for permanent contraception method and willingness to be randomized for a hypothetical trial. Contraception 99:56–60, 2019.

129. **Chene G, Rahimi K, Mes-Masson AM, Provencher D,** Surgical implications of the potential new tubal pathway for ovarian carcinogenesis, J Minim Invasive Gynecol 20:153–159, 2013.

130. **Oskowitz S, Haverkamp AD, Freedman WL,** Experience in a series of fimbriectomies, Fertil Steril 34:320–323, 1980.

131. **Findley AD, Siedhoff MT, Hobbs KA, Steege JF, Carey ET, McCall CA, et al.,** Short-term effects of salpingectomy during laparoscopic hysterectomy on ovarian reserve: a pilot randomized controlled trial, Fertil Steril 100:1704–1708, 2013.

132. **Almog B, Wagman I, Bibi G, Raz Y, Azem F, Groutz A, et al.,** Effects of salpingectomy on ovarian response in controlled ovarian hyperstimulation for in vitro fertilization: a reappraisal, Fertil Steril 95:2474–2476, 2011.

133. **Venturella R, Lico D, Borelli M, Imbrogno MG, Cevenini G, Zupi E, et al.,** 3 to 5 years later: long-term effects of prophylactic bilateral salpingectomy on ovarian function, J Minim Invasive Gynecol 24:145–150, 2017.

134. **Mohamed AA, Yosef AH, James C, Al-Hussaini TK, Bedaiwy MA, Amer S,** Ovarian reserve after salpingectomy: a systematic review and meta-analysis, Acta Obstet Gynecol Scand 96:795–803, 2017.

135. **Gill SE, Mills BB,** Physician opinions regarding elective bilateral salpingectomy with hysterectomy and for sterilization, J Minim Invasive Gynecol 20:517–521, 2013.

129

136. **Jones NL, Schulkin J, Urban RR, Wright JD, Burke WM, Hou JY, et al.,** Physicians' perspectives and practice patterns toward opportunistic salpingectomy in high- and low-risk women, Cancer Invest 35:51–61, 2017.

137. **American College of Obstetricians and Gynecologists,** Committee Opinion No 695 summary: sterilization of women: ethical issues and considerations, Obstet Gynecol 129:775–776, 2017.

138. **Krashin JW, Edelman AB, Nichols MD, Allen AJ, Caughey AB, Rodriguez MI,** Prohibiting consent: what are the costs of denying permanent contraception concurrent with abortion care?, Am J Obstet Gynecol 211:76.e1–76.e10, 2014.

139. **Costello C, Hillis SD, Marchbanks PA, Jamieson DJ, Peterson HB; Group USCRoSW,** The effect of interval tubal sterilization on sexual interest and pleasure, Obstet Gynecol 100:511–517, 2002.

140. **Smith A, Lyons A, Ferris J, Richters J, Pitts M, Shelley J,** Are sexual problems more common in women who have had a tubal ligation? A population-based study of Australian women, BJOG 117:463–468, 2010.

141. **Peterson HB, Jeng G, Folger SG, Hillis SA, Marchbanks PA, Wilcox LS, et al.,** The risk of menstrual abnormalities after tubal sterilization. U.S. Collaborative Review of Sterilization Working Group, N Engl J Med 343:1681–1687, 2000.

142. **Hillis SD, Marchbanks PA, Tylor LR, Peterson HB,** Tubal sterilization and long-term risk of hysterectomy: findings from the United States collaborative review of sterilization. The U.S. Collaborative Review of Sterilization Working Group, Obstet Gynecol 89:609–614, 1997.

143. **Gentile GP, Helbig DW, Zacur H, Park T, Lee YJ, Westhoff CL,** Hormone levels before and after tubal sterilization, Contraception 73:507–511, 2006.

144. **Fagundes ML, Mendes MC, Patta MC, Rodrigues R, Berezowski AT, de Moura MD, et al.,** Hormonal assessment of women submitted to tubal ligation, Contraception 71:309–314, 2005.

145. **Hillis SD, Marchbanks PA, Tylor LR, Peterson HB,** Poststerilization regret: findings from the United States Collaborative Review of Sterilization, Obstet Gynecol 93:889–895, 1999.

146. **Schmidt JE, Hillis SD, Marchbanks PA, Jeng G, Peterson HB,** Requesting information about and obtaining reversal after tubal sterilization: findings from the U.S. Collaborative Review of Sterilization, Fertil Steril 74:892–898, 2000.

147. **Jamieson DJ, Kaufman SC, Costello C, Hillis SD, Marchbanks PA, Peterson HB, et al.,** A comparison of women's regret after vasectomy versus tubal sterilization, Obstet Gynecol 99:1073–1079, 2002.

148. **Curtis KM, Mohllajee AP, Peterson HB,** Regret following female sterilization at a young age: a systematic review, Contraception 73:205–210, 2006.

149. **Borrero SB, Reeves MF, Schwarz EB, Bost JE, Creinin MD, Ibrahim SA,** Race, insurance status, and desire for tubal sterilization reversal, Fertil Steril 90:272–277, 2008.

150. **Yossry M, Aboulghar M, D'Angelo A, Gillett W,** In vitro fertilisation versus tubal reanastomosis (sterilisation reversal) for subfertility after tubal sterilisation, Cochrane Database Syst Rev (3):CD004144, 2006.

151. **Deffieux X, Morin Surroca M, Faivre E, Pages F, Fernandez H, Gervaise A,** Tubal anastomosis after tubal sterilization: a review, Arch Gynecol Obstet 283:1149–1158, 2011.

152. **Practice Committee of the American Society for Reproductive Medicine,** Committee opinion: role of tubal surgery in the era of assisted reproductive technology, Fertil Steril 97:539–545, 2012.

153. **Malacova E, Kemp-Casey A, Bremner A, Hart R, Stewart LM, Preen DB,** Live delivery outcome after tubal sterilization reversal: a population-based study, Fertil Steril 104:921–926, 2015.

154. **Malacova E, Kemp A, Hart R, Jama-Alol K, Preen DB,** Effectiveness of in vitro fertilization in women with previous tubal sterilization, Contraception 91:240–244, 2015.

155. **Borrero S, Zite N, Creinin MD,** Federally funded sterilization: time to rethink policy?, Am J Public Health 102:1822–1825, 2012.

156. **Borrero S, Zite N, Potter JE, Trussell J,** Medicaid policy on sterilization—anachronistic or still relevant?, N Engl J Med 370:102–104, 2014.

157. **Brown BP, Chor J,** Adding injury to injury: ethical implications of the Medicaid sterilization consent regulations, Obstet Gynecol 123:1348–1351, 2014.

158. **Roth R, Ainsworth SL,** "If they hand you a paper, you sign it": a call to end the sterilization of women in prison, Hastings Women's LJ 26:7–50, 2015.

159. **Stulberg DB, Dude, AM, Dahlquist I, Curlin FA,** Obstetrician-gynecologists, religious institutions, and conflicts regarding patient-care policies, Am J Obstet Gynecol 207:73.e1–73.e5, 2012.

160. **Guiahi M, Sheeder J, Teal S,** Are women aware of religious restrictions on reproductive health at Catholic hospitals? A survey of women's expectations and preferences for family planning care, Contraception 90:429–434, 2014.

161. **Moniz MH, Chang T, Heisler M, Admon L, Gebremariam A, Dalton VK, et al.** Inpatient postpartum long-acting reversible contraception and sterilization in the United States, 2008–2013, Obstet Gynecol 129:1078–1085, 2017.

162. **Goodman EJ, Dumas SD,** The rate of successful reactivation of labor epidural catheters for postpartum tubal ligation surgery, Reg Anesth Pain Med 23:258–261, 1998.

163. **Lehn K, Gu L, Creinin MD, Chen MJ,** Successful completion of total and partial salpingectomy at the time of cesarean delivery, Contraception 98:232–236, 2018.

164. **Subramaniam A, Blanchard CT, Erickson BK, Szychowski J, Leath CA, Biggio JR, et al.,** Feasibility of complete salpingectomy compared with standard postpartum tubal ligation at cesarean delivery: a randomized controlled trial, Obstet Gynecol 132:20–27, 2018.

165. **Garcia C, Moskowitz OM, Chisholm CA, Duska LR, Warren AL, Lyons GR, et al.,** Salpingectomy compared with tubal ligation at cesarean delivery: a randomized controlled trial, Obstet Gynecol 132:29–34, 2018.

166. **Shinar S, Blecher Y, Alpern S, Many A, Ashwal E, Amikam U, et al.,** Total bilateral salpingectomy versus partial bilateral salpingectomy for permanent sterilization during cesarean delivery, Arch Gynecol Obstet 295:1185–1189, 2017.

167. **Duncan JR, Schenone MH, Mari G,** Technique for bilateral salpingectomy at the time of cesarean delivery: a case series, Contraception 95:509–511, 2017.

168. **Ganer Herman H, Gluck O, Keidar R, Kerner R, Kovo M, Levran D, et al.,** Ovarian reserve following cesarean section with salpingectomy vs tubal ligation: a randomized trial, Am J Obstet Gynecol 217:472.e1–472.e6, 2017.

169. **Danis RB, Della Badia CR, Richard SD,** Postpartum permanent sterilization: could bilateral salpingectomy replace bilateral tubal ligation?, J Minim Invasive Gynecol 23:928–932, 2016.

170. **American College of Obstetricians and Gynecologists,** Committee opinion no. 530: access to postpartum sterilization, Obstet Gynecol 120:212–215, 2012.

171. **Zite N, Wuellner S, Gilliam M,** Barriers to obtaining a desired postpartum tubal sterilization, Contraception 73:404–407, 2006.

172. **Thurman AR, Harvey D, Shain RN,** Unfulfilled postpartum sterilization requests, J Reprod Med 54:467–472, 2009.

173. **Boardman LA, DeSimone M, Allen RH,** Barriers to completion of desired postpartum sterilization, R I Med J 96:32–34, 2013.

174. **Wolfe KK, Wilson MD, Hou MY, Creinin MD,** An updated assessment of postpartum sterilization fulfillment after vaginal delivery, Contraception 96:41–46, 2017.

175. **Thurman AR, Janecek T,** One-year follow-up of women with unfulfilled postpartum sterilization requests, Obstet Gynecol 116:1071–1077, 2010.

176. **Hernandez IM, Perry G, Katz AR, Held B,** Postabortal laparoscopic tubal sterilization. Results in comparison to interval procedures, Obstet Gynecol 50:356–358, 1977.

177. **Cheng MC, Rochat RW,** The safety of combined abortion-sterilization procedure, Am J Obstet Gynecol 129:548–552, 1977.

131

178. **Cheng MC, Chew SC, Cheong J, Choo HT, Ratnam SS, Belsey MA, et al.,** Safety of postabortion sterilisation compared with interval sterilisation. A controlled study, Lancet 2:682–685, 1979.

179. **Akhter HH, Flock ML, Rubin GL,** Safety of abortion and tubal sterilization performed separately versus concurrently, Am J Obstet Gynecol 152: 619–623, 1985.

180. **Heisterberg L, Jessen P, Schroeder E, Wøhlk P, Pedersen LM,** Comparison of interval and postabortal/puerperal laparoscopic sterilization with the tubal ring procedure, Acta Obstet Gynecol Scand 64:223–225, 1985.

181. **Kaali SG, Szigetvari I, Bartfai G, Feinman M,** Laparoscopic sterilization combined with dilation and evacuation up to 18 weeks' gestation, J Reprod Med 34:463–464, 1989.

182. **Lalonde D,** Regret, shame, and denials of women's voluntary sterilization, Bioethics 32:281–288, 2018.

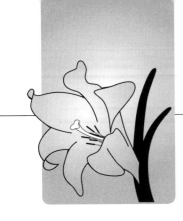

5

Implantable Contraception

Rebecca Cohen, MD, MPH
and Stephanie B. Teal, MD, MPH

The relatively high pregnancy rates with typical use of reversible contraceptive methods indicate the need for long-acting methods that are easier to use, with less dependence on frequent, perfect actions by the user. Implantable, subdermal capsules that release progestins for several years are a response to this need.

Historically, the first widely used contraceptive subdermal implant system was the Norplant levonorgestrel system, consisting of six Silastic (silicone elastomer) tubes containing crystalline levonorgestrel. Although manufacturing of Norplant ceased in 2008, providers may still encounter women using this method. Jadelle is a two-rod levonorgestrel system, which utilizes Silastic rods slightly longer and thicker than those of the six-rod Norplant system. In many parts of the world, Jadelle replaced the use of Norplant. A Chinese version of Jadelle, called Sinoplant II/Levoplant, also consists of levonorgestrel 150 mg contained in two rods. Jadelle is approved by the U.S. Food and Drug Administration but has not been marketed in the United States.

The other widely available implant system is Nexplanon/Implanon NXT, a single-rod implant containing a different gonane progestin, etonogestrel (3-ketodesogestrel) (**Figure 5.1**).[1,2] The implant was originally marketed as Implanon and then Nexplanon/Implanon NXT following changes in the inserter and addition of barium sulfate to make the implant radiopaque (**Figure 5.2**). Like Norplant, Nexplanon has been extensively marketed throughout the world with excellent safety and efficacy and high continuation rates. Contraceptive implants are approved in more than 60 countries and are used by millions of women worldwide. However, use of other methods (permanent contraception, intrauterine device [IUD], or oral contraception) is far more prevalent than implant use in most countries.[3]

The long-acting implantable progestin methods prevent pregnancy at rates similar to permanent contraception and IUDs and more effectively than oral and barrier contraception.[4] An important reason for this high efficacy in actual use is the nature of the delivery systems themselves, which require little effort on the part of the user. Because compliance does not require frequent resupply or instruction in use, as with oral, injectable, or barrier contraception, the actual or typical use effectiveness is very close to the theoretical (highest expected) effectiveness. In developing countries, the single act to

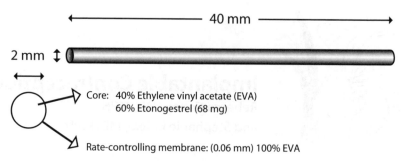

←———————— 40 mm ————————→

2 mm ↕

Core: 40% Ethylene vinyl acetate (EVA)
60% Etonogestrel (68 mg)

Rate-controlling membrane: (0.06 mm) 100% EVA

Figure 5.1 Etonogestrel Single-Rod Implant.

provide years of contraception also eliminates supply chain issues related to ensuring repeated availability of shorter-acting contraceptives.

Sustained-release methods require less of the user but demand more of the clinician. The implant is relatively new compared to other methods, and women may be hesitant to consider its use. Implants involve minor procedures for placement and removal. Clinicians have a special responsibility to become skillful in the operations required to place and remove implants and to be available to women when those skills are required to discontinue use. Disturbances of menstrual patterns and other side effects may require more counseling and follow-up than other contraceptive methods.[5,6]

Implant Systems

Levonorgestrel

Norplant was developed by the Population Council and first approved in 1983 in Finland, where it was manufactured. It was approved in the United

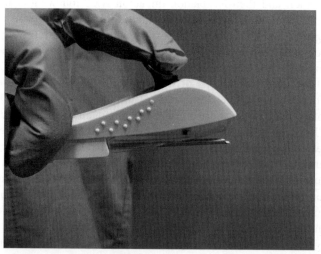

Figure 5.2 Nexplanon inserter.

States in 1990, marketed in 1991, and withdrawn from the U.S. market in a 2002 business decision dictated by profit and liability despite the fact that it provided an excellent option for contraception. In 2008, manufacturing of Norplant ceased.

Jadelle was also developed by the Population Council and manufactured in Finland. It was approved in the United States in 1996, but never marketed. The thin, flexible Jadelle rods are wrapped in Silastic tubing, 43 mm in length and 2.5 mm in diameter.[7] Each rod contains 75 mg levonorgestrel for a total of 150 mg. Whereas Norplant contained crystalline levonorgestrel inside a silicone capsule, the core of the Jadelle rod is a mixture of levonorgestrel and an elastic polymer (dimethylsiloxane/methylvinylsiloxane). The initial levonorgestrel release rate is 100 µg daily, which decreases to 40 µg daily at 1 year and 30 µg daily at 2 years, rates similar to Norplant.[7] Long-term clinical trials indicate that the performance and side effects are similar to Norplant, but insertion and removal are faster.[8,9] Because the release rates with the two levonorgestrel systems are comparable, it is reasonable to conclude that the results from clinical studies with Norplant and Jadelle should be considered interchangeable.

Etonogestrel

Implanon is a single flexible rod, 4 cm long and 2 mm in diameter, that contains 3-ketodesogestrel (etonogestrel, the active metabolite of desogestrel) 68 mg dispersed in a core of ethylene vinyl acetate wrapped with a 0.6-mm-thick membrane of the same material. It was introduced in 1998 and approved in the United States in 2006. Nexplanon/Implanon NXT (approved in the United States in 2011) is bioequivalent to Implanon.[10] There is no evidence that either ethylene vinyl acetate or Silastic has toxic effects when implanted.[11] The hormone is released at an initial rate of about 67 µg/d decreasing to 30 µg after 2 years; concentrations that inhibit ovulation are achieved within 8 hours of insertion.[12] A steady state is achieved after 4 months, after which there is a gradual decline.[12] Side effects are similar to those of the levonorgestrel implants, except for less bleeding and a higher rate of amenorrhea with the etonogestrel implant.[13,14]

In the United States, the etonogestrel implant is FDA approved for up to 3 years of use as a contraceptive method.[15] The etonogestrel implant suppresses ovulation for at least 2.5 years and provides effective contraception for much longer. Among more than 300 women using etonogestrel implants for at least 5 years in research settings, there were no additional pregnancies in the 4th or 5th year of use.[16–18] Women and providers can be reassured that an "expired" implant (used beyond 3 years' duration) can provide effective contraception for several additional months. For women who desire contraception for more than 3 years, extended use of the implant could improve safety (fewer removals/insertions), decrease annual cost of use, and lessen burden on health care systems.[18]

Indications

Contraceptive implants are a good choice for reproductive age women who desire highly effective user-independent reversible contraception. Women who cannot use estrogen (due to medical comorbidities or unacceptable side effects) and those who have difficulty with correct consistent use of user-dependent methods may find the contraceptive implant particularly suitable. Overall, there are few contraindications to implant use.[19] Absolute contraindications include known or suspected pregnancy, undiagnosed genital bleeding suspicious for malignancy, severe decompensated liver disease,[20] benign or malignant liver tumors (except focal nodular hyperplasia), and known or suspected breast cancer.

Mechanism of Action

Hormone release rates from contraceptive implants are determined by total surface area and the progestin density of the polymer. The progestin diffuses from the implant into the surrounding tissues where it is absorbed by the circulatory system and distributed systemically. Within 8 hours after etonogestrel implant insertion, etonogestrel plasma concentrations are about 300 ng/mL, high enough to prevent ovulation.[21] About 90% of women will demonstrate

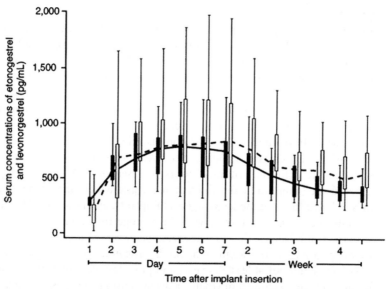

Figure 5.3   Variation in serum levels seen with use of contraceptive implants. Serum concentrations of etonogestrel (*solid line*) and levonorgestrel (*dashes*) during the first 4 weeks after implant insertion. Boxes represent the P25–P75 range; T bars represent the minimum and maximum concentrations. Median values are connected. (From **Makarainen L, van Beek A, Tuomivaara L, Asplund B, Coelingh Bennink H,** Ovarian function during the use of a single contraceptive implant: Implanon compared with Norplant, Fertil Steril 69(4):714–721, 1998. Copyright © 1998 Elsevier. With permission.)

136

unfavorable cervical mucus preventing sperm penetration within 3 days when the levonorgestrel implant is inserted just prior to ovulation (during days 8 to 13 of the menstrual cycle)[22]; however, this is not a reliable marker of in vivo contraceptive effect.[23] There are no in-depth studies of timing of cervical mucus changes after etonogestrel implant insertion.[23] Throughout the duration of implant use, serum levonorgestrel concentrations show much wider within-group variation than serum etonogestrel concentrations **(Figure 5.3)**.[21]

The etonogestrel implant releases 60 μg per 24 hours at 3 months of use. This rate declines gradually to 40 to 50 μg daily by 12 months and 30 μg/d by 2 years of use.[21] The two-rod levonorgestrel implant releases 100 μg daily during the first few months of use, about equivalent to the daily dose of levonorgestrel delivered by the progestin-only oral contraceptive and 25% to 50% of the dose delivered by low-dose combined oral contraceptives (see Figure 2.13 in Chapter 2). After 6 months of use, daily levonorgestrel concentrations are about 0.35 ng/mL; at 5 years, the levels decrease to 0.29 ng/mL.[24] Until the 8-year mark, mean levels remain above 0.25 ng/mL.[25]

Drug Interactions

We do not recommend the use of implants with any of the following drugs that induce microsomal liver enzymes (cytochrome P-450 pathway) because of a likely or hypothetical increased risk of pregnancy due to lower blood levels of the progestin.

> Carbamazepine (Tegretol)[26]
> Efavirenz[27-29]
> Felbamate
> Oxcarbazepine
> Phenobarbital[30]
> Phenytoin (Dilantin)[30]
> Primidone (Mysoline)
> Rifabutin
> Rifampicin (rifampin)[31]
> St. John's wort
> Topiramate
> *Possibly* griseofulvin and troglitazone as failures have been noted with combined estrogen-progesterone contraceptives

Nevirapine is not associated with increased rates of levonorgestrel implant failure.[28,32] Non–enzyme-inducing antiepileptic drugs such as lamotrigine, valproic acid, ethosuximide, and vigabatrin are not expected to decrease the efficacy of the implant.[33] Unlike estrogen-containing methods, the progestin-only implant does not affect lamotrigine levels.[34]

Body weight affects circulating levonorgestrel levels; the greater the weight of the user, the lower the levonorgestrel concentrations at any time during use. The greatest decrease over time occurs in women weighing more than 70 kg (154 lb), but even for heavy women, the release rate is high enough to prevent pregnancy, at least as reliably as oral contraceptives. In early clinical trials, etonogestrel implant failure rates did not increase with increasing body weight in the small numbers of overweight women studied.[35] A pharmacokinetic study showed etonogestrel levels between 31% and 54% lower in obese women compared to normal-weight women within the first 6 months of use, although all users had levels above the threshold of 90 pg/mL needed to prevent ovulation.[36] A 3-year study of over 1,000 etonogestrel implant users showed no difference in failures rates across BMI categories.[37] Levonorgestrel levels can also be affected by the circulating sex hormone–binding globulin (SHBG) levels. Levonorgestrel has a higher affinity for SHBG than etonogestrel.[21] In the week after levonorgestrel implant insertion, SHBG levels decline rapidly and then return to approximately half of preinsertion levels by 1 year of use. This effect on SHBG is not uniform and may account for some of the individual variations in circulating progestin concentrations.[21] Etonogestrel does not cause a decrease in SHBG levels.[38]

Implants are highly effective contraceptives with two modes of action. The progestin suppresses, at both the hypothalamus and the pituitary, the luteinizing hormone (LH) surge necessary for ovulation. As determined by progesterone levels in many users over several years, approximately one third of cycles in levonorgestrel implant users were ovulatory.[39,40] During the first 2 years of use, only about 10% of women are ovulatory, but by 5 years of use, more than 50% are. In those cycles that are ovulatory, there is a high incidence of luteal insufficiency. The etonogestrel implant inhibits ovulation throughout a 3-year period, accounting for almost all of the contraceptive effect.[41,42] However, follicular development does occur, avoiding the problem of clinically significant hypoestrogenemia, and in the last 6 months of the 3rd year with etonogestrel implant use, ovulation occurs occasionally.[21,41] Ovarian cysts, actually persistent follicles, are common and do not require treatment or surveillance if asymptomatic; these occur with low progesterone levels and do not indicate ovulation.[43] The second mechanism of contraceptive action is due to the prolonged effect on the cervical mucus from the steady release of progestin. The mucus thickens and decreases in amount, forming a barrier to sperm penetration.[41,44] The progestin suppresses the estradiol-induced cyclic maturation of the endometrium and eventually causes atrophy, which has been thought of historically as a method of action, preventing implantation should fertilization occur. However, since cervical mucus effects would be present coincident with endometrial atrophy, sperm would not penetrate the mucus at a time when the lining would be hospitable for implantation; thus, fertilization could not occur, making any endometrial change unnecessary for a contraceptive effect. The suppression of ovulation and thickening of cervical mucus appear to be the strongly predominant contraceptive mechanisms.[41]

Advantages

Implants provide a safe, highly effective, continuous method of contraception that requires little user effort. Because this is a progestin-only method, it can be used by women who have contraindications for the use of estrogen-containing contraceptives. The sustained release of low doses of progestin avoids the high initial dose delivered by injectables and the daily hormone surge associated with oral contraceptives. Another advantage of the implant method is that it allows women to plan their pregnancies precisely; return of fertility occurs rapidly; etonogestrel serum levels are undetectable within 1 week after removal of the implant, and ovulation can be expected in the 1st month after discontinuation.[12,21]

One of the major advantages of sustained-release methods is the high degree of efficacy, nearly equivalent to the theoretical limit of effectiveness. In couples for whom elective abortion is unacceptable in the event of an unplanned pregnancy or for women who are at high risk of medical complications with pregnancy, the high efficacy rate is especially important. There are no forgotten pills, broken condoms, lost diaphragms, expelled rings or IUDs, or missed injections.

Exposure of endometriosis to systemic progestin-only contraceptive methods is an effective method to manage the pain associated with this condition. Nexplanon, along with other progestin-containing methods, can improve symptoms of endometriosis.[45–47] Nexplanon may have an advantage over levonorgestrel intrauterine systems for women who benefit from ovulation suppression, such as those with severe premenstrual dysphoric syndrome, menstrual migraines, or catamenial seizures.

Disadvantages

Implants cause disruption of bleeding patterns (see Menstrual Effects section), especially during the first year of use, and some women or their partners find these changes unacceptable.[48] Cultural factors can influence the acceptability of menstrual changes. Some cultures restrict a woman from participating in religious activity, household activities, or sexual intercourse while menstruating. All users must be aware of the possible menstrual changes. It is important to stress that menstrual changes are expected, that they do not cause or represent illness, and that many women revert back to a more normal pattern with increasing duration of use.

Women cannot initiate or discontinue implants without the assistance of a trained clinician. Women also need to understand that implants may be noticed under the skin of the upper arm when elevated and externally rotated or when the area is touched. This sign of the use of contraception may be unacceptable for some women and for some partners.[6,49] However, we strongly recommend against deep placement to hide contraceptive use, due to the potential for neurovascular injury, migration away from the insertion site, or difficulty removing a deeply placed implant.

Like other hormonal methods, implants do not provide protection against sexually transmitted infections (STIs) such as herpes, human papillomavirus, HIV, gonorrhea, or chlamydia. Implant users may be less likely to use condoms because they do not see a need for additional contraceptive protection due to the high efficacy of the implants[50–53]; those at risk for STI acquisition should be reminded to use condoms to prevent infection.

Because the insertion and removal of implants require minor procedures, initiation and discontinuation costs are higher than with oral contraceptives or barrier methods. The cost of implants plus fees for insertion may seem high to patients unless they compare it with the total cost of using other methods for up to 5 years.[54,55] Many women do not use long-acting methods for their full duration of action, for reasons ranging from personal preference to desire for pregnancy and to dissatisfaction with side effects. Short-term implant use is expensive compared with the relatively low initial costs of other reversible methods; however, the etonogestrel implant is cost-effective at nearly all time points when the cost of unintended pregnancy is considered.[56,57] Clinicians should offer the full range of contraceptive options for women and support policies that remove the cost barrier to long-acting reversible contraceptive (LARC) methods.

Insertion and removal of implants will be a new experience for most women. As with any new experience, women may approach it with varying degrees of apprehension. We encourage prospective users to see and touch models of implants. Women should be told that an implant is not inserted with an incision, just a very small needle entry site that heals quickly, leaving small scars that are usually difficult to see because of their location and size. Women can be reassured that the implant will not be damaged or move if the skin above the implant is accidentally injured. Normal activity will not damage or displace the implants. Most women become unaware of their presence. A few women report sensing the implants if they have been touched or manipulated for a prolonged period of time or after vigorous exercise. The implants are more visible in slender women with good muscle tone. Darker-skinned users may notice further darkening of the skin directly over the implants; this resolves after removal. Implants may rarely break after excessive manipulation. This does not change efficacy and does not necessitate removal.

Efficacy

Contraceptive implants provide highly effective birth control. In 2- and 3-year studies in 11 international clinical trials of 942 women using the etonogestrel implant, no pregnancies occurred.[35] In studies of Norplant conducted in 11 countries, totaling 12,133 woman-years of use, the pregnancy rate was 0.2 pregnancies per 100 woman-years of use.[58] If luteal phase insertions are excluded from analysis, the first-year pregnancy rate drops to 0.01 per 100 woman-years. In adolescents, implants provide better protection against unwanted pregnancy than do oral contraceptives.[59–61]

There are no weight restrictions for levonorgestrel implant users, but heavier women (more than 70 kg) may experience slightly higher pregnancy rates in the later years of use compared with lighter women. The differences in pregnancy rates by weight are probably due to the dilutional effect of larger body size on the low, sustained serum levels of levonorgestrel. Heavier women should not rely on Jadelle beyond the 5-year limit. For slender women, the duration of efficacy extends well past the 5th year of use. In an extended-use trial, rare pregnancies were reported into the 7th year.[62]

The contraceptive efficacy of the etonogestrel implant surpasses that of Norplant, Jadelle, and permanent contraception using occlusive or partial salpingectomy procedures.[2] Pregnancy rarely occurs, resulting in a Pearl Index of less than 0.01.[42,63] In over 70,000 cycles, no pregnancies were recorded because of total inhibition of ovulation until the last 6 months of the 3-year period.[41,64] Postmarketing surveillance of pregnancies in Australia, where nearly one quarter of contraceptors relied on Implanon in 2004, revealed that of 218 pregnancies, only 13 could *possibly* have been failures of the method.[65] Instead, pregnancies had occurred before insertion or resulted from failure to correctly insert the implant. While pregnancy in implant users is rare, it should be considered if there are concerns for an early (undetected) pregnancy at the time of implant insertion, if there is suspicion for improper insertion or noninsertion of the implant (i.e., if implant is not palpable immediately after insertion), or if the patient is taking a medication that can reduce the effectiveness of the implant. A sensitive urine pregnancy test should be obtained in these settings or if a woman reports symptoms consistent with pregnancy. Women who remain amenorrheic throughout their use of implants are unlikely to become pregnant.[66]

Ectopic Pregnancy

Due to the fact that overall pregnancy rates among contraceptive implant users are so low, ectopic pregnancies are extremely rare. Studies of levonorgestrel two-rod systems have found ectopic pregnancy rates of 0.2 to 0.8 per 1,000 women-years. Ectopic pregnancies represent around 20% of all pregnancies reported.[67] There are fewer studies including etonogestrel implant users; because pregnancies are exceedingly rare, there are no stable estimates of the risk of ectopic pregnancy should pregnancy occur. Should a pregnancy occur in a woman using the etonogestrel implant, we recommend ruling out ectopic pregnancy.[65,67]

Menstrual Bleeding Effects

Menstrual bleeding patterns are highly variable among users of implant contraception. The simple and concise caveats are that all progestin implants cause unpredictable/irregular bleeding. With levonorgestrel implants, the bleeding generally becomes more regular over time for many women. With the etonogestrel implant, bleeding usually remains irregular over the course of use but tends to be light and tolerable. Women using the etonogestrel implant who initially experience amenorrhea or infrequent bleeding are very likely to maintain a good pattern over the ensuing year.

Among levonorgestrel implant users, the changes include alterations in the interval between bleeding, the duration and volume of menstrual flow, and spotting. About 10% of users experienced amenorrhea for at least 90 consecutive days in the first year of use, and about 20% reported normal menstrual bleeding patterns. Users reported a mean of 20 days of bleeding or spotting per 90 days of use in the first year.[68] After 2 years, ovulation occurs in about half of the menstrual cycles among levonorgestrel implant users,[21] so bleeding may become more regular. Although bleeding problems occur much less frequently after the 2nd year, they can occur at any time.[66,69]

141

With continued use, the endometrium of implant users becomes atrophic with enlarged fragile venous sinusoids.[70] In a study of 60 levonorgestrel and etonogestrel implant users, none showed hyperplastic or metaplastic changes.[71] Within weeks after insertion, the density of endometrial small blood vessels increases, and the endometrium regresses to an atrophic state.[72] Abnormal bleeding may result from decreased endometrial perfusion causing proliferation of less-stable, highly permeable endometrial vessels.[73]

The etonogestrel implant alters bleeding patterns in an unpredictable manner. In a large clinical study that assessed bleeding across several 90-day "reference periods," women experienced a median 13 to 16 days of bleeding or spotting per reference period, with no consistent improvement or worsening over time. Women who experienced favorable bleeding patterns early in use (0 to 28 bleeding or spotting days in the reference period beginning 1 month after implant initiation) were likely to continue with a favorable bleeding pattern. Women with unfavorable bleeding patterns had approximately a 50% chance of attaining a favorable bleeding pattern if they did not discontinue use.[5] A single etonogestrel implant suppresses ovulation reliably for most women for 2.5 years, and, therefore, menses do not become more regular over time. Bleeding is lighter and less frequent among etonogestrel implant users than among levonorgestrel implant users because more profound ovarian suppression results in less follicular estrogen production and less endometrial stimulation; nevertheless, irregular bleeding continues to be a major reason for discontinuation.[5,74]

Despite an increase in the number of spotting and bleeding days over preinsertion menstrual patterns, hemoglobin concentrations do not decrease in etonogestrel or levonorgestrel implant users because of a decrease in the average amount of menstrual blood loss.[75-77]

If a woman presents with concerns of heavy or otherwise concerning bleeding, we recommend ruling out other potential causes of bleeding such as pregnancy, infection, fibroid/polyp, and anticoagulation. Those at risk of STIs (e.g., in a new relationship and not using a barrier method) should be appropriately evaluated. Women due for cervical cytology screening should receive this testing as part of the evaluation of unscheduled bleeding.[78]

Implant users who can no longer tolerate bothersome bleeding may benefit from a short course of estrogen to stabilize the endometrium, although bleeding typically returns quickly after pills are stopped.[79,80] The irregular bleeding patterns noted in implant users confound investigation of effective therapies for bleeding, as many women who received placebo rather than estrogen-progestin oral contraceptives in a randomized controlled trial also experienced improvement of bothersome bleeding within 1 month.[80] For women without contraindications to estrogen, we recommend use of a combined oral contraceptive pill for short-term treatment (10 to 20 days).[81] No specific formulation has been shown to be superior, but we recommend starting with a pill that contains ethinyl estradiol 30 or 35 µg. If women desire longer-term bleeding control, combined oral contraceptives can be used along with the implant continuously (with typically fewer overall bleeding days but less predictability) or with a placebo week to allow for more predictable withdrawal bleeding. In a prospective cohort study of 20 women using the etonogestrel implant as backup to combined oral contraceptives, most participants reported infrequent or irregular bleeding.[82] By 6 months after initiation, two women requested implant removal (not for bleeding complaints) and seven women had discontinued use of oral contraceptives; of participants continuing concurrent use of both methods, most reported unchanged or improved bleeding patterns.[82] Nonsteroidal anti-inflammatory drugs can improve bleeding by inhibiting cyclooxygenase.[83] Mefenamic acid 500 mg orally three times daily for 5 to 7 days decreased subsequent bleeding over the next 28 days in etonogestrel implant users (10.5 bleeding days vs. 16.8 bleeding days in women who received placebo).[84] In levonorgestrel implant users, celecoxib 200 mg orally daily led to both faster cessation of a bleeding episode (70% stopped bleeding within 7 days vs. 0% in the placebo group) and a longer bleeding-free interval after cessation (24 vs. 10 days).[85] As both of these medications require a prescription for use, providers can also consider use of over-the-counter alternatives ibuprofen (800 mg three times daily for 5 days) or naproxen (500 mg twice daily for 5 days).[83] Tamoxifen[86] and tranexamic acid[83] (used separately) each show promise as a method of improving implant-related bleeding patterns in the short term. In the randomized trial of tamoxifen, women who received 10 mg twice daily for 7 days reported 5 fewer days of bleeding/spotting over 30 days (95% confidence interval [CI] −9.9 to −0.05), and 15.2 more continuous bleeding-free days (95% CI 2.8–27.5 days) after first use of study drug.[86] Results of using doxycycline (as a matrix metalloproteinase inhibitor) to improve bleeding have been mixed, and mifepristone can improve bleeding but is difficult to obtain and may compromise contraceptive efficacy.[83] A small study of ulipristal acetate versus placebo (used daily for 7 days) showed increased satisfaction and decreased bleeding in the 30 days following use (median 12 days of bleeding for placebo and 7 days for ulipristal acetate).[87]

Metabolic Effects

Exposure to the sustained, low doses of progestin delivered by the implants is not associated with significant metabolic changes. Studies of liver function,[88–90] blood coagulation,[91] immunoglobulin levels,[92,93] serum cortisol levels,[38,94,95] lipoprotein profile,[77,90,96–98] carbohydrate metabolism and insulin sensitivity,[90,97–99] inflammatory markers,[100] thyroid and adrenal function,[101] and blood chemistries[102,103] have failed to detect clinically significant changes outside of normal ranges in healthy levonorgestrel or etonogestrel implant users. Blood pressure does not change significantly with implant use.[98] Insulin-treated diabetics did not show worsening of carbohydrate metabolism, lipid metabolism, or microvascular lesions during 2 years of etonogestrel implant use.[104]

Implant contraception is a good choice for a woman at risk for estrogen-associated thromboembolism. In large studies, use of implants was not associated with increased risk of thrombosis.[105,106]

Measurements of bone density in young women reveal that neither the etonogestrel nor the levonorgestrel implant affects the teenage gain in bone; similar gains in bone were recorded in implant users and control subjects over 18 years of age.[107,108] The American Academy of Pediatrics notes that the impact of implant use on bone health in adolescents, while presumed to be limited, has not been adequately assessed.[109] In adult women, changes in bone mineral density after 1 year of use were small and did not differ from a control group of copper IUD users.[110] In a comparative study, two-rod levonorgestrel and etonogestrel implant users showed similar decreases in the forearm, but central bone density was not evaluated.[111,112] In older women, an increase in forearm, spine, and femur bone density has been documented after 6 and 12 months of levonorgestrel implant use.[113,114] An international cross-sectional study reported a small loss in bone density with levonorgestrel implant use that was rapidly regained after discontinuation.[115] No studies have assessed fracture risk with implant use.[116]

Effects on Future Fertility

Most women resume normal ovulatory cycles during the first month after implant removal.[21] The pregnancy rates during the first year after removal are comparable with those of women not using contraceptive methods and trying to become pregnant.[117] There are no long-term effects on future fertility, nor are there any effects on sex ratios, rates of ectopic pregnancy, spontaneous miscarriage, stillbirth, or congenital malformations.[117] The rate and outcome of subsequent pregnancies are not influenced by duration of use, apart from age-related declines in fertility.

For women who are spacing their pregnancies and considering nondaily systemic progestin methods, the difference between implants and depot-medroxyprogesterone acetate (DMPA) in the timing of the return to fertility can be critical. Implants allow more consistent timing of pregnancy because the return of ovulation after removal is prompt, in contrast to the 6- to 18-month delay in ovulation that can follow DMPA injections.[117-119]

Side Effects

The occurrence of serious side effects, such as those seen with estrogen-containing methods, is rare and not different in incidence than background rates observed in the general population.

In addition to menstrual changes, implant users have reported the following side effects: headache, acne, weight change, mastalgia, hyperpigmentation over the implants, hirsutism, depression, mood changes, anxiety, nervousness, ovarian cyst formation, and galactorrhea.[63,102,120] Side effect profiles do not differ appreciably between levonorgestrel and etonogestrel implants.[14,121]

It is difficult, of course, to be certain which of these effects were actually caused by the progestin. Although most of these side effects are minor in nature, they can cause patients to discontinue the method. Patients often find common side effects tolerable after assurance that they do not represent a health hazard.[6] Many complaints respond to reassurance; others can be treated with simple therapies. Headache is the most common nonmenstrual side effect experienced by users (16% of etonogestrel implant users), but only 1.6% of women who discontinued the etonogestrel implant cited headache as the reason for discontinuation.[63] Studies have not shown a significant relationship between implant use and depressive symptoms.[122] Implant use may benefit women with migraine headaches through suppression of ovulation and the avoidance of estrogen withdrawal symptoms.[123]

Weight Change

Women using implants more frequently complain of weight gain than of weight loss, but findings are variable.[98,124,125] Assessment of weight change in implant users is confounded by changes in exercise, diet, and aging, and it is unclear whether perceived weight change correlates with objective weight change. In a prospective study where women were assigned to initiate levonorgestrel implant use immediately upon enrollment (implant group) or after a 3-month delay (control group), median weight gain at 1 and 3 months did not differ although more women in the implant group perceived weight gain over time.[126] In another prospective study of contraceptive users (including implant users), perceived weight gain had a strong correlation with objective weight gain.[127] As part of a large prospective study in which neither group received diet or exercise counseling, 130 etonogestrel implant users and 100 copper IUD users recorded baseline weight and weight at 12 months of use.[125] Mean weight gain over 12 months was 2.1 kg (range −16.3 to 32.7) for etonogestrel implant users and 0.2 kg (range −16.3 to 16.3) for copper IUD users ($p = 0.01$). After adjusting for confounders, weight change over time was not significantly different between the two groups.[125] In the first year of use, changes in body fat percentage and lean body mass did not differ significantly between 33 etonogestrel implant and 31 copper IUD users who had maintained stable weight for 6 months prior to contraceptive initiation.[128]Although an increase in appetite can be attributed to the androgenic activity of progestins, it is unlikely that the low levels with implants have any clinical impact. Counseling for weight management focuses best on activity level and dietary changes, although no interventions have been studied in implant users.

Acne

Acne, with or without an increase in oil production, is the most common skin complaint among contraceptive implant users.[102] As many users are switching to the implant from estrogen-containing methods that can improve acne, it is difficult to separate the effects of implant initiation and cessation of exogenous estrogen. For levonorgestrel implant users, the acne is caused by the androgenic activity of the levonorgestrel that produces a direct impact and also causes a decrease in SHBG levels leading to an increase in free steroid levels (both levonorgestrel and testosterone).[129] Etonogestrel is less androgenic than levonorgestrel[120] and does not significantly decrease SHBG levels.[130] However, users of etonogestrel and levonorgestrel implants reported similar rates of acne.[121] Common therapies for complaints of acne include dietary change, practice of good skin hygiene with the use of soaps or skin cleansers, and application of topical antibiotics (e.g., 1% clindamycin solution or gel or topical erythromycin). Additionally, using combined oral contraceptive pills with the implant will not only help bleeding patterns and continuation rates but can improve acne.[131,132]

Ovarian Cysts

Unlike combined hormonal contraception, the low serum levels of progestin-only maintained by implants do not suppress follicle-stimulating hormone (FSH), which continues to stimulate ovarian follicle growth in most users. The LH peak during the first 2 years of use, on the other hand, is usually abolished so that these follicles do not ovulate.[133] Symptomatic ovarian cysts, while rare, were approximately four times more frequent in Norplant users compared with women using nonhormonal contraception.[134] In clinical trials, investigators also assessed prevalence of ovarian cysts among asymptomatic women using bimanual exam and ultrasound. At 12 months of use, 26.7% of etonogestrel implant users and 14.6% of levonorgestrel users had follicles $\geq$25 mm in diameter.[43] In asymptomatic women, because these are persistent follicles (and most regress spontaneously within 1 to 2 months of detection), they need not be sonographically or laparoscopically evaluated.[14,43] Further evaluation is indicated if they became large and painful or fail to regress.

Reasons for Discontinuation

Implant discontinuation occurs at a rate of 10% to 15% yearly, about the same as for intrauterine contraception, but lower than for barrier or oral contraception.[74] Menstrual changes are the most common reason; an unspoken concern for many patients and their partners is the fact that bleeding irregularity interferes with sexual interactions. Other cited reasons for discontinuation include desire for pregnancy as well as a range of side effects including headache, acne, mood change, and perceived weight gain.[6,74] While headaches are frequently experienced, headache is a rare reason for discontinuation compared to changes in bleeding.[63,120] Most women who discontinued use due to side effects reported that their symptoms resolved after discontinuation.[6]

Cancer

The risk of endometrial cancer is likely reduced. Studies of the endometrial effects of the levonorgestrel and etonogestrel implants failed to find any evidence of hyperplasia, even when progestin levels were low and endogenous estradiol production was normal.[71,135] Among women with normal cervical cytology at baseline, no abnormalities developed over 24 months in 60 users of levonorgestrel or etonogestrel implants.[71] Risk of precancerous cervical lesions did not differ between women using the copper IUD and women using progestogen-only contraceptives (Norplant, DMPA, or progestin-only pills).[136] The risk of ovarian cancer is also probably reduced, and we would expect a potentially greater effect with etonogestrel because it more effectively suppresses ovulation. Confounding variables limit the evaluation of breast cancer risk with implants. The low progestin dose of implants, however, would be unlikely to have effects different from other hormonal contraceptives. In a very large case-control study, neither DMPA nor implants were associated with an increase in the risk of breast cancer.[137] Current or past implant use was not associated with an increased risk of breast cancer in a recent database study from Denmark.[138]

Insertion and Removal

Prior to implant initiation, clinicians should obtain a detailed personal and family medical history and review the World Health Organization (international)[139] or Centers for Disease Control and Prevention (United States)[19] Medical Eligibility Criteria or other similar appropriate guidelines if medical comorbidities or significant family health concerns exist. If a patient elects to use a contraceptive implant, a detailed description of the method, including effectiveness, side effects (including a detailed discussion of expected bleeding), risks, benefits, as well as insertion and removal procedures, should be provided. Before insertion, the patient is asked to read and sign a written consent for the surgical placement of the implants. The consent reviews the potential complications of the procedure that include reaction to the local anesthetic, infection, expulsion of the implants, superficial phlebitis, bruising, and the possibility of a subsequent difficult removal. In addition, in the United States, the FDA requires the clinician to provide the patient information sheet that is part of the package insert and review and sign a consent indicating that she had a chance to read this information prior to insertion.

Patients should be questioned about allergies to local anesthetics, antiseptic solutions, and tape. A discussion about the technique of insertion and anticipated sensations is an important part of preparing the patient for the experience. Many women report that fear of pain or needles can dissuade them from initiating an implant.[140,141] Clinicians should provide reassurance that most women experience little pain with placement.[142]

Implant insertion can be performed at any time during the menstrual cycle as long as the provider is reasonably certain that a woman is not pregnant.[81] If placement occurs after Day 5 of the menstrual cycle, a barrier method or abstinence should be used for 7 days after insertion.

How to Be Reasonably Certain a Woman Is Not Pregnant

A health care provider can be reasonably certain that a woman is not pregnant if she has no symptoms or signs of pregnancy and meets any one of the following criteria:[81]

- Is ≤7 days after the start of normal menses
- Has not had sexual intercourse since the start of last normal menses
- Has been correctly and consistently using a reliable method of contraception
- Is ≤7 days after spontaneous or induced abortion
- Is within 4 weeks postpartum

■ Is fully or nearly fully breastfeeding (exclusively breastfeeding or the vast majority [≥85%] of feeds are breastfeeds), amenorrheic, and less than 6 months postpartum

Using these criteria and negative pregnancy testing, Nexplanon can be safely placed without increasing the risk of luteal phase pregnancies over the manufacturer's more stringent protocol of placement within 5 days of the last menstrual period.[143] While studies of cervical mucus suggest that a 3-day use of backup method is sufficient,[22] given the uncertainty associated with this assessment, we usually recommend 7 days of alternative protection.[23] Implants can be inserted immediately postpartum or postabortion with no change in insertion technique.

Insertion Technique

Selection of the site for placement of implants is based on both functional and esthetic factors. Various sites (the upper leg, forearm, and upper arm) have been used in clinical trials. The nondominant, upper, inner arm is the typically used site. This area is easily accessible to the clinician with minimal exposure of the patient, well protected during most normal activities, and not highly visible. The risk of implant migration from the insertion site is minimal when the implant is properly placed.[144] The site of placement does not affect circulating progestin levels.

Insertion is carried out under local anesthesia in the office or clinic by a trained health care provider. In the United States, providers must complete a manufacturer-provided clinical training course before inserting Nexplanon and to become eligible to order product for their office.[145] Many practice groups require this training for insertion privileges. Outside of the United States, manufacturer training is not required to insert any implant. A multi-site study showed median insertion times of 40 seconds for the etonogestrel implant and 70 seconds for the two-rod levonorgestrel implant, with 98% of insertions rated as easy by providers.[142]

Required equipment for implant insertion:

2.5-mL syringe
0.5-in, 25-gauge needle for injecting the anesthetic
1% chloroprocaine or lidocaine with epinephrine
Antiseptic solution
Adhesive strip for puncture closures
Pressure bandage

POSITIONING THE PATIENT. The patient is placed in a flat supine position with the full length of her arm exposed. Typically, the nondominant arm is chosen. The upper inner arm is positioned by bending the elbow so that her hand is underneath her head or close to the head. Adequate support under the arm should be provided to ensure comfort. To minimize the risk of infection, strict aseptic technique should be maintained throughout the procedure.

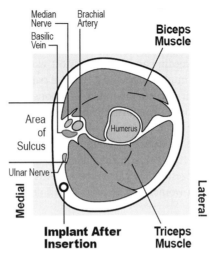

Figure 5.4 Cross-sectional anatomy of upper arm. (Used by permission from Merck & Co., Inc., Whitehouse Station, NJ, USA.)

Identify the insertion site, which is at the inner side of the nondominant upper arm, approximately 8 to 10 cm (3 to 4 in) proximal to the medial epicondyle of the humerus. The groove between the biceps and the triceps muscles should be identified. Nexplanon should be placed 3 to 5 cm dorsomedial to the sulcus, that is, in the skin overlying the triceps muscle, away from the groove to minimize risk of neurovascular injury **(Figure 5.4)**.[15,146] We recommend making a mark with a pen at the insertion site, and a second mark a few centimeters proximal to the first, to guide the direction of the insertion **(Figure 5.5)**. Avoid injecting the lidocaine or placing the inserter through the pen mark as this may permanently stain the skin. A sterile drape is placed under the arm, and the insertion site on the arm is cleaned with an antiseptic such as povidone-iodine.

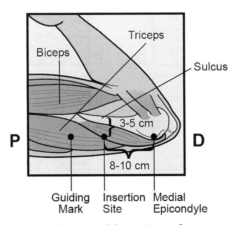

Figure 5.5 Correct marking and location of etonogestrel implant placement. (Used by permission from Merck & Co., Inc., Whitehouse Station, NJ, USA.)

ANESTHESIA. Local anesthesia for the incision is obtained by raising a wheal of anesthetic using a 25-gauge needle and injecting 2 to 3 mL under the skin along the full length of the implant insertion path. Use of epinephrine in the anesthetic block may reduce bleeding and bruising. Most women experience little pain during or following implant placement,[142] but if pain occurs afterwards, it can be relieved with aspirin, acetaminophen, or a nonsteroidal anti-inflammatory agent. The most commonly reported discomfort is a burning sensation during the injection of the local anesthetic. This effect of local anesthetic can be eliminated for most patients by adding sodium bicarbonate 1 mEq to each 10 mL of anesthetic (this shortens shelf life to 24 hours).[147] Alternatively, ethyl chloride topical analgesic spray can be used.[148] After the onset of anesthesia in 2 to 3 minutes, most women feel no more than a pressure sensation.

PLACEMENT (FIGURE 5.6). Although the Nexplanon inserter was theoretically designed to minimize the risk of deep placement, providers are still able to place the implant deeply if proper technique is not followed. *Verify the presence of Nexplanon* after removing the needle cap by looking carefully at the tip of the needle. If the implant (a white rod) is not visible, insertion should not be attempted. Keep the applicator sterile.

The insertion needle should be pushed directly through the skin at no greater than a 30-degree angle without making an incision. Applying countertraction to the skin at the entry site facilitates advancement of the needle. Insert the needle through the skin until the bevel is just under the skin; if inserted past the bevel, the needle should be withdrawn until only

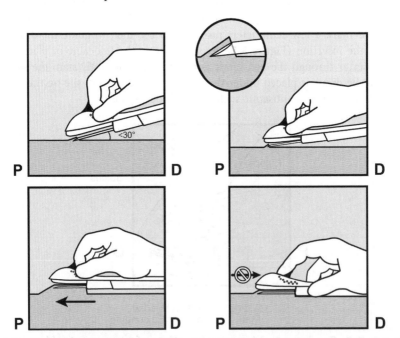

Figure 5.6 Technique for Nexplanon placement. P, proximal; D, distal. (Used by permission from Merck & Co., Inc., Whitehouse Station, NJ, USA.)

the bevel is beneath the skin. To minimize the chance of deep insertion, lift or tent the skin with the tip of the needle as you advance the trocar while maintaining countertraction to the skin and keeping the back end of the applicator slightly higher than the front end. If the skin dimples, the needle is too superficial. Pull the needle back and redirect.

Once the needle has been fully advanced, pull back on the purple slider while maintaining gentle forward pressure on the inserter. This action causes the needle to retract. Once the purple slider is fully retracted, lift the inserter away from the patient's arm, leaving the implant behind under the skin. If the purple slider is moved prior to fully inserting the needle, it will retract the needle and the implant will release prematurely.

Immediately after insertion, palpate the implant to verify correct insertion (both ends should be palpable). Look for the purple tip of the obturator, near the retracted needle site on the inserter. If the implant is not palpable and has been released from the inserter, it must be located before contraception can be assured. If placement is in doubt, another contraceptive method must be used.[149] Nexplanon is radiopaque and can be located with x-ray, computed tomography (CT) scan, high-frequency ultrasound, or magnetic resonance imaging (MRI).[15]

The two rods of the Jadelle or Sino-implant are placed in a V shape with the insertion site 8 to 10 cm proximal to the medial epicondyle of the humerus (same insertion site as Nexplanon). Sterility of the two rods should be maintained throughout. First clean the insertion site and inject 3 to 5 mL of 1% lidocaine (with or without epinephrine) along the insertion paths. Introduce the disposable trocar beneath the skin and advance to the mark nearest to the inserter handle. Next, remove the obturator, load the first implant, and then replace the obturator. Hold the obturator steady and retract the trocar to the mark near the tip without removing the trocar from the arm. Move the trocar slightly to form a narrow V shape and advance the trocar to the mark nearest to the inserter handle, remove the obturator, load the second implant, and then replace the obturator. Hold the obturator steady and pull the trocar back to fully remove the trocar from the arm. Palpate the implants and place a skin closure (e.g., Steri-Strip) over the insertion site.[150] Jadelle is also radiopaque and can be located with imaging if rods are not palpable.

After insertion, show the patient how to palpate the implants. Place an adhesive closure or bandage over the insertion site. A pressure dressing may be used to try to decrease bruising.

COMPLICATIONS OF INSERTION. Potential complications include improper placement, infection, hematoma formation, local irritation or rash over the implants, expulsion of the implant, and allergic reactions to adhesives of the dressing.[14] In a voluntary postmarketing surveillance program of Implanon, providers described more than 20,000 insertions. They reported "difficult insertion" in 0.8% of cases and deep insertion (in muscle or deep in fat tissue) in 0.2% of cases.[151] A U.S. prospective post-marketing surveillance study of Nexplanon included data on 7364 insertion and 5159 removal procedures. Deep placement was reported in 0.9%. Among reported removals, four

(0.08%) women with deep implants required surgery for removal.[152] The incidence of complications is minimized by clinician training and experience and the use of strict aseptic technique. Postinsertion pregnancies reported with Implanon were commonly due to a failure to insert the implant, usually when clinicians inadvertently allowed the implant to fall out of the inserter prior to placement.[65] While the Nexplanon inserter was designed to minimize the risk of improper insertion or insertion failure,[153,154] the clinician must still make sure the implant is visualized in the trocar prior to insertion and confirm correct position by palpation under the skin after placement.

INFECTION. The insertion site rarely becomes infected. In a study of 997 Jadelle users and 997 Implanon users, one infection was reported by a Jadelle user and none among Implanon users.[142] Infection can be treated either by the removal of the implant or the administration of oral antibiotics, while the implant remains in place. If the infection does not resolve with antibiotic treatment or patient shows signs of systemic infection, consider implant removal. There have been no reports of infections leading to serious injury. Rarely, a superficial phlebitis develops. If it resolves over 1 to 2 weeks with heat and elevation of the arm, the implants need not be removed.

EXPULSION. Expulsion of a contraceptive implant is rare, and the majority of expulsions are associated with concurrent infection at the insertion site. Another cause of expulsion is failure to advance the implants far enough from the incision, causing pressure on the incision by the distal tip of the implant. One expulsion of Jadelle was noted in an early clinical trial of nearly 600 women.[8] In 11 large trials of Implanon, no expulsions occurred[63]; however, rare cases have been noted in postmarketing surveillance.[65] Immediately after placement, the implant can be pushed back out through the insertion site. We caution patients who may be enthusiastic about showing friends and family a new device to avoid manipulation for the first week.

LOCAL REACTIONS. Bruising is common after placement, and use of a pressure dressing for 24 hours is recommended. Although not common, hematomas can form; continued use of a pressure dressing for 72 hours should prevent enlargement. Application of an ice pack for 30 minutes immediately after insertion also helps. Local irritation, rash, pruritus, swelling, and pain occur in 4.7% of Norplant users, usually during the first month of use.[155] Allergies to skin closure strip adhesives or to latex gloves account for some reactions.[156] These problems resolve spontaneously, but itching can be relieved by topical corticoid steroids.

Removal Techniques

Although implant removal is an office procedure requiring only a small amount of local anesthesia and a few simple instruments, instruction and practice are necessary. Simulation training may be helpful but evidence is lacking.[157] The patient should undergo appropriate counseling and informed consent procedures.

Most problems with removal occur in the setting of deep placement. The incidence of complicated removals was approximately 5% for Norplant or Jadelle and 1.4% for Nexplanon, an incidence that can be best minimized by good training and careful insertion.[158] A voluntary postmarketing surveillance study of 5,700 Implanon removals described a 5.9% incidence of difficult removals, including unsuccessful attempts, or removal requiring additional time or a larger incision.[151] Eight patients (0.1%) required referral to a surgeon or interventional radiologist for Implanon removal.[151] Proper positioning of the implant at the time of insertion is the most important factor influencing ease of removal. Insertion of an implant deep to the fascia of the muscle increases the risk of nerve injury[159] and may require additional testing or referral to other specialists for localization or management of complications.[160,161] Deeply placed implants can be more challenging to remove and may require additional equipment or a larger incision. Complex removal should not be attempted unless the provider is certain of the implant's location and is comfortable with advanced removal techniques. For providers who lack experience in removal of nonpalpable implants (discussed in detail below), we recommend confirming the location of the implant in the arm using x-ray (for Nexplanon or Jadelle) or ultrasound (any implant). If the implant is in the arm, refer the patient to an experienced colleague or a removal center of experience (contact the manufacturer at 877-888-4231). If the implant is not in the arm, obtain an etonogestrel blood level and refer the patient for further assessment if etonogestrel is detected. If the etonogestrel level is below the detection threshold, this indicates inadvertent failure to initially insert the implant.

REMOVAL OF A PALPABLE IMPLANT. Most removals are not painful (95% of patients reported no or mild discomfort), and systemic analgesia is not required.[162] In a study directly comparing the single rod and the two-rod levonorgestrel systems, mean duration of removal time was 78 seconds for the single rod, and 149 seconds for the two-rod system although technique was not described.[18] In that study, providers rated 98% of single-rod removals and 91% of two-rod system removals as easy.[18] The most common cause of discomfort during the procedure is injection of the local anesthetic. Patients may feel pressure or tugging from manipulation of the fibrous sheaths and the implants, but these sensations are not severe if the clinician waits a few minutes after injection of the local anesthetic.

First, confirm that the woman does not have allergies to be antiseptic or anesthetic to be used. Remove the implant under aseptic conditions. The following equipment is needed for removal of the implant:

- An examination table for the woman to lie on
- Sterile surgical drapes, sterile gloves, antiseptic solution
- Local anesthetic, needles, and syringe
- Sterile scalpel, forceps (straight and curved mosquito)
- Skin closure, sterile gauze, adhesive bandage, and pressure bandages

The patient is placed in a supine position with her arm flexed and externally rotated to expose the area of the arm with the implant. After palpation of the implant, some providers mark the distal implant end (end closest to the elbow). In some cases, the entry incision may provide a mark for removal. Cleaning a wide area above and below the planned incision site with an antiseptic solution increases the likelihood of maintaining asepsis during manipulations. Next, an anesthetic such as 1% lidocaine 1 to 2 mL with epinephrine 1:100,000 should be infiltrated under the implant tips. *Placing the anesthetic under the tip of an implant raises it up closer to the skin surface, facilitating removal. Using the smallest amount of local anesthetic possible reduces the chance that tissue edema will make an implant tip difficult to feel.* We find that depressing the proximal tip of the implant with the nondominant forefinger and elevating the distal tip with the thumb ("pop-up") stabilizes the implant in a position such that the tip is easily visible through the skin.

Incisions can be made transversely, which is common for levonorgestrel two-rod implant removal (approximately 4-mm incision slightly distal to the narrow end of the "V") or longitudinally in line with the long axis of the implant, which is common for the etonogestrel implant (approximately 2-mm longitudinal incision directly over the raised tip). In many cases, this will lead to delivery of the implant tip directly through the incision. In such cases, the fibrous sheath needs to be gently dissected with the knife blade or a gauze sponge to free the implant enough for removal without the need to grasp the tip with instruments ("pop-out" technique).[163] If the implant does not present through the incision, gently push the implant toward the incision until the tip is visible and can be grasped with a curved mosquito forceps. If the implant is not visible in the incision, the curved or straight forceps can be introduced into the incision to grasp it. The implant is quite flexible. After grasping, the forceps can be flipped over 180° to expose the underside of the implant, which can then be freed of the fibrous tissue in the usual fashion.

Be sure the entire implant is removed. The etonogestrel implant is 40 mm in length and the levonorgestrel two-rod implants are 43 mm long. After removal, we show the woman the complete implant so that she has no doubts that it has been completely removed. The incision should be closed with Steri-Strips, and a pressure bandage can be applied to minimize bruising.

PROCEDURE FOR REMOVAL OF A NONPALPABLE IMPLANT
LOCALIZATION

A nonpalpable implant must always be located prior to attempting removal. There is no value in making an incision at the insertion scar to "see" if the implant is there. If the implant cannot be felt, imaging should be performed to help localize the device. Migration of implants greater than 2 cm from the insertion site is rare; however, there have been reported cases, often associated with inadvertent deep placement.[164,165] The radiopaque Nexplanon can be demonstrated on plain radiographs if it has migrated; clinicians should consider chest imaging in the case of nonpalpable implants. An implant that has been too deeply inserted or has migrated significantly (e.g., to the axilla) may need to be localized using imaging procedures. Both Nexplanon and the two-rod levonorgestrel systems are radiopaque and easily located on two-dimensional x-ray or CT. High-frequency linear array ultrasound transducers (typically 10 MHz or greater), CT, or MRI can be used to evaluate the location of deeply placed implants, whether the implant is supra- or subfascial and the distance from the skin and to important neurovascular structures. If the implant cannot be found in the arm after these localization attempts, we recommend a chest x-ray, as there have been rare reports of implant migration to the pulmonary vasculature, probably from inadvertent placement into the brachial vein.[166,167]

REMOVAL

The key to removing nonpalpable implants is a precise understanding of the exact position of the implant in three dimensions, which can be achieved by careful skin marking and depth measurement by a radiology technician followed by removal in a clinic setting,[168] by removal under real-time ultrasound guidance,[169] or through interventional radiology techniques.[161] The technique is quite different from the usual removal of palpable implants, in that we attempt to grasp the implant with an atraumatic modified vasectomy (modification is a narrower tip) forceps rather than using a sharp mosquito clamp (to avoid injury to the neurovascular bundle) **(Figure 5.7)**. Since the modified vasectomy forceps does not crush the implant but rather fits carefully around it, the implant should be grasped closer to its midpoint and brought up through the incision **(Figure 5.8)**. The fibrous tissue can then be removed with careful use of the scalpel in the longitudinal fashion or with sterile gauze. The implant can easily bend almost in half during this procedure; as long as the implant is not nicked with the scalpel, it will not break. Once the fibrous sheath has been opened, the exposed bend of the implant can be grasped with a straight or curved mosquito clamp, and the entire device can be removed Link to a video of non-palpable implant removal using the modified vasectomy forceps at https://www.youtube.com/watch?v=kBzsoXv8hPI. We must emphasize that complicated removal should not be attempted by clinicians with limited experience with these techniques.

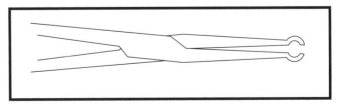

Figure 5.7 Modified vasectomy forceps.

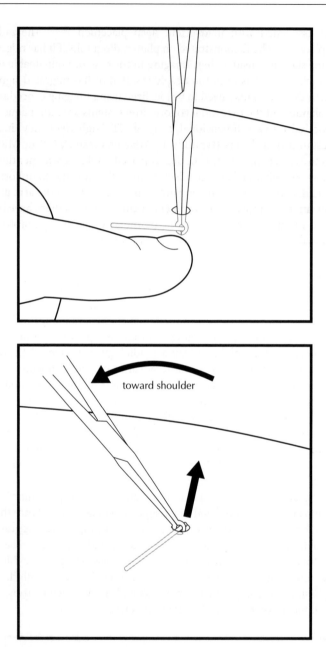

toward shoulder

Figure 5.8 Removal technique using modified vasectomy forceps.

Reinsertion

A new implant can be inserted immediately through the same incision used to remove the old implant, or a new implant can be placed in the other arm. The implant can be positioned in the same direction as the original device.

User Acceptance of Contraceptive Implants

Overall, women worldwide perceive sustained-release methods as highly acceptable methods of contraception.[170-173] In the United States, the primary motivations for implant use have been problems with previous contraceptive methods and ease of implant use. Although fear of pain during implant insertion is a prominent source of anxiety for many women, the actual pain experienced does not match the expectations. The level of satisfaction has been high when barriers to access are removed.[174] Teenagers provide an example of well-documented success. Their 1-year pregnancy rates are much lower and continuation rates much higher than that with oral contraceptives.[59,175] However, adolescents are more likely to discontinue a LARC method than adult women.[176] The lower rate of irregular bleeding with the etonogestrel implant contributes to higher patient acceptability, but irregular bleeding continues to be the major reason for discontinuation.[177,178]

Counseling Women

Frank information about negative factors such as irregular bleeding will avoid surprise and disappointment and encourage women to continue use long enough to enjoy the positive attributes such as convenience, safety, and efficacy. Open discussion of side effects will lead to public and media awareness of the disadvantages as well as the advantages of these methods. Helping women decide if they are good candidates for use of implants before they invest too much time and money in long-acting contraception is a very important objective of good counseling.

Common patient questions regarding contraceptive implants are as follows:

- Is it effective?
- How is it inserted and removed; how long do these procedures take; does it hurt, and will it leave scars?
- Will the implants be visible under the skin?
- Will the implants be uncomfortable or restrict movement of the arm?
- Will the implants move in the body?
- Will the implants be damaged if they are touched or bumped?
- Will this contraceptive change sexual drive and enjoyment?
- What are the short- and long-term side effects?
- Are there any effects on future fertility?
- What do the implants look and feel like?
- What happens if pregnancy occurs during use?
- How long will it take for the method to be effective after insertion?
- Can a partner tell if this method is being used?

Clinicians can provide reassurance that the implant is more than 99% effective at preventing pregnancy and that fertility returns rapidly after removal. They should review the insertion and removal processes with patients, often with the help of models or diagrams, and reinforce that the implant will not interfere with arm movement or regular activity. Clinicians can review that a properly placed implant has a very low risk of migration or of being damaged. Patients should be properly advised of side effects (primarily irregular bleeding) and encouraged to return to discuss management of these side effects. Clinicians should ensure that a patient has all questions answered before proceeding with insertion and should explicitly state that the implant can be removed if the patient requests this for any reason.

Postpartum and Postabortal Use

Immediate postpartum use of etonogestrel implants is a cost-effective strategy that results in high long-term continuation and successful birth spacing.[56,179-181] Implants offer an excellent choice for a breastfeeding woman and can be inserted immediately postpartum. There are no effects on breast milk quality or quantity, and infants grow normally.[182-184]

Women have similar rates of continuation when implants are initiated immediately postabortion versus interval placement.[185,186] Additionally, women who initiated a levonorgestrel implant[187] or etonogestrel implant[188] immediately after surgical abortion had significantly lower rates of pregnancy in the next 24 months compared to women who initiated shorter-acting methods. Inserting an etonogestrel implant at the time of initiating medication abortion with mifepristone does not increase medication abortion failure rates.[189,190]

References

1. **Edwards JE, Moore A,** Implanon. A review of clinical studies, Br J Fam Plann 24:3–16, 1999.

2. **Meirik O, Fraser IS, d'Arcangues C; WHO Consultation on implantable contraceptives for women,** Implantable contraceptives for women. Hum Reprod Update 9:49–59, 2003.

3. **United Nations, Department of Economic and Social Affairs, Population Division, ed.,** Trends in Contraceptive Use Worldwide 2015, 2015.

4. **Sundaram A, Vaughan B, Kost K, Bankole A, Finer L, Singh S, et al.,** Contraceptive failure in the United States: estimates from the 2006-2010 National Survey of Family Growth. Perspect Sex Reprod Health 49:7–16, 2017.

5. **Mansour D, Korver T, Marintcheva-Petrova M, Fraser IS,** The effects of implanon on menstrual bleeding patterns, Eur J Contracept Reprod Health Care 13:13–28, 2008.

6. **Darney PD, Atkinson E, Tanner S, Macpherson S, Hellerstein S, Alvarado A,** Acceptance and perceptions of Norplant among users in San-Francisco, USA, Stud Fam Plann 21:152–160, 1990.

7. **Sivin I, Nash H, Waldman S,** Jadelle® Levonorgestrel Rod Implants: A Summary of Scientific Data and Lessons Learned from Programmatic Experience, 2002.

8. **Sivin I, Alvarez F, Mishell DR Jr, Darney P, Wan L, Brache V, et al.,** Contraception with two levonorgestrel rod implants. A 5-year study in the United States and Dominican Republic, Contraception 58:275–282, 1998.

9. **Wan LS, Stiber A, Lam LY,** The levonorgestrel two-rod implant for long-acting contraception: 10 years of clinical experience, Obstet Gynecol 102:24–26, 2003.

10. **Schnabel P, Merki-Feld GS, Malvy A, Duijkers I, Mommers E, van den Heuvel MW,** Bioequivalence and x-ray visibility of a radiopaque etonogestrel

implant versus a non-radiopaque implant: a 3-year, randomized, double-blind study, Clin Drug Investig 32:413–422, 2012.

11. **Shastri PV,** Toxicology of polymers for implant contraceptives for women, Contraception 65:9–13, 2002.

12. **Huber J, Wenzl R,** Pharmacokinetics of Implanon. An integrated analysis, Contraception 58:85S–90S, 1998.

13. **Affandi B,** An integrated analysis of vaginal bleeding patterns in clinical trials of Implanon, Contraception 58:99S–107S, 1998.

14. **Brache V, Faundes A, Alvarez F, Cochon L,** Nonmenstrual adverse events during use of implantable contraceptives for women: data from clinical trials, Contraception 65:63–74, 2002.

15. Nexplanon Prescribing Information. [cited 2018 March 20]. https://www. merck.com/product/usa/pi_circulars/n/ nexplanon/nexplanon_pi.pdf

16. **McNicholas C, Maddipati R, Zhao QH, Swor E, Peipert JF,** Use of the etonogestrel implant and levonorgestrel intrauterine device beyond the US Food and Drug Administration-approved duration, Obstet Gynecol 125:599–604, 2015.

17. **McNicholas C, Swor E, Wan LP, Peipert JF,** Prolonged use of the etonogestrel implant and levonorgestrel intrauterine device: 2 years beyond Food and Drug Administration-approved duration. Am J Obstet Gynecol 216:586.e1–586.e6, 2017.

18. **Ali M, Akin A, Bahamondes L, Brache V, Habib N, Landoulsi S, et al.,** Extended use up to 5 years of the etonogestrel-releasing subdermal contraceptive implant: comparison to levonorgestrel-releasing subdermal implant. Hum Reprod 31:2491–2498, 2016.

19. US Medical Eligibility Criteria for Contraceptive Use: Classifications for Progestin-Only Contraceptives. [cited 2018 November 10]. https://www.cdc. gov/reproductivehealth/contraception/ mmwr/mec/appendixc.html

20. **Kapp N,** WHO provider brief on hormonal contraception and liver disease, Contraception 80:325–326, 2009.

21. **Makarainen L, van Beek A, Tuomivaara L, Asplund B, Coelingh Bennink H,** Ovarian function during the use of a single contraceptive implant: Implanon compared with Norplant, Fertil Steril 69:714–721, 1998.

22. **Dunson TR, Blumenthal PD, Alvarez F, Brache V, Cochon L, Dalberth B, et al.,** Timing of onset of contraceptive effectiveness in Norplant implant users. Part I. Changes in cervical mucus, Fertil Steril 69:258–266, 1998.

23. **Han L, Taub R, Jensen JT,** Cervical mucus and contraception: what-we know and what we don't, Contraception 96:310–321, 2017.

24. **Croxatto HB, Diaz S, Miranda P, Elamsson K, Johansson EDB,** Plasma-levels of levonorgestrel in women during longterm use of Norplants, Contraception 22:583–596, 1980.

25. **Croxatto HB,** Progestin implants. Steroids 65:681–685, 2000.

26. **Lazorwitz A, Davis A, Swartz M, Guiahi M,** The effect of carbamazepine on etonogestrel concentrations in contraceptive implant users, Contraception 95:571–577, 2017.

27. **Chappell CA, Lamorde M, Nakalema S, Chen BA, Mackline H, Riddler SA, et al.,** Efavirenz decreases etonogestrel exposure: a pharmacokinetic evaluation of implantable contraception with anti-retroviral therapy, AIDS 31:1965–1972, 2017.

28. **Scarsi KK, Darin KM, Nakalema S, Back DJ, Byakika-Kibwika P, Else LJ, et al.,** Unintended pregnancies observed with combined use of the levonorgestrel contraceptive implant and efavirenz-based antiretroviral therapy: a three-arm pharmacokinetic evaluation over 48 weeks, Clin Infect Dis 62:675–682, 2016.

29. **Leticee N, Viard JP, Yamgnane A, Karmochkine M, Benachi A,** Contraceptive failure of etonogestrel implant in patients treated with antiretrovirals including efavirenz, Contraception 85:425–427, 2012.

30. **Gaffield ME, Culwell KR, Lee CR,** The use of hormonal contraception among women taking anticonvulsant therapy, Contraception 83:16–29, 2011.

31. **Patni S, Ebden P, Kevelighan E, Bibby J,** Ectopic pregnancy with Implanon, J Fam Plann Reprod Health Care 32:115, 2006.

32. **Perry SH, Swamy P, Preidis GA, Mwanyumba A, Motsa N, Sarero HN,** Implementing the Jadelle implant for women living with HIV in a resource-limited setting: concerns for drug interactions leading to unintended pregnancies, AIDS 28:791–793, 2014.

33. **Lange J, Teal S, Tocce K,** Decreased efficacy of an etonogestrel implant in a woman on antiepileptic medications: a case report, J Med Case Reports 8: 43, 2014.

34. **Reimers A, Helde G, Brodtkorb E,** Ethinyl estradiol, not progestogens, reduces lamotrigine serum concentrations, Epilepsia 46:1414–1417, 2005.

35. **Darney P, Patel A, Rosen K, Shapiro LS, Kaunitz AM,** Safety and efficacy of a single-rod etonogestrel implant (Implanon): results from 11 international clinical trials, Fertil Steril 91:1646–1653, 2009.

36. **Mornar S, Chan LN, Mistretta S, Neustadt A, Martins S, Gilliam M,** Pharmacokinetics of the etonogestrel contraceptive implant in obese women, Am J Obstet Gynecol 207:110e1–116e1, 2012.

37. **Xu H, Wade JA, Peipert JF, Zhao Q, Madden T, Secura GM,** Contraceptive failure rates of etonogestrel subdermal implants in overweight and obese women, Obstet Gynecol 120:21–26, 2012.

38. **Biswas A, Viegas OA, Bennink HJ, Korver T, Ratnam SS,** Effect of Implanon use on selected parameters of thyroid and adrenal function, Contraception 62:247–251, 2000.

39. **Brache V, Alvarez-Sanchez F, Faundes A, Tejada AS, Cochon L,** Ovarian endocrine function through five years of continuous treatment with NORPLANT subdermal contraceptive implants, Contraception 41:169–177, 1990.

40. **Alvarez F, Brache V, Tejada AS, Faundes A,** Abnormal endocrine profile among women with confirmed or presumed ovulation during long-term Norplant use, Contraception 33:111–119, 1986.

41. **Croxatto HB,** Mechanisms that explain the contraceptive action of progestin implants for women, Contraception 65:21–27, 2002.

42. **Croxatto HB, Makarainen L,** The pharmacodynamics and efficacy of Implanon (R)—an overview of the data, Contraception 58:91s–97s, 1998.

43. **Hidalgo MM, Lisondo C, Juliato CT, Espejo-Arce X, Monteiro I, Bahamondes L,** Ovarian cysts in users of Implanon and Jadelle subdermal contraceptive implants, Contraception 73:532–536, 2006.

44. **Croxatto HB, Diaz S, Salvatierra AM, Morales P, Ebensperger C, Brandeis A,** Treatment with Norplant subdermal implants inhibits sperm penetration through cervical mucus in vitro, Contraception 36:193–201, 1987.

45. **Walch K, Unfried G, Huber J, Kurz C, van Trotsenburg M, Pernicka E, et al.,** Implanon versus medroxyprogesterone acetate: effects on pain scores in patients with symptomatic endometriosis—a pilot study, Contraception 79:29–34, 2009.

46. **Yisa SB, Okenwa AA, Husemeyer RP,** Treatment of pelvic endometriosis with etonogestrel subdermal implant (Implanon), J Fam Plann Reprod Health Care 31:67–70, 2005.

47. **Fraser IS,** Added health benefits of the levonorgestrel contraceptive intrauterine system and other hormonal contraceptive delivery systems, Contraception 87:273–279, 2013.

48. **Berenson AB, Tan A, Hirth JM,** Complications and continuation rates associated with 2 types of long-acting contraception, Am J Obstet Gynecol 212:761 e1–768 e1, 2015.

49. **Frank ML, Ditmore JR, Ilegbodu AE, Bateman L, Poindexter AN,** Characteristics and experiences of American women electing for early removal of contraceptive implants, Contraception 52:159–165, 1995.

50. **Bastow B, Sheeder J, Guiahi M, Teal S,** Condom use in adolescents and young women following initiation of long- or short-acting contraceptive methods, Contraception 97:70–75, 2018.

51. **Lemoine J, Teal SB, Peters M, Guiahi M,** Motivating factors for dual-method contraceptive use among adolescents and young women: a qualitative investigation, Contraception 96:352–356, 2017.

52. **McNicholas CP, Klugman JB, Zhao QH, Peipert JF,** Condom use and incident sexually transmitted infection after initiation of long-acting reversible

contraception, Am J Obstet Gynecol 217:672.e1–672.e6, 2017.

53. **Rattray C, Wiener J, Legardy-Williams J, Costenbader E, Pazol K, Medley-Singh N, et al.,** Effects of initiating a contraceptive implant on subsequent condom use: a randomized controlled trial, Contraception 92:560–566, 2015.

54. **Trussell J,** Update on and correction to the cost-effectiveness of contraceptives in the United States, Contraception 85:611, 2012.

55. **Dusetzina SB, Dalton VK, Chernew ME, Pace LE, Bowden G, Fendrick AM,** Cost of contraceptive methods to privately insured women in the United States, Women's Health Issues 23: e69–e71, 2013.

56. **Han L, Teal SB, Sheeder J, Tocce K,** Preventing repeat pregnancy in adolescents: is immediate postpartum insertion of the contraceptive implant cost effective?, Am J Obstet Gynecol 211: 24 e1–27 e1, 2014.

57. **Lipetz C, Phillips CJ, Fleming CF,** The cost-effectiveness of a long-acting reversible contraceptive (Implanon) relative to oral contraception in a community setting, Contraception 79:304–309, 2009.

58. **Sivin I,** International experience with NORPLANT and NORPLANT-2 contraceptives, Stud Fam Plann 19:81–94, 1988.

59. **Secura GM, Madden T, McNicholas C, Mullersman J, Buckel CM, Zhao Q, et al.,** Provision of no-cost, long-acting contraception and teenage pregnancy, N Engl J Med 371:1316–1323, 2014.

60. **Winner B, Peipert JF, Zhao Q, Buckel C, Madden T, Allsworth JE, et al.,** Effectiveness of long-acting reversible contraception, N Engl J Med 366:1998–2007, 2012.

61. **Rosenstock JR, Peipert JF, Madden T, Zhao Q, Secura GM,** Continuation of reversible contraception in teenagers and young women, Obstet Gynecol 120:1298–1305, 2012.

62. **Sivin I, Wan L, Ranta S, Alvarez F, Brache V, Mishell DR, et al.,** Levonorgestrel concentrations during 7 years of continuous use of Jadelle contraceptive implants, Contraception 64:43–49, 2001.

63. **Blumenthal PD, Gemzell-Danielsson K, Marintcheva-Petrova M,** Tolerability and clinical safety of Implanon, Eur J Contracept Reprod Health Care 13:29–36, 2008.

64. **Croxatto HB, Urbancsek J, Massai R, Bennink HC, van Beek A, Group IS,** A multicentre efficacy and safety study of the single contraceptive implant Implanon (R), Hum Reprod 14:976–981, 1999.

65. **Harrison-Woolrych M, Hill R,** Unintended pregnancies with the etonogestrel implant (Implanon): a case series from postmarketing experience in Australia, Contraception 71:306–308, 2005.

66. **Shoupe D, Mishell DR Jr, Bopp BL, Fielding M,** The significance of bleeding patterns in Norplant implant users, Obstet Gynecol 77:256–260, 1991.

67. **Callahan R, Yacobson I, Halpern V, Nanda K,** Ectopic pregnancy with use of progestin-only injectables and contraceptive implants: a systematic review, Contraception 92:514–522, 2015.

68. **Hubacher D, Lopez L, Steiner MJ, Dorflinger L,** Menstrual pattern changes from levonorgestrel subdermal implants and DMPA: systematic review and evidence-based comparisons, Contraception 80:113–118, 2009.

69. **Sivin I, Diaz S, Holma P, Alvarez-Sanchez F, Robertson DN,** A four-year clinical study of NORPLANT implants, Stud Fam Plann 14:184–191, 1983.

70. **Dinh A, Sriprasert I, Williams AR, Archer DF,** A review of the endometrial histologic effects of progestins and progesterone receptor modulators in reproductive age women, Contraception 91:360–367, 2015.

71. **Mascarenhas L, van Beek A, Bennink HC, Newton J,** A 2-year comparative study of endometrial histology and cervical cytology of contraceptive implant users in Birmingham, UK, Hum Reprod 13:3057–3060, 1998.

72. **Hickey M, Simbar M, Young L, Markham R, Russell P, Fraser IS,** A longitudinal study of changes in endometrial microvascular density in Norplant implant users, Contraception 59:123–129, 1999.

73. **Hickey M, Krikun G, Kodaman P, Schatz F, Carati C, Lockwood CJ,** Long-term progestin-only contraceptives result in reduced endometrial blood flow and oxidative stress, J Clin Endocrinol Metab 91:3633–3638, 2006.

74. **Diedrich JT, Zhao Q, Madden T, Secura GM, Peipert JF,** Three-year continuation of reversible contraception, Am J Obstet Gynecol 213:662 e1–668 e1, 2015.

75. **Zheng SR, Zheng HM, Qian SZ, Sang GW, Kaper RF,** A randomized multicenter study comparing the efficacy and bleeding pattern of a single-rod (Implanon) and a six-capsule (Norplant) hormonal contraceptive implant, Contraception 60:1–8, 1999.

76. **Fakeye O, Balogh S,** Effect of Norplant contraceptive use on hemoglobin, packed cell-volume and menstrual bleeding patterns, Contraception 39:265–274, 1989.

77. **Dilbaz B, Ozdegirmenci O, Caliskan E, Dilbaz S, Haberal A,** Effect of etonogestrel implant on serum lipids, liver function tests and hemoglobin levels, Contraception 81:510–514, 2010.

78. **Mansour D, Bahamondes L, Critchley H, Darney P, Fraser IS,** The management of unacceptable bleeding patterns in etonogestrel-releasing contraceptive implant users, Contraception 83: 202–210, 2011.

79. **Guiahi M, McBride M, Sheeder J, Teal S,** Short-term treatment of bothersome bleeding for etonogestrel implant users using a 14-day oral contraceptive pill regimen: a randomized controlled trial, Obstet Gynecol 126:508–513, 2015.

80. **Hou MY, McNicholas C, Creinin MD,** Combined oral contraceptive treatment for bleeding complaints with the etonogestrel contraceptive implant: a randomised controlled trial, Eur J Contracept Reprod Health Care 21:361–366, 2016.

81. **Curtis KM, Jatlaoui TC, Tepper NK, Zapata LB, Horton LG, Jamieson DJ, et al.,** US selected practice recommendations for contraceptive use, 2016. MMWR Recomm Rep 65:3–68, 2016.

82. **Chen MJ, Hsia JK, Creinin MD,** Etonogestrel implant use in women primarily choosing a combined oral contraceptive pill: a proof-of-concept trial, Contraception 97:533–537, 2018.

83. **Zigler RE, McNicholas C,** Unscheduled vaginal bleeding with progestin-only contraceptive use, Am J Obstet Gynecol 216:443–450, 2017.

84. **Phaliwong P, Taneepanichskul S,** The effect of mefenamic acid on controlling irregular uterine bleeding second to Implanon use, J Med Assoc Thai 87:S64–S68, 2004.

85. **Buasang K, Taneepanichskul S,** Efficacy of celecoxib on controlling irregular uterine bleeding secondary to Jadelle use, J Med Assoc Thai 92:301–307, 2009.

86. **Simmons KB, Edelman AB, Fu R, Jensen JT,** Tamoxifen for the treatment of breakthrough bleeding with the etonogestrel implant: a randomized controlled trial, Contraception 95:198–204, 2017.

87. **Zigler RE, Madden T, Ashby C, Wan L, McNicholas C,** Ulipristal acetate for unscheduled bleeding in etonogestrel implant users: a randomized controlled trial, Obstet Gynecol 132:888–894, 2018.

88. **Biswas A, Biswas S, Viegas OAC,** Effect of etonogestrel subdermal contraceptive implant (Implanon®) on liver function tests—a randomized comparative study with Norplant® implants, Contraception 70:379–382, 2004.

89. **Nasr A, Nafeh HM,** Effect of etonogestrel contraceptive implant (Implanon) on portal blood flow and liver functions, Contraception 79:236–239, 2009.

90. **Guazzelli CA, de Queiroz FT, Barbieri M, Barreiros FA, Torloni MR, Araujo FF,** Metabolic effects of contraceptive implants in adolescents, Contraception 84:409–412, 2011.

91. **Vieira CS, Ferriani RA, Garcia AA, Pintao MC, Azevedo GD, Gomes MKO, et al.,** Use of the etonogestrel-releasing implant is associated with hypoactivation of the coagulation cascade, Hum Reprod 22:2196–2201, 2007.

92. **Shaaban MM, Elwan SI, el-Sharkawy MM, Farghaly AS,** Effect of subdermal levonorgestrel contraceptive implants, Norplant, on liver functions, Contraception 30:407–412, 1984.

93. **Croxatto HB, Diaz S, Robertson DN, Pavez M,** Clinical chemistry in women treated with levonorgestrel

implants (Norplant) or a TCu 200 IUD, Contraception 27:281–288, 1983.

94. **Diaz S, Pavez M, Brandeis A, Cardenas H, Croxatto HB,** A longitudinal study on cortisol, prolactin and thyroid hormones in users of Norplant subdermal implants or a copper T device, Contraception 40:505–517, 1989.

95. **Toppozada MK, Ramadan M, el-Sawi M, Mehanna MT, Khamis Y, Marzouk S,** Effect of Norplant implants on the pituitary-adrenal axis function and reserve capacity, Contraception 55:7–10, 1997.

96. **Biswas A, Viegas OA, Roy AC,** Effect of Implanon and Norplant subdermal contraceptive implants on serum lipids—a randomized comparative study, Contraception 68:189–193, 2003.

97. **Araujo FF, de Lima GR, Guazzelli CAF, Barbieri M, Vigorito NM, Lindsey PC, et al.,** Long-term evaluation of lipid profile and oral glucose tolerance test in Norplant (R) users, Contraception 73:361–363, 2006.

98. **Villas-Boas J, Vilodre LC, Malerba H, Salcedo MP, Jimenez MF, El Beitune P,** Metabolic safety of the etonogestrel contraceptive implant in healthy women over a 3-year period, Eur J Obstet Gynecol Reprod Biol 202:51–54, 2016.

99. **Oderich CL, Wender MC, Lubianca JN, Santos LM, de Mello GC,** Impact of etonogestrel-releasing implant and copper intrauterine device on carbohydrate metabolism: a comparative study, Contraception 85:173–176, 2012.

100. **Hernandez-Juarez J, Sanchez-Serrano JC, Moreno-Hernandez M, Alvarado-Moreno JA, Hernandez-Lopez JR, Isordia-Salas I, et al.,** Effects of the contraceptive skin patch and subdermal contraceptive implant on markers of endothelial cell activation and inflammation, J Clin Pharmacol 55:780–786, 2015.

101. **Inal MM, Yildirim Y, Ertopcu K, Avci ME, Ozelmas I, Tinar S,** Effect of the subdermal contraceptive etonogestrel implant (Implanon) on biochemical and hormonal parameters (three years follow-up). Eur J Contracept Reprod Health Care 13:238–242, 2008.

102. **Funk S, Miller MM, Mishell DR Jr, Archer DF, Poindexter A, Schmidt J, et al.,** Safety and efficacy of Implanon, a single-rod implantable contraceptive containing etonogestrel, Contraception 71:319–326, 2005.

103. **Molland JR, Morehead DB, Baldwin DM, Castracane VD, Lasley B, Bergquist CA,** Immediate postpartum insertion of the Norplant contraceptive device, Fertil Steril 66:43–48, 1996.

104. **Vicente L, Mendonca D, Dingle M, Duarte R, Boavida JM,** Etonogestrel implant in women with diabetes mellitus, Eur J Contracept Reprod Health Care 13:387–395, 2008.

105. **Bergendal A, Persson I, Odeberg J, Sundstrom A, Holmstrom M, Schulman S, et al.,** Association of venous thromboembolism with hormonal contraception and thrombophilic genotypes, Obstet Gynecol 124:600–609, 2014.

106. **Lidegaard O,** Venous thrombosis in users of non-oral hormonal contraception: follow-up study, Denmark 2001-10, BMJ 344:e2990, 2012.

107. **Cromer BA, Blair JM, Mahan JD, Zibners L, Naumovski Z,** A prospective comparison of bone density in adolescent girls receiving depot medroxyprogesterone acetate (Depo-Provera), levonorgestrel (Norplant), or oral contraceptives, J Pediatr 129:671–676, 1996.

108. **Beerthuizen R, van Beek A, Massai R, Makarainen L, Hout J, Bennink HC,** Bone mineral density during long-term use of the progestagen contraceptive implant Implanon compared to a non-hormonal method of contraception, Hum Reprod 15:118–122, 2000.

109. **Ott MA, Sucato GS,** Contraception for adolescents, Pediatrics 134:e1257–e1281, 2014.

110. **Modesto W, DalAva N, Monteiro I, Bahamondes L,** Body composition and bone mineral density in users of the etonogestrel-releasing contraceptive implant, Arch Gynecol Obstet 292:1387–1391, 2015.

111. **Bahamondes L, Monteiro-Dantas C, Espejo-Arce X, Fernandes AMD, Lui-Filho JF, Perrotti M, et al.,** A prospective study of the forearm bone density of users

of etonorgestrel- and levonorgestrel-releasing contraceptive implants, Hum Reprod 21:466–470, 2006.

112. **Monteiro-Dantas C, Espejo-Arce X, Lui-Filho JF, Fernandes AM, Monteiro I, Bahamondes L,** A three-year longitudinal evaluation of the forearm bone density of users of etonogestrel- and levonorgestrel-releasing contraceptive implants, Reprod Health 4:11, 2007.

113. **Naessen T, Olsson SE, Gudmundson J,** Differential-effects on bone-density of progestogen-only methods for contraception in premenopausal women, Contraception 52:35–39, 1995.

114. **Di XO, Li YH, Zhang CH, Jiang JW, Gu SJ,** Effects of levonorgestrel-releasing subdermal contraceptive implants on bone density and bone metabolism, Contraception 60:161–166, 1999.

115. **Petitti DB, Piaggio G, Mehta S, Cravioto MC, Meirik O,** Steroid hormone contraception and bone mineral density: a cross-sectional study in an international population. The WHO Study of Hormonal Contraception and Bone Health, Obstet Gynecol 95: 736–744, 2000.

116. **Lopez LM, Grimes DA, Schulz KF, Curtis KM, Chen M,** Steroidal contraceptives: effect on bone fractures in women, Cochrane Database Syst Rev (6):CD006033, 2014.

117. **Mansour D, Gemzell-Danielsson K, Inki P, Jensen JT,** Fertility after discontinuation of contraception: a comprehensive review of the literature, Contraception 84:465–477, 2011.

118. **Glasier A,** Implantable contraceptives for women: effectiveness, discontinuation rates, return of fertility, and outcome of pregnancies, Contraception 65:29–37, 2002.

119. **Schwallie PC, Assenzo JR,** The effect of depo-medroxyprogesterone acetate on pituitary and ovarian function, and the return of fertility following its discontinuation: a review, Contraception 10:181–202, 1974.

120. **Urbancsek J,** An integrated analysis of nonmenstrual adverse events with Implanon, Contraception 58:109S–115S, 1998.

121. **Bahamondes L, Brache V, Meirik O, Ali M, Habib N, Landoulsi S, et al.,** A 3-year multicentre randomized controlled trial of etonogestrel- and levonorgestrel-releasing contraceptive implants, with non-randomized matched copper-intrauterine device controls, Hum Reprod 30:2527–2538, 2015.

122. **Worly BL, Gur TL, Schaffir J,** The relationship between progestin hormonal contraception and depression: a systematic review, Contraception 97: 478–489, 2018.

123. **Nappi RE, Merki-Feld GS, Terreno E, Pellegrinelli A, Viana M,** Hormonal contraception in women with migraine: is progestogen-only contraception a better choice?, J Headache Pain 14: 66, 2013.

124. **Sivin I, Campodonico I, Kiriwat O, Holma P, Diaz S, Wan L, et al.,** The performance of levonorgestrel rod and Norplant contraceptive implants: a 5 year randomized study, Hum Reprod 13:3371–3378, 1998.

125. **Vickery Z, Madden T, Zhao Q, Secura GM, Allsworth JE, Peipert JF,** Weight change at 12 months in users of three progestin-only contraceptive methods, Contraception 88:503–508, 2013.

126. **Gallo MF, Legardy-Williams J, Hylton-Kong T, Rattray C, Kourtis AP, Jamieson DJ, et al.,** Association of progestin contraceptive implant and weight gain, Obstet Gynecol 127:573–576, 2016.

127. **Nault AM, Peipert JF, Zhao Q, Madden T, Secura GM,** Validity of perceived weight gain in women using long-acting reversible contraception and depot medroxyprogesterone acetate, Am J Obstet Gynecol 208:48.e1–48.e8, 2013.

128. **dos Santos PDS, Madden T, Omvig K, Peipert JF,** Changes in body composition in women using long-acting reversible contraception, Contraception 95:382–389, 2017.

129. **Affandi B, Cekan SZ, Boonkasemsanti W, Samil RS, Diczfalusy E,** The interaction between sex hormone binding globulin and levonorgestrel released from Norplant, an implantable contraceptive, Contraception 35:135–145, 1987.

130. **Davies GC, Feng LX, Newton JR, Vanbeek A, Coelinghbennink HJT,** Release characteristics, ovarian activity and menstrual bleeding pattern with a single contraceptive implant releasing 3-ketodesogestrel, Contraception 47:251–261, 1993.

131. **Arowojolu AO, Gallo MF, Lopez LM, Grimes DA,** Combined oral contraceptive pills for treatment of acne, Cochrane Database Syst Rev (7):CD004425, 2012.

132. **Trivedi MK, Shinkai K, Murase JE,** A Review of hormone-based therapies to treat adult acne vulgaris in women, Int J Womens Dermatol 3:44–52, 2017.

133. **Alvarez F, Brache V, Faundes A, Tejada AS, Thevenin F,** Ultrasonographic and endocrine evaluation of ovarian function among Norplant(R) implants users with regular menses, Contraception 54:275–279, 1996.

134. **International Collaborative Post-Marketing Surveillance of Norplant,** Post-marketing surveillance of Norplant contraceptive implants: I. Contraceptive efficacy and reproductive health, Contraception 63:167–186, 2001.

135. **Darney PD, Taylor RN, Klaisle C, Bottles K, Zaloudek C,** Serum concentrations of estradiol, progesterone, and levonorgestrel are not determinants of endometrial histology or abnormal bleeding in long-term Norplant implant users, Contraception 53:97–100, 1996.

136. **Darwish A, Labeeb S, Galal M, Rashad H, Hassan S,** Cervical changes associated with progestagen-only contraceptives: a team approach, Contraception 69:121–127, 2004.

137. **Strom BL, Berlin JA, Weber AL, Norman SA, Bernstein L, Burkman RT, et al.,** Absence of an effect of injectable and implantable progestin-only contraceptives on subsequent risk of breast cancer, Contraception 69:353–360, 2004.

138. **Mørch LS, Skovlund CW, Hannaford PC, Iversen L, Fielding S, Lidegaard Ø,** Contemporary hormonal contraception and the risk of breast cancer. N Engl J Med 377:2228–2239, 2017.

139. World Health Organization Medical Eligibility Criteria for Contraceptive Use, 2015. [cited 2018 November 18]; 5th. http://apps.who.int/iris/bitstream/handle/10665/181468/9789241549158_eng.pdf;jsessionid=686D163E4A46D62F9ED804E9D11B0042?sequence=1

140. **Bharadwaj P, Akintomide H, Brima N, Copas A, D'Souza R,** Determinants of long-acting reversible contraceptive (LARC) use by adolescent girls and young women, Eur J Contracept Reprod Health Care 17:298–306, 2012.

141. **Bracken J, Graham CA,** Young women's attitudes towards, and experiences of, long-acting reversible contraceptives, Eur J Contracept Reprod Health Care 19:276–284, 2014.

142. **Meirik O, Brache V, Orawan K, Habib NA, Schmidt J, Ortayli N, et al.,** A multicenter randomized clinical trial of one-rod etonogestrel and two-rod levonorgestrel contraceptive implants with nonrandomized copper-IUD controls: methodology and insertion data, Contraception 87:113–120, 2013.

143. **Richards M, Teal SB, Sheeder J,** Risk of luteal phase pregnancy with any-cycle-day initiation of subdermal contraceptive implants, Contraception 95:364–370, 2017.

144. **Ismail H, Mansour D, Singh M,** Migration of Implanon (R), J Fam Plann Reprod Health Care 32:157–159, 2006.

145. **Merck,** Request Training: Nexplanon. [cited 2018 March 7]; http://www.nexplanon-usa.com/en/hcp/services-and-support/request-training/

146. **Iwanaga J, Fox MC, Rekers H, Schwartz L, Tubbs RS,** Neurovascular anatomy of the adult female medial arm in relationship to potential sites for insertion of the etonogestrel contraceptive implant, Contraception 100:26–30, 2019. doi: 10.1016/j.contraception.2019.02.007.

147. **Nelson AL,** Neutralizing Ph of lidocaine reduces pain during Norplant(R) system insertion procedure, Contraception 51:299–301, 1995.

148. **Shefras J, Forsythe A, Nathani F, Hoffman D,** An alternative method of anaesthesia for implant insertion: description of a clinical initiative in contraceptive care, J Fam Plann Reprod Health Care 40:226–228, 2014.

149. **Shulman LP, Gabriel H,** Management and localization strategies for the non-palpable Implanon rod, Contraception 73:325–330, 2006.

150. Jadelle Insertion. [cited]. http://www.jadelle.com/static/documents/Jadelle_PosterInsertion.pdf

151. **Creinin MD, Kaunitz AM, Darney PD, Schwartz L, Hampton T, Gordon K, et al.,** The US etonogestrel implant

mandatory clinical training and active monitoring programs: 6-year experience, Contraception 95:205–210, 2017.

152. **Reed S, Do Minh T, Lange JA, Koro C, Fox M, Heinemann K,** Real world data on Nexplanon® procedure-related events: final results from the Nexplanon Observational Risk Assessment study (NORA), Contraception 100:31–36, 2019. doi: 10.1016/j.contraception.2019.03.052.

153. **Mansour D, Mommers E, Teede H, Sollie-Eriksen B, Graesslin O, Ahrendt HJ, et al.,** Clinician satisfaction and insertion characteristics of a new applicator to insert radiopaque Implanon: an open-label, noncontrolled, multicenter trial, Contraception 82:243–249, 2010.

154. **Mansour D,** Nexplanon(®): what Implanon (®) did next, J Fam Plann Reprod Health Care 36:187–189, 2010.

155. **Klavon SL, Grubb GS,** Insertion site complications during the first year of NORPLANT use, Contraception 41:27–37, 1990.

156. **Blain S, Oloto E, Meyrick I, Bromham D,** Skin reactions following Norplant(R) insertion and removal-possible causative factors, Br J Fam Plann 21:130–132, 1996.

157. **Goldthwaite LM, Tocce K,** Simulation training for family planning procedures, Curr Opin Obstet Gynecol 29:437–442, 2017.

158. **Rowlands S,** Legal aspects of contraceptive implants, J Fam Plann Reprod Health Care 36:243–248, 2010.

159. **Laumonerie P, Blasco L, Tibbo ME, Leclair O, Kerezoudis P, Chantalat E, et al.,** Peripheral nerve injury associated with a subdermal contraceptive implant: illustrative cases and systematic review of literature, World Neurosurg 111:317–325, 2018.

160. **Odom EB, Eisenberg DL, Fox IK,** Difficult removal of subdermal contraceptive implants: a multidisciplinary approach involving a peripheral nerve expert, Contraception 96:89–95, 2017.

161. **Guiahi M, Tocce K, Teal S, Green T, Rochon P,** Removal of a Nexplanon implant located in the biceps muscle using a combination of ultrasound and fluoroscopy guidance, Contraception 90:606–608, 2014.

162. **del Carmen Cravioto M, Alvarado G, Canto-de-Cetina T, Bassol S, Oropeza G, Santos-Yung R, et al.,** A multicenter comparative study on the efficacy, safety, and acceptability of the contraceptive subdermal implants Norplant and Norplant-II, Contraception 55:359–367, 1997.

163. **Pymar HC, Creinin MD, Schwartz JL,** "Pop-out" method of levonorgestrel implant removal. Contraception 59:383–387, 1999.

164. **Diego D, Tappy E, Carugno J,** Axillary migration of Nexplanon (R): case report, Contraception 95:218–220, 2017.

165. **Kang S, Niak A, Gada N, Brinker A, Jones SC,** Etonogestrel implant migration to the vasculature, chest wall, and distant body sites: cases from a pharmacovigilance database, Contraception 96:439–445, 2017.

166. **Rowlands S, Mansour D, Walling M,** Intravascular migration of contraceptive implants: two more cases, Contraception 95:211–214, 2017.

167. **Heudes P-M, Laigle Querat V, Darnis E, Defrance C, Douane F, Frampas E,** Migration of a contraceptive subcutaneous device into the pulmonary artery. Report of a case, Case Rep Womens Health 8:6–8, 2015.

168. **Chen MJ, Creinin MD,** Removal of a nonpalpable etonogestrel implant with preprocedure ultrasonography and modified vasectomy clamp, Obstet Gynecol 126:935–938, 2015.

169. **Persaud T, Walling M, Geoghegan T, Buckley O, Stunell H, Torreggiani WC,** Ultrasound-guided removal of Implanon (TM) devices, Eur Radiol 18:2582–2585, 2008.

170. **Ortayli N,** Users' perspectives on implantable contraceptives for women, Contraception 65:107–111, 2002.

171. **Madden T, Secura GM, Nease RF, Politi MC, Peipert JF,** The role of contraceptive attributes in women's contraceptive decision making, Am J Obstet Gynecol 213:46.e1–46.e6, 2015.

172. **Donnelly KZ, Foster TC, Thompson R,** What matters most? The content and concordance of patients' and providers' information priorities for contraceptive decision making, Contraception 90:280–287, 2014.

173. Secura GM, Allsworth JE, Madden T, Mullersman JL, Peipert JF, The Contraceptive CHOICE Project: reducing barriers to long-acting reversible contraception, Am J Obstet Gynecol 203:115.e1–115.e7, 2010.

174. Diedrich JT, Desai S, Zhao Q, Secura G, Madden T, Peipert JF, Association of short-term bleeding and cramping patterns with long-acting reversible contraceptive method satisfaction, Am J Obstet Gynecol 212:50.e1–50.e8, 2014.

175. Berenson AB, Wiemann CM, Use of levonorgestrel implants versus oral contraceptives in adolescence: a case-control study, Am J Obstet Gynecol 172:1128–1135; discussion 35–37, 1995.

176. O'Neil-Callahan M, Peipert JF, Zhao Q, Madden T, Secura G, Twenty-four-month continuation of reversible contraception, Obstet Gynecol 122:1083–1091, 2013.

177. Bitzer J, Tschudin S, Alder J; Swiss Implanon Study Group, Acceptability and side-effects of Implanon in Switzerland: a retrospective study by the Implanon Swiss Study Group, Eur J Contracep Reprod Health Care 9:278–284, 2004.

178. Modesto W, Bahamondes MV, Bahamondes L, A randomized clinical trial of the effect of intensive versus non-intensive counselling on discontinuation rates due to bleeding disturbances of three long-acting reversible contraceptives, Hum Reprod 29:1393–1399, 2014.

179. Cohen R, Sheeder J, Arango N, Teal SB, Tocce K, Twelve-month contraceptive continuation and repeat pregnancy among young mothers choosing postdelivery contraceptive implants or postplacental intrauterine devices, Contraception 93:178–183, 2016.

180. Tocce K, Sheeder J, Python J, Teal SB, Long acting reversible contraception in postpartum adolescents: early initiation of etonogestrel implant is superior to IUDs in the outpatient setting, J Pediatr Adolesc Gynecol 25:59–63, 2012.

181. Gariepy AM, Duffy JY, Xu X, Cost-effectiveness of immediate compared with delayed postpartum etonogestrel implant insertion, Obstet Gynecol 126:47–55, 2015.

182. Phillips SJ, Tepper NK, Kapp N, Nanda K, Temmerman M, Curtis KM, Progestogen-only contraceptive use among breastfeeding women: a systematic review, Contraception 94:226–252, 2016.

183. Braga GC, Ferriolli E, Quintana SM, Ferriani RA, Pfrimer K, Vieira CS, Immediate postpartum initiation of etonogestrel-releasing implant: a randomized controlled trial on breastfeeding impact, Contraception 92:536–542, 2015.

184. Carmo L, Braga GC, Ferriani RA, Quintana SM, Vieira CS, Timing of etonogestrel-releasing implants and growth of breastfed infants: a randomized controlled trial, Obstet Gynecol 130:100–107, 2017.

185. Madden T, Eisenberg DL, Zhao Q, Buckel C, Secura GM, Peipert JF, Continuation of the etonogestrel implant in women undergoing immediate postabortion placement, Obstet Gynecol 120:1053–1059, 2012.

186. Mark A, Sonalkar S, Borgatta L, One-year continuation of the etonogestrel contraceptive implant in women with postabortion or interval placement, Contraception 88:619–623, 2013.

187. Rose SB, Garrett SM, Stanley J, Immediate postabortion initiation of levonorgestrel implants reduces the incidence of births and abortions at 2 years and beyond, Contraception 92:17–25, 2015.

188. Cameron ST, Glasier A, Chen ZE, Johnstone A, Dunlop C, Heller R, Effect of contraception provided at termination of pregnancy and incidence of subsequent termination of pregnancy, BJOG 119:1074–1080, 2012.

189. Raymond EG, Weaver MA, Tan YL, Louie KS, Bousieguez M, Lugo-Hernandez EM, et al., Effect of immediate compared with delayed insertion of etonogestrel implants on medical abortion efficacy and repeat pregnancy: a randomized controlled trial, Obstet Gynecol 127:306–312, 2016.

190. Hognert H, Kopp Kallner H, Cameron S, Nyrelli C, Jawad I, Heller R, et al., Immediate versus delayed insertion of an etonogestrel releasing implant at medical abortion-a randomized controlled equivalence trial, Hum Reprod 31:2484–2490, 2016.

167

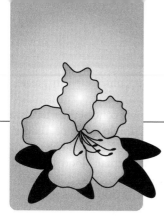

6

Intrauterine Contraception

Jennifer E. Kaiser, MD, MSCI
and David K. Turok, MD, MPH

Nomenclature
For consistency throughout this chapter authors use the term "intrauterine device (IUD)" when referring generically to all intrauterine methods of contraception. We acknowledge intrauterine contraceptive nomenclature can be confusing. For the subset of hormone-releasing devices, we use the term intrauterine system (IUS) to distinguish them and their resultant cervical mucous thickening from others.

Over 200 million women worldwide use intrauterine contraceptives (**Table 6.1**). All currently available IUDs were not marketed prior to 1988. In the United States, IUD use with older products peaked in the mid-1970s with around 2.5 million users, representing about 10% of all contraceptors. These rates declined rapidly through the 1980s, falling by two thirds from 1982 (7.1%) to 1988 (2.0%), reaching a nadir of 0.8% of contraceptive users in 1995.[4] With the introduction of the first levonorgestrel (LNG) IUS in 2000, their popularity in the United States has grown considerably.[6,7] By 2014, 12% of contracepting women used an IUD, and the rate is still climbing.[5] New safety data over the past two decades have driven enthusiasm among reproductive health professionals. The favorable effects on bleeding patterns seen with the new LNG devices and growing interests

Table 6.1 Use of the IUD in the United States, China, and the World[1–5]

	United States	**China**	**Total World**
1981	2.2 million women	42 million	60 million
1988	0.7 million women	59 million	83 million
1995	0.3 million women	75 million	106 million
2007	0.7 million women	>115 million	>180 million
2015	>7.2 million women	>120 million	>219 million

in nonhormonal methods, like copper IUDs, has contributed to greater acceptance by women.

IUDs provide women with the ability to reversibly control their fertility for years following a single placement during a simple office procedure. Current options include the hormone-free copper IUD and LNG IUS; the latter results in significant reductions in menstrual blood loss and discomfort.

Fewer than 1 in 100 women using a modern IUD over many years will experience pregnancy, and unlike short-acting methods like the pill, this success is not altered by user characteristics that affect compliance. Data from the CHOICE study and the Colorado Family Planning initiative (see Chapter 1) demonstrate that offering no cost availability of IUDs increases uptake and improves outcomes. While these data support offering IUDs to all women, clinicians should also recognize that acceptance or continuation of an IUD requires an active choice by the individual. We support a reproductive justice–centered approach to contraceptive counseling and recommendation of IUDs that empowers woman to choose the best method and timing of use for her instead of placing undue emphasis on methods and times deemed "best" by the medical profession.[8,9] No woman should experience coercion to accept or continue with use of an IUD.

History of Modern IUDs

The use of IUDs has a long and colorful history.[10] See the supplemental history chapter for details. Enthusiasm for the first oral contraceptive pills led to the introduction of a variety of mostly inert plastic IUDs of various designs with general good performance and acceptability.

Jaime Zipper of Chile initially suggested the addition of copper to the IUD. His experiments with metals indicated that copper acted locally on the endometrium.[11] Howard Tatum in the United States combined Zipper's suggestion with the development of the T shape to diminish the uterine reaction to the structural frame and produced the copper T. The addition of copper conferred several benefits: (1) the device could be smaller than inert IUDs and still provide effective contraception, (2) a spermicidal effect that resulted in an increase in contraceptive efficacy, and (3) a decrease in removals for pain and bleeding due to the reduction in the size and structure of the frame. The Cu-7 with a copper wound stem was developed in 1971 and quickly became the most popular device in the United States.

In 1970, AH Robbins introduced the Dalkon Shield, a small plastic device and promoted use of the product in young nulliparous women. Within 3 years, reports of serious pelvic infections began to appear in the literature prompting widespread concern about the overall safety of IUDs. These concerns eroded consumer and health care provider confidence in IUD safety and led to a significant decline in IUD use and the withdrawal of all but one device (Progestasert™) from the United States (U.S.) market by the mid-1980s.

We must credit the efforts of investigators who worked to point out the unique problems with the Dalkon Shield and reestablish the overall safety of IUDs that led to the current renaissance in use. Tatum and colleagues[12] pointed out that a serious design flaw (a multifilament removal thread) of the Shield predisposed women to the risk of pelvic infection. Lee and colleagues[13] published the first study that compared PID risk among IUD users to an appropriate control group using nonhormonal methods. They found an increased risk (RR = 8.3, 95% CI = 4.7 to 14.5) of PID confined to Dalkon Shield users, with risk for other devices small and isolated to the first 4 months following placement. In a landmark case-control study assessing infectious antibodies, Hubacher et al.[14] showed that the risk of tubal infertility in nulliparous women was not associated with prior use of a copper IUD.

Although both the Cu-7 and the Tatum-T were withdrawn from the U.S. market in 1986 by G. D. Searle and Company in response to the Dalkon Shield controversy, IUD development continued. More copper was added to the Tatum-T frame by Population Council investigators, leading to the TCu380A (380 mm^2 of exposed copper surface area) with copper wound around the stem plus a copper sleeve on each horizontal arm.[15] The "A" in TCu380A is for "arms," indicating the importance of the copper sleeves. Making the copper solid and tubular increased effectiveness and the lifespan of the IUD. The TCu380A has been in use in more than 30 countries since 1982, and in 1988, it was marketed in the United States as Paragard®.

Although bleeding profiles improved with a smaller device, the copper IUD did not solve the issue of heavy uterine bleeding. In an effort to decrease uterine bleeding, Dr. Tapani Luukkainen developed a long-acting progestin-releasing system by replacing the copper on a Nova-T copper IUD with LNG to create the first LNG-IUS, the Nova-T LNG.[16] This LNG-IUS, containing LNG 52 mg, was first approved in Europe in 1990 for a 5-year duration. In the United States, it was introduced and marketed as the Mirena® IUS in 2000 by Berlex. Since that time, Bayer acquired Mirena and has developed smaller, lower-dose LNG-containing IUSs (Kyleena®, Skyla/Jaydess®). In addition, Medicines360, a nonprofit company, brought an LNG-IUS product of the same size and dose as Mirena to market in the United States (Liletta®) with the goal of ensuring a lower price in the U.S. public sector market and providing LNG-IUS access in the developing world. This same product is comarketed around the world by various companies with names including Levosert® and Avibela®.

Types of IUDs

As we consider the variety of IUDs used over time, it is worth considering two characteristics: shape and component materials. IUDs have been developed in dozens of shapes and variations including rings, coils, Ts, and many other configurations **(Figure 6.1)**. Currently, most common forms use a T shape. The two most common T forms are the Tatum-T whose arms are bent toward the stem to load into the inserter (like a person standing

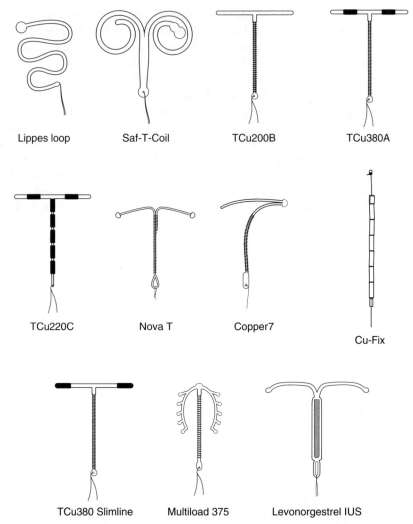

Figure 6.1 Selected IUDs available throughout the world.

with the hands in the front pockets) and the Nova-T whose arms are placed above the stem in the inserter (like a diver with arms above the head). Device component materials can be divided into the following groups: inert, copper, and hormone.

Inert Devices

Inert IUDs generate a local inflammatory reaction. Globally, women used inert steel and plastic IUDs in a range of shapes and sizes for contraception. The Lippes Loop was one popular inert IUD made of polyethylene impregnated with barium sulfate for radiographic identification. Removal of the Dalkon Shield from the U.S. market and data supporting greater efficacy for medicated (e.g., copper and levonorgestrel-containing) devices gradually and completely replaced inert IUDs.

Copper Devices

Since the 1980s, women's health care providers in the United States have had access to only one copper IUD, the T380A (Paragard). The name emphasizes the components: T is the T shape, 380 is the amount of exposed surface area of copper on the polyethylene frame (380 mm^2), and the A stresses the importance of the copper bands on the arms. The bands are why this design has a longer duration of action compared to other available copper IUDs with just copper wire wrapped tightly around the stem. The Food and Drug Administration (FDA) approved the T380A for 10 years although efficacy has been demonstrated up to 12 years[17] and in a limited population up to 20 years.[18]

Over the last three decades, the U.S. market offered one copper IUD from one company. During this same time period, with greater competition and fewer barriers to regulatory approval, the European market provided over 30 different copper IUDs from several companies. These include different shaped devices with different copper quantities. In Europe, copper IUDs are considered devices and not drugs and must only demonstrate safety and not efficacy for approval.

Other TCu380 devices are also available. The TCu380Ag, approved in Finland, is identical to the TCu380A except that the copper wire on the stem has a silver core to prevent fragmentation and extend the lifespan of the copper. The TCu380 Slimline, approved in Canada and the United Kingdom, has tapered copper sleeves flush at the ends of the horizontal arms to facilitate easier loading and insertion. The performance of the TCu380Ag and the TCu380 Slimline is equal to that of the TCu380A.[19,20] Other copper-laden devices used worldwide include the TCu220C, the Nova-T, the Multiload-375, and the Sof-T. The TCu220C has a lower copper load on the Tatum-T frame. The Multiload-375 uses a unique frame that has 375 mm^2 of copper wire wound around its stem. Product developers proposed that the flexible arms with multiple projections to contact the endometrium would minimize expulsions. This is a popular device in many parts of the world though it has similar efficacy and performance compared to the TCu380A.[21] The copper Nova-T uses the same 32 × 32-mm frame as does the LNG-IUS, with 380 mm^2 of copper on the stem only. The Mona Lisa® NT Mini IUD, currently approved in Europe and Canada, uses a smaller (22 × 30 mm) Nova-T frame permitting use of a narrower insertion tube, which could ease placement in some women; this system also wraps 380 mm^2 of copper on the stem only. This device is being compared to the TCu380A in a U.S. randomized controlled trial (ClinicalTrials.gov NCT03124160).

A frameless IUD, the GyneFix® (also known as the Cu-Fix or the FlexiGard) consists of six copper sleeves (330 mm^2 of copper) strung on a surgical nylon (polypropylene) thread that is knotted at one end. Lacking cross-arms, they minimally distort the uterine cavity. The knot is pushed into the myometrium during insertion with a notched needle that works like a miniature harpoon. GyneFix is available in Mexico, Mongolia, Vietnam, Bolivia, Europe, China, Kenya, and Indonesia. Research demonstrated comparable efficacy to the TCu380A IUD over 8 years though more insertion failures, expulsions, and pregnancies in the first year of use.[22,23]

A novel approach to address the increased menstrual pain and bleeding frequently occurring with the TCu380A IUD is the addition of indomethacin in five different Chinese copper IUDs.[24,25] Models of note include the Medicated Gamma Cu380, the Medicated Gamma Cu200, and the Active-γ-IUD. Chinese data demonstrate reduced bleeding and comparable efficacy of these devices when compared to other copper IUDs.[24]

The VeraCept IUD (Sebela Pharmaceuticals, Inc.) is a novel copper IUD on a flexible nickel and titanium alloy frame thought to better accommodate the uterine contour. The insertion tube diameter is narrower than the TCu380A, and the 175 mm² of copper surface area, less than half of the TCu380A, is located just inside the cervical os and bilaterally at the tubal ostia. A randomized control trial (RCT) comparing VeraCept and TCu380A IUD users reported less insertion discomfort, fewer expulsions, and fewer pain or bleeding removals than copper T380A users.[26] A U.S. phase 3 FDA study of this device is under way (ClinicalTrials.gov NCT03633799).

The Hormone-Releasing Intrauterine Systems (IUS)

Hormonal IUDs were developed in the 1970s in Chicago based on the discovery that administering progesterone inside the uterus could have contraceptive benefits. A Finnish doctor, Tapani Luukkainen, created the Progestasert IUS in 1976, which had a 1-year lifespan and never achieved widespread popularity. Sales of the Progestasert were discontinued in 1988.

The use of LNG in a capsule on an IUS stem provides extremely effective and safe contraception while reliably decreasing or eliminating menstrual bleeding. The first LNG-IUS, Mirena, was approved in 1991 in Europe and 2000 in the United States. This T-shaped device has a steroid-releasing reservoir covered by a rate-limiting membrane attached to the vertical stem, which contains LNG 52 mg dispersed in a polydimethylsiloxane capsule. It releases initially at a rate of 20 µg/d in vivo, progressively declining (reaching half of the initial rate after 5 years).[27,28] The European Medicines Agency approved Levosert, another LNG 52 mg IUS made of similar components with reproducible clinical effects, in 2012. In 2015, the U.S. FDA approved its use with the product name Liletta. The FDA currently approves Mirena and Liletta for 5 years, but consistent evidence demonstrates contraceptive efficacy for at least 7 years.[29,30] Manufacturers of both of these LNG-IUS systems have clinical trials in progress seeking to extend the approved duration of use for contraception beyond 5 years, with the Medicines360 study planned for 10 years (ClinicalTrials.gov NCT00995150, NCT02985541).

The LNG-IUS has multiple noncontraceptive benefits. Among these benefits is the ability of the LNG 52 mg IUS to treat heavy menstrual bleeding (HMB), endometrial hyperplasia, and dysmenorrhea. Treatment of HMB is an approved indication throughout the world for Mirena and in every country outside the United States for Liletta[31,32]; a HMB trial for Liletta to have this approval in the United States is currently under way (ClinicalTrials.gov NCT03642210). The LNG 52 mg IUS is about as effective as endometrial ablation for HMB treatment.[33-35] The high local levels of LNG at the endometrium provide strong suppression of proliferation useful for a variety of gynecologic conditions, and the literature supports off-label use for endometrial protection in women using tamoxifen, for postmenopausal women receiving estrogen therapy, for treatment of endometrial hyperplasia, and for dysmenorrhea.[36-43]

Two lower-dose LNG-IUSs are also available. Both have narrower diameter insertion tubes (1 mm narrower) which may facilitate insertion for nulliparous women and cause less initial discomfort with insertion compared to LNG 52 mg IUSs.[44] The FDA approved the LNG 13.5 mg IUS (Skyla) in 2013, which releases 14 µg/d after 24 days and declines to 5 µg/d after 3 years.[45] The FDA approved the LNG 19.5 mg IUS (Kyleena) in 2016. This product releases 17.5 µg/d after 24 days and declines to 7.4 µg/d after 5 years.[45] These lower-dose LNG-IUSs provide lower LNG serum concentrations, lower rates of anovulation, and less amenorrhea at 1 and 3 years compared to LNG 52 mg IUSs **(Table 6.2)**.[45] This may be a benefit for women who desire less bleeding but do not desire amenorrhea; however, users need to be aware that the bleeding is infrequently regular and clinical trials demonstrate discontinuation for bleeding complaints around 5% over 3 years of use for both lower-dose products (compared to 2% for the LNG 52 mg IUS).[51,53] The reduction in insertion discomfort with the lower-dose devices should be weighed against less of a decline in bleeding and amenorrhea without a reduction in cost.[44,51] It is worth noting that the FDA phase 3 ACCESS IUS study for the Liletta 52 mg IUS included 1,011 nulliparous women, 57.7% of participants. The trial demonstrated high efficacy, safety, and continuation among nulliparous women supporting that almost all women are candidates for the larger device.[53] The LNG 52 mg IUS is further distinguished from

175

Table 6.2 Clinical Trial Experience of IUD Use[30,46-52]

	Event Rates (%)				
	Pregnancy	Expulsion	Removal	Amenorrhea	
Device	**1 Year**	**1 Year**	**1 Year**	**1 Year**	**3 Years**
TCu380A	0.5–0.8	5	14	0.05	0.06
LNG 52 mg	0.1–0.2	6	17	19–20	36–37
LNG 19.5 mg	0.2	4	19	12	20
LNG 13.5 mg	0.4	5	22	6	12

lower-dose LNG IUSs as it is approved for treatment of HMB and endo-metrial protection during hormone replacement therapy in many countries (but not the United States). Though we lack comparative studies, the higher local and systemic levels with the 52 mg IUS appear a more sensible choice than lower-dose IUSs for hyperestrogenic situations such as treatment of endometrial hyperplasia, treatment of HMB, and pelvic pain. Still, many women of all ages have concerns about hormonal dose, and counseling for IUD choice should include the pros and cons of the lower-dose systems. While not an approved option for HMB, the lower-dose LNG-IUS offers an alternative to a copper IUD in women with concerning menstrual bleeding or pain histories who would prefer to minimize hormonal dose.

Several companies produce and investigate LNG-IUSs that do not use the Nova-T frame. Available in Europe but not the United States are the 5-year Femilis® LNG 60 mg IUS with a cross-arm width of 28 mm and the 3-year Femilis 40 mg Slim with a width of 24 mm.[24,54] Both of these systems use a novel frame with a solid flexible upper arm design that permits "push-in technique" of the inserter.[55] Developers of the GyneFix and VeraCept copper IUDs are also applying their unique frame designs and inserters to LNG-containing IUSs. The frameless LNG device, called Fibroplant, con-tinues development, and LevoCept, an LNG 52 mg IUS that uses the modi-fied VeraCept (with a minimally wider inserter to accommodate the LNG capsule) has completed a phase 2 study (ClinicalTrials.gov NCT02882191).

IUD Evidence Versus Myths

Over time, conventional wisdom of appropriate IUD usage and practice has changed dramatically. Although the myths below no longer seem relevant given the high acceptance of intrauterine contraception, these misconcep-tions remain in the literature and the minds of some clinicians and women. Very strong evidence now exists to assure the safety of the listed practices. Specific rebuttals to each myth listed below follow in this chapter. We hope this information will lay to rest specific myths associated with IUDs. For reference, the following list includes evidence-based statements addressing some (outdated) common misconceptions among clinicians:

1. IUDs are *NOT* abortifacients.[56-58]
2. IUDs do *NOT* increase the risk of pelvic infection including PID.[19,59]
3. IUDs *CAN* be inserted at the time of screening for gonorrhea and chlamydia.[60-62]
4. IUD use *DOES NOT* increase the risk of infertility.[63-69]
5. IUDs *DO NOT* increase the risk of ectopic pregnancy and *CAN* be used by women with a previous ectopic.[69-76]
6. IUDs *CAN* be used by nulliparous women and adolescents.[53,77-79]
7. IUDs *CAN* be inserted immediately postpartum, including after first- and second-trimester abortions.[80-87]
8. IUDs *CAN* be inserted in HIV-positive women.[88-92]
9. Prophylactic antibiotics are *NOT* necessary prior to IUD insertion.[93]
10. Women at risk for STIs *CAN* use IUDs.[60]

Mechanism of Action

Clinicians require a firm understanding of IUD mechanisms of action to inform potential users and avoid misconceptions, which limit access. Like many drugs, the precise mechanism of action of IUDs is not completely understood. However, strong clinical evidence in aggregate informs us that the timing of IUD effect is almost entirely prefertilization, by preventing sperm-egg union (e.g., contraception). No scientific human data support a postimplantation effect. The American College of Obstetricians and Gynecologists (ACOG) agrees with the biologic definition that pregnancy begins with the implantation of a fertilized egg.[94] As such, IUDs are not abortifacients.[56–58] However, it is unclear if in exceptional situations IUD alterations of the endometrium prevent a fertilized egg from implanting.[95] The correct term for inhibition of implantation is contragestion (contragestation) and not abortion. Here, we review the objective scientific data explaining critical components of IUD action. The high efficacy of modern IUDs suggests multiple mechanisms at play, and these may vary by several factors including IUD type and time that the IUD is in place relative to last act of intercourse. For the interested reader, we recommend Ortiz and Croxatto's rigorous review of the objective data on this subject.[57]

All IUD types create inflammatory, spermicidal environments in the endometrial cavity that prevent fertilization.[57,96] Inert IUDs significantly increase the number of inflammatory cells in the uterine cavity, which release cytotoxic substances. The increased protein content in the endometrium of inert IUD users reflects cellular degradation from neutrophils and macrophages. These inflammatory cells have been shown to phagocytize sperm.[97] While these inflammatory cells may also create a hostile uterine environment to negatively affect implantation, we lack direct evidence of this effect. High failure rates with inert devices likely occur due to more fertilizations. This led to the development of medicated IUDs.

The addition of copper to IUDs provides a release of free copper and copper salts that have spermicidal effect. Copper also has both a biochemical and morphologic impact on the endometrium and cervix producing alterations in cervical mucus and endometrial secretions. These include a sterile inflammatory response, marked by production in the endometrium of cytokine peptides known to be cytotoxic to sperm and inhibition of various endometrial enzymes.[98] Direct evidence from detailed clinical experiments has shown that very few, if any, sperm reach the ovum in the fallopian tube. In women using copper IUDs, sensitive assays for human chorionic gonadotropin do not find evidence of fertilization.[99,100] This is consistent with the fact that the copper IUD protects against both intrauterine and ectopic pregnancies.

The LNG-IUSs add the endometrial action of the progestin to the foreign body reaction. This hormonal action leads to endometrial decidualization, deceased response to estrogen through down-regulation of progesterone receptors, and atrophy of the glands causing a predictable decrease in bleeding frequency and intensity. We do not have evidence that these endome-

177

trial changes provide a primary contraceptive effect.[101] The available data strongly support prevention of fertilization via thickened mucus as the primary mechanism of action in LNG-IUS users. The high local release of LNG leads to the development of a progestin-mediated thickening of cervical mucus. This was demonstrated by light microscopy of cervical mucus, which showed a barrier to sperm penetration in LNG-IUS users compared to nonhormonal users (**Figure 6.2**).[102] The high efficacy of the LNG-IUS in preventing pregnancy is incontrovertible. This is most likely due to lack of sperm penetration through highly unfavorable cervical mucus. Limitations of the certainty of this statement come from the lack of scientific data demonstrating the quantity, motility, and function of sperm with LNG-IUS use. However, high levels of local LNG may have deleterious effects on sperm-egg interaction through interference with sperm transport, capacitation, and the acrosome reaction.[103] In addition, LNG delivered from the IUD may impair oviduct transport via an effect on tubal motility.[104-106] Efficacy may also be augmented by modest decreases in ovulatory function during early use of the LNG-IUS. After the first year, cycles are ovulatory in 50% to 75% of women, regardless of their bleeding patterns.[107]

Several studies have flushed the uterine cavity through the cervix or an excised portion of the fallopian tube at the time of surgery to assess for the presence of sperm and fertilized ova. The most robust clinical data come from a 1988 prospective assessment by Alvarez et al. In this study, researchers flushed the uterus and fallopian tubes of two groups of women undergoing

Figure 6.2 Effect of intrauterine delivery of levonorgestrel on cervical mucus. *In vitro* sperm penetration through cervical mucus obtained at midcycle from women using a LNG 52 mg IUS (*left panel*) and from controls using no hormonal method (*right panel*). The thick wall of mucus created in response to the presence of the LNG-IUS demonstrates its primary mechanism of action. Sperm (*small white dots*) is present throughout the control sample and absent from the thick mucus produced in users of the LNG-IUS. (Reprinted from **Lewis RA, Taylor D, Natavio MF, Melamed A, Felix J, Mishell D Jr,** Effects of the levonorgestrel-releasingintrauterine system on cervical mucus quality and sperm penetrability, Contraception 82(6):491–496, 2010. Copyright © 2010 Elsevier. With permission.)

salpingectomy within 132 hours of the LH peak. The experimental group included 56 women with a variety of inert, copper and hormonal IUDs. Their tubal flushings were compared to 115 women using no contraception. The tubal flushings returned eggs from 39% of IUD users and 56% of control participants. The uterine flushing returned no eggs from IUD users and 4 from the 115 control subjects. A subset of participants with retrieved eggs reported intercourse from 70 hours before to 11 hours after the LH peak and had evidence of spermatozoa in their cervical mucus. None of the 14 IUD users had eggs with evidence of fertilization versus 10 of 20 control participants whose eggs showed 2- to 8-cell postfertilization development.[108]

The accumulation of data demonstrates that sperm transport to the potential site of fertilization is severely compromised in IUD users. The lack of sperm and egg interaction explains the vast majority of IUD efficacy. Although pregnancies uncommonly occur in IUD users, the methods are not 100% effective. This provides strong evidence against a hostile endometrial environment that prevents implantation as a primary mechanism for the contraceptive effect. Our best evidence supports that in general use, an IUD functions as a contraceptive and prevents fertilization. When this primary mechanism fails, the fertilized egg has the opportunity to implant in the fallopian tube or uterine cavity, or fail to implant. While the presence of an IUD may reduce the potential of a fertilized egg to successfully implant, we lack direct experimental evidence of this effect.

Emergency Contraception

Under typical use, IUDs prevent fertilization and have a contraceptive mechanism of action. However, copper IUDs appear to have a contragestive effect when placed during the preimplantation window. This allows use of a copper IUD for emergency contraception up to 5 days after ovulation following unprotected intercourse. High levels of copper, present due to burst release following copper IUD placement, likely contribute to this enhanced effect.[109] The fact that copper IUDs function well for emergency contraception does not support an effect on implantation as a primary mechanism of action during regular contraception. We have no evidence for use of the LNG-IUS for emergency contraception. (see discussion of clinical use of IUDs for emergency contraception on page 201).

Noncontraceptive Benefits of the IUD

The LNG-IUS and the copper IUD both provide many noncontraceptive benefits (**Box 6.1**). The LNG 52 mg IUS is an effective treatment for heavy uterine and abnormal uterine bleeding (AUB). Through down-regulation of endometrial estrogen receptors, the endometrium becomes inactive with decreased proliferation and bleeding. The effect of local LNG is more effective than the administration of oral progestins, combined hormonal contraceptives, or inhibitors of prostaglandin synthesis and compares favorably with surgical treatment (hysterectomy or endometrial ablation).[33,110–119]

Box 6.1 Summary of Noncontraceptive Benefits of the IUD (Approved Indications in the United States Noted Where Applicable)

- Reduction of heavy menstrual bleeding (FDA approved for Mirena), abnormal uterine bleeding, and improvement of related anemia (LNG 52 mg)[33,72–85]
- Reduction of menstrual bleeding in women with hemostatic disorders and in anticoagulated women (LNG 52 mg)[87–93]
- Treatment of primary dysmenorrhea (LNG 52 mg)[116]
- Reduction of myoma prevalence as well as uterine volume and bleeding associated with myomas (LNG 52 mg)[94,98–101]
- Treatment of endometriosis and pain associated with endometriosis (LNG 52 mg)[52,53,117–124]
- Suppression of endometriosis (LNG 52 mg)[43,106–108,110–114]
- Decrease in uterine volume and pain associated with adenomyosis (LNG 52 mg)[115]
- Protection against polyps associated with postmenopausal estrogen therapy or tamoxifen treatment (LNG 52 mg)[36,38–42,117–119]
- Reduction of endometrial cancer risk (copper and LNG)[125–128]
- Conservative treatment of endometrial hyperplasia or low-risk endometrial cancer (LNG 52 mg)[52,120–124,129]
- Prevention of ectopic pregnancy (copper and LNG)[130–135]
- Protection against pelvic infection (LNG 52 mg)[57,136,137]

Initial clinical observations that users of the LNG 52 mg IUS for contraception experienced high rates of discontinuation for amenorrhea led to clinical studies designed to evaluate this as a health benefit and improve counseling regarding expected bleeding patterns. The LNG 52 mg IUS rapidly decreases dysmenorrhea and menstrual blood loss (about 40% to 50%). Bleeding over time can be reduced by 90%, with 1 in 5 women becoming amenorrheic 1 year after insertion (actually this rate is achieved by 9 months) and 1 in 3 by 3 years **(Table 6.2)**.[120–122,138] Amenorrhea rates remain around 40% through 5 years of use.[123] Average long-term hemoglobin and iron levels increase compared with preinsertion values.[123] The LNG 19.5 mg IUS and LNG 13.5 mg IUS result in lower rates of amenorrhea at 1 and 3 years **(Table 6.2)**.[139] Bleeding patterns for all LNG-IUSs improve over time with decreases in the number of spotting and bleeding days.[51,52]

Additionally, the LNG 52 mg IUS can be safely and effectively used in women with inherited bleeding disorders and in women using anticoagulation therapy to reduce heavy bleeding. In small retrospective studies, women with inherited bleeding disorders (von Willebrand's disease being the most common) saw a significant decrease in the amount of bleeding and an amenorrhea rate of 56% at 9 months.[124] In a study of women on warfarin therapy, 87% experienced a reduction in menstrual blood loss with the

LNG-IUS.[129] However, these women may require earlier replacement (e.g., before 5 years) of the LNG-IUS if heavy bleeding returns.[124–127,129,140,141]

The LNG 52 mg IUS also reduces bleeding in the presence of leiomyomas.[128,142–145] Limited evidence supports that the LNG-IUS reduces the prevalence of leiomyomas and decreases uterine volume.[19,128,142,143,146] The presence of uterine leiomyomas may also lead to higher IUD expulsion rates. However, use of the LNG-IUS should be considered in women with fibroids due to the benefit of achieving reduced blood flow in up to 90% and amenorrhea in up to 44.5%.[143,147,148] The presence of a submucosal leiomyoma is a relative contraindication to use of the LNG-IUS, as these women may not respond favorably to treatment and placement may be more difficult.[149]

The LNG 52 mg IUS has been used successfully to treat endometriosis and especially pelvic pain and dysmenorrhea associated with endometriosis.[43,150–154] Results appear similar to those achieved with gonadotropin-releasing hormone agonist treatment for pain, and the IUS provides long-lasting benefit.[155] The advantages of LNG-IUS treatment of endometriosis include many years of efficacy, fewer side effects, and contraception. The LNG-IUS also effectively reduces uterine volume and relieves dysmenorrhea secondary to adenomyosis.[130,131,156] Likewise, the 52 mg LNG-IUS decreases the severity of primary dysmenorrhea.[132] The LNG 52 mg IUS effectively protects the endometrium against hyperplasia and polyps in women using tamoxifen or postmenopausal estrogen therapy.[36,38–42,133–135] In addition, this IUS can be used to treat endometrial hyperplasia and low-risk endometrial cancer in patients desiring conservative management.[157–163] Comparison studies indicate that the LNG-IUS is as effective as, and probably better than, standard treatment with an oral progestin.[161,164,165] However, clinicians should keep in mind that these represent off-label indications in the United States, and the use of an LNG-IUS is contraindicated in women with breast cancer though clinical judgement and user preference could prompt use in progestin receptor negative disease.

The lower-dose LNG-IUS should also provide endometrial protection during estrogen replacement therapy, but clinicians should keep in mind the differences between the systems and expected duration of action. The LNG 52 mg IUS initial release rate of approximately 20 µg/d declines to about 10 µg/d after 5 years; the 19.5 mg IUS starts at 17.5 µg/d and decreases to 7.4 µg/d after 5 years; and the 13.5 mg IUS initially releases 12.6 µg/d and decreases to 5 µg/d after 3 years.[28,166] Raudaskoski and colleagues[167] randomized women taking oral estradiol valerate to either oral medroxyprogesterone acetate (MPA) or one of two LNG-IUSs; the standard LNG 52 mg IUS with an initial LNG release of 20 µg/d or a prototype "menopausal levonorgestrel system (MLS)" with an initial release of 10 µg/d system on a small Nova-T frame. None of the women treated with the 52 mg IUS showed proliferative endometrium at 1 year, compared to 2.1% in the MLS and 38% in the MPA group.

The copper IUD may likewise reduce the risk of endometrial cancer based on epidemiologic data.[168–171] In studies from the 1980s and 1990s, the use of copper IUDs was associated with a 30% reduced risk of invasive cervical cancer.[172] Studies have not evaluated the effects of the LNG-IUS on cervical cancer risk.

Although the LNG-IUS reliably provides good protection against endometrial hyperplasia, clinicians should maintain a high degree of suspicion when unusual bleeding occurs and consider assessing the endometrium. Rare cases of endometrial adenocarcinoma have been reported in users of the LNG-IUS.[173,174] As noted, however, many studies have documented protection against and even regression of endometrial hyperplasia. While the presence of the IUD makes assessment of the endometrial thickness by ultrasound challenging, in our experience, a reliable measurement is possible in most cases.

Lastly, the LNG-IUS may protect against pelvic infection. In a randomized 5-year trial comparing a copper IUD with the LNG 52 mg IUS, the pelvic infection rate was lower than the incidence in the general population with both devices, but the rate with the LNG-IUS was significantly lower compared with the copper IUD.[59] A 7-year randomized trial comparing a copper IUD and LNG 52 mg IUS found declining pelvic inflammatory disease (PID) rates with long-term use of both devices, but selection bias likely influenced this result.[19]

Efficacy of IUDs

Intrauterine Pregnancy

The TCu380A is approved for use in the United States for 10 years. However, this device has been demonstrated to maintain its efficacy over at least 12 years of use.[17] Use through 20 years was associated with a very low risk of pregnancy in a small number of users.[18] The LNG 52 mg IUS (Mirena and Liletta) is FDA approved for 5 years, but can be used for at least 7 years and possibly longer.[21,175] The American College of Obstetricians and Gynecologists (ACOG) supports a 2-year extension beyond FDA approval for maximum use of both the copper T380 IUD and the LNG 52 mg IUS to 12 and 7 years, respectively.[79]

The extension to 7 years of use for the LNG 52 mg IUS is based on a WHO randomized trial that allocated women to either a copper IUD or LNG 52 mg IUS with 7 years' follow-up. In the LNG-IUS group, 1,884 women had IUS placement; 398 completed the 7 years of follow-up with the remainder either discontinuing the method or lost to follow-up. Pregnancy rate at 7 years for the LNG-IUS was 0.53 per 100 women with no pregnancies occurring in the years 6 and 7.[21] Study limitations include the low proportion of women contributing 7 years of data. Additional data supporting 7 years of use for the LNG 52 mg IUS come from prospective clinical data demonstrating continued low pregnancy risk and sustained LNG effect with a thin endometrial stripe (2.8 ± 0.1 mm) and continued amenorrhea for 42% of users.[29] Hormonal IUSs will retain similar efficacy to inert devices even after the cessation of hormone release (failure rate of 1 to 4.8 per 100 woman-years).[176] Clinicians should also be aware that decreasing fecundity with increasing patient age may also contribute to the prolonged efficacy beyond FDA approval of these devices. Therefore, clinicians should take an individualized approach to counseling women about prolonged use.

Pregnancy and expulsion rates at 1 year of use are low for both types of IUDs and removal rates at 1 year are similar (**Tables 6.2 and 6.3**). With increasing duration of use and increasing age, failure rate decrease, as do removals for pain and bleeding (**Table 6.3**). Women use IUDs longer than other reversible methods of contraception. In a 3-year follow-up of contraceptive users, 70% of LNG-IUS and copper IUD users were still using

Table 6.3 Seven-Year Experience with the TCu380A and the LNG 52 mg IUS

	Cumulative Rates per 100 Users per Year			
	Year			
	1	3	5	7
Copper IUD				
Pregnancy	0.4	1.5	1.9	2.5
Expulsion	3.5	5.6	7.3	8.8
Increased bleeding removal	2.4	4.6	7.4	9.9
Pain removal	1.7	3.6	5.0	7.4
All IUD discontinuations	9.9	20.5	30.8	40.8
Number starting each year	1,871	1,587	1,270	989
LNG 52 mg IUS				
Pregnancy	0.1	0.4	0.5	0.5
Expulsion	2.9	5.2	6.3	8.2
Increased bleeding removal	2.8	3.7	4.3	6.0
Pain removal	2.1	4.0	5.3	6.1
All IUD discontinuations	16.5	38.2	52.5	70.6
Number starting each year	1,884	1,491	1,000	717

From **Rowe P, Farley T, Peregoudov A, Piaggio G, Boccard S, Landoulsi S, et al.,** Safety and efficacy in parous women of a 52-mg levonorgestrel-medicated intrauterine device: a 7-year randomized comparative study with the TCu380A, Contraception 93(6):498–506, 2016.

their method at 3 years compared to 31% of users of short-acting reversible contraceptives.[177]

Expulsion

Approximately 3% to 4% of patients spontaneously expel the LNG 52 mg IUS and TCu380A within the first year.[30] Women younger than age 20 may have a higher expulsion rate than older women, although more recent studies have not borne this out.[178-180] A range of expulsion rates are reported for adolescents. A recent systematic review and meta-analysis found that 8% of adolescents completed their IUD use with an expulsion. This included expulsion rates as low as 2% to 4% with interval insertions and as high as 21% with postpartum insertion.[181] An expulsion event typically presents with cramping, vaginal discharge, or uterine bleeding. However, in some cases, the only observable change is lengthening or absence of the IUD removal threads. Patients with symptoms suggestive of expulsion should be seen urgently, preferably by a clinician experienced in the management of IUD problems. Partial expulsion is diagnosed by presence of the IUD stem in the cervix by ultrasound or visualization of the IUD stem protruding through the cervix on speculum exam. If pregnancy or infection is not present and the patient desires to continue intrauterine contraception, then a new IUD can be inserted immediately.[182] If an IUD is not replaced, alternative contraception must be provided. If ultrasound findings demonstrate an IUD is in the endometrial cavity above the cervix but not at the fundus, an LNG IUS can remain in place. Management is less clear with a copper IUD. Efficacy may be affected, and consideration for removal and new contraception provision should be given.

Ectopic Pregnancy

The previous use of an IUD does not increase the risk of a subsequent ectopic pregnancy and the history of a prior ectopic is not a contraindication for IUD use.[69,70,73,76] The current use of an IUD offers some protection against ectopic pregnancy.[70-75] A WHO multicenter study concluded that IUD users were 50% less likely to have an ectopic pregnancy when compared with women using no contraception.[70] This is due to the exceedingly low number of fertilizations that occur with use of an IUD.

The lowest ectopic pregnancy rates are seen with the most effective IUDs, like the TCu380A and LNG-IUS. Users of the LNG-IUS are 90% less likely than noncontraceptors to experience an ectopic pregnancy **(Table 6.4)**.[184] In a prospective cohort study comparing the copper IUD and LNG-IUS, the proportion of ectopic pregnancies among all contraceptive failures was 15% and 27%, respectively. As reviewed under mechanisms of action, reduction in tubal motility by the LNG-IUS may lead to this increased ectopic rate over the copper IUD. However, as the overall risk of failure is much lower among LNG-IUS users, the adjusted hazard ratio for ectopic pregnancy among LNG-IUS users compared to copper IUD users was 0.26 (95% CI = 0.10 to 0.66).[185] In addition, the lower rate of ectopic among copper IUD

Table 6.4 Ectopic Pregnancy Rates per 1,000 Woman-Years

	Rate per 1,000 Woman-Years
Noncontraceptive users, all ages	3.00–4.50
LNG 52 mg IUD	0.20
TCu380A IUD	0.20–0.8

From **Sivin I,** Dose- and age-dependent ectopic pregnancy risks with intrauterine contraception, Obstet Gynecol 78:291, 1991; **Heinemann K, Reed S, Moehner S, Minh TD,** Comparative contraceptive effectiveness of levonorgestrel-releasing and copper intrauterine devices: the European Active Surveillance Study for Intrauterine Devices, Contraception 91(4):280–283, 2015; **Franks AL, Beral V, Cates W, Hogue CJR,** Contraception and ectopic pregnancy risk, Am J Obstet Gynecol 163:1120, 1990.[183]

users suggests that postfertilization interruption is not a major mechanism of action by which the copper IUD prevents pregnancy during typical use.

The risk of ectopic pregnancy does not increase with increasing duration of use with the TCu380A or the LNG-IUS.[19,186] In a 7-year prospective study, not a single ectopic pregnancy was encountered with the LNG-IUS, and in a 5-year study, only one.[19,59] In 8,000 woman-years of experience in randomized multicenter trials, there was only a single ectopic pregnancy reported with the TCu380A.[19] Therefore, the risk of ectopic pregnancy during the use of the copper IUD or the LNG-IUS is much lower compared with noncontraceptive users; however, if pregnancy occurs, the likelihood of an ectopic pregnancy is high.[185] Thus, if a pregnancy is diagnosed with either type of IUD in place, an ultrasound should be obtained immediately to confirm location. The protection against ectopic pregnancy provided by the overall high contraception effect of the TCu380A and the LNG-IUS makes these IUDs acceptable choices for contraception in women with previous ectopic pregnancies.

Side Effects

Significant side effects with use of either the copper or LNG IUD are rare. The symptoms most often responsible for IUD discontinuation are increased uterine bleeding and increased menstrual pain. Both LNG and copper IUDs produce predictable patterns of increased bleeding with early use that improve over time. For LNG 52 mg IUS users frequent and prolonged bleeding occurs in the first 3 months that dramatically declines by the second 3 months of use with one fifth (19%) having amenorrhea by a year and over one third (36%) by 3 years.[53] These patterns are similar with lower-dose LNG-IUSs, but amenorrhea by 1 year is less frequent (12% for LNG 19.5 mg IUS).[187] Cu T380A users continue to have regular menses throughout use with bleeding and cramping increasing with insertion and gradually decreasing over the first 6 months.[188]

Over 3 years of follow-up, the rate of premature discontinuation for pain or bleeding was higher among women choosing a copper IUD (35% bleeding, 17% pain) compared with the LNG 52 mg IUS (19% and 11%).[177] Bleeding and cramping are most severe in the first 3 months after IUD insertion. In a survey of self-reported bleeding and pain at 3 months post insertion, 15% of LNG 52 mg IUS users and 70% of copper IUD users reported heavier bleeding. Similarly, 32% of LNG 52 mg IUS and 63% of copper IUD users experienced increased cramping. Although women reported similar rates of cramping for each type of IUD at 6 months, 62% of LNG 52 mg IUS users reported lighter bleeding, and 55% reported less frequent bleeding at 6 months compared to 3 months. Among copper IUD users, 72% reported no change of bleeding frequency between 3 and 6 months.[189] Based on these data, women with prolonged, HMB or significant dysmenorrhea may not be able to tolerate a copper IUD but may benefit from an LNG IUS.[120]

Because bleeding and cramping are most severe in the first few months after IUD insertion, treatment with a nonsteroidal anti-inflammatory drug (NSAID, an inhibitor of prostaglandin synthesis) during early IUD use can be beneficial for copper and LNG users. For LNG IUS users, an RCT showed that naproxen 500 mg twice daily for the first week of each of the first 3 months of use was superior to estradiol and placebo for control of irregular bleeding following LNG-IUS initiation, but no intervention was highly effective.[190] For copper IUD users NSAIDs are modestly effective in reducing pain and bleeding with early use in the first 6 months though they are not effective in reducing pain with insertion or decreasing IUD discontinuation.[191,192]

Following insertion of a modern copper IUD, measured menstrual blood loss increases by about 55%, and this level of bleeding may continue for the duration of IUD use.[193] However, a more recent study from China showed a mean increase in bleeding of 25% confined to the first year of copper IUD use.[194] Women typically experience a slight (1 to 2 day) prolongation of menstruation and/or use of an additional pad or tampon each day. Over a year's time, this amount of blood loss does not result in changes indicative of iron deficiency (e.g., serum ferritin), but with longer use, ferritin levels decline suggesting a depletion of iron stores.[195] Assessment for iron depletion and anemia should be considered in long-term users of copper IUDs and in women susceptible to iron deficiency anemia. In populations with a high prevalence of anemia, these changes occur more rapidly, and iron supplementation is recommended.[196] While most women tolerate this amount of menstrual blood loss, women with baseline heavy bleeding require more diligent monitoring.

Because of the antiproliferative effect on the endometrium, amenorrhea can develop over time with the LNG-releasing IUS. With the LNG 52 mg IUS, 70% of patients are oligomenorrheic and 30% to 40% are amenorrheic within 2 years.[122,197] In a group of women who used the LNG 52 mg IUS in consecutive 5-year cycles for more than 12 years, 60% were amenorrheic; 12% experienced infrequent, scanty bleeding; and 28% had regular but light bleeding.[123] This effect on menstruation contributes to an increase in blood hemoglobin levels and no adverse health effects.[19,198] However, not all women desire or tolerate amenorrhea, so this possibility must be discussed in counseling for the device.

Progestin-related side effects such as acne, hirsutism, weight gain, and mood changes can occur with use of the LNG IUSs. Women who use combined hormonal products typically have reduced symptoms of acne in part due to the increase in sex hormone–binding globulin (SHBG) induced by ethynyl estradiol. This effect rapidly decreases after discontinuation of a combined method. The low levels of circulating LNG in users of the IUS do not suppress SHBG, but the androgenic properties of LNG may affect some users.[199] Circulating plasma levels of LNG in LNG-IUS users are one half those in contraceptive implant users and ten times less than those in progestin-only pill users.[200,201] There are no significant metabolic effects, including changes in glucose, insulin sensitivity, and lipids.[202] In a large postmarketing survey, the incidence of breast cancer in users of the LNG-IUS was equivalent to that in the general population.[203] The combination of the LNG-IUS and estrogen therapy in postmenopausal women did not increase breast density.[204]

Some women report increased vaginal discharge while using an IUD. A small prospective study found no difference in the vaginal microbiome of users of the LNG 52 mg IUS.[205] Another study demonstrated an increased association of IUD use with bacterial vaginosis (BV), but that the risk was confined to women experiencing irregular bleeding.[206] Vaginal complaints deserve examination for the presence of vaginal or cervical infection. Treatment can be provided with the IUD remaining in place.

Long-term use of the IUD is associated with impressive safety and lack of serious side effects. In a 7-year prospective study, the use of either the copper IUD or the LNG 52 mg IUS beyond 5 years led to no increase in pelvic infection, no increase in ectopic pregnancy rates, no increase in anemia, and no increase in abnormal Pap tests.[19]

The copper IUD is not affected by magnetic resonance imaging (MRI), and therefore, the copper IUD need not be removed before MRI, and neither patients nor workers need be excluded from MRIs or the MRI environment.[207,208]

Complications

Infections

The concern over the association of IUDs and PID has waned greatly since the era of the Dalkon Shield. Multiple studies show the protective benefit of the LNG IUS and copper IUD against PID, as well as the rare occurrence of PID in long-term users.[13,59,136,209,210] In a randomized, 5-year trial comparing a copper IUD with the LNG IUS, pelvic infection was lower than the incidence in a general population, but the rate with the LNG-IUS was significantly lower compared with the copper IUD.[59] IUD-related bacterial infection may rarely occur due to contamination of the endometrial cavity at the time of insertion. Mishell and colleagues[211] classic study indicated that the uterus is routinely contaminated by bacteria at insertion but that this rarely results in infection. In a WHO study of over 22,000 IUD insertions, the risk of infection was six times higher during the 20 days after insertion compared to a later time (9.7 vs. 1.4 per 1,000 woman-years).[212] The background rate of sexually transmitted infections (STIs) influenced the risk as did the study location. Based on these data and a Cochrane review, prophylactic antibiotics at time of IUD placement are not recommended.[93]

Older recommendations included use of prophylactic antibiotics and completion of *Neisseria gonorrhoeae* (GC) and *Chlamydia trachomatis* (CT) screening prior to insertion. In a prospective cohort study of over 1,700 LNG 52 mg IUS insertions, screening was completed in 80% and 63% of women for CT and GC, respectively, at the time of insertion. The overall risk of PID was 0.2%.[62] A retrospective study of nearly 58,000 IUD insertions (of both types of IUDs) found an overall risk of PID of 0.5% whether patients were screened on the same day of insertion, within 3 months of insertion, or never screened.[61] Lastly, a prospective study of 5,000 insertions of both types of IUDs found that adopting a risk-based strategy for GC/CT screening (age ≤ 25, multiple sexual partners, inconsistent condom use, and/or history of an STI) at the time of IUD insertion will miss approximately 0.7% of infections.[60] In light of this evidence, current guidelines for STI screening should be followed, and if chlamydia and gonorrhea screenings are indicated they should be performed at the time of insertion.[213,214] Despite low rates of PID among IUD users, at-risk women should still be counseled on continued dual use of condoms for the prevention of STIs as part of their routine preventive health care.

Asymptomatic IUD users whose genital testing demonstrates gonorrhea or Chlamydia infection should receive Centers for Disease Control–recommended treatments without removal of the IUD. In IUD users diagnosed with PID or tubal infection (as evidenced by cervical motion tenderness, abdominal rebound tenderness, adnexal tenderness or masses, or elevated white blood count and sedimentation rate), prompt initiation of appropriate antibiotic coverage should initially occur with the device in place **(Box 6.2)**. Based on consensus recommendations, if no clinical improvement is noted within 48 to 72 hours of treatment initiation, removal of the IUD should be considered.[88] Data are currently lacking to guide management of tubo-ovarian abscess with an IUD in situ. An acceptable management protocol, again based on consensus recommendations, would be to treat with intravenous antibiotics and consider IUD removal if no clinical improvement.[215]

Vaginal infections such as BV, vaginal *Candida* infection, and trichomoniasis should be treated appropriately with the IUD remaining in place. There is conflicting evidence that IUDs increase the prevalence of BV; however, in one longitudinal study comparing IUD users to combined hormonal contraceptive users (pills, patch, vaginal ring), there was no difference in rates of BV after adjusted analysis.[206,216–220] Another coloniz-

---

> ### Box 6.2 Centers for Disease Control PID Treatment Guidelines[214]
>
> *Appropriate outpatient management of less severe infections:*
>
> Ceftriaxone (250 mg intramuscularly once) plus doxycycline (100 mg orally twice daily), for 14 days
> Cefoxitin (2 g intramuscularly once) plus probenecid (1 g orally once) plus doxycycline (100 mg orally twice daily), for 14 days
> Metronidazole (500 mg orally twice daily) for 14 days may be added to either above regimen
>
> *Severe infections require hospitalization and treatment with:*
>
> Cefoxitin (2 g intravenous every 6 hours) or cefotetan (2 g intravenous every 12 hours)
> Plus doxycycline (100 mg every 12 hours orally or intravenous)
> Clindamycin (900 mg intravenous every 8 hours) plus gentamicin (intravenous loading dose 2 mg/kg followed by 1.5 mg/kg every 8 hours)
> Followed by 14 days of doxycycline (100 mg orally twice daily)
>
> *The following is an alternative regimen:*
>
> Ampicillin-sulbactam (3 g intravenous every 6 hours) plus doxycycline (100 mg twice daily)

ing microbe of the vagina is the gram-positive bacilli *Actinomyces*. This organism is most frequently detected on routine cervical cytology. Prior literature has cited the prevalence of *Actinomyces*-like organisms in the vagina at 7%; however, more recent studies indicate a prevalence closer to 0.26%, which may vary by geographic location.[221,222] When found in the absence of symptoms, patients do not require treatment or removal of their IUD.[79,222] If signs or symptoms of PID are present in the setting of detected *Actinomyces*, IUD removal should be considered.

For suspected simple endometritis, in which uterine tenderness is the only physical finding, one treatment approach is doxycycline (100 mg b.i.d. for 14 days).[223] Again, leave the IUD in place for initial treatment.

There was a suggestion (in cross-sectional studies) that IUD use (type of IUD unspecified in the studies) increased the risk of human immunodeficiency virus (HIV) transmission from man to woman, especially when the IUD was inserted or removed during exposure to the infected man.[224,225] However, this is not a strong suggestion, because the risk with IUD use was ascertained compared with other contraceptive methods (which can protect against transmission) and the many and various influencing factors are difficult to adjust and control. In a randomized trial of almost 8,000 African women at risk for HIV infection, there was no difference in the prevalence of new HIV infection among those who received depot medroxyprogesterone acetate injection, the copper IUD, or the LNG contraceptive implant.[226] In the only study assessing, female-to-male HIV transmission with IUD use no evidence of transmission was detected.[227] HIV-infected women who utilize IUDs for contraception *do not* have a greater incidence of complications (including PID), and genital shedding of HIV is not affected.[89-92] The CDC Medical Eligibility Criteria for Contraception provides a "2" recommendation (advantages outweigh potential risks) for initiation or continuation of either an LNG or a copper IUD in women with HIV.

Hepatitis C virus is believed to be transmitted with sexual contact. A cross-sectional study in Turkey indicated that Cu IUD use by women in stable, monogamous relationships did not increase the incidence of hepatitis C seropositivity.[228]

Pregnancy with an IUD In Situ

Spontaneous Miscarriage

Spontaneous miscarriage occurs more frequently among women who become pregnant with IUDs in place, a rate of approximately 40% to 75%. If the IUD is removed, the miscarriage rate falls to 8% to 27%.[229] Therefore, IUDs should always be removed if pregnancy is diagnosed and the string is visible. When strings are not visible, the use of sonographic guidance and alligator forceps, Bozeman packing forceps, or a curved Kelly forceps is reasonable. In a case series of 82 pregnancies with IUDs in situ with no strings visible, sonographic guidance resulted in the successful removal of 81 of the 82 IUDs with comparable rates of miscarriage and preterm birth to studies where strings were visible.[229,230] Hysteroscopy provides an alternative to ultrasound guidance when the IUD is below the implanted gestation.

Septic Abortion

In the past, if the IUD could not be easily removed from a pregnant uterus, the patient was offered induced abortion because it was believed that the risk of life-threatening septic, spontaneous miscarriage in the second trimester was increased 20-fold if the pregnancy continued with the IUD in utero. However, this belief was derived from experiences with the Dalkon Shield. There is no evidence that there is an increased risk of septic abortion if pregnancy occurs with an IUD in place other than the Shield.[231,232] There were no deaths in the United States from 1977 to 1993 among women pregnant with an IUD.[233] While septic abortion is no longer the concern with an IUD in situ, other complications still support removal of the device even if continuation of pregnancy desired.

If a patient plans to terminate a pregnancy that has occurred with an IUD in place, the IUD should be removed immediately. If there is no evidence of infection, the IUD can safely be removed in a clinic or office.

If an IUD is in an infected, pregnant uterus, removal of the device should be undertaken only after antibiotic therapy has been initiated, and equipment for cardiovascular support and resuscitation is immediately available. These precautions are necessary because removal of an IUD from an infected, pregnant uterus can lead to septic shock.

Congenital Anomalies

There is no evidence that exposure of a fetus to medicated IUDs is harmful. The risk of congenital anomalies is not increased among infants born to women who become pregnant with an IUD in place.[231,234] A case-control study did not find an increased incidence of IUD use in pregnancies resulting in limb-reduction deformities.[235] There is theoretical concern of exposure of the fetus to LNG in a pregnancy with a retained LNG-IUS. As levels of LNG are high in the uterus and potentially within the amniotic fluid, this could lead to exposure during critical times of fetal development. Although there is insufficient evidence to describe any potential negative effects from intrauterine LNG exposure, counseling should include the potential risk of congenital anomalies with a retained LNG-IUS. There is not an association between oral LNG used as emergency contraception and adverse physical or mental development.[236]

Preterm Labor and Birth

The risk of preterm delivery is increased when conception occurs with an IUD in place. Preterm birth rates range from 7% to 25% in pregnancies with a retained IUD and from 2% to 17% in pregnancies where the IUD is removed.[229]

Chorioamnionitis and Placental Abruption

The presence of an IUD during pregnancy increases the risk of chorioamnionitis and abruption. Similar to preterm delivery, the increased risk of chorioamnionitis and abruption may persist even with removal of the IUD.[237,238]

IUD Placement

Patient Selection and Counseling

Few women have contraindications to use of the IUD. Patient selection for successful IUD use requires attention to menstrual history and the contraceptive needs specific to each patient (see **Box 6.3** for further counseling points). The Centers for Disease Control Medical Eligibility Criteria clearly defines levels of risk in different medical conditions for copper IUD and LNG-IUS use. Nonmonogyny or the presence of risk factors for STIs is not a contraindication to IUD use, although recent or recurrent PID requires a discussion of risks and benefits with the patient and current PID should be treated fully prior to insertion.

Box 6.3 Key Points in Patient Counseling

1. Protection against unwanted pregnancy begins immediately after insertion with a copper IUD.
2. Menses can be longer and heavier with the copper IUD.
3. Irregular spotting can occur over the first 3–6 months of use with the LNG-IUS.
4. Tampons can be used.
5. Protection against infections transmitted through the vaginal mucosa requires the use of condoms.
6. Ectopic pregnancies can still occur.
7. The IUD can be spontaneously expelled; if the patient sees the device or feels something hard (suggestive of the IUD frame), a clinician should be notified as soon as possible. Backup contraception should be provided until the patient can be examined.

Nulliparous and nulligravid women and adolescents can safely use the IUD.[53] The LNG-IUS performs well when used by young women with higher continuation rates than all short-acting methods (82.1% vs. 48.5% for all other methods at 1 year).[137,177,239] Complications, including expulsion, perforation, infection, heavy bleeding, or removals for bleeding, are rare among young women and adolescents.[178,240,241] In a retrospective review of nearly 1,200 IUD insertions in women aged 13 to 24, there was no difference in success of first-attempt IUD placement between nulliparous and parous young women (95.8% vs. 96.7%, respectively).[242] The American Academy of Pediatricians and ACOG support IUDs as a first-choice contraceptive for adolescents and nulliparous women.[77–79]

Patients with heavy menstrual periods should be cautioned regarding the increase in menstrual bleeding associated with the copper IUD. Women who are anticoagulated or have a bleeding disorder are obviously not good candidates for the copper IUD, but they might benefit from the LNG-IUS.

There are other conditions that can compromise successful placement and use of IUDs. Women who have abnormalities of uterine anatomy (bicornuate uterus, submucous myoma, cervical stenosis) may not accommodate an IUD though case reports of successful use with uterine anomalies exist.[243] Neither a copper IUD nor an LNG-IUS is a good choice when the uterine cavity is severely distorted by leiomyomas, and an LNG-IUS would be favored in women with HMB from uterine myomas that do not severely distort the cavity or have a submucous location (see section on Noncontraceptive Benefits). According to conventional wisdom, the few individuals who have allergies to copper or have Wilson's disease (a prevalence of about 1 in 200,000) should not use copper IUDs; however, no cases of difficulty have ever been recorded and it is doubtful, considering the low exposure to copper, that there would be a problem. The amount of copper released into the circulation per day is less than that consumed in a normal diet.[244] Nevertheless, long-acting progestin-only methods are recommended for individuals with Wilson's disease.[245]

Immunosuppressed patients and those with treated or untreated HIV can use IUDs.[88] Cervical dysplasia with our without the presence of HIV does not preclude IUD insertion or continued use.

The American Heart Association no longer recommends antibiotic prophylaxis for prevention of bacterial endocarditis in women with heart disease prior to IUD insertion or removal.[246] The bacteriologic contamination of the uterine cavity at insertion is short lived.[211] Four studies have attempted to document bacteremia during IUD insertion or removal, and only one of the three could find blood culture evidence of bacteremia, and it was present transiently and rarely.[247–250]

It is worth emphasizing that no increase in adverse events has been observed with copper IUD or LNG-IUS use in women with either insulin-dependent or non–insulin-dependent diabetes.[251–254] Indeed, the IUD can be an ideal choice for a woman with diabetes, especially if vascular disease is present, minimizing risk of thromboembolism with combined hormonal contraception.

As mentioned previously, all women should receive counseling regarding expected bleeding pattern changes with IUD use. Women who accept a copper IUD need to understand that they may experience heavier bleeding, but no overall change to cyclicity. Women choosing the LNG-IUS will typically experience irregular bleeding for 3 months, followed by light and/or irregular bleeding. While most women using the LNG 52 mg IUS will experience amenorrhea at some point during use, this does not occur in all users and may be of variable duration. Women using lower-dose LNG-IUS products are less likely to experience amenorrhea and may have longer irregular bleeding. Research has demonstrated that counseling can improve acceptability of bleeding patterns and reduces discontinuation.[255]

Insertion of the IUD/IUS

A careful bimanual examination is essential prior to IUD insertion. It is important to know the position of the uterus; undetected extreme posterior uterine position is the most common reason for perforation at the time of IUD insertion. However, perforation is rare; in a prospective study of nearly 62,000 IUD insertions (both copper and LNG), the overall perforation rate was 1.4 per 1,000 insertions for LNG-IUSs and 1.1 per 1,000 insertions for copper IUDs.[256] While this study confirmed the low risk of perforation, several important risk factors for perforation deserve mention. Breast-feeding at the time of placement increased the risk of perforation sixfold, and placement by a less experienced clinician (fewer than 50 devices/year) nearly doubled the risk. A very small or large uterus, determined by examination and sounding, deserves attention and strong consideration for use of ultrasound guidance to assure insertion occurs at the fundus. The ACCESS IUS study used a minimum cutoff for uterine sound depth of 5.5 cm; of the 1,910 women enrolled, this resulted in the exclusion of only two participants.[53]

193

Our clinical experience with trainees supports the use of ultrasound to evaluate uterine size in the setting of an unsuspected sound depth of under 6 cm. A frequent problem is significant ante- or retroflexion. Knowledge of the true cavity size can aid in successful placement.

Chlamydia and gonorrhea screening can be performed per recommended guidelines at the time of insertion. However, if the speculum exam reveals mucopurulent discharge from the cervix at time of planned placement, the insertion should be delayed until after appropriate workup and treatment.

Insertion at any point in the menstrual cycle can be undertaken if there is reasonable certainty that the patient is not pregnant. The CDC has created specific guidelines for determining reasonable certainty **(Box 6.4)**.[88] In the past, many references suggested scheduling insertion during menses or at midcycle to reduce complications. In a systematic review of insertion at different times in the menstrual cycle, timing had no effect on continuation, efficacy, or safety.[257] An additional concern has been difficulty of insertion in nulliparous patients, with many trials focusing on methods to ease the insertion procedure. These trials primarily involve administration of misoprostol prior to IUD insertion. A Cochrane review determined patients given misoprostol prior to insertion report higher levels of pain with insertion.[258] A subsequent systematic review of 15 RCTs determined that there is no significant difference in ease of insertion between women receiving and not receiving medications.[259]

Pain Management at Time of Insertion

Multiple studies have investigated the use of different analgesic medications for the reduction of pain associated with IUD insertion. A 2015 Cochrane review pooled trials on medications to reduce insertion-related pain including topical lidocaine preparations, misoprostol, various NSAIDs, and tramadol. Lidocaine 2% gel and misoprostol did not reduce pain scores. Of the NSAIDs included in trials, oral naproxen was associated with reduced pain

---

Box 6.4 CDC Recommendations to be Reasonably Certain a Woman Is Not Pregnant[88]

- Is ≤7 days after the start of normal menses
- Has not had sexual intercourse since the start of last normal menses
- Has been correctly and consistently using a reliable method of contraception
- Is ≤7 days after spontaneous or induced abortion
- Is within 4 weeks postpartum
- Is fully or nearly fully breast-feeding (exclusively breast-feeding or the vast majority [≥85%] of feeds are breast-feeds), amenorrheic, and less than 6 months postpartum

scores in one out of two trials and oral ibuprofen did not reduce pain in four trials (including a trial of 800 mg). Intramuscular ketorolac reduced pain for nulliparous women but not for multiparous women. Although the evidence is conflicting about insertion-related pain reduction, naproxen use has been associated with decreased pain at 5 and 15 minutes post insertion.[258,260]

The use of a paracervical lidocaine block has also been studied with conflicting results.[258] In one RCT of 50 women undergoing IUD insertion, 26 received a 10 mL 1% lidocaine paracervical block and 24 received no block. There was no statistical difference between groups; however, the study is likely underpowered as women with a block reported a median visual analogue scale (0 mm = no pain, 100 mm = worst pain possible) of 24.0 versus 62.0 mm in the no block group.[261] A second single-blind, sham-controlled randomized trial of LNG 13.5 mg IUS insertion in 95 young women and adolescents found a 10-mL 1% lidocaine paracervical block reduced pain scores compared to the sham block (30.0 vs. 71.5 mm).[262] These studies suggest that some women may benefit from a paracervical block. However, because the injection can be painful, providers should counsel women about the positives and negatives associated with paracervical block administration, including prolongation of the procedure. Routine provision for patients in which IUD insertion is anticipated to be difficult, such as one requiring cervical dilation, is a reasonable consideration.

A phase II trial of LNG 13.5 and 19.5 mg IUSs, which have smaller IUS frames and narrower insertion tubes, versus the LNG 52 mg IUS did show less pain with insertion when evaluating no pain or mild pain reporting (72.3% vs. 57.9% of users reporting "no" or "mild" pain with insertion, respectively, $p < 0.001$).[44] However, the proportion of women with severe pain did not differ between the groups (6.7% vs. 4.3%, respectively, $p = 0.22$).

Insertion Technique

Inserting an IUD requires only a few minutes, has few complications, and is rarely painful, but preoperative examination, medication, and the right equipment will ensure a good experience for your patient. After introducing a vaginal spectrum, the cervix is cleaned with chlorhexidine or povidone-iodine. It is important to maintain sterile tip (no-touch) technique where any instrument to be passed into the uterine cavity (uterine sound, dilators, and IUD inserter) does not touch any nonsterile area. Insertion does not require use of sterile gloves when no-touch technique is employed. Grasp the anterior cervical lip with the tenaculum ratcheting it only to the first position in a slow, deliberate fashion. Some clinicians find that positioning the tenaculum on the posterior cervix improves the ease of insertion for a retroverted uterus. Some providers recommend the use of local anesthetic prior to tenaculum placement, but the evidence for routine use is not conclusive.[263] As an alternative, many clinicians ask the patient to produce a constant cough, sing, hum, or grunt during tenaculum placement for distraction as a strategy to reduce discomfort. Sound and measure the depth of the uterus. The device should not be opened from the protective package until after the clinician verifies that the sound can be passed to the fundus. This may require cervical dilation in select cases. Following manufacturer directions, load the IUD into the inserter and position the flange on the insertion tube at the sounded distance.

There are two general ways that T-shaped IUDs are loaded, and the technique depends on the IUD frame type. Tatum-T devices, like the TCu380A **(Figure 6.3)**, are loaded by folding the arms downward into the end of the insertion tube. An obturator keeps the IUD stem in the correct position in the insertion tube. For deployment in the uterine cavity, the insertion tube is advanced until the flange contacts the cervix to position the device at the fundus and the insertion tube is then pulled back (pull technique) to release the arms as the obturator remains stabilized to maintain the fundal position. In contrast, devices with a Nova-T frame **(Figures 6.4 and 6.5)** are loaded by pulling the device into the insertion tube and therefore folding the arms upward. The inserter is only advanced until the flange is within 1.5 to 2 cm of the cervix, and the arms are then unfolded in the midcavity by pulling back on a sliding lever on the insertion device handle (slightly different technique for each manufacturer). Once the arms are deployed, the IUS is then advanced until the flange touches the cervix to position the IUS at the uterine fundus. High fundal placement is key for avoiding expulsions or incorrectly positioned devices. Remove the inserter and trim the IUD strings to 2 to 3 cm in length.

In some counties, Nova-T frame devices are packaged with a basic insertion system that more closely resembles those used for Tatum-T devices. In these cases, the clinician pulls on the removal thread to withdraw the arms into the insertion tube, stabilizing the device with an obturator. However, in contrast to the Tatum-T insertion process, the device is positioned in

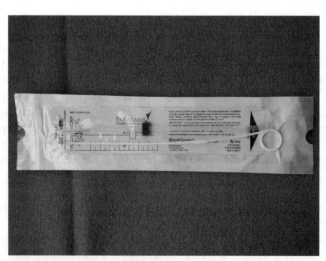

Figure 6.3 The Paragard inserter.

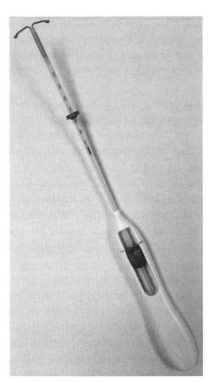 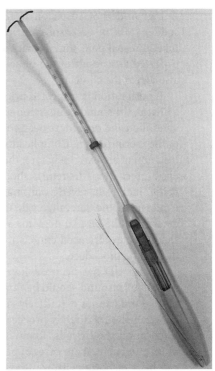

Figure 6.4 The Mirena inserter.   **Figure 6.5 The Liletta inserter.**

a Nova-T fashion advancing the tube until the flange is 1.5 to 2 cm from the cervix and then releasing the arms prior to advancing the device to the fundus.

We anticipate new devices will enter the market. Clinicians should always carefully review and follow manufacturer recommendations prior to placement of any IUD.

Management of Suspected Perforation at Time of Placement

Although rare, uterine perforation represents a serious complication during IUD placement. Perforation may occur without symptoms and be recognized only as a result of absent IUD threads or pregnancy. In a retrospective study of 75 women referred to a tertiary center, 29% were completely asymptomatic with the diagnosis made during routine follow-up (21%) or because of pregnancy (8%).[264] Among the women with known timing of insertion, about half reported having experienced immediate symptoms of pain within 5 days. Bleeding complaints occurred less commonly. Although cramping pain and bleeding may occur following uncomplicated placement, women who call with these complaints following IUD placement deserve evaluation.

Since perforation most frequently occurs in the midline due to anteflexion or retroflexion, unusual bleeding may not be evident to the clinician.

A high index of suspicion is required. Clues for perforation include a sudden loss of resistance during placement of the sound or insertion tube, unusual pain, and a cavity depth out of range (>9 cm) or proportion expected as a result of the bimanual exam. Sudden brisk bleeding should also alarm the clinician.

If perforation is suspected prior to the deployment of the IUD (e.g., with a dilator, the sound or insertion tube), the placement attempt should be discontinued and procedure delayed for 2 to 6 weeks to allow complete healing of the uterine defect. Complications from a uterine perforation with a blunt instrument are extremely rare; therefore, the women can be sent home with basic precautions to return should she develop unusual symptoms (e.g., abdominal pain, fever, vomiting). Provide alternative contraception. The clinician should carefully evaluate the circumstances of the perforation to determine the best strategy for a repeat attempt. This may involve referral to a more experienced clinician, cervical dilation, or ultrasound guidance during the procedure.

If the IUD has been deployed and perforation is suspected, a transvaginal ultrasound should be immediately done to confirm position. If the ultrasound cannot definitively confirm correct position of the device, the clinician should directly proceed to remove the device by applying gentle traction on the threads. Removal generally occurs without complication or unusual pain. As in cases of perforation with the sound only, the patient can be sent home with routine precautions and return for repeat placement attempt after the uterine wound has healed. If removal is difficult or painful, anesthesia may be indicated, but laparoscopy would rarely be required.

In practice settings where high-quality transvaginal ultrasound is not immediately available, if perforation is suspected following release of the IUD, the device threads should be immediately grasped and the device removed. Referral for ultrasound in this setting may result in the withdrawal of the removal threads into the abdominal cavity such that vaginal removal is no longer possible. The potential harms associated with the need for laparoscopic removal of an intra-abdominal IUD far outweigh the harm of unnecessary removal of a correctly positioned IUD in the uterine cavity.

Follow-Up After Insertion

A 1-month follow-up visit and monthly string checks by IUD users are no longer recommended as no data exist to support these practices.[265] The CDC Selected Practice Recommendations advise clinicians to counsel IUD users to return for a follow-up visit should they experience side effects, have concerns about the IUD, or wish to change methods.[88] Although not evidence based, the rationale for monthly "string checks" still makes sense for copper IUD users who experience heavy bleeding or clotting. A silent expulsion can occur during passage of a clot. Reassessing that the IUD remains in place following menses will increase confidence in the contraceptive protection.

IUD Removal

Removal of an IUD can usually be accomplished by grasping the string with a ring forceps or uterine dressing (Bozeman) forceps and exerting firm traction. If strings cannot be seen, they can sometimes be extracted from the cervical canal by rotating two cotton-tipped applicators or a cytobrush in the endocervical canal. If further maneuvers are required, the cervix should be cleansed with chlorhexidine or povidone-iodine and a paracervical block should be considered.

If IUD strings cannot be identified or extracted from the endocervical canal, the clinician should first confirm that the IUD is actually in the uterus. Prior to instrumentation, an ultrasound should be done to confirm intrauterine placement. See below for guidance on workup of a missing IUD. Commercially available devices (Emmett IUD Thread Retriever; Retrievette IUCD Thread Retriever) designed to snare the IUD threads in the cervix or uterine cavity provide a simple approach to remove most devices without exploratory instrumentation of the uterine cavity. Facit polyp or alligator-type forceps can be used to identify and grasp strings within the cervical canal to facilitate removal. If this maneuver is not successful, these same forceps provide tactile feedback as to the location of the device within the uterus and for removal. Take care to open the forceps widely immediately on passing it through the internal cervical os so that the IUD can be caught between the jaws. Sometimes, it is necessary to advance the forceps to the fundus to grasp the arms of the device. Only clinicians skilled at intrauterine procedures should attempt these maneuvers. If removal is not easily accomplished using these steps, ultrasound-guided removal will assist localization. Although transvaginal ultrasonography provides the best image to confirm the location of an IUD, transabdominal sonography should be used to guide retrieval. In a prospective case series of 29 LNG 52 mg IUS removals without visible strings, all 29 were successfully removed in clinic on the first visit through this technique with or without the use of ultrasonography.[266]

Occasionally, the IUD threads will break during an attempt at removal. The same general approach to removal with instruments as described above is generally successful. If removal attempts result in unusual pain, embedment should be considered (see below).

Fertility returns promptly and pregnancies after removal of an IUD occur at a normal rate, sooner than after oral contraception.[63–65,67–69] Pregnancy outcome after IUD removal is associated with a normal incidence of spontaneous miscarriage and ectopic pregnancy.[65]

If a patient wishes to continue use of an IUD, a new device can be placed immediately after removal of the old one.

Embedded IUDs

Ultrasonography done for other gynecologic indications or to workup suspected IUD problems sometimes identifies a portion of the IUD frame within the myometrium (partial embedment). In rare cases, the entire device may be located within the uterine wall (complete embedment). Embedment likely occurs as a complication of device placement due to partial perforation or as a consequence of uterine muscular contractions during chronic expulsion. If partial embedment is suspected in an asymptomatic patient, no action is required. In a patient with bleeding or pain, removal should be considered. We recommend removal of a device that appears more than 25% embedded (e.g., more than one arm and/or a portion of the stem) even in an asymptomatic woman, due to concerns regarding contraceptive effects. Repeat imaging including 3D ultrasound may improve diagnostic certainty.

If upon transvaginal sonography myometrial embedment is suspected, in-office removal should still be attempted first as described above. In a case series of 157 women with failed in-office removals, only 10% of IUDs diagnosed as embedded on presurgical imaging were confirmed to be embedded hysteroscopically.[267] In another case series report of failed IUD removals referred to a specialty clinic for ultrasound-guided removal, 19 of 23 (83%) were successfully removed in clinic. The remaining 4 were removed hysteroscopically in the operating room.[268] If in-office removal fails, hysteroscopy is indicated. Should the IUD prove to be embedded in the myometrium at the time of hysteroscopy, hysteroscopic forceps can be used to grasp the device. Sometimes, grasping the device and moving the forceps cephalad will affect removal of a stubborn embedded fragment angled away from the cervix. Use a closed hysteroscopic grasper to dissect out any embedded portions of the IUD. If on ultrasonography the IUD is suspected of being embedded in the myometrium but protruding through the uterine serosa, operative laparoscopy may be necessary.

Occasionally, when removing an embedded IUD, the removal threads may break off the device or the device itself may break, leaving a retained fragment behind. In the instance of broken removal threads, the approach to IUD removal would be the same as above with ultrasound guidance in clinic and hysteroscopy if the device is not successfully removed in-office. In the case of a fragmented device, a transvaginal ultrasound should be performed to precisely locate the retained fragment. An MRI may be considered if ultrasound is inconclusive. Although a kidney, ureter, and bladder (KUB) x-ray can also be performed as an inexpensive imaging modality to confirm that a fragment is actually in the body for general localization (along with a lateral view of the pelvis), this will not precisely locate the fragment in the uterus.[269] The office-based removal procedures described above should be attempted first. Additional options include a manual vacuum aspirator (MVA) or IUD hook. Should these attempts prove unsuccessful, hysteroscopic guided retrieval may be necessary in the operating room. The patient should be counseled prior to attempted removal in the operating room that if the fragment cannot be visualized with hysteroscopy, it might not be possible to remove.[269]

Thorough counseling should be undertaken, and an attempt at fragment removal made if a woman desires future fertility or is having pain or heavy bleeding. If a fragment cannot be identified on hysteroscopy, waiting 2 to 3 months may improve visualization. Use of a GnRH agonist for several months may decrease myometrial thickness and increase the opportunity to remove the fragment hysteroscopically. In an asymptomatic woman who has completed childbearing, a retained IUD fragment in the myometrium does not necessarily require removal. Little is known about the impact of a retained fragment on a future pregnancy should the woman desire continued fertility.

The Missing IUD

When an IUD cannot be found with ultrasonography, in addition to expulsion, one has to consider perforation of the uterus into the abdominal cavity (1/1,000 risk). Perforation must be considered in all cases when a woman does not provide a direct confirmation of device removal or expulsion. All IUDs are radiopaque, but localization requires a radiograph abdominal film that includes both diaphragmatic borders and the complete pelvis. This may require more than one view. If the IUD is identified in the abdominal cavity, but not in the uterus, it should be removed using operative laparoscopy. Copper in the abdominal cavity can lead to adhesion formation, making laparoscopic removal difficult.[270] Although inert perforated devices without closed loops were previously allowed to remain in the abdominal cavity, current practice is to remove any perforated IUD, including the LNG system.

This problem should be put into perspective. With the new generation of IUDs (copper and levonorgestrel), adhesion formation appears to be an immediate reaction that does not progress and rarely leads to serious complications.[271] In appropriate situations (in which the risk of surgery is considerable), clinician and patient may elect not to remove the translocated IUD in the absence of concerning symptoms.[272] However, a case has been reported of sigmoid perforation occurring 5 years after insertion, and the general consensus continues to favor removal of a perforated IUD immediately on diagnosis.[273]

Emergency Contraception

Use of a copper IUD for emergency contraception (EC) is an opportunity to provide the most effective form of EC (0.1% risk of pregnancy) while providing ongoing contraception.[274] Chapter 12 provides additional data on the use of copper IUDs for EC. There is accumulating evidence that with a negative pregnancy test, an IUD can be used for EC regardless of timing in the menstrual cycle or days since unprotected intercourse.[275] One barrier to IUD insertion for EC is the preference by many women for a hormonal IUS, such as the LNG 52 mg IUS, over the copper T380 IUD.[276] A recent study found a low risk of pregnancy with combined use of oral

LNG for EC and immediate placement of the LNG 52 mg IUS, the study was underpowered to assess the effectiveness of the approach for emergency contraception.[276] Although the use of the LNG-IUS makes sense to provide ongoing protection against pregnancy, we do not recommend use of the LNG-IUS alone for emergency contraception. However, ongoing studies are collecting data regarding pregnancy risk with use of the LNG-IUS alone for EC (ClinicalTrials.gov NCT02175030, NCT 02076217, and NCT01539720). These include RCTs of the LNG-IUS versus the T380 Cu IUD and versus ulipristal acetate. These studies should provide additional guidance.

Postabortion and Postpartum Use of IUDs

Post Abortion

An IUD can be inserted immediately after a first-trimester or second-trimester abortion or at the time of follow-up after successful medication abortion.[80,81,84,86] Two retrospective cohort studies demonstrated a significant reduction in repeat abortion among women receiving immediate postabortion IUDs. Women with immediate IUD placement were up to 20 times less likely to return for a subsequent termination.[277,278]

A randomized noninferiority trial of immediate versus delayed postabortion IUD placement after a first-trimester procedure evaluated the risk of expulsion. Of the 575 women randomized, 100% in the immediate insertion group and 71% in the delayed insertion group were using the IUD at 6 months (RR = 1.40, 95% CI = 1.31 to 1.50). Although more expulsions occurred in the immediate group (5% vs. 2.7%), this elevation was within the predefined noninferiority limit (RR = 1.90, CI = 0.73 to 4.91). Infection rates were low (<1%) and not different between groups. No perforations were reported.[80]

Initially, concern over higher expulsion and perforation rates led to caution over immediate IUD insertion following second-trimester abortions. However, two RCTs of second-trimester postabortion IUD placement have demonstrated the safety and efficacy of immediate placement.[84,86]

Studies have also demonstrated safety and efficacy of IUD placement following medical abortion.[81,279] In a prospective observational study, women receiving an IUD at medical abortion follow-up 7-10 days after treatment had low rates of expulsions (4.1% in 3 months of follow-up), no perforations or pelvic infections, and a high continuation rate at 3 months of 80%.[81]

Postpartum Use: Immediate Postplacental Insertion and Delayed Insertion

Both copper IUDs and LNG-IUSs can be safely placed immediately (<10 minutes following placental delivery) after a vaginal or cesarean delivery. Immediate placement is not associated with an increased risk of infection, uterine perforation, postpartum bleeding, or uterine subinvolution.[82,83,85,87] Postdelivery insertion is not recommended if intrauterine infection is present.

A systematic review and meta-analysis evaluated postpartum IUD expulsion risk following postpartum device placement as a function of timing of placement, IUD type, and delivery method. They classified immediate placement as 10 minutes or less after placental delivery and early placement as greater than 10 minutes to less than 4 weeks postpartum. Immediate and early postpartum placements had a greater than sixfold increased risk of expulsion relative to interval placement (more than 4 weeks postpartum). Relative to cesarean delivery, immediate and early placement following vaginal delivery had a fivefold higher rate of expulsion (RR = 5.19, 95% CI = 3.85 to 6.99). Placement of the LNG-IUS was associated with an almost twofold higher expulsion risk than the CuT380A when inserted less than 4 weeks postpartum (aRR = 1.91, 95% CI = 1.50 to 2.43).[280]

Concerns have been raised over the effect of immediate postplacental insertion of an LNG-IUS on breast-feeding. A RCT of breast-feeding and immediate postplacental LNG 52 mg IUS placement versus delayed placement demonstrated noninferiority in time to lactogenesis or continuation of breast-feeding at 8 weeks.[281]

When placing an IUD immediately postpartum, placement should occur within 10 minutes of delivery of the placenta. High fundal placement is key in reducing rates of expulsion. Insertion can be achieved manually by placing the device with a hand or with the use of ring forceps or Kelly placental forceps. If forceps are used, care should be taken to not crush the device. A guiding hand placed at the fundus on the abdomen can ensure proper positioning, and bedside ultrasonography during and after placement should be used without reservation to confirm high fundal placement.

Delayed postpartum placement, within 2 to 4 weeks, can also be undertaken safely with low rates of infection and perforation.[282-284] Expulsion rates during this period are also lower than immediate postpartum placement.[87,284]

203

References

1. **Population Crisis Committee,** Access to birth control: a world assessment, In: Population Briefing Paper. Washington, DC, 1986.

2. **United Nations,** World Contraceptive Use 2007, 2009. http://www.un.org/esa/population/publications/contraceptive2007/contraceptive_2007_table.pdf

3. **United Nations Department of Economic and Social Affairs, Population Division,** Trends in Contraceptive Use Worldwide 2015, 2015. [cited 2018 May 4]. http://www.un.org/en/development/desa/population/publications/pdf/family/trendsContraceptiveUse2015Report.pdf

4. **Piccinino LJ, Mosher WD,** Trends in Contraceptive Use in the United States: 1982-1995, Fam Plann Perspect 30:4, 1998.

5. **Kavanaugh ML, Jerman J,** Contraceptive method use in the United States: trends and characteristics between 2008, 2012 and 2014, Contraception 97:14–21, 2018.

6. **Mosher WD, Jones J,** Use of contraception in the United States: 1982-2008, Vital Health Stat 23:1–44, 2010.

7. **Hubacher D, Finer LB, Espey E,** Renewed interest in intrauterine contraception in the United States: evidence and explanation, Contraception 83:291–294, 2011.

8. **Gubrium AC, Mann ES, Borrero S, Dehlendorf C, Fields J, Geronimus AT, et al.,** Realizing reproductive health equity needs more than Long-acting reversible contraception (LARC), Am J Public Health 106:18–19, 2016.

9. **Higgins JA,** Celebration meets caution: LARC's boons, potential busts, and the benefits of a reproductive justice approach, Contraception 89:237–241, 2014.

10. **Tone A,** Devices and Desires: A History of Contraceptives in America, Hill and Wang, New York, 2001.

11. **Zipper J, Medel M, Prager R,** Suppression of fertility by intrauterine copper and zinc in rabbits. A new approach to intrauterine contraception, Am J Obstet Gynecol 105:529–534, 1969.

12. **Tatum HJ, Schmidt FH, Phillips D, McCarty M, O'Leary WM,** The Dalkon Shield controversy. Structural and bacteriological studies of IUD tails, JAMA 231:711–717, 1975.

13. **Lee NC, Rubin GL, Ory HW, Burkman RT,** Type of intrauterine device and the risk of pelvic inflammatory disease, Obstet Gynecol 62:1, 1983.

14. **Lopez LM, Bernholc A, Hubacher D, Stuart G, Van Vliet HA,** Immediate postpartum insertion of intrauterine device for contraception, Cochrane Database Syst Rev (6):CD003036, 2015.

15. **Sivin I, Tatum HJ,** Four years of experience with the TCu 380A intrauterine contraceptive device, Fertil Steril 36:159, 1981.

16. **Thiery M,** Intrauterine contraception: from silver ring to intrauterine contraceptive implant, Eur J Obstet Gynecol Reprod Biol 90:145–152, 2000.

17. **United Nations Development Programme,** Long-term reversible contraception. Twelve years of experience with the TCu380A and TCu220C, Contraception 56:341–352, 1997.

18. **Sivin I,** Utility and drawbacks of continuous use of a copper T IUD for 20 years, Contraception 75:S70, 2007.

19. **Sivin I, Stern J,** Health during prolonged use of levonorgestrel 20 µg/d and the Copper TCu 380Ag intrauterine contraceptive devices: a multicenter study, Fertil Steril 61:70, 1994.

20. **Sivin I, Diaz S, Pavez M, Alvarez F, Brache V, Diaz J, et al.,** Two-year comparative trial of the Gyne T* 380 slimline and Gyne T* 380 extrauterine copper devices, Contraception 44:481, 1991.

21. **Chi IC,** The TCu-380A (Ag), MLCu375, and Nova-T LUDs and the IUD daily releasing 20 µg levonorgestrel-four pillars of IUD contraception for the nineties and beyond? Contraception 47:325, 1993.

22. **O'Brien PA, Marfleet C,** Frameless versus classical intrauterine device for contraception, Cochrane Database Syst Rev (1):CD003282, 2005.

23. **Meirik O, Rowe PJ, Peregoudov A, Piaggio G, Petzold M,** The frameless copper IUD (GyneFix) and the TCu380A IUD: results of an 8-year multicenter randomized comparative trial, Contraception 80:133–141, 2009.

24. **Hsia JK, Creinin MD,** Intrauterine Contraception, Semin Reprod Med 34:175–182, 2016.

25. **Zhang S, Li Y, Yu P, Chen T, Zhou W, Zhang W, et al.,** In vitro release of cupric ion from intrauterine devices: influence of frame, shape, copper surface area and indomethacin, Biomed Microdevices 17:19, 2015.

26. **Reeves MF, Katz BH, Canela JM, Hathaway MJ, Tal MG,** A randomized comparison of a novel nitinol-frame low-dose-copper intrauterine contraceptive and a copper T380S intrauterine contraceptive, Contraception 95:544–548, 2017.

27. **Luukkainen T, Allonen H, Haukkamaa M, Lähteenmäki P, Nilsson CG, Toivonen J,** Five years' experience with levonorgestrel-releasing IUDs, Contraception 33:139, 1986.

28. **Creinin MD, Jansen R, Starr RM, Gobburu J, Gopalakrishnan M, Olariu A,** Levonorgestrel release rates over 5 years with the Liletta® 52-mg intrauterine system, Contraception 94:353–356, 2016.

29. **McNicholas C, Swor E, Wan L, Peipert JF,** Prolonged use of the etonogestrel implant and levonorgestrel intrauterine device: 2 years beyond Food and Drug Administration-approved duration, Am J Obstet Gynecol 216:586.e1–586.e6, 2017.

30. **Rowe P, Farley T, Peregoudov A, Piaggio G, Boccard S, Landoulsi S, et al.,** Safety and efficacy in parous women of a 52-mg levonorgestrel-medicated

intrauterine device: a 7-year randomized comparative study with the TCu380A, Contraception 93:498–506, 2016.

31. **Kaunitz AM, Bissonnette F, Monteiro I, Lukkari-Lax E, Muysers C, Jensen JT,** Levonorgestrel-releasing intrauterine system or medroxyprogesterone for heavy menstrual bleeding: a randomized controlled trial, Obstet Gynecol 116:625–632, 2010.

32. **Mawet M, Nollevaux F, Nizet D, Wijzen F, Gordenne V, Tasev N, Segedi D, Marinescu B, Enache A, Parhomenko V, Frankenne F, Foidart JM,** Impact of a new levonorgestrel intrauterine system, Levosert(®), on heavy menstrual bleeding: results of a one-year randomised controlled trial, Eur J Contracept Reprod Health Care 19:169–179, 2014.

33. **Wildemeersch D, Janssens D, Andrade A,** The Femilis® LNG-IUS: contraceptive performance–an interim analysis, Eur J Contracept Reprod Health Care 14:103, 2009.

34. **Crosignani P, Vercellini P, Mosconi P, Oldani S, Cortesi I, Degiorgi O,** Levonorgestrel-releasing intrauterine device versus hysteroscopic endometrial resection in the treatment of dysfunctional uterine bleeding, Obstet Gynecol 90:257, 1997.

35. **Kaunitz AM, Meredith S, Inki P, Kubba A, Sanchez-Ramos L,** Levonorgestrel-releasing intrauterine system and endometrial ablation in heavy menstrual bleeding, Obstet Gynecol 113:1104, 2009.

36. **Silva-Filho AL, Pereira Fde A, de Souza SS, Loures LF, Rocha AP, Valadares CN, et al.,** Five-year follow-up of levonorgestrel-releasing intrauterine system versus thermal balloon ablation for the treatment of heavy menstrual bleeding: a randomized controlled trial, Contraception 87:409–415, 2013.

37. **Gardner FJE, Konje JC, Abrams KR, Brown LJR, Khanna S, Al-Azzawi F, et al.,** Endometrial protection from tamoxifen-stimulated changes by a levonorgestrel-releasing intrauterine system: a randomised controlled trial, Lancet 356:1711, 2000.

38. **Hampton NRE, Rees MCP, Lowe DG, Rauramo I, Barlow D, Guillebaud J,** Levonorgestrel intrauterine system (LNG-IUS) with conjugated oral equine estrogen: a successful regimen for HRT in perimenopausal women, Hum Reprod 20:2653, 2005.

39. **Raudaskoski T, Tapanainen J, Tomas E, Luotola H, Pekonen F, Ronni-Sivula H, et al.,** Intrauterine 10 microg and 20 microg levonorgestrel systems in postmenopausal women receiving oral oestrogen replacement therapy: clinical, endometrial and metabolic response, Br J Obstet Gynaecol 109:136, 2002.

40. **Raudaskoski TH, Lahti EI, Kauppila AJ, Apaja-Sarkkinen MA, Laatikainen TJ,** Transdermal estrogen with a levonorgestrel-releasing intrauterine device for climacteric complaints: clinical and endometrial responses, Am J Obstet Gynecol 172:114–119, 1995.

41. **Suhonen S, Holmström T, Lähteenmäki P,** Three-year follow-up of the use of a levonorgestrel-releasing intrauterine system in hormone replacement therapy, Acta Obstet Gynecol Scand 76:145, 1997.

42. **Suvanto-Luukkonen E, Kauppila A,** The levonorgestrel intrauterine system in menopausal hormone replacement therapy: five-year experience, Fertil Steril 72:161, 1999.

43. **Varila E, Wahlström T, Rauramo I,** A 5-year follow-up study on the use of a levonorgestrel intrauterine system in women receiving hormone replacement therapy, Fertil Steril 76:969, 2001.

44. **Vercellini P, Aimi G, Panazza S, De Giorgi O, Pesole A, Crosignani PG,** A levonorgestrel-releasing intrauterine system for the treatment of dysmenorrhea associated with endometriosis: a pilot study, Fertil Steril 72:505, 1999.

45. **Gemzell-Danielsson K, Schellschmidt I, Apter D,** A randomized, phase II study describing the efficacy, bleeding profile, and safety of two low-dose levonorgestrel-releasing intrauterine contraceptive systems and Mirena, Fertil Steril 97:616-22.e1-3, 2012.

46. **Apter D, Gemzell-Danielsson K, Hauck B, Rosen K, Zurth C,** Pharmacokinetics of two low-dose levonorgestrel-releasing intrauterine systems and effects on ovulation rate and cervical function: pooled analyses of phase II and III studies, Fertil Steril 101:1656-62.e1-4, 2014.

47. **Bayer Healthcare,** [cited 2018 May 4]. https://labeling.bayerhealthcare.com/html/products/pi/Mirena_PI.pdf

48. **Bayer Healthcare,** [cited 2018 May 3]. https://labeling.bayerhealthcare.com/html/products/pi/Kyleena_PI.pdf

49. **Bayer Healthcare,** [cited 2018 May 2]. http://labeling.bayerhealthcare.com/html/products/pi/Skyla_PI.pdf

50. **Meirik O, Farley TMM, Sivin I,** Safety and efficacy of levonorgestrel implant, intrauterine device, and sterilization, Am J Obstet Gynecol 97:539, 2001.

51. **Sivin I, Mahgoub SE, McCarthy T, Mishell DR, Shoupe D, Alvarez F, et al.,** Long-term contraception with the levonorgestrel 20 mcg/day (LNg 20) and the Copper T 380Ag intrauterine devices: a five-year randomized study, Contraception 42:361, 1990.

52. **Nelson A, Apter D, Hauck B, Schmelter T, Rybowski S, Rosen K, et al.,** Two low-dose levonorgestrel intrauterine contraceptive systems: a randomized controlled trial, Obstet Gynecol 122:1205–1213, 2013.

53. **Schreiber CA, Teal SB, Blumenthal PD, Keder LM, Olariu AI, Creinin MD,** Bleeding patterns for the Liletta® levonorgestrel 52 mg intrauterine system, Eur J Contracept Reprod Health Care 23:116–120, 2018.

54. **Eisenberg DL, Schreiber CA, Turok DK, Teal SB, Westhoff CL, Creinin MD,** Three-year efficacy and safety of a new 52-mg levonorgestrel-releasing intrauterine system, Contraception 92:10–16, 2015.

55. **Turok D,** The quest for better contraception: future methods, Obstet Gynecol Clin North Am 34:137–166, x, 2007.

56. **Ortiz ME, Croxatto HB,** The mode of action of IUDs, Contraception 36:37, 1987.

57. **Ortiz ME, Croxatto HB,** Copper-T intrauterine device and levonorgestrel intrauterine system: biological bases of their mechanism of action, Contraception 75:S16, 2007.

58. **Sivin I,** IUDs are contraceptives, not abortifacients: a comment on research and belief, Stud Fam Plann 20:355, 1989.

59. **Andersson K, Odlind V, Rybo G,** Levonorgestrel-releasing and copper-releasing (Nova T) IUDs during five years of use: a randomized comparative trial, Contraception 49:56, 1994.

60. **Grentzer JM, Peipert JF, Zhao Q, McNicholas C, Secura GM, Madden T,** Risk-based screening for Chlamydia trachomatis and Neisseria gonorrhoeae prior to intrauterine device insertion, Contraception 92:313–318, 2015.

61. **Sufrin CB, Postlethwaite D, Armstrong MA, Merchant M, Wendt JM, Steinauer JE,** Neisseria gonorrhea and Chlamydia trachomatis screening at intrauterine device insertion and pelvic inflammatory disease, Obstet Gynecol 120:1314–1321, 2012.

62. **Turok DK, Eisenberg DL, Teal SB, Keder LM, Creinin MD,** A prospective assessment of pelvic infection risk following same-day sexually transmitted infection testing and levonorgestrel intrauterine system placement, Am J Obstet Gynecol 215:599.e1–599.e6, 2016.

63. **Belhadj H, Sivin I, Diaz S, Pavez M, Tejada A-S, Brache V, et al.,** Recovery of fertility after use of the Levonorgestrel 20 mcg/d or copper T 380 Ag intrauterine device, Contraception 34:261, 1986.

64. **Sivin I, Stern J, Diaz J, Diaz MM, Faundes A, El Mahgoub S, et al.,** Two years of intrauterine contraception with levonorgestrel and with copper: a randomized comparison of the TCu 380Ag and levonorgestrel 20 mcg/day device, Contraception 35:245, 1987.

65. **Sivin I, Stern J, Diaz S, Pavéz M, Alvarez F, Brache V, et al.,** Rates and outcomes of planned pregnancy after use of Norplant capsules, Norplant II rods, or levonorgestrel-releasing or copper TCu 380Ag intrauterine contraceptive devices, Am J Obstet Gynecol 166:1208, 1992.

66. **Skjeldestad F, Bratt H,** Fertility after complicated and non-complicated use of IUDs. A controlled prospective study, Adv Contracept 4:179, 1988.

67. **Skjeldestad FE, Bratt H, Molne K,** [Fertility after complications with intrauterine devices. A prospective study], Tidsskr Nor Laegeforen 108:1112–1114, 1988.

68. **Vessey MP, Lawless M, McPherson K, Yeates D,** Fertility after stopping use of intrauterine contraceptive device, Br Med J 283:106, 1983.

69. **Wilson JC,** A prospective New Zealand study of fertility after removal of copper intrauterine contraceptive devices for conception and because of complications: a four-year study, Am J Obstet Gynecol 160:391, 1989.

70. A multinational case-control study of ectopic pregnancy. The World Health Organization's Special Programme of Research, Development and Research Training in Human Reproduction: Task Force on Intrauterine Devices for Fertility Regulation, Clin Reprod Fertil 3:131–143, 1985.

71. **Edelman DA, Porter CW,** The intrauterine device and ectopic pregnancy, Contraception 36:85, 1987.

72. **Mäkinen JI, Erkkola RU, Laippala PJ,** Causes of the increase in the incidence of ectopic pregnancy: a study on 1017 patients from 1966 to 1985 in Turku, Finland, Am J Obstet Gynecol 160:642, 1989.

73. **Marchbanks PA, Annegers J, Coulam C, Strathy J, Kurland L,** Risk Factors for ectopic pregnancy, JAMA 259:1823, 1985.

74. **Ory HW,** Ectopic pregnancy and intrauterine contraceptive devices: new perspectives. The Women's Health Study, Obstet Gynecol 57:137–144, 1981.

75. **Skjeldestad FE,** How effectively do copper intrauterine devices prevent ectopic pregnancy? Acta Obstet Gynecol Scand 76:684, 1997.

76. **Zhang D, Shi W, Li C, Yuan JJ, Xia W, Xue RH, et al.,** Risk factors for recurrent ectopic pregnancy: a case-control study, BJOG 123:82–89, 2016.

77. Contraception for adolescents, Pediatrics 134:e1244–e1256, 2014.

78. ACOG Committee Opinion No. 735: Adolescents and long-acting reversible contraception: implants and intrauterine devices, Obstet Gynecol 131:e130–e139, 2018.

79. **Committee on Practice Bulletins-Gynecology Long-Acting Reversible Contraception Work Group,** Practice Bulletin No. 186: long-acting reversible contraception: implants and intrauterine devices, Obstet Gynecol 130:e251–e269, 2017.

80. **Bednarek PH, Creinin MD, Reeves MF, Cwiak C, Espey E, Jensen JT,** Immediate versus delayed IUD insertion after uterine aspiration, N Engl J Med 364:2208–2217, 2011.

81. **Betstadt SJ, Turok DK, Kapp N, Feng KT, Borgatta L,** Intrauterine device insertion after medical abortion, Contraception 83:517–521, 2011.

82. **Çelen Ş, Möröy P, Sucak A, Aktulay A, Danışman N,** Clinical outcomes of early postplacental insertion of intrauterine contraceptive devices, Contraception 69:279, 2004.

83. **Chi IC, Farr G,** Postpartum IUD contraception—a review of an international experience, Adv Contracept 5:127, 1989.

84. **Cremer M, Bullard KA, Mosley RM, Weiselberg C, Molaei M, Lerner V, et al.,** Immediate vs. delayed postabortal copper T 380A IUD insertion in cases over 12 weeks of gestation, Contraception 83:522–527, 2011.

85. **Eggebroten JL, Sanders JN, Turok DK,** Immediate postpartum intrauterine device and implant program outcomes: a prospective analysis, Am J Obstet Gynecol 217:51.e1–51.e7, 2017.

86. **Hohmann HL, Reeves MF, Chen BA, Perriera LK, Hayes JL, Creinin MD,** Immediate versus delayed insertion of the levonorgestrel-releasing intrauterine device following dilation and evacuation: a randomized controlled trial, Contraception 85:240–245, 2012.

87. **Whitaker AK, Chen BA,** Society of Family Planning Guidelines: postplacental insertion of intrauterine devices, Contraception 97:2–13, 2018.

88. **Curtis KM, Tepper NK, Jatlaoui TC, Berry-Bibee E, Horton LG, Zapata LB, et al.,** U.S. medical eligibility criteria for contraceptive use, 2016, MMWR Recomm Rep 65:1–103, 2016.

89. **Heikinheimo O, Lehtovirta P, Suni J, Paavonen J,** The levonorgestrel-releasing intrauterine system (LNG-IUS) in HIV-infected women—effects on bleeding patterns, ovarian function and genital shedding of HIV, Hum Reprod 21:2857, 2006.

90. **Lehtovirta P, Paavonen J, Heikinheimo O,** Experience with the levonorgestrel-releasing intrauterine system among HIV-infected women, Contraception 75:37, 2007.

91. **Sinei SK, Morrison CS, Sekadde-Kigondu C, Allen M, Kokonya D,** Complications of use of intrauterine

207

devices among HIV-1-infected women, Lancet 351:1238, 1998.

92. **Stringer EM, Kaseba C, Levy J, Sinkala M, Goldenberg RL, Chi BH, et al.,** A randomized trial of the intrauterine contraceptive device vs hormonal contraception in women who are infected with the human immunodeficiency virus, Am J Obstet Gynecol 197:144, 2007.

93. **Grimes DA, Schulz KF,** Antibiotic prophylaxis for intrauterine contraceptive device insertion, Cochrane Database Syst Rev (2):CD001327, 2001.

94. **The American College of Obstetricians and Gynecologists,** Facts Are Important Emergency Contraception (EC) and Intrauterine devices (IUDs) Are Not Abortifacients, 2014. [cited 2018 November 30]. https://www.acog.org/-/media/Departments/Government-Relations-and-Outreach/FactsAreImportantEC.pdf

95. **Rivera R, Yacobson I, Grimes D,** The mechanism of action of hormonal contraceptives and intrauterine contraceptive devices, Am J Obstet Gynecol 181:1263–1269, 1999.

96. **Johannisson E,** Mechanism of action of intrauterine devices: biochemical changes, Contraception 36:11–22, 1987.

97. **Sagiroglu N, Sagiroglu E,** Intrauterine contraceptive devices and their biological effect, Hacettepe Bull Med Surg 2:179–214, 1969.

98. **Ämmälä M, Nyman T, Strengell L, Rutanen E-M,** Effect of intrauterine contraceptive devices on cytokine messenger ribonucleic acid expression in the human endometrium, Fertil Steril 63:773, 1995.

99. **Segal SJ, Alvarez-Sanchez F, Adejuwon CA, de Mejia VB, Leon P, Faundes A,** Absence of chorionic gonadotropin in sera of women who use intrauterine devices, Fertil Steril 44:214, 1985.

100. **Wilcox AJ, Weinberg CR, Glenn Armstrong E, Canfield RE,** Urinary human chorionic gonadotropin among intrauterine device users: detection with a highly specific and sensitive assay, Fertil Steril 47:265, 1987.

101. **Critchley HO, Wang H, Jones RL, Kelly RW, Drudy TA, Gebbie AE, et al.,** Morphological and functional features of endometrial decidualization following long-term intrauterine levonorgestrel delivery, Hum Reprod 13:1218, 1998.

102. **Lewis RA, Taylor D, Natavio MF, Melamed A, Felix J, Mishell D Jr,** Effects of the levonorgestrel-releasing intrauterine system on cervical mucus quality and sperm penetrability, Contraception 82:491–496, 2010.

103. **Tamburrino L, Marchiani S, Minetti F, Forti G, Muratori M, Baldi E,** The CatSper calcium channel in human sperm: relation with motility and involvement in progesterone-induced acrosome reaction, Hum Reprod 29:418–428, 2014.

104. **Bylander A, Nutu M, Wellander R, Goksor M, Billig H, Larsson DG,** Rapid effects of progesterone on ciliary beat frequency in the mouse fallopian tube, Reprod Biol Endocrinol 8:48, 2010.

105. **Mahmood T, Saridogan E, Smutna S, Habib AM, Djahanbakhch O,** The effect of ovarian steroids on epithelial ciliary beat frequency in the human Fallopian tube, Hum Reprod 13:2991–2994, 1998.

106. **Nutu M, Weijdegard B, Thomas P, Thurin-Kjellberg A, Billig H, Larsson DG,** Distribution and hormonal regulation of membrane progesterone receptors beta and gamma in ciliated epithelial cells of mouse and human fallopian tubes, Reprod Biol Endocrinol 7:89, 2009.

107. **Barbosa I, Olsson SE, Odlind V, Goncalves T, Coutinho E,** Ovarian function after seven years' use of a levonorgestrel IUD, Adv Contracept 11:85, 1995.

108. **Alvarez F, Brache V, Fernandez E, Guerrero B, Guiloff E, Hess R, et al.,** New insights on the mode of action of intrauterine contraceptive devices in women, Fertil Steril 49:768, 1988.

109. **Gemzell-Danielsson K, Berger C, GLL P,** Emergency contraception—mechanisms of action, Contraception 87:300–308, 2013.

110. **Brown PM, Farquhar CM, Lethaby A, Sadler LC, Johnson NP,** Cost-effectiveness analysis of levonorgestrel intrauterine system and thermal balloon ablation for heavy menstrual bleeding, Br J Obstet Gynaecol 113:797, 2006.

111. **Busfield RA, Farquhar CM, Sowter MC, Lethaby A, Sprecher M, Yu Y, et al.,** A randomised trial comparing the levonorgestrel intrauterine system and thermal balloon ablation for heavy menstrual bleeding, Br J Obstet Gynaecol 113:257, 2006.

208

112. **Hurskainen R, Teperi J, Rissanen P, Aalto A-M, Grenman S, Kivelä A, et al.**, Clinical outcomes and costs with the levonorgestrel-releasing intrauterine system or hysterectomy for treatment of menorrhagia, JAMA 291:1456, 2004.

113. **Irvine GA, Campbell-Brown MB, Lumsden MA, Heikkila A, Walker JJ, Cameron IT,** Randomised comparative trial of the intrauterine system and norethisterone levonorgestrel for treatment of idiopathic menorrhagia, Br J Obstet Gynaecol 105:592, 1998.

114. **Istre O, Trolle B,** Treatment of menorrhagia with the levonorgestrel intrauterine system versus endometrial resection, Fertil Steril 76:304, 2001.

115. **Milsom I, Andersson K, Andersch B, Rybo G,** A comparison of flurbiprofen, tranexamic acid, and a levonorgestrel-releasing intrauterine contraceptive device in the treatment of idiopathic menorrhagia, Am J Obstet Gynecol 164:879, 1991.

116. **Reid PC, Virtanen-Kari S,** Randomised comparative trial of the levonorgestrel intrauterine system and mefenamic acid for the treatment of idiopathic menorrhagia: a multiple analysis using total menstrual fluid loss, menstrual blood loss and pictorial blood loss assessment charts, Br J Obstet Gynaecol 112:1121, 2005.

117. **Römer T,** Prospective comparison study of levonorgestrel IUD versus Roller-Ball endometrial ablation in the management of refractory recurrent hypermenorrhea, Eur J Obstet Gynecol Reprod Biol 90:27, 2000.

118. **Shaw RW, Symonds IM, Tamizian O, Chaplain J, Mukhopadhyay S,** Randomised comparative trial of thermal balloon ablation and levonorgestrel intrauterine system in patients with idiopathic menorrhagia, Aust N Z J Obstet Gynaecol 47:335, 2007.

119. **Tang GWK, Lo SST,** Levonorgestrel intrauterine device in the treatment of menorrhagia in chinese women: efficacy versus acceptability, Contraception 51:231, 1995.

120. **Andersson JK, Rybo G,** Levonorgestrel-releasing intrauterine device in the treatment of menorrhagia, Br J Obstet Gynaecol 97:690, 1990.

121. **Baldaszti E, Wimmer-Puchinger B, Löschke K,** Acceptability of the long-term contraceptive levonorgestrel-releasing intrauterine system (Mirena®): a 3-year follow-up study, Contraception 67:87, 2003.

122. **Hidalgo M, Bahamondes L, Perrotti M, Diaz J, Dantas-Monteiro C, Petta C,** Bleeding patterns and clinical performance of the levonorgestrel-releasing intrauterine system (Mirena) up to two years, Contraception 65:129, 2002.

123. **Ronnerdag M, Odlind V,** Health effects of long-term use of the intrauterine levonorgestrel-releasing system. A follow-up study over 12 years of continuous use, Acta Obstet Gynecol Scand 78:716, 1999.

124. **Kingman CEC, Kadir RA, Lee CA, Economides DL,** The use of levonorgestrel-releasing intrauterine system for treatment of menorrhagia in women with inherited bleeding disorders, Br J Obstet Gynaecol 111:1425, 2004.

125. **Kilic S, Yuksel B, Doganay M, Bardakci H, Akinsu F, Uzunlar O, et al.,** The effect of levonorgestrel-releasing intrauterine device on menorrhagia in women taking anticoagulant medication after cardiac valve replacement, Contraception 80:152, 2009.

126. **Lukes A, Reardon B, Arepally G,** Use of the levonorgestrel-releasing intrauterine system in women with hemostatic disorders, Fertil Steril 90:673, 2007.

127. **Schaedel ZE, Dolan G, Powell MC,** The use of the levonorgestrel-releasing intrauterine system in the management of menorrhagia in women with hemostatic disorders, Am J Obstet Gynecol 193:1361, 2005.

128. **Fong Y-F, Singh K,** Effect of the levonorgestrel-releasing intrauterine system on uterine myomas in a renal transplant patient, Contraception 60:51, 1999.

129. **Pisoni CN, Cuadrado MJ, Khamashta MA, Hunt BJ,** Treatment of menorrhagia associated with oral anticoagulation: efficacy and safety of the levonorgestrel releasing intrauterine device (Mirena coil), Lupus 15:877, 2006.

130. **Cho S, Nam A, Kim H, Chay D, Park K, Cho DJ, et al.,** Clinical effects of the levonorgestrel-releasing intrauterine device in patients with adenomyosis, Am J Obstet Gynecol 198:373, 2008.

209

131. **Imai A, Matsunami K, Takagi H, Ichigo S,** Levonorgestrel-releasing intrauterine device used for dysmenorrhea: five-year literature review, Clin Exp Obstet Gynecol 41:495–498, 2014.

132. **Lindh I, Milsom I,** The influence of intrauterine contraception on the prevalence and severity of dysmenorrhea: a longitudinal population study, Hum Reprod 28:1953–1960, 2013.

133. **Chan SSC, Tam WH, Yeo W, Yu MMY, Ng DPS, Wong AWY, et al.,** A randomised controlled trial of prophylactic levonorgestrel intrauterine system in tamoxifen-treated women, Br J Obstet Gynaecol 114:1510, 2007.

134. **Gardner FJE, Konje JC, Bell SC, Abrams KR, Brown LJR, Taylor DJ, et al.,** Prevention of tamoxifen induced endometrial polyps using a levonorgestrel releasing intrauterine system: long-term follow-up of a randomised control trial, Gynecol Oncol 114:452, 2009.

135. **Kesim MD, Aydin Y, Atis A, Mandiraci G,** Long-term effects of the levonorgestrel-releasing intrauterine system on serum lipids and the endometrium in breast cancer patients taking tamoxifen, Climacteric 11:252, 2008.

136. **Toivonen J, Luukkainen T, Allonen H,** Protective effect of intrauterine release of levonorgestrel on pelvic infection: three years' comparative experience of levonorgestrel- and copper-releasing intrauterine devices, Obstet Gynecol 77:261–264, 1991.

137. **Suhonen S, Haukkamaa M, Jakobsson T, Rauramo I,** Clinical performance of a levonorgestrel-releasing intrauterine system and oral contraceptives in young nulliparous women: a comparative study, Contraception 69:407, 2004.

138. **Teal SB, Turok DK, Chen BA, Kimble T, Olariu AI, Creinin MD,** Five-year contraceptive efficacy and safety of a levonorgestrel 52-mg intrauterine system, Obstet Gynecol 133:63–70, 2019.

139. **Goldthwaite LM, Creinin MD,** Comparing bleeding patterns for the levonorgestrel 52 mg, 19.5 mg, and 13.5 mg intrauterine systems, Contraception 100:128–131, 2019.

140. **Kadir RA, Chi C,** Levonorgestrel intrauterine system: bleeding disorders and anticoagulant therapy, Contraception 75:S123–S129, 2007.

141. **Chi C, Huq FY, Kadir RA,** Levonorgestrel-releasing intrauterine system for the management of heavy menstrual bleeding in women with inherited bleeding disorders: long-term follow-up, Contraception 83:242–247, 2011.

142. **Grigorieva V, Chen-Mok M, Tarasova M, Mikhailov A,** Use of a levonorgestrel-releasing intrauterine system to treat bleeding related to uterine leiomyomas, Fertil Steril 79:1194, 2003.

143. **Magalhães J, Aldrighi JM, de Lima GR,** Uterine volume and menstrual patterns in users of the levonorgestrel-releasing intrauterine system with idiopathic menorrhagia or menorrhagia due to leiomyomas, Contraception 75:193, 2007.

144. **Mercorio F, De Simone R, Di Spiezio Sardo A, Cerrota G, Bifulco G, Vanacore F, et al.,** The effect of a levonorgestrel-releasing intrauterine device in the treatment of myoma-related menorrhagia, Contraception 67:277, 2003.

145. **Soysal S, Soysal ME,** The efficacy of levonorgestrel-releasing intrauterine device in selected cases of myoma-related menorrhagia: a prospective controlled trial, Gynecol Obstet Invest 59:29, 2005.

146. **Tasci Y, Caglar GS, Kayikcioglu F, Cengiz H, Yagci B, Gunes M,** Treatment of menorrhagia with the levonorgestrel releasing intrauterine system: effects on ovarian function and uterus, Arch Gynecol Obstet 280:39, 2009.

147. **Sayed GH, Zakherah MS, El-Nashar SA, Shaaban MM,** A randomized clinical trial of a levonorgestrel-releasing intrauterine system and a low-dose combined oral contraceptive for fibroid-related menorrhagia, Int J Gynaecol Obstet 112:126–130, 2011.

148. **Zapata LB, Whiteman MK, Tepper NK, Jamieson DJ, Marchbanks PA, Curtis KM,** Intrauterine device use among women with uterine fibroids: a systematic review, Contraception 82:41–55, 2010.

149. **Rizkalla HF, Higgins M, Kelehan P, O'Herlihy C,** Pathological findings associated with the presence of a Mirena intrauterine system at hysterectomy, Int J Gynecol Pathol 27:74, 2008.

150. **Bahamondes L, Petta CA, Fernandes A, Monteiro I,** Use of the levonorgestrel-releasing intrauterine system in women with endometriosis, chronic pelvic

pain and dysmenorrhea, Contraception 75:S134, 2007.

151. **Gomes MKO, Ferriani RA, Rosa e Silva JC, Japur de Sá Rosa e Silva AC, Vieira CS, Cândido dos Reis FJ,** The levonorgestrel-releasing intrauterine system and endometriosis staging, Fertil Steril 87:1231, 2007.

152. **Lockhat FB, Emembolu J, Konje J,** The evaluation of the effectiveness of an intrauterine-administered progestogen (levonorgestrel) in the symptomatic treatment of endometriosis and in the staging of the disease, Hum Reprod 19:179, 2004.

153. **Lockhat FB, Emembolu JO, Konje JC,** The efficacy, side-effects and continua-tion rates in women with symptomatic endometriosis undergoing treatment with an intra-uterine administered progestogen (levonorgestrel): a 3 year follow-up, Hum Reprod 20:789, 2005.

154. **Petta CA, Ferriani RA, Abrao MS, Hassan D, Rosa e Silva JC, Podgaec S, et al.,** Randomized clinical trial of a levonorgestrel-releasing intrauterine system and a depot GnRH analogue for the treatment of chronic pelvic pain in women with endometriosis, Hum Reprod 20:1993, 2005.

155. **Petta CA, Ferriani RA, Abrão MS, Hassan D, Rosa e Silva JC, Podgaec S, et al.,** A 3-year follow-up of women with endometriosis and pelvic pain users of the levonorgestrel-releasing intrauterine system, Eur J Obstet Gynecol Reprod Biol 143, 2009.

156. **Sheng J, Zhang WY, Zhang JP, Lu D,** The LNG-IUS study on adenomyosis: a 3-year follow-up study on the efficacy and side effects of the use of levonorgestrel intrauterine system for the treatment of dysmenorrhea associated with adenomyo-sis, Contraception 79:189, 2009.

157. **Bahamondes L, Ribeiro-Huguet P, de Andrade KC, Leon-Martins O, Petta CA,** Levonorgestrel-releasing intrauter-ine system (Mirena®) as a therapy for endometrial hyperplasia and carcinoma, Acta Obstet Gynecol Scand 82:580, 2003.

158. **Haimovich S, Checa MA, Mancebo G, Fusté P, Carreras R,** Treatment of endometrial hyperplasia without atypia in peri- and postmenopausal women with a levonorgestrel intrauterine device, Menopause 15:1002, 2008.

159. **Pal N, Broaddus RR, Urbauer DL, Balakrishnan N, Milbourne A, Schmeler KM, et al.,** Treatment of Low-Risk Endometrial Cancer and Complex Atypical Hyperplasia with the levo-norgestrel-releasing intrauterine device, Obstet Gynecol 131:109–116, 2018.

160. **Varma R, Soneja H, Bhatia K, Ganesan R, Rollason T, Clark TJ, et al.,** The effectiveness of a levonorgestrel-releasing intrauterine system (LNG-IUS) in the treatment of endometrial hyperplasia—A long-term follow-up study, Eur J Obstet Gynecol Reprod Biol 139:169, 2008.

161. **Vereide AB, Kaino T, Sager G, Arnes M, Ørbo A,** Effect of levonorgestrel IUD and oral medroxyprogesterone acetate on glan-dular and stromal progesterone receptors (PRA and PRB), and estrogen receptors (ER-α and ER-β) in human endometrial hyperplasia, Gynecol Oncol 101:214, 2006.

162. **Wheeler DT, Bristow RE, Kurman RJ,** Histologic alterations in endometrial hyperplasia and well-differentiated carci-noma treated with progestins, Am J Surg Pathol 31:988, 2007.

163. **Wildemeersch D, Rowe PJ,** Assessment of menstrual blood loss in women with ideopathic menorrhagia using the frame-less levonorgestrel-releasing intrauterine system, Contraception 70:165, 2004.

164. **Ørbo A, Arnes M, Hancke C, Vereide AB, Pettersen I, Larsen K,** Treatment results of endometrial hyperplasia after prospective D-score classification, Gynecol Oncol 111:68, 2008.

165. **Vereide AB, Arnes M, Straume B, Maltau JM, Ørbo A,** Nuclear morpho-metric changes and therapy monitoring in patients with endometrial hyper-plasia: a study comparing effects of intrauterine levonorgestrel and systemic medroxyprogesterone, Gynecol Oncol 91:526, 2003.

166. Product labeling for Mirena, Kyleena, and Skyla http://labeling.bayerhealthcare.com/html/products/pi/Mirena_PI.pdf; http://labeling.bayerhealthcare.com/html/products/pi/Kyleena_PI.pdf; http://labeling.bayerhealthcare.com/html/products/pi/Sklya_PI.pdf

167. **Raudaskoski T, Tapanainen J, Tomas E, Luotola H, Pekonen F, Ronni-Sivula H, et al.,** Intrauterine 10 microg and 20 microg levonorgestrel systems in postmenopausal women receiving oral

oestrogen replacement therapy: clinical, endometrial and metabolic response, BJOG 109:136–144, 2002.

168. **Benshushan A, Paltiel O, Rojansky N, Brzezinski A, Laufer N,** IUD use and the risk of endometrial cancer, Eur J Obstet Gynecol Reprod Biol 105:166, 2002.

169. **Castellsagué X, Thompson WD, Dubrow R,** Intra-uterine contraception and the risk of endometrial cancer, Int J Cancer 54:911, 1993.

170. **Hill DA, Weiss NS, Voigt LF, Beresford SAA,** Endometrial cancer in relation to intra-uterine device use, Int J Cancer 70:278, 1997.

171. **Sturgeon S, Brinton L, Berman M, Mortel R, Twiggs L, Barrett R, et al.,** Intrauterine device use and endometrial cancer risk, Int J Epidemiol 26:496, 1997.

172. **Cortessis VK, Barrett M, Brown Wade N, Enebish T, Perrigo JL, Tobin J, et al.,** Intrauterine device use and cervical cancer risk: a systematic review and meta-analysis, Obstet Gynecol 130:1226–1236, 2017.

173. **Abu J, Brown L, Ireland D,** Endometrial adenocarcinoma following insertion of the levonorgestrel-releasing intrauterine system (mirena) in a 36-year-old woman, Int J Gynecol Cancer 16:1445, 2006.

174. **Kresowik J, Ryan GL, Van Voorhis BJ,** Progression of atypical endometrial hyperplasia to adenocarcinoma despite intrauterine progesterone treatment with the levonorgestrel-releasing intrauterine system, Obstet Gynecol 111:547, 2008.

175. **Hidalgo MM, Hidalgo-Regina C, Bahamondes MV, Monteiro I, Petta CA, Bahamondes L,** Serum levonorgestrel levels and endometrial thickness during extended use of the levonorgestrel-releasing intrauterine system, Contraception 80:84, 2009.

176. **Lippes J,** Contraception with intrauterine plastic loops, Am J Obstet Gynecol 93:1024–1030, 1965.

177. **Diedrich JT, Zhao Q, Madden T, Secura GM, Peipert JF,** Three-year continuation of reversible contraception, Am J Obstet Gynecol 213:662.e1–662.e8, 2015.

178. **Aoun J, Dines VA, Stovall DW, Mete M, Nelson CB, Gomez-Lobo V,** Effects of age, parity, and device type on complications and discontinuation of intrauterine devices, Obstet Gynecol 123:585–592, 2014.

179. **Rivera R, Chen-Mok M, McMullen S,** Analysis of client characteristics that may affect early discontinuation of the TCu-380A IUD, Contraception 60:155, 1999.

180. **Sivin I, Stern J, Coutinho E, Mattos CER, El Mahgoub S, Diaz S, et al.,** Prolonged intrauterine contraception: a seven-year randomized study of the levonorgestrel 20 mcg/day (LNg 20) and the Copper T380 Ag IUDS, Contraception 44:473, 1991.

181. **Diedrich JT, Klein DA, Peipert JF,** Long-acting reversible contraception in adolescents: a systematic review and meta-analysis, Am J Obstet Gynecol 216:364.e1–364.e12, 2017.

182. **Thonneau P, Almont T, de La Rochebrochard E, Maria B,** Risk factors for IUD failure: results of a large multicentre case-control study, Hum Reprod 21:2612, 2006.

183. **Franks AL, Beral V, Cates W, Hogue CJR,** Contraception and ectopic pregnancy risk, Am J Obstet Gynecol 163:1120, 1990.

184. **Sivin I,** Dose- and age-dependent ectopic pregnancy risks with intrauterine contraception, Obstet Gynecol 78:291, 1991.

185. **Heinemann K, Reed S, Moehner S, Minh TD,** Comparative contraceptive effectiveness of levonorgestrel-releasing and copper intrauterine devices: the European Active Surveillance Study for Intrauterine Devices, Contraception 91:280–283, 2015.

186. The TCu380A, TCu220C, multiload 250 and Nova T IUDS at 3,5 and 7 years of use—results from three randomized multicentre trials. World Health Organization. Special Programme of Research, Development and Research Training in Human Reproduction: Task Force on the Safety and Efficacy of Fertility Regulating Methods, Contraception 42:141–158, 1990.

187. **Gemzell-Danielsson K, Apter D, Dermout S, Faustmann T, Rosen K, Schmelter T, et al.,** Evaluation of a new, low-dose levonorgestrel intrauterine contraceptive system over 5 years of use, Eur J Obstet Gynecol Reprod Biol 210:22–28, 2017.

188. **Sanders JN, Adkins DE, Kaur S, Storck K, Gawron LM, Turok DK,** Bleeding, cramping, and satisfaction among new copper IUD users: a prospective study, PLoS One 13:e0199724, 2018.

189. **Diedrich JT, Desai S, Zhao Q, Secura G, Madden T, Peipert JF,** Association of short-term bleeding and cramping patterns with long-acting reversible contraceptive method satisfaction, Am J Obstet Gynecol 212:50.e1–50.e8, 2015.

190. **Madden T, Proehl S, Allsworth JE, Secura GM, Peipert JF,** Naproxen or estradiol for bleeding and spotting with the levonorgestrel intrauterine system: a randomized controlled trial, Am J Obstet Gynecol 206:129.e1-8, 2012.

191. **Friedlander E, Kaneshiro B,** Therapeutic options for unscheduled bleeding associated with long-acting reversible contraception, Obstet Gynecol Clin North Am 42:593–603, 2015.

192. **Grimes DA, Hubacher D, Lopez LM, Schulz KF,** Non-steroidal anti-inflammatory drugs for heavy bleeding or pain associated with intrauterine-device use, Cochrane Database Syst Rev 18:CD006034, 2006.

193. **Milsom I, Andersson K, Jonasson K, Lindstedt G, Rybo G,** The influence of the Gyne-T 380S IUD on menstrual blood loss and iron status, Contraception 52:175, 1995.

194. **Zhuang L, Yang B, Yuan H,** [Medicated stainless steel ring-165, medicated gamma-intrauterine devices and TCu220C: a multicenter comparative study], Zhonghua Fu Chan Ke Za Zhi 32:97–101, 1997.

195. Effects of contraceptives on hemoglobin and ferritin. Task Force for Epidemiological Research on Reproductive Health, United Nations Development Programme/United Nations Population Fund/World Health Organization/World Bank Special Programme of Research, Development and Research Training in Human Reproduction, World Health Organization, Geneva, Switzerland, Contraception 58:262–273, 1998.

196. **Hassan EO, El-Husseini M, El-Nahal N,** The effect of 1-year use of the CuT 380A and oral contraceptive pills on hemoglobin and ferritin levels, Contraception 60:101, 1999.

197. **Backman T, Huhtala S, Blom T, Luoto R, Rauramo I, Koskenvuo M,** Length of use and symptoms associated with premature removal of the levonorgestrel intrauterine system: a nation-wide study of 17,360 users, Br J Obstet Gynaecol 107:335, 2000.

198. **Sivin I, Schmidt F,** Effectiveness of IUDs: a review, Contraception 36:55, 1987.

199. **Pakarinen P, Lähteenmäki P, Rutanen E-M,** The effect of intrauterine and oral levonorgestrel administration on serum concentrations of sex hormone-binding globulin, insulin and insulin-like growth factor binding protein-1, Acta Obstet Gynecol Scand 78:423, 1999.

200. **Orme ML, Back DJ, Breckenridge AM,** Clinical pharmacokinetics of oral contraceptive steroids, Clin Pharmacokinet 8:95–136, 1983.

201. **Sivin I, Lahteenmaki P, Ranta S, Darney P, Klaisle C, Wan L, et al.,** Levonorgestrel concentrations during use of levonorgestrel rod (LNG ROD) implants, Contraception 55:81–85, 1997.

202. **Morin-Papunen L, Martikainen H, McCarthy MI, Franks S, Sovio U, Hartikainen A-L, et al.,** Comparison of metabolic and inflammatory outcomes in women who used oral contraceptives and the levonorgestrel-releasing intrauterine device in a general population, Am J Obstet Gynecol 199:529, 2008.

203. **Backman T, Rauramo I, Jaakkola K, Inki P, Vaahtera K, Launonen A, et al.,** Use of the levonorgestrel-releasing intrauterine system and breast cancer, Obstet Gynecol 106:813, 2005.

204. **Lundström E, Söderqvist G, Svane G, Azavedo E, Olovsson M, Skoog L, et al.,** Digitized assessment of mammographic breast density in patients who received low-dose intrauterine levonorgestrel in continuous combination with oral estradiol valerate: a pilot study, Fertil Steril 85:989, 2006.

205. **Jacobson JC, Turok DK, Dermish AI, Nygaard IE, Settles ML,** Vaginal microbiome changes with levonorgestrel intrauterine system placement, Contraception 90:130–135, 2014.

206. **Madden T, Grentzer JM, Secura GM, Allsworth JE, Peipert JF,** Risk of bacterial vaginosis in users of the intrauterine

device: a longitudinal study, Sex Transm Dis 39:217–222, 2012.

207. **Mark AS, Hricak H,** Intrauterine contraceptive devices: MR imaging, Radiology 162:311, 1987.

208. **Pasquale SA, Russer TJ, Foldesy R, Mezrich RS,** Lack of interaction between magnetic resonance imaging and the copper-T380A IUD, Contraception 55:169, 1997.

209. **Lee NC, Rubin GL, Borucki R,** The intrauterine device and pelvic inflammatory disease revisited: new results from the Women's Health Study, Obstet Gynecol 72:1–6, 1988.

210. **Mehanna MTR, Rizk MA, Ramadan M, Schachter J,** Chlamydial serologic characteristics among intrauterine contraceptive device users: does copper inhibit chlamydial infection in the female genital tract? Am J Obstet Gynecol 171:691, 1994.

211. **Mishell DR, Bell JH, Good RG, Moyer DL,** The intrauterine device: a bacteriologic study of the endometrial cavity, Am J Obstet Gynecol 96:119, 1966.

212. **Farley TMM, Rowe PJ, Meirik O, Rosenberg MJ, Chen JH,** Intrauterine devices and pelvic inflammatory disease: an international perspective, Lancet 339:785, 1992.

213. **LeFevre ML,** Screening for Chlamydia and gonorrhea: U.S. Preventive Services Task Force recommendation statement, Ann Intern Med 161:902–910, 2014.

214. **Workowski KA, Bolan GA,** Sexually transmitted diseases treatment guidelines, 2015. MMWR Recomm Rep 64:1–137, 2015.

215. **American College of Obstetricians and Gynecologists' Committee on Gynecologic Practice: Long-Acting Reversible Contraceptive Expert Work Group,** Committee Opinion No 672: clinical challenges of long-acting reversible contraceptive methods, Obstet Gynecol 128:e69–e77, 2016.

216. **Donders GG, Berger J, Heuninckx H, Bellen G, Cornelis A,** Vaginal flora changes on Pap smears after insertion of levonorgestrel-releasing intrauterine device, Contraception 83:352–356, 2011.

217. **Joesoef MR, Karundeng A, Runtupalit C, Moran JS, Lewis JS, Ryan CA,** High rate of bacterial vaginosis among women with intrauterine devices in Manado, Indonesia, Contraception 64:169–172, 2001.

218. **Lessard T, Simoes JA, Discacciati MG, Hidalgo M, Bahamondes L,** Cytological evaluation and investigation of the vaginal flora of long-term users of the levonorgestrel-releasing intrauterine system (LNG-IUS), Contraception 77:30–33, 2008.

219. **Moi H,** Prevalence of bacterial vaginosis and its association with genital infections, inflammation, and contraceptive methods in women attending sexually transmitted disease and primary health clinics, Int J STD AIDS 1:86–94, 1990.

220. **Shoubnikova M, Hellberg D, Nilsson S, Mårdh P-A,** Contraceptive use in women with bacterial vaginosis, Contraception 55:355, 1997.

221. **Kim YJ, Youm J, Kim JH, Jee BC,** Actinomyces-like organisms in cervical smears: the association with intrauterine device and pelvic inflammatory diseases, Obstet Gynecol Sci 57:393–396, 2014.

222. **Westhoff C,** IUDs and colonization or infection with Actinomyces, Contraception 75:S48–S50, 2007.

223. **Johnston-MacAnanny EB, Hartnett J, Engmann LL, Nulsen JC, Sanders MM, Benadiva CA,** Chronic endometritis is a frequent finding in women with recurrent implantation failure after in vitro fertilization, Fertil Steril 93:437–441, 2010.

224. Risk factors for male to female transmission of HIV. European Study Group, BMJ 298:411–415, 1989.

225. **Musicco M, Nicolosi A, Saracco A, Lazzarin A,** IUD use and man to woman sexual transmission of HIV-1, In: Bardin C, Mishell D Jr, eds. Proceedings from the Fourth International Conference on IUDs, Butterworth-Heinemann, Boston, 1994.

226. **Evidence for Contraceptive Options and HIV Outcomes (ECHO) Trial Consortium,** HIV incidence among women using intramuscular depot medroxyprogesterone acetate, a copper intrauterine device, or a levonorgestel iimplant for contraception: a randomised, multicentre, open-label trial. Lancet. Epub ahead of print. June 13, 2019.

227. Comparison of female to male and male to female transmission of HIV in 563

stable couples. European Study Group on Heterosexual Transmission of HIV, BMJ 304:809–813, 1992.

228. **Ozgun MT, Batukan C, Mazicioglu MM, Serin IS, Baskol M, Ozturk A,** Intrauterine device use does not increase the incidence of anti-hepatitis C seropositivity among monogamous women in Turkey, Contraception 80:261, 2009.

229. **Brahmi D, Steenland MW, Renner RM, Gaffield ME, Curtis KM,** Pregnancy outcomes with an IUD in situ: a systematic review, Contraception 85:131–139, 2012.

230. **Schiesser M, Lapaire O, Tercanli S, Holzgreve W,** Lost intrauterine devices during pregnancy: maternal and fetal outcome after ultrasound-guided extraction. An analysis of 82 cases, Ultrasound Obstet Gynecol 23:486–489, 2004.

231. **Family UK, Planning Research Network,** Pregnancy outcome associated with the use of IUDs, Br J Fam Plann 15, 1989.

232. **Williams P, Johnson B, Vessey M,** Septic abortion in women using intrauterine devices, Br Med J iv:263, 1975.

233. **Atrash HK, Frye AA, Hogue C,** Incidence of morbidity and mortality with IUD in situ in the 1980s and 1990s, In: Bardin C, Mishell D Jr, eds. Proceedings from the Fourth International Conference on IUDs, Butterworth-Heinemann, Boston, 1994. p 76.

234. **Guillebaud J,** Letter: IUD and congenital malformation, Br Med J i:1016, 1975.

235. **Layde PM, Goldberg MF, Safra MJ, Oakley GP,** Failed intrauterine device contraception and limb reduction deformities: a case-control study, Fertil Steril 31:18, 1979.

236. **Zhang L, Ye W, Yu W, Cheng L, Shen L, Yang Z,** Physical and mental development of children after levonorgestrel emergency contraception exposure: a follow-up prospective cohort study, Biol Reprod 91:27, 2014.

237. **Ganer H, Levy A, Ohel I, Sheiner E,** Pregnancy outcome in women with an intrauterine contraceptive device, Am J Obstet Gynecol 201:381.e1-5, 2009.

238. **Kim SK, Romero R, Kusanovic JP, Erez O, Vaisbuch E, Mazaki-Tovi S, et al.,** The prognosis of pregnancy conceived despite the presence of an intrauterine device (IUD), J Perinat Med 38:45–53, 2010.

239. **Usinger KM, Gola SB, Weis M, Smaldone A,** Intrauterine contraception continuation in adolescents and young women: a systematic review, J Pediatr Adolesc Gynecol 29:659–667, 2016.

240. **Jatlaoui TC, Riley HE, Curtis KM,** The safety of intrauterine devices among young women: a systematic review, Contraception 95:17–39, 2017.

241. **Veldhuis H, Vos A, Lagro-Janssen A,** Complications of the intrauterine device in nulliparous and parous women, Eur J Contracept Reprod Health Care 10:82, 2004.

242. **Teal SB, Romer SE, Goldthwaite LM, Peters MG, Kaplan DW, Sheeder J,** Insertion characteristics of intrauterine devices in adolescents and young women: success, ancillary measures, and complications, Am J Obstet Gynecol 213:515.e1-5, 2015.

243. **Espey E, Ogburn T, Hall R, Byrn F,** Use of intrauterine device in the setting of uterus didelphys, Obstet Gynecol 108:774–776, 2006.

244. **Newton J, Tacchi D,** Long-term use of copper intrauterine devices, Br J Fam Plann 16:116, 1990.

245. **Haimov-Kochman R, Ackerman Z, Anteby EY,** The contraceptive choice for a Wilson's disease patient with chronic liver disease, Contraception 56:241, 1997.

246. **Wilson W, Taubert KA, Gewitz M, Lockhart PB, Baddour LM, Levison M, et al.,** Prevention of infective endocarditis: guidelines from the American Heart Association: a guideline from the American Heart Association Rheumatic Fever, Endocarditis, and Kawasaki Disease Committee, Council on Cardiovascular Disease in the Young, and the Council on Clinical Cardiology, Council on Cardiovascular Surgery and Anesthesia, and the Quality of Care and Outcomes Research Interdisciplinary Working Group, Circulation 116:1736–1754, 2007.

247. **Everett ED, Reller LB, Droegemueller W, Greer BE,** Absence of bacteremia after insertion or removal of intrauterine devices, Obstet Gynecol 47:207–209, 1976.

248. **Hall SM, Jamieson JR, Witcomb MA,** Letter: Bacteraemia after insertion

of intrauterine devices, S Afr Med J 50:1232, 1976.

249. **Murray S, Hickey JB, Houang E,** Significant bacteremia associated with replacement of intrauterine contraceptive device, Am J Obstet Gynecol 156:698, 1987.

250. **Suri V, Aggarwal N, Kaur R, Chaudhary N, Ray P, Grover A,** Safety of intrauterine contraceptive device (copper T 200 B) in women with cardiac disease, Contraception 78:315, 2008.

251. **Kimmerle R, Weiss R, Berger M, Kurz KH,** Effectiveness, safety, and acceptability of a copper intrauterine device (CU Safe 300) in type I diabetic women, Diabetes Care 16:1227, 1993.

252. **Kjos SL, Ballagh SA, La Cour M, Xiang A, Mishell DR Jr,** The copper T380A intrauterine device in women with type II diabetes mellitus, Obstet Gynecol 84:1006–1009, 1994.

253. **Skouby SO, Mølsted-Pedersen L, Kosonen A,** Consequences of intrauterine contraception in diabetic women, Fertil Steril 42:568, 1984.

254. **Visser J, Snel M, Van Vliet HA,** Hormonal versus non-hormonal contraceptives in women with diabetes mellitus type 1 and 2, Cochrane Database Syst Rev (3):CD003990, 2013.

255. **Modesto W, Bahamondes MV, Bahamondes L,** A randomized clinical trial of the effect of intensive versus non-intensive counselling on discontinuation rates due to bleeding disturbances of three long-acting reversible contraceptives, Hum Reprod 29:1393–1399, 2014.

256. **Barnett C, Moehner S, Do Minh T, Heinemann K,** Perforation risk and intra-uterine devices: results of the EURAS-IUD 5-year extension study, Eur J Contracept Reprod Health Care 22:424–428, 2017.

257. **Whiteman MK, Tyler CP, Folger SG, Gaffield ME, Curtis KM,** When can a woman have an intrauterine device inserted? A systematic review, Contraception 87:666–673, 2013.

258. **Lopez LM, Bernholc A, Zeng Y, Allen RH, Bartz D, O'Brien PA, et al.,** Interventions for pain with intrauterine device insertion, Cochrane Database Syst Rev (7):CD007373, 2015.

259. **Zapata LB, Jatlaoui TC, Marchbanks PA, Curtis KM,** Medications to ease intrauterine device insertion: a systematic review, Contraception 94:739–759, 2016.

260. **Ngo LL, Braaten KP, Eichen E, Fortin J, Maurer R, Goldberg AB,** Naproxen sodium for pain control with intrauterine device insertion: a randomized controlled trial, Obstet Gynecol 128:1306–1313, 2016.

261. **Mody SK, Kiley J, Rademaker A, Gawron L, Stika C, Hammond C,** Pain control for intrauterine device insertion: a randomized trial of 1% lidocaine paracervical block, Contraception 86:704–709, 2012.

262. **Akers AY, Steinway C, Sonalkar S, Perriera LK, Schreiber C, Harding J, et al.,** Reducing pain during intrauterine device insertion: a randomized controlled trial in adolescents and young women, Obstet Gynecol 130:795–802, 2017.

263. **Goldthwaite LM, Baldwin MK, Page J, Micks EA, Nichols MD, Edelman AB, et al.,** Comparison of interventions for pain control with tenaculum placement: a randomized clinical trial, Contraception 89:229–233, 2014.

264. **Kaislasuo J, Suhonen S, Gissler M, Lahteenmaki P, Heikinheimo O,** Uterine perforation caused by intrauterine devices: clinical course and treatment, Hum Reprod 28:1546–1551, 2013.

265. **Steenland MW, Zapata LB, Brahmi D, Marchbanks PA, Curtis KM,** The effect of follow-up visits or contacts after contraceptive initiation on method continuation and correct use, Contraception 87:625–630, 2013.

266. **Swenson C, Royer PA, Turok DK, Jacobson JC, Amaral G, Sanders JN,** Removal of the LNG IUD when strings are not visible: a case series, Contraception 90:288–290, 2014.

267. **Turok DK, Gurtcheff SE, Gibson K, Handley E, Simonsen S, Murphy PA,** Operative management of intrauterine device complications: a case series report, Contraception 82:354–357, 2010.

268. **Verma U, Astudillo-Davalos FE, Gerkowicz SA,** Safe and cost-effective ultrasound guided removal of retained

intrauterine device: our experience, Contraception 92:77–80, 2015.

269. **Wilson S, Tan G, Baylson M, Schreiber C,** Controversies in family planning: how to manage a fractured IUD, Contraception 88:599–603, 2013.

270. **Gorsline JC, Osborne NG,** Management of the missing intrauterine contraceptive device: report of a case, Am J Obstet Gynecol 153:228, 1985.

271. **Adoni A, Ben Chetrit A,** The management of intrauterine devices following uterine perforation, Contraception 43:77, 1991.

272. **Markovitch O, Klein Z, Gidoni Y, Holzinger M, Beyth Y,** Extrauterine mislocated IUD: is surgical removal mandatory? Contraception 66:105, 2002.

273. **Grønlund B, Blaabjerg J,** Serious intestinal complication five years after insertion of a Nova-T, Contraception 44:517, 1991.

274. **Cleland K, Zhu H, Goldstuck N, Cheng L, Trussell J,** The efficacy of intrauterine devices for emergency contraception: a systematic review of 35 years of experience, Hum Reprod 27:1994–2000, 2012.

275. **Turok DK, Godfrey EM, Wojdyla D, Dermish A, Torres L, Wu SC,** Copper T380 intrauterine device for emergency contraception: highly effective at any time in the menstrual cycle, Hum Reprod 28:2672–2676, 2013.

276. **Turok DK, Sanders JN, Thompson IS, Royer PA, Eggebroten J, Gawron LM,** Preference for and efficacy of oral levonorgestrel for emergency contraception with concomitant placement of a levonorgestrel IUD: a prospective cohort study, Contraception 93:526–532, 2016.

277. **Goodman S, Hendlish SK, Reeves MF, Foster-Rosales A,** Impact of immediate postabortal insertion of intrauterine contraception on repeat abortion, Contraception 78:143–148, 2008.

278. **McNicholas C, Peipert JF,** Initiation of long-acting reversible contraceptive methods (IUDs and implant) at pregnancy termination reduces repeat abortion, Evid Based Med 18:e29, 2013.

279. **Pohjoranta E, Suhonen S, Mentula M, Heikinheimo O,** Intrauterine contraception after medical abortion: factors affecting success of early insertion, Contraception 95:257–262, 2017.

280. **Jatlaoui TC, Whiteman MK, Jeng G, Tepper NK, Berry-Bibee E, Jamieson DJ, et al.,** Intrauterine device expulsion after postpartum placement: a systematic review and meta-analysis, Obstet Gynecol 132:895–905, 2018.

281. **Turok DK, Leeman L, Sanders JN, Thaxton L, Eggebroten JL, Yonke N, et al.,** Immediate postpartum levonorgestrel intrauterine device insertion and breast-feeding outcomes: a noninferiority randomized controlled trial, Am J Obstet Gynecol 217:665.e1–665.e8, 2017.

282. **Baldwin MK, Edelman AB, Lim JY, Nichols MD, Bednarek PH, Jensen JT,** Intrauterine device placement at 3 versus 6 weeks postpartum: a randomized trial, Contraception 93:356–363, 2016.

283. **Chen MJ, Hou MY, Hsia JK, Cansino CD, Melo J, Creinin MD,** Long-acting reversible contraception initiation with a 2- to 3-week compared with a 6-week postpartum visit, Obstet Gynecol 130:788–794, 2017.

284. **Zerden ML, Stuart GS, Charm S, Bryant A, Garrett J, Morse J,** Two-week postpartum intrauterine contraception insertion: a study of feasibility, patient acceptability and short-term outcomes, Contraception 95:65–70, 2017.

217

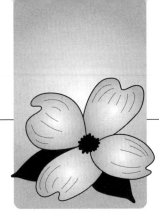

7

Combined Hormonal Contraception

Carolyn L. Westhoff, MD, MSc, Surya Cooper, MD, MPH, and Ian Joseph Bishop, MD, MPH

Types of Combined Hormonal Contraception

Combination hormonal contraceptives (CHCs) include pills, rings, patches, and injections and contain, by definition, an estrogen and a progestin. The mainstay of combined hormonal contraceptives for the first decades was a combination estrogen/progestin oral tablet. A fixed combination of mestranol 150 μg/norethynodrel 9.85 mg was developed as a combination oral contraceptive but first approved in 1957 as a treatment for menstrual disorders and infertility. The combination, marketed as Enovid®, was approved by the U.S. FDA as an oral contraceptive pill (OCP) in 1960 with a regimen of 21 consecutive days of active pills with a 7-day break between cycles. The 7-day break was designed to induce a withdrawal bleed that would mimic menses, resulting in 13 artificial cycles per year. As the original pills contained a substantial hormone dose, the hypothalamic-pituitary axis remained suppressed during the 7-day break, thus maintaining effectiveness. Innovations from this prototype include decreases in dose, changes in specific hormonal constituents, deviations from the fixed combination, and increases in the number of active tablets with concomitant decreases in the number of inert tablets per cycle. In the United States, at least 20 distinct formulations of combined oral contraceptives (COCs) are FDA approved and available, most of which contain ethinyl estradiol (EE) as the estrogen component. COCs are marketed as both branded and therapeutic equivalent (generic) products; the generic versions are also given distinct product names creating a market with an appearance of dozens of different formulations. The U.S. FDA approved a combination estrogen/progestin injection in 2000; such injections are not currently available in the United States but are widely used elsewhere (see Chapter 8). The U.S. FDA approved the first transdermal and transvaginal contraceptive delivery systems in 2001. The first non-EE containing COCs became available in Europe in 2009 and the United States in 2010.

Following their approval in 1960, oral contraceptive use increased rapidly in the United States and Europe. Case reports of pulmonary embolism in oral contraceptive users led to hearings on the cardiovascular safety by the FDA in 1963.[1] In 1968, Vessey and Doll[2] published a large case-control study of thrombosis risk in U.K. pill users, reporting a 9-fold risk increase. Due to this serious risk and other side effects, lower dose formulations rapidly emerged and dominated the market worldwide. Today's oral contraceptives have approximately 90% lower progestin doses than Enovid. However, with so many different progestins in use, each having different affinities for steroid hormone receptors, one cannot make simple dose comparisons between progestins based on their weight alone. Similarly, the estrogen content of COCs has declined. Mestranol is a prodrug of EE, and 150 μg of mestranol is roughly equivalent to 105 μg of EE. Most of today's oral contraceptives have daily EE doses ranging from 10 to 35 μg; the disadvantage of using lower EE doses (or estradiol at any dose) is more spotting or unpredictable bleeding,[3] which may contribute to user dissatisfaction. Importantly, it remains controversial whether COCs with EE doses below 35 μg are actually safer or otherwise more acceptable to users. Such results indicate that improving safety related to the estrogen component of oral contraceptives may require new estrogens or different delivery systems.

Several combined hormonal contraceptives already in use or under study contain estrogens other than EE. Estradiol 2.5 mg combined with the progestin nomegestrol acetate 1.5 mg (sold under the brand names Naemis and Zoely® among others) has a cycle with 24 active tablets and 4 placebo tablets; this product is available in Europe but not in the United States. A multiphasic oral contraceptive containing estradiol valerate (E2V) 1 to 3 mg per tablet and dienogest (DNG) 2 to 3 mg per tablet (sold as Natazia® and Qlaira®) has a cycle with 26 active tablets and 2 placebo tablets. Estradiol valerate circulates as estradiol. Products under development include pills that contain estetrol (E4), an estrogen with four hydroxyl side chains, and vaginal rings with estradiol (E2) instead of EE.

While the search for a safer pill has driven most dose reductions and other innovations in oral contraceptive regimens, the desire for a more favorable side effect profile has been another key motivator. Other changes in the past few decades have been non–science based; patent expiration and industry competition for marketing advantage has driven a number of minor and generally unimportant OC formulation changes. While many of these factors have led to dramatic decreases in estrogen doses, EE remains the most commonly used estrogen in oral contraceptives (and in the transdermal patch and the vaginal ring) worldwide. EE is a potent estrogen that is easily absorbed orally and that provides excellent cycle control.[3]

As we move forward in our discussion of CHCs, it is important to remember the concepts of "high-dose" and "low-dose" COC formulations that were introduced in Chapter 2. This "dose" refers to the estrogen content, specifically EE. High-dose COCs contain EE 50 μg or more, whereas low-dose products contain EE doses less than 50 μg.

Variations in Oral Formulations

Throughout the 1960s and still today, monophasic formulations (every tablet contains the same estrogen-progestin dose) dominate the market for combined hormonal products. Although the original 21-day active hormone and 7-day pill-free interval remains the most common COC regimen, alterations in drug delivery over 4-week or longer time periods have increased the options available to women today.

Phasic Regimens

Phased pill products emerged in the late 1970s with both sequential (biphasic) regimens and multiphasic regimens; some only altered the progestin doses and others varied both the estrogen and progestin doses throughout a single cycle. Today, multiphasic products include even more variations. The general aim of this approach is to lessen total dosage and minimize metabolic changes, spotting, breakthrough bleeding, or other annoying side effects (if any) while maintaining efficacy. Some products were developed simply to provide patent protection for a company for their hormonal product line. Overall, metabolic studies of multiphasic preparations indicate no differences or very slight improvements over the metabolic effects of low-dose monophasic products, and no difference in efficacy. Multiphasic products have efficacy similar to monophasic products, but evidence that multiphasic products have less breakthrough bleeding than do their monophasic counterparts is weak.[4,5] Thus, starting hormonal contraception with a monophasic product is reasonable.

Extended Regimens

The term "extended regimen" refers to combined hormonal administration for more than 21 days in a 28-day cycle. With a traditional 21/7 regimen, the hypothalamic-pituitary-ovarian (HPO) axis returns to near-normal activity quickly after the last dose. In an evaluation of 15 premenopausal women using 30 to 50 μg EE pills combined with levonorgestrel (LNG) or norgestrel, the investigators found follicle-stimulating hormone (FSH) and luteinizing hormone (LH) concentrations and pulse frequency, fully suppressed on the first day of the hormone-free interval (HFI), increased to levels similar to values obtained on cycle day 2 to 11 from controls with regular cycles not using an OC. Thus, HPO axis activation occurs by the end of a 7-day hormone-free week. Killick et al.[6] evaluated extending the HFI to 9 or 11 days in women using 30 to 40 μg EE pills combined with either LNG or gestodene (GSD). They used a crossover design, so each of the 28 subjects had a cycle of observation with a 7-, 9-, and 11-day HFI. Although none of the women ovulated, the investigators found significant variation in follicle growth between subjects with the longer intervals raising concern that reactivation of the HPO axis presents a mechanism for failure.

Given the importance of estrogen feedback on suppression of FSH, lowering the dose of EE below 30 μg may allow more rapid follicle development. van Heusden and Fauser[7] compared hormone profiles and follicle growth during the 7-day HFI between users of 20 and 30 μg EE pills with similar (gonane) progestins. Median follicle diameters at the beginning and at the end of the HFI were statistically significantly smaller in the 30 μg EE group, with a dominant follicle (defined as greatest follicle diameter ≥10 mm) observed at the end of the HFI in 22% of women using 20 μg compared to none among women using 30 µg EE pills. Consistent with greater follicle activity, the area under the curve (AUC) for E2 during the HFI was higher in users of the 20 µg EE pills and correlated with a more rapid rise of FSH than among users of the higher EE dose. Thus, the hormone-free week may allow a dominant follicle to develop, and any delay in beginning, or improper use (e.g., missed pill, ring removal) during the subsequent cycle may increase the risk of ovulation and pregnancy.

Studies evaluating the pharmacodynamics of a shorter HFI have not consistently shown a reduction in follicle growth or pituitary suppression.[8,9] The best data supporting the benefit of a reduced HFI come from a large prospective cohort study involving over 52,000 women conducted in Europe and the United States. This study found significantly lower failure rates associated with using 24-day regimens of EE combined with either drospirenone (DRSP) or norethindrone (NET) compared to 21-day formulation.[10]

Whether reducing the HFI improves breakthrough bleeding associated with initiation of low EE pills remains controversial, as most studies do not compare results with a common formulation.[11,12] However, reducing the HFI does seem to decrease the number of days of withdrawal bleeding.[11]

Trials comparing 21/7 and 24/4 products with the same hormones provide clarity about the differences with these regimens. A randomized open-label, 6-month study of an EE 20 µg/NET acetate 1 mg pill enrolled 938 women in a 4:1 ratio with 705 women receiving the 24/4 regimen and 181 in the 21/7 regimen in the final analysis.[13] The study was not large enough to determine a significant difference in efficacy comparing the two products. The number of days with breakthrough bleeding or spotting was comparable between the groups, but the 24-day group demonstrated a steady decline in breakthrough bleeding/spotting days, so that in cycle 6, the mean number of bleeding days was lower in the 24-day group (0.95 vs. 1.63). Additionally, each cycle with the 24-day product demonstrated a shorter duration of withdrawal bleeding (bleeding beginning after the last day of active drug intake), achieving statistical significance in the second cycle. On average, women using the 24/4 regimen experienced one less day of bleeding per month. Thus, if both products are available, the 24/4 regimen has slightly better cycle control; whether this translates to increased compliance or continuation is unknown.

A 3-cycle treatment study compared ovarian activity with 24/4 and 21/7 regimens of an EE 20 µg/DRSP 3 mg pill.[14] In the third cycle, the first 3 tablets were substituted with placebo to identify what would happen with noncompliance when starting a new pill pack (in essence, the 21/7 group had a 10-day pill-free interval and the 24/4 had a 7-day pill-free interval). The 24/4 schedule was associated with greater follicular suppression and only one ovulation in cycle 3 compared with four ovulations in the 21/7 regimen. A study of 12 women using this formulation for either 23 or 24 hormone days documented greater suppression of FSH, LH, inhibin B, and estradiol during the pill-free interval when compared to women using the same product with 21 hormone days.[8]

This latter study demonstrates the concept of "escape" follicular activity, which is decreased in women using a 24/4-day regimen, even with lower hormone doses. In general, ovarian follicular activity is greater with products containing less EE, and the maximal follicular size reached is larger. In one study, approximately 30% of women using an EE 20 µg product achieved follicular diameters of 15 mm or greater compared to only 15% of women using an EE 35 µg product when the pill-free interval was extended from 7 to 9 days.[15] Once follicles achieve a diameter greater than 10 mm, an increasing percentage will ovulate even in the presence of oral contraceptive treatment.[16] Lower-dose EE formulations produce less suppression of gonadotropin secretion; users of a 20 µg EE product have higher FSH, LH, and estradiol blood levels.[15] Thus, increasing the number of active hormone days to 24 in a 28-day cycle overcomes the risk of escape ovulation. Bear in mind that with correct daily COC use, a pharmacodynamics trial found no differences in follicular development between women assigned to an OC with EE 20 µg versus an OC with EE 30 µg.[17]

Another approach to reducing reactivation of the HPO axis during the HFI involves the addition of a low EE dose given alone to replace inert pills for several days (e.g., Mircette® has 21 EE/desogestrel [DSG] tablets, two placebo tablets, and 5 EE-only tablets; Lo Loestrin® Fe has 24 EE/NET tablets, two EE-only tablets, and two hormone-free iron tablets). The rationale for this approach is that EE should result in suppression of FSH secretion and prevent follicle growth. A randomized study that compared women using either a 21-day EE 20 µg/LNG 100 µg pill followed by a 7-day HFI or a 24/4 regimen of EE 20 µg/DRSP 3 mg to an experimental regimen of EE 20 µg with DSG 150 µg followed by EE 10 µg for 7 days found no difference in follicle activity between formulations.[18] However, the different progestins used make interpretation of results challenging. A study that evaluated the effects of EE during the HFI among women using EE 30 µg/LNG 150 µg did show a beneficial effect on suppression of FSH, E2, and inhibin B.[19]

Extended Cycles

"Extended cycle" refers to the continuous use of a combined hormonal product beyond 28 days without an HFI. Three approaches are in common use: tricycle extended cycles, continuous cycles, and flexible cycles. The tricycle regimen provides a convenient approach to reduce the number of withdrawal bleeds to four times per year. Each blister pack includes 84 active combined pills followed by 7 days of placebo pills (Seasonale® EE 30 µg/LNG 150 µg) or 7 days of EE 10 µg (Seasonique® EE 30 µg/LNG 150 µg; LoSeasonique® EE 20 µg/LNG 100 µg). For continuous cycles, women use the active combined hormonal product every day without any hormone-free interruption. A formulation of EE 20 µg/LNG 90 µg is approved for 1-year continuous use by the U.S. FDA; however, any low-dose monophasic pill is suitable for continuous doing. A potential disadvantage of continuous use is breakthrough bleeding particularly in early cycles of use, but this seems to improve over time.[20] A small randomized study that compared 21/7 cycles or continuous use of a EE 20 µg/LNG 100 µg pill found more overall bleeding and spotting days in the continuous group but significantly fewer bleeding days that required protection.[21] Women randomized to continuous use were also more likely to have amenorrhea and reported significantly fewer days of bloating and menstrual pain.

Flexible cycle refers to an extended cycle of variable length. With flexible use, the woman decides when to initiate a 4-day HFI. Typically, this decision is prompted by an episode of breakthrough bleeding. Only one 4-day HFI is permitted every 28 days. The rationale for a flexible 4-day HFI comes from a study that demonstrated that initiation of a 4-day pill break improved bleeding patterns in women using continuous pills.[22] A formulation of EE 20 µg/DRSP 3 mg designed for flexible use with a novel electronic tablet dispensing device is approved in Australia but not in the United States.[23] A 1-year open-label phase 3 study conducted in the United States randomized women to one of two flexible extended regimens or the conventional 24/4 regimen, and found a bleeding-signal flexible approach was associated with good contraceptive efficacy and fewer bleeding/spotting days than the conventional 24/4 regimen.[24]

Taking active pills continuously can more fully suppress ovulation and can suppress menses and other cyclic symptoms like dysmenorrhea, mood changes, headaches, and bloating.[22] For years, clinicians have prescribed unlimited daily oral contraceptives to treat conditions such as endometriosis, bleeding disorders, menstrual seizures, and menstrual migraine headaches, as well as to avoid bleeding in athletes and busy individuals. Many women do not require the periodic experience of vaginal bleeding to assure themselves that they are not pregnant. Monthly bleeding, periodic bleeding, or no bleeding—this is an individual woman's choice. Any combination oral contraceptive can be used on a daily basis; even the lowest estrogen dose formulations provide excellent bleeding and side effect profiles in a continuous regimen.[20,21,25] As with the extended regimen, continuous dosing provides greater ovarian suppression, reducing the potential for breakthrough and escape ovulations.[26] A further benefit of continuous use is simplification of the pill-taking schedule with the potential of better compliance and a lower failure rate. The return of ovulation and achievement of pregnancy are not delayed after discontinuation of continuous dosing.[26,27] Extended cycling to suppress menses is increasingly acceptable.[28,29]

Variations in Oral Contraceptives Unrelated to Hormonal Content

Some products replace the inert tablets with either iron or folate or even add folate to the active hormonal component of each pack. Because reproductive age women may develop iron deficiency secondary to heavy menses, adding some iron may be beneficial, but since any combined hormonal contraceptive use tends to reduce menstrual blood loss, the benefit of adding iron is modest. The goal of adding folate is to help women maintain folate sufficiency, so that if they become pregnant immediately on stopping the

OC, this folate sufficiency may help to prevent a neural tube defect in that pregnancy.[30,31] The benefits of adding minerals or vitamins to contraceptive formulations have yet to be proven and mostly serve as a patent modifier related to marketing.

In the United States, pill packs usually contain 28 tablets with 7 inert tablets during the 7-day break; including these inert tablets was intended to help women maintain their pill-taking routine. In many other countries, a 21-day blister pack (without any inert tablets) is routine.

Nonoral Formulations

In addition to pills, CHC is also available in a monthly vaginal ring formulation, weekly transdermal adhesive patch formulation, and monthly combined injections—most of these are provided in 4-week cycles. A vaginal ring (Annovera™) designed for use for 13 consecutive 21/7 cycles was approved in the United States in 2018. The hormones in the rings and patch are also available in oral formulations. While the ring, patch, and injections have been less well studied than pills, the risks and benefits are likely similar. The main benefit of using a ring, patch, or injection (where available) is that less frequent dosing may help to support more consistent use; however, evidence for that benefit is inconsistent.[32,33] Using a ring or an injection may also be more discreet, a benefit for some adults and adolescents who do not want partners or parents to know about their contraceptive use.

Transdermal Contraceptives

The U.S. FDA-approved transdermal contraceptives include a 20-cm^2 patch that releases EE 20 μg/day and norelgestromin (NLGM, the primary active metabolite of norgestimate [NGM]) 150 μg/day. The product was originally marketed as the branded product Evra®, but now is only available as the generic Xulane®. Three weekly patches are used consecutively (thus for 21 days) after which scheduled withdrawal bleeding will occur during a patch-free week. The overall 1-year Pearl Index from the pivotal trials ranged between 0.7 and 1.24.[34-36] At that time, most women in clinical trials were required to be at or close to normal weight and thus only 10% of the participants in the pivotal trials had a weight greater than 90 kg; these heavier study participants experienced one third of the on-treatment pregnancies.[37] The patch label therefore carries a warning about lesser effectiveness in heavier women, and these results led to extensive evaluation of the possible relation between weight and effectiveness for many other hormonal contraceptives.[38]

A 4-month U.S. trial randomized 500 COC users who were content with their COC but willing to try a nondaily option to use either the EE/NLGM patch or the 1-month vaginal ring contraceptive; at the end of the study, most patch users preferred to resume the oral contraceptive while ring users preferred the ring.[39]

A randomized pharmacokinetic study compared this EE/NLGM patch to an EE 30 μg/LNG 150 μg oral contraceptive and the EE/etonogestrel (ENG) contraceptive vaginal ring.[40] The 21-day AUC for EE was 50% greater among the women who used the patch compared to those who used the oral contraceptive, and 300% greater than contraceptive ring users; even with just eight women in each group, these results were highly statistically significant. The higher-than-expected EE AUC may explain side effects (breast tenderness) and greater hepatic globulin induction with patch use compared to use of oral contraceptives of the same dose,[41] which could translate to higher venous thromboembolism (VTE) risk.

Concerns over EE exposure have led to the development of other patches. Alternatives to the EE/NLGM patch under investigation include a weekly formulation designed to deliver EE 30 µg/day and LNG 120 µg/day and EE 20 µg/day and GSD 60 µg/day.

A large trial that randomized women to either the EE/LNG patch or an EE 20 µg/day LNG 100 µg/day COC showed comparable 6-month Pearl Indexes (4.45 [patch] and 4.02 [COC]),[42] bleeding patterns, safety, and acceptability.[43,44] The study population included a large proportion of obese women, but an analysis stratified by obesity found minimal difference in Pearl Indices. The U.S. FDA did not approve the EE/LNG patch based upon this Pearl Index despite the comparable result in the COC group. Data from other recent studies of hormonal contraceptives has shown a trend toward rising Pearl Indexes with more recent COC clinical trials of the same products (See Chapter 2 for discussion of the "Creeping Pearl").[38,45]

The weekly EE/GSD patch containing EE 0.55 mg and GSD 2.1 mg provides similar daily systemic exposure to EE and GSD as an oral contraceptive containing EE 20 µg/day and GSD 60 µg/day; in contrast, the EE systemic exposure with the EE/NLGM patch was at least 200% greater than an oral comparator.[46] An analysis of ovulation inhibition in 173 women using the EE/GSD patch showed no differences by body mass index (BMI), even among women with a BMI greater than 35 kg/m^2.[47] The bleeding pattern with this patch was comparable to an EE 20 µg/LNG 100 µg oral contraceptive.[48] Results from a 13-cycle phase 3 open-label study in Europe yielded an adjusted Pearl Index of 0.81 with favorable bleeding patterns and a low rate of adverse events.[49] However, results from a large multicenter U.S. study of this patch that began in 2009 have not been reported (ClinicalTrials.gov NCT00910637), suggesting that the development program has been halted.

Extended use of the existing combined hormonal patch may be associated with some estrogen accumulation; as this patch already yields higher systemic hormone levels than most current CHC, extended use seems unwise.[40] A small randomized study comparing a 12-week regimen of continuous use of the EE/NGM patch followed by a 1-week HFI to the standard cycles showed high acceptability of both use patterns. Because the release system for each patch is different, any new patches that enter the market will require evaluation of extended use.

Vaginal Hormonal Contraception

The original CHC vaginal ring, 52 mm in diameter, 4 mm in cross section, and made of ethylene vinyl acetate (EVA), releases EE 15 µg/day and etonogestrel (ENG, which is the active metabolite of DSG) 120 μg/day (NuvaRing® and bioequivalent rings including MyRing™ and Ornibel®). The hormones are embedded with EVA in a core that has a thin EVA outer release-controlling membrane. These rings are approved for single-cycle use for 21 days, but ovarian suppression continues even with 6 or more weeks of use.[50] Four efficacy studies showed pregnancy rates of less than 1%, similar to the pregnancy rates in contemporary studies of COCs.[51] In a crossover study, ovarian suppression was substantially greater when using the ring than when using a monophasic EE 20 or 30 μg oral contraceptive with LNG.[52] Despite the low EE dose and the consequent low EE systemic exposure,[40] bleeding and spotting days are somewhat less with this ring than with an EE 30 μg/day oral contraceptive.[53] In a U.S. trial that evaluated 500 COC users interested in switching methods, most of those who were randomly assigned to this vaginal ring were highly satisfied and preferred to continue the ring after the study ended.[39]

A novel CHC ring, FDA designated as a "contraceptive vaginal system," releases EE 13 μg/day and segesterone acetate (SA) 150 μg/day (Annovera). SA, also known as Nestorone®, is a potent progestin not used in pills as it is not orally active. This ring is also intended for cyclic use (21 days in, 7 days out), but it is unique in that a single ring is reusable for up to 1 year or 13 cycles.[54,55] Prolonged use of the same ring does not increase the risk of vaginal infection and does not disrupt the vaginal ecosystem.[56]

Contraceptive vaginal rings delivering estradiol are under investigation. A dose-finding study evaluated six 21-day rings designed to release E2 300 μg/day along with various doses of ENG or nomegestrol acetate.[57] Results demonstrated excellent ovulation suppression and cycle control with most of the six rings. Merck Sharp & Dohme Corp. initiated a U.S. phase 3 clinical trial program with a vaginal ring releasing estradiol 300 μg/day and ENG 125 μg/day in 2015 but terminated the study prematurely for business reasons (ClinicalTrials.gov NCT02524288). Fortunately, development of a combined E2/SA ring continues through the efforts of the Population Council and National Institute of Child Health and Human Development. Dose-finding studies have evaluated rings designed for 90 days of continuous use releasing E2 (in a range of doses) and SA 200 μg/day and found excellent ovulation suppression.[58] A phase 2B study currently in progress is evaluating the efficacy, safety, and cycle control of a 3-month E2/SA vaginal ring (ClinicalTrials.gov NCT03432416).

Studies support using the EE/ENG contraceptive ring continuously[50,59] albeit with a similar spotting profile as that seen with extended-cycle COCs. With continuous use, the ring can be prescribed monthly rather than every 4 weeks. One approach for continuous use of the ring involves changing on a standard day each month (such as the first of the month, or any date significant to the woman), rather than every 28 days as the ring contains sufficient hormone release for this interval.

Injectable Combination Hormonal Contraception

Two monthly CHC injections are widely available around the world. Combined injections are highly effective reversible methods with failure rates less than 1%; in randomized trials, they have higher continuation rates than do progestin-only injections due to more predictable bleeding patterns.[3]

Cyclofem® contains 5 mg estradiol cypionate and 25 mg medroxyprogesterone acetate (E2-C/MPA); this formulation was studied and FDA approved as Lunelle in the United States in 2000, but was withdrawn due to manufacturing challenges. A large 60-week U.S. clinical trial with a COC comparison group demonstrated high efficacy and safety. Withdrawal bleeding starts about 22 days after the injection, lasts an average of 6 days, and tends to be consistent during the first year of use.[60] Amenorrhea incidence is 1% to 4% per cycle. Acceptability and satisfaction were similar between COC and injections.[61] Pharmacokinetic-pharmacodynamic studies reported contraceptive concentrations of MPA and found that ovulation remained suppressed for at least 2 months after the third injection. Injection site (arm, hip, or leg) and body weight had no important effects on MPA concentrations.[62,63]

Another CHC injection is Mesigyna®, which contains 5 mg estradiol valerate and 50 mg norethisterone enanthate (E2-V/NET-EN). Estradiol valerate is rapidly metabolized to yield estradiol (E2) after injection.

The progestin components of these combined injections differ, but both are widely used at higher doses in progestin-only injectables. A large randomized trial with 5,680 women in China compared efficacy, side effects, and bleeding patterns of Mesigyna, Cyclofem, and a third investigational injectable.[64,65] Mesigyna and Cyclofem had low (<1%) 1-year failure rates. Discontinuations for bleeding complaints were lower for Mesigyna than for Cyclofem (0.6% vs. 3.7%). Overall discontinuation rates were lower for Mesigyna than for Cyclofem (14% vs. 19%).

Pharmacodynamics

Contraceptive Effects

The primary mechanism of action of CHCs is suppression of the HPO axis, limiting gonadotropin release and thus inhibiting follicular development and ovulation. Progestins alone suppress LH release and thus can be highly effective contraceptives. The estrogen component of CHC contributes to suppressing FSH, thus attenuating follicle development, and the estrogen also potentiates the progestin actions. This estrogen function has allowed reduction of the progestin dose in the pill. The mechanism for this action is probably estrogen's effect in increasing the concentration of intracellular progestin receptors. Therefore, a minimal level of estrogen enhances CHC efficacy. The estrogen component also balances the progestin effect on the endometrium, reducing breakthrough bleeding as compared to progestin-only systemic contraception. The effects of estrogens and progestins on ovulation are well documented, and ultrasound assessment of follicle growth and rupture combined with serum hormone evaluation to document progesterone production by the corpus luteum provide reliable surrogates of a contraceptive effect.

Because the progestin will always take precedence over estrogen (unless the estrogen dose is increased many, many fold), changes in the endometrium, cervical mucus, and perhaps tubal function reflect progestin stimulation. The contribution of contraceptive mechanisms other than ovulation inhibition has not been conclusively demonstrated. Although the progestin in the CHC produces an endometrium considered not receptive to ovum implantation (decidualized bed with exhausted and atrophied glands) and cervical mucus thick and impervious to sperm transport, both of these potential mechanisms become moot when ovulation does not occur. In the setting of ovulation, ovarian steroids may lead to more favorable endometrial and cervical changes. Therefore, while the product labeling for CHCs suggest endometrial or cervical mechanisms, these are largely theoretical. Chapter 2 reviews contraceptive mechanisms of steroid hormones in more detail.

Hepatic Effects

Contraceptive steroids affect numerous organs and systems separate from the reproductive system or from the mechanism of action. These effects vary based on the type of estrogen and progestin; future development of novel agonists and antagonists will likely result in products with differential effects on various organ systems. Today, most products contain EE. Key EE effects include stimulation of hepatic proteins through both first- and second-pass metabolism. Use of a CHC releasing EE increases sex hormone–binding globulin (SHBG), corticotropin-binding globulin (CBG), and thyroid-binding globulin (TBG), with maximal levels by day 7 to 10 of each cycle regardless of the route of administration. These changes are so characteristic that they can reveal, in COC users, whether an individual has been taking the pill (somewhat analogous to measuring HgA1C among people with diabetes to evaluate treatment success).[66] The magnitude of binding globulin increases is directly related to the estrogen dose. These EE-induced increases are generally mitigated by the progestin, and this effect varies greatly by progestin type and dose. The more androgenic progestins, such as LNG decrease these changes, while newer progestins, such as DRSP, that do not stimulate the androgen receptor, allow the largest estrogen-induced increases to occur. In essence, these "androgenic" effects are actually "antiestrogenic." Increases in these binding globulins do not have direct clinical effects, but they do lead to changes in the circulating levels of their ligands. For instance, among pill users, the circulating total thyroid levels will be higher due to the increases in TBG, but these levels do not signify thyroid dysfunction. Estradiol delivered transdermally or vaginally in physiologic doses does not stimulate the liver.

229

Metabolic Effects

Weight Gain

Many women believe weight gain is a common side effect of CHCs.[67,68] COC users who attribute weight gain to their contraceptive are more likely to discontinue use by 6 months.[69] However, available data from clinical trials contradict this belief.[70-75] Results from two multicenter randomized double-blind placebo-controlled randomized clinical trials designed to evaluate the efficacy of triphasic EE/NGM in the treatment of moderate acne vulgaris provide insight into commonly reported side effects.[54,70] Over 500 women took part in these 6-month studies, and only 18 (7.9%) EE/NGM subjects and 9 (3.8%) placebo subjects discontinued because of adverse experiences. Notably, three of the nine discontinuations in the placebo group occurred due to weight gain, compared to only one in the EE/NGM group (the additional discontinuations in the OC group occurred primarily due to nuisance side effects such as nausea), and the incidence of weight gain (2%) did not differ between the groups.

A Swedish longitudinal study from 1986 to 2006, including over 600 women, reported no difference in weight/BMI increase between women who had used COCs at some time and women who had never used COCs. Further, a longitudinal analysis to assess any association between COC use and weight gain, which evaluated age, COC use, children, smoking, and exercise, found the only predictor for weight increase was age (gain of 0.45 kg/year).[76] A Cochrane review that included 49 trials did not find evidence supporting a causal relationship between CHC and weight gain.[77] The majority of trials that compared pill types and doses found little difference in weight gain between groups, contradicting the myth that weight gain is dose related.

Fewer studies have evaluated the effect of CHCs on weight gain in obese women, as most CHC studies have excluded this population. A study that randomized women to use of either an EE 30 μg/LNG 150 μg or EE 20 μg/LNG 100 μg COC for 3 to 4 months found no difference in the pattern of weight gain between the cohorts of normal weight ($n = 96$) and obese ($n = 54$) women with either OC formulation.[78] A Swedish randomized, multicenter, open-label trial of 983 women treated with the EE/ENG vaginal ring or a COC for 13 cycles saw relatively small changes in baseline mean body weight and body composition for both groups with no notable between-group differences.[79] Although these data support lack of a causal relationship between CHC use and weight gain, clinicians need to approach the discussion of weight gain with sensitivity. Clinicians need to carefully reinforce the lack of association between oral contraceptives and weight gain and focus the patient on the real culprits: diet and level of exercise. Most women gain a moderate amount of weight as they age, whether they use CHCs or not. However, if a woman strongly believes her CHC is causing weight gain, she is at high risk for discontinuation and requires counseling on alternative contraceptive strategies.

Lipoproteins and Oral Contraception

In women who use CHC for at least 3 months, the estrogen component of CHC lowers low-density lipoprotein cholesterol (LDL) and increases high-density lipoprotein cholesterol (HDL).[80] These changes occur due to first-pass hepatic effects with all orally administered estrogens, and as a result of secondary pass of EE. The progestin component antagonizes estrogen-induced beneficial lipid changes, modulated by the progestin's effect on androgenicity. Oral contraceptives with relatively high doses of progestins (doses not used in today's low-dose formulations) do produce unfavorable lipoprotein changes.[81] Formulas with less androgenic progestins generally show more favorable effects on lipids compared to more androgenic progestins, such as LNG.[82] The magnitude of change is related to the EE dose, the progestin type, and the woman's weight (i.e., normal weight vs. obese).

EE causes a dose-related increase in triglycerides. Oral, but not transdermal, estradiol also increases triglyceride levels. Although COC formulations containing EE 35 µg increase triglyceride-rich very low-density lipoprotein (VLDL) levels by 2.2-fold, these estrogen-induced triglyceride particles are different in size than endogenously produced triglycerides and do not appear to increase a woman's risk for atherosclerosis.[83]

Animal studies have indicated a protective action of estrogen against atherosclerosis. Oral administration of combination estrogen/progestin to monkeys being fed a high-cholesterol, atherogenic diet decreased the extent of coronary atherosclerosis.[84-86] In similar experiments, estrogen treatment markedly prevented arterial lesion development in rabbits.[87-89] These animal studies help explain why older, higher dose combinations, which had an adverse impact on the lipoprotein profile, did not increase subsequent cardiovascular disease.[90,91]

Similarly, in a prospective study of normal-weight and obese women randomly assigned to one of two lose-dose 21-day COC formulations (either EE 30 µg/LNG 150 µg or EE 20 µg/LNG 100 µg), no changes in mean total cholesterol or triglycerides were observed in the overall group or in either BMI subgroup. There was a 5.7% reduction in HDL in the overall group; in the BMI subgroups, this reduction was somewhat greater in the normal weight group and in all women assigned to the EE 30 µg/LNG 150 µg pill. These small changes in lipid markers are not clinically significant and are unlikely to impact cardiovascular risk. These findings provide evidence to support that low-dose CHCs do not have an important effect on lipid profiles of women with higher BMIs.[92]

Unless a patient has a strong family history of cardiovascular disease or preexisting hyperlipidemia, routine screening for lipid levels is not necessary before prescribing CHC. In past decades, considerable marketing hype emphasized the importance of the impact of CHCs on the cholesterol-lipoprotein profile. If indeed certain CHCs had a negative relevant impact on the lipoprotein profile, one would expect to find evidence of atherosclerosis as a cause of an increase in subsequent cardiovascular disease. There is no such evidence.[91,93] Thus, the mechanism of the cardiovascular complications during CHC use is likely a short-term acute mechanism related to thrombosis, an estrogen-related effect.

Low androgenic progestins do not adversely affect the cholesterol-lipoprotein profile. One must be cautious regarding the clinical significance of subtle lipoprotein changes, and as with the older progestins and adverse changes in lipoproteins, it seems unlikely that oral contraceptives will have a clinically meaningful beneficial or adverse effect on the incidence of coronary heart disease.

Carbohydrate Metabolism

Insulin sensitivity is affected mainly by the progestin component of CHCs.[94] Progesterone is a competitive inhibitor of the insulin receptor, and estrogen increases the release of insulin from the pancreatic islet cells and decreases insulin sensitivity. The glucose intolerance is dose related, and effects are minimal with the low-dose formulations. With the older high-dose oral contraceptives, many women experienced marked impairment of glucose tolerance and impaired insulin secretion.[95] But modern low-dose CHCs currently available in the United States do not have any clinically significant adverse effects on carbohydrate metabolism and do not increase the incidence of diabetes.[96] CHC may produce an increase in peripheral resistance to insulin action. Most women can meet this challenge by increasing insulin secretion, and there is no change in the glucose tolerance test. In the CARDIA Study, which included 1,940 women aged 18 to 30 years, use of low-dose COCs was associated with lower glucose levels and with a lower odds ratio (OR) for the development of diabetes.[97] Further, obesity has little effect on any CHC-induced changes in carbohydrate metabolism: obese and normal-weight women experience similar changes in glucose and insulin, all too small to be clinically significant.[92] Long-term use (up to 7 years) of low-dose COCs did not increase the risk of type 2 diabetes compared with use of nonhormonal contraception in women with a history of prior gestational diabetes mellitus.[98] Further, women with polycystic ovarian syndrome and insulin resistance do not report increased insulin resistance.[99]

Long-term follow-up studies of large populations have failed to detect any increase in the incidence of diabetes mellitus or impaired glucose tolerance (even in past and current users of high-dose pills).[100–102] Oral contraceptive use does not produce an increase in diabetes mellitus.[101–104] The minor hyperglycemia associated with oral contraception is not deleterious and is completely reversible. Even women who have risk factors for diabetes in their history are not affected. Use of low-dose monophasic and multiphasic oral contraceptives in women with recent gestational diabetes does not significantly impact glucose tolerance over 6 to 13 months does not increase the risk of overt diabetes mellitus during long-term follow-up.[98,105] Women with previous gestational diabetes often develop overt diabetes and its associated vascular complications. Until overt diabetes develops, these patients can still appropriately use low-dose CHC. The contraindication to use reflects the cardiovascular risk.

In clinical practice, it may be necessary to prescribe CHC for the overtly diabetic patient. Historically, women with diabetes were denied CHC due to concerns about the effect on carbohydrate and lipid metabolism. Recent data and the CDC MEC emphasize the safety of CHC for women with diabetes without complications (category 2 applies for CHC for any diabetic patient without cardiovascular or microvascular complications associated with diabetes). No effect on insulin requirement is expected with low-dose formulations.[106] This effect in women under age 35 who are otherwise healthy and do not smoke is probably very minimal with low-dose CHC. Reliable protection against pregnancy is a benefit for these patients that outweighs the small risk. In a 1-year study of women with insulin-dependent diabetes mellitus who were using a low-dose oral contraceptive, no deterioration could be documented in lipoprotein or hemostatic biochemical markers for cardiovascular risk.[107] A case-control study could find no evidence that oral contraceptive use by young women with insulin-dependent diabetes mellitus increased the development of retinopathy or nephropathy.[108] Finally, no effect of oral contraceptives on cardiovascular mortality could be detected in a group of women with diabetes mellitus.[109] Although the CDC MEC states that the advantages of using CHC in the overt diabetic without complications outweigh the theoretical or proven risks (category 2), there still remains a need for clinical judgment as directly relevant studies are not available.[110]

Cardiovascular Effects

Venous Thromboembolism

Coagulation Biomarkers

Administration of EE at pharmacologic levels causes an increase in the production of procoagulant factors such as factor V, factor VIII, factor X, and fibrinogen.[111] In addition, anticoagulant factors and proteins significantly decrease. The progestin component modulates the EE-induced clotting factor responses.[112] The net effects depend upon the estrogen used and route of administration (see Chapter 2). EE-containing contraceptives rapidly cause prothrombotic changes in the coagulation system manifested by immediate downstream effects such as increased prothrombin fragment 1 + 2, increased D-dimer, and changes in endogenous thrombin potential, a global marker of thrombophilia.[112,113] Studies that have tried to differentiate the effects of different HC formulations on thrombophilia have had mixed results.[112,114–118] The coagulation system changes in a procoagulant direction with CHC use, but the average changes are small and values tend to remain with normal ranges. Which changes are clinically important is not entirely clear.[112] Changes in individual factors have weak or unknown relationships to VTE risk, and thus one must be cautious about overinterpreting the clinical importance of the any laboratory changes, as none are validated surrogates or proven predictors for VTE risk.

Pharmacodynamic studies of EE-containing contraceptives are consistent in showing procoagulant effects. E2-containing oral contraceptives are less well studied but have similar or slightly less effect on the coagulation system compared to EE-containing contraceptives.[119,120]

Whether the various progestins paired with EE modulate the procoagulant effect of estrogen is controversial with studies reporting small differences of uncertain clinical relevance.[121,122] Studies that evaluated a specific measure of thrombin generation, the activated protein C sensitivity ratio, have reported that CHCs containing EE and low-androgenic gonanes or DRSP cause more thrombin generation than older CHCs.[123] This research test is a global measure of coagulation system activation, and studies show that greater activation is directly related to VTE risk in individuals with hereditary thrombophilias.[124,125] However, this test has not been validated as a surrogate for VTE risk associated with different CHC formulations.

Estetrol (E4) is another estrogen being studied as an oral contraceptive. A detailed hematologic study demonstrated that E4 combined with DRSP caused little or no procoagulant changes from baseline, while the comparison oral contraceptive containing EE/DRSP led to substantial changes from baseline.[126] Current experience with this agent is limited to clinical trials; we will not be able to learn if the favorable laboratory results will translate into lower VTE risk until this combination comes into widespread clinical use.

Transdermal and transvaginal CHC delivery systems avoid hepatic first-pass effects. As such, initial hopes were that these nonoral contraceptives would have less effect on coagulation and on VTE risk than EE-containing oral contraceptives. However, in actuality, the second-pass metabolism of EE when delivered via a nonoral route is quite extensive. A randomized crossover study found that patch and ring use were associated with greater increases in the activated protein C sensitivity ratio than with an EE/LNG oral contraceptive.[127] Another crossover study showed similar adverse changes of multiple coagulation factors when comparing the EE/NLGM patch and an EE/NGM oral contraceptive.[128] These results suggested that using the patch or ring would not avoid the VTE risks of EE-containing COCs.

The monthly contraceptive injections are less studied; a WHO randomized trial published in 2003 compared the hemostasis effects among 259 women using two monthly injectables to the effects of an EE/NET oral contraceptive among 119 women.[129] In the 9-month study, the injection users had slightly smaller unfavorable changes in their coagulation system than did the oral contraceptive users. While that study measured many individual factors, it did not assess the more global measures of coagulation system activation such as thrombin generation (measured by APCsr) or D-dimer or fragment 1+2.

Epidemiologic Studies of CHC and Thrombosis

Older epidemiologic evaluations of oral contraceptives and vascular disease indicated that venous thrombosis was an effect of estrogen, limited to current users, with a disappearance of the risk by 3 months after discontinuation.[130,131] Thromboembolic disease was believed to be a consequence of EE administration with the level of risk related only to the EE dose.[132-134] In the first years of oral contraception, the available products, containing high doses of EE or mestranol, were associated with a 4- to 6-fold increased risk of venous thrombosis.[135] Smoking was documented to produce an additive increase in the risk of arterial thrombosis[136-138] but had no effect on the risk of VTE.[139,140]

Because of the increased risks for venous thrombosis, myocardial infarction (MI), and stroke, lower dose formulations (<50 µg estrogen) came to dominate the market, and clinicians became more careful in their screening of patients and prescribing of oral contraception. Two forces, therefore, were at work simultaneously to bring greater safety to women utilizing oral contraception: (1) the use of lower dose formulations and (2) the avoidance of COCs by high-risk patients. Because of these two forces, the Puget Sound study in the United States documented a reduction in venous thrombosis risk to 2-fold greater than nonusers.[141]

Is there still a risk of VTE with the current low-dose oral contraceptive formulations and nonoral CHC? Epidemiologic studies have included case-control studies, very large multiyear prospective trials, and even larger database evaluations (**Table 7.1**).

Each study type has its strengths and weaknesses. VTE is fortunately rare, with about 1 event per 1,000 CHC users per year, but this relative rarity makes comparator studies difficult. The very large studies that use data directly from existing databases are often the only quick and cost-efficient way to evaluate the associations between various CHC types and these outcomes. Despite these advantages, database studies usually cannot evaluate important confounding factors (for VTE, these may include family history, obesity, smoking, and other risk factors not captured by insurance claims or registries). Database studies also have only indirect measures of the CHC exposure—that is, they typically know about prescriptions, but do not have direct information about whether and when a woman actually used the CHC. The incidence of VTE in database studies is usually lower than that found in other study types.[142-144]

In contrast, case-control studies may be disadvantaged by recall bias[145-147] while the smaller number of VTEs available for analysis typically hamper prospective cohort studies, as seen with Dinger et al.[148]

Dramatic changes in CHC availability and in clinical practice frequently can occur during the time frame of any study, which can create analytical challenges. Thus, the differences in results across studies remain a topic for vigorous methodologic discussion. Keeping these limitations in mind, we present some of the key papers below.

The World Health Organization (WHO) Collaborative Study of Cardiovascular Disease and Steroid Hormone Contraception was a hospital-based, case-control study with subjects collected from 21 centers in 17 countries in Africa, Asia, Europe, and Latin America.[145] A subevaluation of data from 10 centers in 9 countries assessed the risk of

Table 7.1 Epidemiologic Studies of CHC and VTE Risk

Exposure	Range of Effect Estimates		
	Database Studies (Relative Risks)	Prospective Studies (Hazard Ratios)	Case-Control Studies (Odds Ratios)
Oral EE with levonorgestrel (reference)	1.0	1.0	1.0
Oral EE with desogestrel/gestodene	1.8–2.1	—	1.4–2.2
Oral EE with drospirenone	1.6–2.1	0.8–1.0	1.0
Oral E2 valerate with dienogest	—	0.5	—
Vaginal EE with etonogestrel	1.1–1.9	0.8	—
Transdermal EE with norelgestromin	1.1–2.4	—	—

See text for details of individual studies.

idiopathic VTE associated with a formulation containing EE 30 µg and LNG (doses ranging from 125 to 250 µg) compared to the risk associated with preparations containing EE 20 or 30 µg and either DSG or GSD.[149] The OR for VTE, adjusted for body weight and height, for EE-LNG formulation users compared with nonusers was 3.5. Compared to nonusers, the OR for EE-DSG and EE-GSD products were 9.1. Thus, the risk of VTE with EE-LNG use was 2.6 times lower than with EE-DSG and EE-GSD use.

The Transnational Study of Oral Contraceptives and the Health of Young Women analyzed 471 cases of deep vein thrombosis and/or VTE from the United Kingdom and Germany.[146] These investigators found an OR of 3.2 for VTE among women using CHC containing EE 35 µg or less and a progestin other than DSG or GSD. They reported that the OR was 1.5-fold greater for women using EE-DSG and EE-GSD products than other products.

In Denmark, Lidegaard et al.[150] performed a hospital-based, case-control study of women with confirmed diagnoses of VTE in 1994 and 1995 (in Denmark, all women with this diagnosis are hospitalized, and therefore, very few, if any, cases were missed). They identified a 2-fold increased VTE risk in current oral contraceptive users, across EE doses ranging from 20 to 50 μg. The increased risk was concentrated in the first year of use. Because there were more short-term users of the new progestins and more long-term users of the older progestins, adjustment for duration of use resulted in no significant differences between the progestin types. Factors associated with an increased VTE risk included coagulation disorders, treated hypertension during pregnancy, family history of VTE, and a greater BMI. Notably, conditions not associated with an increased risk of VTE included smoking, migraine, diabetes, hyperlipidemia, parity, or age at first birth. This study could not establish the absence or presence of a dose-response relationship comparing the EE 20 μg dose to higher doses. However, a 5-year update reported that EE 20 μg had a lower risk than did products with EE 30 to 40 μg.[151] Additionally, this update found that the risk of venous thrombosis associated with current COC use declined with increasing duration of use, VTE risk was slightly lower with EE/LNG than EE/DSG or EE/GSD oral contraceptives, smoking more than 10 cigarettes per day increased VTE risk, and progestin-only contraceptive products did not increase VTE risk.

Case-control studies using VTE cases derived from the computer records of general practices in the United Kingdom concluded that the increased risk associated with oral contraceptives was the same for all types, and that the pattern of risk with specific oral contraceptives suggested confounding because of "preferential prescribing" (defined later).[152,153] In these studies, matching cases and controls by year of birth eliminated differences between different types of oral contraceptives. A similar analysis based on 42 cases from a German database also found no difference between new progestin and older progestin oral contraceptives.[154] Thus, in these two studies, more precise adjustments for age eliminated a confounding bias. An assessment of the incidence of VTE in the United Kingdom before and after the decline in EE/DSG and EE/GSD product use could detect no impact on the statistics (neither an increase nor a decrease).[155]

A reanalysis of the Transnational Case-Control Study considered the duration and patterns of oral contraceptive use, focusing on first-time users of oral contraceptives with EE doses less than 50 μg.[156,157] Statistical analysis with adjustment for duration of use in the 105 cases who were first-time users could find no differences between different progestin products. A similar reanalysis of the United Kingdom General Practice Database could demonstrate no difference between different oral contraceptive formulations.[157]

A case-control study in Germany assessed the outcome when the cases were restricted to hospitalized patients compared to results when all cases, both in-hospital and out-of-hospital, were considered.[158] The conclusion indicated that hospital-based studies overestimated the risk of VTE, and that there was no difference comparing progestins when all cases were included.

Former users discontinue oral contraceptives for a variety of reasons and often are switched to what clinicians perceive to be "safer" products, a practice called "preferential prescribing."[159–161] Individuals who do well with a product tend to remain with that product. Thus, at any one point in time, individuals on an older product will be relatively healthy and free of side effects—the "healthy user effect." This is also called attrition of susceptibles because higher risk individuals with problems are gradually eliminated from the group.[162] Comparing users of older and newer CHC products requires careful analysis to adjust for important differences between these individuals.

Because EE/DSG and EE/GSD products were marketed as less andro-genic and therefore "better" (a marketing claim not substantiated by epide-miologic studies), clinicians chose to provide these products to higher risk patients and older women.[159,160] In addition, clinicians switched patients perceived to be at greater VTE risk from older oral contraceptives to the newer formulations with EE/DSG and EE/GSD. Furthermore, these prod-ucts were prescribed more often to young women who were starting oral contraception for the first time (these young women will not have expe-rienced the test of pregnancy or previous oral contraceptive use to help identify those who have an inherited predisposition to venous thrombosis). These changing practice patterns exert different effects over the lifetime of a product, and meaningful analytical adjustments are extremely difficult to achieve.

The initial VTE risk epidemiologic studies were impressive in their agreement. All indicated increased relative risks (RRs) or ORs associ-ated with EE/DSG and EE/GSD compared with EE/LNG. Nevertheless, results of the early studies may have been influenced by the same unrec-ognized biases. Consistent conclusions may be the result of consistent errors.

Shortly after the first oral contraceptive with DRSP (EE 30 μg/DRSP 3 mg) was marketed, 40 VTE cases in DRSP users (2 of which were fatal) were reported in Europe in 2002.[163] The Dutch College of General Practitioners issued a statement encouraging clinicians not to prescribe the EE-DRSP product. However, this story is similar to that reported with EE/DSG and EE/GSD ("third-generation" progestins), only to learn that preferential prescribing and the healthy user effect probably biased the early studies. In postmarketing surveillance of EE 30 μg/DRSP 3 mg, only one VTE case occurred in a million cycles compared with five among users of other oral contraceptives.[163] In a subsequent monitoring study, the VTE incidence in new DRSP users was comparable to that seen in users of other low-dose oral contraceptives.[164] The prospective European Active Surveillance (EURAS) cohort study (see below) enrolled only new OC users containing a variety of progestins, including DRSP and LNG.[165] The cardiovascular event incidence was similar for all progestins. An American cohort study also focused on new OC users and found that VTE occurred at a similar low rate when comparing DRSP users to other oral contraceptives.[166]

The Danish investigators have continued their interest in hormonal contraception and venous thrombosis and performed a national database study using the reliable Danish national registries of events from 1995 to 2005.[143] As in the earlier Danish case-control study,[151] the VTE risk in current COC users decreased with duration of use and with EE dose and was slightly higher with EE/DSG, EE/GSD, EE/DRSP, and EE-cyproterone acetate (CPA) products. Did this study escape the problems of preferential prescribing and the healthy user effect (attrition of susceptibles)? The incidence of thrombotic events in the comparator group (EE-LNG users) was lower than that reported in other studies, possibly because this group did demonstrate a healthy user effect, but also because database studies often ascertain fewer cases than studies that use active surveillance. The study was not limited to new users. This study was unable to control for BMI or family history of thrombosis, two important markers for women at high risk of venous thrombosis. Preferential prescribing may be a confounder in the Danish database studies; however, the problem of a healthy user effect is also possible.

A case-control study from the Netherlands also reported higher risks of venous thrombosis in EE/DSG, EE/GSD, EE/DRSP, and EE/CPA users compared with EE-LNG users.[147] The authors supported their results by citing findings from their own institution that users of oral contraceptives containing EE/DRSP and EE/CPA had lower levels of free protein S and free tissue factor pathway inhibitor associated with greater resistance to activated protein C compared with EE/LNG users.[118] The RRs in that study were surprisingly high, more so than all other reports involving low-dose oral contraceptives. Once again, the healthy user effect is a possible confounder because the study was not limited to new users. The authors claimed to mitigate any attrition of susceptibles by analyzing only short-term users. Even though the validity of this approach can be debated, the results indicated nonsignificant increased risks with EE/DRSP and EE/CPA compared with EE/LNG, and any conclusion was limited by a small number of short-term users. In that study, the risk associated with products containing EE 20 μg was not increased compared to nonusers.

In an effort to better ascertain risk, several true prospective studies have compared the thrombosis effects of various CHC formulations. Strengths of these studies include the ability to adjust for baseline confounding and rigorous adjudication of outcome with published methodology. The European Active Surveillance (EURAS) study enrolled 58,674 European women initiating a new prescription for combined oral contraception and contacted subjects every 6 months to assess safety outcomes and found no significant difference in VTE risk between DRSP and LNG COCs (hazard ratio [HR], 1.0; 95% confidence interval [CI], 0.6 to 1.8) and DRSP with

239

other oral contraceptives (HR, 0.8; 95% CI, 0.5 to 1.3).[165] The subsequent International Surveillance Study of Women Taking Oral Contraceptives (INAS-OC) study followed more than 85,000 women in the United States and Europe and found no increased risk of VTE in DRSP users compared with LNG users (HR, 0.8; 95% CI, 0.4 to 1.3).[167] The Transatlantic Active Surveillance on Cardiovascular Safety of NuvaRing study used a similar design and found no significant difference in the risk of VTE between women using the EE/ENG contraceptive vaginal ring compared with combined OCPs users (adjusted HR, 0.8; 95% CI, 0.5 to 1.5).[168] Most recently, the International Active Surveillance study "Safety of Contraceptives: Role of Estrogens" (INAS-SCORE) investigated the cardiovascular risks associated with the use of estradiol-containing pills and found an adjusted HR of 0.5 (95% CI, 0.2 to 1.5) for a COC-containing E2V and DNG compared to EE/LNG pills.[148]

Several studies have compared VTE risk between oral and nonoral contraceptive users.[169] Six studies assessing the contraceptive patch had mixed results with two studies suggesting a VTE risk among patch users about double the risk in EE/LNG oral contraceptive users, but the other such studies found similar VTE risks among patch and oral contraceptive users. Only three studies assessed VTE risk among vaginal contraceptive users; one of these found a doubling of risk and the others found no increase in risk compared to COC users. While excess VTE risk among patch and ring users (compared to COC users) is uncertain, it is clear that the patch and ring are not safer than oral contraceptives for VTE. A 2017 systematic review did not identify any studies of VTE risk among women using monthly injectable CHC.[169]

Conclusion: The venous thrombosis risk associated with modern EE-containing hormonal contraceptives is increased about 2-fold and is greatest in the first year of use.[165,170,171] VTE risk increases with increasing body weight and age and increases with EE dose. The contribution of different progestins to the VTE risk seems to be small; studies of different design find different progestin effects, which may reflect bias and unmeasured confounding. The important takeaway is that EE increases venous thrombosis risk; the impact of progestins remains controversial. Although progestins may modulate the hepatic effects of estrogens, prospective studies fail to show any significant differential effect on thrombosis risk. Thus far, a single prospective study suggests that estradiol-containing oral contraceptives may have slightly lower VTE risk than EE-containing contraceptives.

The general population incidence of VTE is higher than previously estimated; this may be due to obesity and other lifestyle changes as well as the prevalence of sensitive diagnostic methods. VTE risk associated with low-dose oral and nonoral CHCs is lower than previously reported and concentrated among high-risk individuals (e.g., obesity and inherited or acquired thrombophilias). Because women over 40 and women with a BMI greater than 30 kg/m^2 have higher baseline VTE risks, CHC is not a first-choice contraceptive for them.

Venous Thromboembolism and Inherited Thrombophilias

An inherited resistance to activated protein C, the factor V Leiden mutation, is common in European populations with as much as 5% to 7% having this single gene mutation. The mutation is much less prevalent (<1%) in Africans, Asians, and other populations.[172] The factor V Leiden mutation is the most common inherited coagulation problem transmitted in an autosomal-dominant fashion.[173,174] Heterozygotes have a 6- to 8-fold increased risk of VTE, and homozygotes an 80-fold increased risk. This mutation accounts for a significant portion of VTE in European populations, including among women who experience VTE while taking CHC.

CHC users who have this mutation will thus experience an independent increased VTE risk from both risk factors (i.e., a multiplicative increase in risk). The VTE risk in EE CHC users with this mutation may be 15- to 30-fold greater than women who do not use CHC and do not have the mutation.[175-177] The risk of VTE is greatest in the initial months of CHC use, and it has been suggested that VTE occurring in the first month of exposure should make the clinician suspect the presence of a clotting disorder.[178]

The second most prevalent inherited thrombophilia is the prothrombin gene *20210A* mutation. A combination of the prothrombin gene mutation and the Leiden mutation is found in about 2% of VTE cases[179]; the prothrombin gene mutation leads to smaller increases in VTE risk than the factor V Leiden mutation. Although genetic defects in the coagulation inhibitors antithrombin, protein C, and protein S are less frequent, they still carry a substantial increase in risk. Acquired thrombophilias include the presence of antiphospholipid antibodies (lupus anticoagulant and anticardiolipin) usually associated with autoimmune diseases.

Should screening for the factor V Leiden mutation (or for other inherited clotting disorders) be routine prior to prescribing contraceptives? Given the ethnic mix in the United States, of the approximately 12 million women currently using oral contraceptives, about one-half million are likely to carry the factor V Leiden mutation. Most experts believe that screening for inherited disorders should be pursued only in women with a family history (in a parent or sibling) of VTE or, perhaps, in obese women. Calculations of the number needed to screen (NNS) to prevent one VTE and the cost for selective screening using contemporary testing modalities are not available at this time. Women who have an inherited disorder of the coagulation system, whether this is known due to screening or case finding, should not use CHC.

The inherited and acquired thrombophilias predispose to VTE independently from the increased risk associated with estrogen-containing contraceptives. Even among women with a thrombophilia, VTE is uncommon, and identification of a thrombophilia does not predict a clinical event. **Table 7.2** synthesizes many risk estimates to give an approximation of the VTE risks in different population subgroups. We know that VTE generally occurs among people who have multiple risk factors; even women experiencing a VTE during CHC use usually have multiple risk factors,[113] and

Table 7.2 Relative Risk and Approximate Incidence of Venous Thromboembolism

Population	Relative Risk	Approximate Incidence per 10,000 Women-Year
Young women— general population	1	5–10
Pregnant women	6	30–60
High-dose COC users	6–10	30–100
Low-dose COC users	2–3	10–30
Leiden mutation carrier	6–8	30–80
Leiden carrier and COC	10–15	50–100
Leiden mutation— homozygous	80	400–800

COC, combined oral contraceptive (data regarding nonoral HC are limited); High-dose oral contraceptive, ethinyl estradiol 50 μg or higher; Low-dose oral contraceptive, ethinyl estradiol less than 50 μg.

From **Dinger JC, Heinemann LA, Kuhl-Habich D,** The safety of a drospirenone-containing oral contraceptive: final results from the European Active Surveillance Study on oral contraceptives based on 142,475 women-years of observation, Contraception 75(5): 344–354, 2007, Ref.[165]; **Heinemann LA, Dinger JC,** Range of published estimates of venous thromboembolism incidence in young women, Contraception 75:328–336, 2007, Ref.[170]; **Pomp ER, le Cessie S, Rosendaal FR, Doggen CJ,** Risk of venous thrombosis: obesity and its joint effect with oral contraceptive use and prothrombotic mutations, Br J Haematol 139:289–296, 2007, Ref.[171]

thus clinicians should avoid prescribing CHC to women who have multiple VTE risk factors.

Hypertension

Hormonal contraceptive–induced hypertension was observed in approximately 5% of users of high-dose pills. More recent evidence indicates that small increases in blood pressure can be observed even with EE 30 μg pills.[180–183] The lack of clinical hypertension in most studies may be due to the rarity of its occurrence. The Nurses' Health Study reported an increased risk of clinical hypertension in current users of low-dose COCs, with an incidence of 41.5 cases per 10,000 women per year.[184] Therefore, an initial and a periodic blood pressure assessment is still an important element of clinical surveillance, even when low-dose oral contraceptives are used. Postmenopausal women in the Rancho Bernardo Study who had previously used oral contraceptives (probably high-dose products) had slightly higher (2 to 4 mm Hg) diastolic blood pressures.[100] Because past users do not demonstrate differences in incidence or risk factors for cardiovascular disease, it is unlikely this blood pressure difference has an important clinical effect.

The mechanism for an effect of CHC on blood pressure is thought to be related to the effect of EE on the renin-angiotensin system. The most consistent finding is a marked increase in plasma angiotensinogen, the renin substrate, up to 8-fold normal values (on high-dose EE pills). In nearly all women, excessive vasoconstriction is prevented by a compensatory decrease in plasma renin concentration. If hypertension does develop, the renin-angiotensinogen changes may take 3 to 6 months to disappear after CHC discontinuation. Changes in angiotensinogen are less pronounced with E4-containing COCs.[106]

One must also consider the effects of CHCs in patients with preexisting hypertension or cardiac disease. Women with uncontrolled hypertension using a CHC have an increased risk of arterial thrombosis.[185-187] Some women with treated hypertension using CHCs have been reported to have poor control of blood pressure with higher diastolic pressures.[188] With successful medical control of blood pressure and close follow-up (e.g., every 3 months), the clinician and the nonsmoking patient who is under age 35 and otherwise healthy may choose low-dose CHC, but with each additional cardiovascular risk factor, other contraceptives become preferred choices. Closer follow-up is also indicated in women with renal disease or a strong family history of hypertension or cardiovascular disease.

Arterial Thrombosis (Myocardial Infarction and Stroke)

Because death and disability can follow stroke and MI, these are the most important potential CHC adverse effects. A relative increase in incidence of stroke or MI in young women carries little increase in absolute risk because the baseline incidence is so low. However, the incidence of stroke and MI increase dramatically with age; thus, CHC use should be avoided among women 35 years and older with any significant cardiovascular disease risk factors including hypertension, diabetes, metabolic syndrome, migraine, smoking, and obesity. Careful patient selection is the key to avoiding MI and stroke.

It has been difficult to establish a dose-response relationship between contraceptive estrogens and arterial thrombosis because these events are so rare. Nevertheless, EE dose appears to be important for the risk of MI and stroke.[189,190] Thus, a rationale for advocating low-dose CHCs (i.e., those with EE < 50 μg) continues to be valid.

Myocardial Infarction

Myocardial infarction is a rare event in healthy reproductive age women (**Table 7.3**). In a WHO multicenter case-control study that included 368 cases of acute MI in COC users, factors associated with an increased risk included smoking, history of hypertension (including hypertension in

Table 7.3 Incidence of Myocardial Infarction in Reproductive Age Women

Overall	5/100,000/y
Younger than age 35	
Nonsmokers	4/100,000/y
Nonsmokers and CHC (data mostly from COC)	4/100,000/y
Smokers	8/100,000/y
Smokers and CHC (data mostly from COC)	43/100,000/y
35 years old and older	
Nonsmokers	10/100,000/y
Nonsmokers and CHC (data mostly from COC)	40/100,000/y
Smokers	88/100,000/y
Smokers and CHC (data mostly from COC)	485/100,000/y

From **WHO Collaborative Study of Cardiovascular Disease and Steroid Hormone Contraception,** Acute myocardial infarction and combined oral contraceptives: results of an international multicentre case-control study, Lancet 349:1202–1209, 1997, Ref.[185] and **Petitti DB, Sidney S, Quesenberry CP Jr, Bernstein A,** Incidence of stroke and myocardial infarction in women of reproductive age, Stroke 28(2):280–283, 1997, Ref.[191]

pregnancy), diabetes, rheumatic heart disease, abnormal blood lipids, and a family history of stroke or MI.[185] Duration of use and past use of CHC did not affect risk. Although there was about a 5-fold overall increased odds of MI in current COC users, essentially all cases occurred in women with cardiovascular risk factors. A population-based, case-control study published in 1996 analyzed 187 cases of MI in low-dose CHC users in the Kaiser Permanente Medical Care Program.[192] The MI incidence among CHC users was 5.2 per 100,000 woman-years for an OR of MI among current CHC users of 1.65 (95% CI, 0.45 to 6.06) compared with past or never users. Current CHC users who experienced an MI had more risk factors than the CHC users in the control group. A European case-control study including 182 MI cases found that 77% of the MIs had occurred among women aged 35 or older. That study reported an overall OR of 2.34 for current CHC users with MI risk concentrated among smokers and women with hypertension, diabetes, obesity, and a family history of MI.[193,194] These results are consistent with other studies of MI and CHC[195–197] and emphasize the great importance of carefully assessing CV risk factors before prescribing CHC. The lower odds of MI reported in the more contemporary studies (compared to the earliest studies of this association) reflects both lower CHC dose and the benefits of more careful screening prior to CHC prescription. Case-control studies of oral low-dose EE oral contraceptives consistently show that MI and stroke in HC users are concentrated among women who have hypertension or are smokers.[91,111,198-200] The cohort studies are somewhat less helpful because their numbers of cases are too small for definitive analyses of subgroups.

Stroke

Both case-control and cohort studies indicate an increased risk of stroke among current high-dose COC users and a lesser risk (with ORs around 2) among women using lower doses.[138,201-203] Thrombotic stroke is extremely rare in healthy, nonsmoking, normotensive women with the use of COCs containing EE doses less than 50 μg (**Table 7.4**). A study of all 408 strokes identified among 1.1 million reproductive age women enrolled in the California Kaiser Permanente Medical Care Program yielded an incidence rate of 11.3 strokes per 100,000 woman-years. In a case-control analysis, the adjusted OR for current CHC use was 1.18 for ischemic stroke and 1.14 for hemorrhagic stroke, both estimates with

Table 7.4 Incidence of Stroke in Reproductive Age Women

Incidence of ischemic stroke	
Overall	5/100,000/y
Younger than 35 year	1–3/100,000/y
35 years and older	10/100,000/y
Incidence of hemorrhagic stroke	
Overall	6/100,000/y
Excess cases per year due to COCs, including smokers and hypertensives	
Overall	2/100,000/y
Low-dose OC users younger than 35 years	1/100,000/y
High-dose OC users overall	8/100,000/y

From **WHO Collaborative Study of Cardiovascular Disease and Steroid Hormone Contraception,** Ischaemic stroke and combined oral contraceptives: results of an international, multicentre case-control study, Lancet 348:498–505, 1996, Ref.[186]; **WHO Collaborative Study of Cardiovascular Disease and Steroid Hormone Contraception,** Haemorrhagic stroke, overall stroke risk, and combined oral contraceptives: results of an international, multicentre, case-control study, Lancet 348:505–510, 1996, Ref.[187]; **Petitti DB, Sidney S, Quesenberry CP Jr, Bernstein A,** Incidence of stroke and myocardial infarction in women of reproductive age, Stroke 28(2):280–283, 1997, Ref.[191]; **Petitti DB, Sidney S, Bernstein A, Wolf S, Quesenberry C, Ziel HK,** Stroke in users of low-dose oral contraceptives, N Engl J Med 335:8–15, 1996, Ref.[204]

wide confidence intervals overlapping 1.0.[204] Similar to MI, the risk factors for ischemic stroke included smoking, hypertension, diabetes, and elevated body weight. The risk factors for hemorrhagic stroke were similar. The low risk of stroke among CHC users at Kaiser Permanente may partly result from stringent medical criteria regarding who would be eligible to use CHC. A case-control study from Washington State had similar results.[205] A pooled analysis of the data from California and Washington concluded that low-dose oral contraceptives are not associated with an increase in stroke risk.[206]

In contrast, a contemporary European case-control study of 220 women with ischemic strokes[207] found a 3-fold increase in the risk of ischemic stroke associated with the use of COCs with higher risks in smokers (more than 10 cigarettes per day), women with hypertension, and users of higher dose EE products.[186,187] The WHO conducted a hospital-based, case-control study from 21 centers in 17 countries, which accumulated 697 cases of ischemic stroke, 141 from Europe, and 556 from developing countries.[186] The overall OR for ischemic stroke indicated about a 3-fold increased risk with current COC use. The higher risks observed in the studies in Europe and in developing countries are potentially related to use of somewhat higher dose COC formulations and provision to women without a blood pressure reading to exclude hypertension.

A second Danish case-control study, reported in 1998, included thrombotic strokes and transitory cerebral ischemic attacks analyzed together.[189] This study found a dose-response relationship with EE 20, 30 to 40, and 50 μg users, although the number of EE 20 μg users (5 cases, 22 controls) was not sufficient to establish a lower risk at this dose. A 2003 Danish case-control study indicated that the OR of cerebral thrombosis decreased from a high of 4.5 with EE 50 μg pills to 1.6 with EE 20 to 40 μg pills.[208] Hypertension increased the stroke risk 5-fold, migraine 3.2 times, diabetes 5.6 times, and hyperlipidemia and coagulation disorders about 12-fold.

Screening for hypertension before initiating CHC is especially important because hypertension is a major risk factor for stroke associated with CHC use.

Migraine headaches have been evaluated extensively as a risk factor for stroke. True migraine headaches are common in women, while tension headaches (90% of all headaches) occur equally in men and women.[209] No well-done studies have determined the impact of CHC on migraine severity; migraineurs may report that their headaches are worse or better during CHC use. Migraine headaches occur with or without aura. Aura occurs in about 30% of migraineurs with symptoms that begin *before* the headache and resolve with the onset of the headache. Symptoms that occur during headaches, especially photophobia, are not signs of aura. Symptoms that indicate a premonition of a headache such as light or sound sensitivity, poor concentration, and fatigue occurring 1 to 2 days before a headache are not signs of aura.

Migraine with aura symptoms include the following:

- Scotomata (blind spots) or blurred vision
- Bright zig-zag lines
- Episodes of blindness
- Numbness, paresthesias
- Speech difficulties
- Unilateral symptoms, such as weakness

True vascular headaches (migraine with aura) are an indication to avoid or discontinue CHC. CHCs can be considered in women under age 35, who have migraine *without* aura, and who are otherwise healthy and not smokers. Migraine headaches, especially with aura, are a risk factor for stroke.[210] The risk is greater in women with hypertension, in smokers, with a family history of migraine, and in women with a long history of migraine or with more than 12 attacks per year of migraine with aura.[211,212] Studies with COCs containing EE doses of 50 μg or more link migraine headaches to a risk of stroke. More recent studies with EE formulations with less than 50 μg yield mixed results. One failed to find a further increase in stroke in patients with migraine who use oral contraception; another concluded that CHC use by migraineurs was associated with a 4-fold increase of the already increased risk of ischemic stroke.[213,214] The WHO case-control study indicated an increased risk in migraine among COC users who smoked.[211] Because 20% and 30% of women experience migraine headaches, one would expect the study populations in the most recent studies of thrombosis to have included substantial numbers of migraineurs. An adverse effect of low-dose COCs on stroke risk in migraineurs should have manifested itself in the data. The lack of an increased risk of stroke in these studies is reassuring. Nevertheless, it is believed that migraineurs using COCs have an increased stroke risk. The absolute risk in a 20-year-old woman is approximately 10 per 100,000 and for a 40-year-old woman, 100 per 100,000.[215] Because of the small numbers of young women who have strokes, most studies cannot differentiate outcomes between migraine with and without aura. However, in the American Stroke Prevention in Young Women Study, COC use in smokers was associated with an increased risk of stroke only in migraineurs with aura.[216] Calculating the exact additional stroke risk for such women is impossible due to sparse data and varying definitions of headaches in the exiting studies. Even though the magnitude of excess stroke risk in migraineurs is uncertain, stroke morbidity is so great that caution is appropriate.

Conclusion—Myocardial Infarction and Stroke

Oral contraceptives containing EE doses less than 50 μg do not increase the risk of MI or stroke in healthy, nonsmoking women without hypertension, regardless of age. The effect of smoking in women under age 35 is, as long recognized, not detectable in the absence of hypertension. After age 35, increasing age and smoking by themselves have little impact on stroke risk in women using oral contraceptive with EE doses less than 50 μg. The most recent studies looking at the newer oral contraceptives have sparse data, but their estimates regarding MI and CVA are compatible with data from the older studies. *There is no reason to doubt that these conclusions apply as well to the vaginal and transdermal and perhaps the injectable methods of CHC.*

Epidemiologic studies fail to find any substantial risk of ischemic or hemorrhagic stroke with low-dose oral contraceptives in healthy, young women. The WHO study did find evidence for an adverse impact of smoking in women under age 35; the Kaiser study did not. This difference is explained by the confounding effect of hypertension, the major risk factor identified. In the WHO study, a history of hypertension was based on whether a patient reported ever having had high blood pressure (other than in pregnancy) and not validated by medical records. In the Kaiser study, women were classified as having hypertension if they reported using antihypertensive medication (<5% of oral contraceptive users had treated hypertension, and there were no users of higher dose products). In the WHO study, the effect of using oral contraceptives in the presence of a high-risk factor is apparent in the different ORs when European women who received good screening from clinicians were compared with women in developing countries who received little screening; therefore, more women with cardiovascular risk factors in developing countries were using oral contraceptives. *The studies indicate that hypertension should be a major concern (even if treated), especially with regard to the risk of stroke.*

Summary of Cardiovascular Disease Risks

The outpouring of epidemiologic data in the last two decades allows the construction of a clinical formulation that is evidence based. The following conclusions are consistent with the recent reports but are based on COC exposure with few data regarding the nonoral CHC.

CHCs and Thrombosis

- Pharmacologic EE doses increase the production of clotting factors.
- Progestins have no significant direct impact on procoagulant and anticoagulant clotting factors and proteins but may modulate the impact of EE on circulating levels.
- Past users of COCs do not have an increased incidence of cardiovascular disease.
- All low-dose COCs, regardless of progestin type, increase VTE risk, primarily in the first year of use. The actual VTE risk with low-dose oral contraceptives is lower in recent studies compared with previous reports. It is logical that the lower risk results from better patient selection and from lower estrogen doses. The risk increases with increasing age and body weight.
- Smoking yields a large increase in arterial thrombosis risk and has only a small effect on VTE risk.

- Smoking and estrogen (EE by any route and oral E2) have an additive effect on the risk of arterial thrombosis. Why is there a difference between venous and arterial clotting? The venous system has low flow with a state of high fibrinogen and low platelets, in contrast to the high-flow state of the arterial system with low fibrinogen and high platelets. Thus, it is understandable why these two different systems can respond in different ways.
- Hypertension is a very important additive risk factor for stroke in CHC users.
- Low-dose oral contraceptives do not increase the risk of MI or stroke in healthy, nonsmoking women, regardless of age.
- Almost all MIs and strokes in COC users occur with high-dose products or users with cardiovascular risk factors over the age of 35. In the Oxford Family Planning Association cohort, cardiac deaths were concentrated among women who smoked 15 or more cigarettes per day.[217]
- Arterial thrombosis (MI and stroke) has a dose-response relationship with the dose of estrogen, but there are insufficient data to determine whether there is a difference in risk with products that contain EE 20, 30, or 35 μg.

Results from epidemiologic studies reinforce that the risks of arterial and venous thrombosis are a consequence of the estrogen component of combination oral contraceptives. Current evidence does not support an advantage or disadvantage for any particular formulation, except for the greater safety associated with any product containing EE doses less than 50 μg. Although it is logical to expect the greatest safety with the lowest dose of estrogen, the rarity of arterial and venous thrombosis in healthy women makes it unlikely that there will be any measurable differences in the attributable incidence of clinical events with all low-dose products. Similarly, one might hope that newer estrogens will prove to be safer than EE, but again the rarity of arterial thrombosis will make this extremely difficult to evaluate.

Study results support the importance of good patient screening. The occurrence of arterial thrombosis is essentially limited to older women who smoke or have cardiovascular risk factors, especially hypertension. The impact of good screening is evident in the repeated failure to detect an increase in mortality due to MI or stroke in healthy, nonsmoking women.[142,191,217] Although VTE risk is slightly increased in healthy young women, the incidence is still rare. The overall mortality rate with VTE is about 1% and probably less with oral contraceptives because most deaths from thromboembolism occur among those cases associated with trauma, surgery, or a major illness. The minimal risk of venous thrombosis associated with COC use does not justify the cost of routine screening for coagulation deficiencies. Nevertheless, the importance of this issue is illustrated by the increased risk of a very rare event, cerebral sinus thrombosis, in women who have an inherited predisposition for clotting and use oral contraceptives.[218,219]

If a woman seeking to initiate CHC has a close family history (parent or sibling) with an idiopathic thromboembolism, an evaluation to search for an underlying abnormality in the coagulation system is warranted. Family history of VTE itself may have low predictive value.[220] However, another study indicated that testing for thrombophilia did not allow for prediction of recurrent events, but risk factors such as family history did provide prediction.[221] The conservative recommendation for a high-risk woman considering exposure to exogenous estrogen (EE by any route or oral E2) stimulation is to rule out an underlying thrombophilia. The following measurements are recommended, and abnormal results require consultation with a hematologist regarding prognosis and prophylactic treatment (**Table 7.5**). This list of laboratory tests is long and thus expensive, and because this is a dynamic and changing field, the best advice is to consult with a hematologist. If a diagnosis of a congenital deficiency is made, screening should be offered to other family members.

CHCs are contraindicated in women who have a personal history of idiopathic VTE and in women who have a well-documented close family history (parent or sibling) of idiopathic VTE. These women will have a

Table 7.5 Recommended Screening Coagulation Testing for Women at High Risk for Venous Thrombosis

Hypercoagulable Conditions	Thrombophilia Screening
Antithrombin III deficiency	Antithrombin III
Protein C deficiency	Protein C
Protein S deficiency	Protein S
Factor V Leiden mutation	Activated protein C resistance ratio
Prothrombin gene mutation	Activated partial thromboplastin time
Antiphospholipid syndrome	Hexagonal activated partial thromboplastin time
	Anticardiolipin antibodies
	Lupus anticoagulant
	Fibrinogen
	Prothrombin G mutation (DNA test)
	Thrombin time
	Homocysteine level
	Complete blood count

higher incidence of congenital deficiencies in important clotting measurements, especially antithrombin III, protein C, protein S, and resistance to activated protein C.[222] Such a patient who then screens negative for an inherited clotting deficiency might still consider the use of CHCs, but this would be a difficult decision with unknown risks for both patient and clinician, and it is more prudent to consider other contraceptive options. Other risk factors for thromboembolism that clinicians should consider include an acquired predisposition such as the presence of lupus anticoagulant or malignancy, and immobility or trauma. Varicose veins are not a risk factor unless they are very extensive.[135] *Progestin-only methods, including implants, depot medroxyprogesterone acetate, and the LNG-releasing intrauterine system (IUS), are recommended for high-risk women and for women who are anticoagulated.*

Overall, low-dose COCs and other available CHCs are very safe for healthy, young women. By effectively screening older women for the presence of smoking and cardiovascular risk factors, especially hypertension, we can limit, if not eliminate, any increased risk for arterial disease associated with low-dose oral contraceptives. No increased risk of cardiovascular events emerges with duration of use (long term). In large cohort studies, users and nonusers of oral contraceptives have similar overall mortality rates.[91,217,223] While most data come from studies of COCs, these conclusions likely also apply to transdermal and vaginal estrogen-progestin contraception.

Over the years, there has been recurring discussion over whether to provide oral contraceptives over the counter on a nonprescription basis. The WHO report on cardiovascular disease risk makes an impressive argument against such a move. The increased risk of MI was most evident in developing countries where 70% of the cases received their oral contraceptives from a nonclinical source. Absent screening, women with risk factors in developing countries were exposed to greater risk. However, OTC supply of CHC is prevalent globally, and studies support that women can self-screen for these contraindications. How to assure normal blood pressure is a key issue for safe provision of CHC on a nonprescription basis.

Cancer Effects

Breast Cancer

Because of breast cancer's prevalence and its long latent phase, concern over the relationship between CHCs and breast cancer continues to be an issue in the minds of both patients and clinicians. Older studies reported a protective effect of higher dose COCs on benign breast disease. After 2 years, there was a progressive reduction (about 40%) in the incidence of fibrocystic changes in the breast. Women who used COCs were one-fourth as likely to be diagnosed with benign breast disease as nonusers, but this protection was limited to current and recent users.[224–226] In the large Oxford Family Planning Association cohort, the incidence of benign breast disease decreased with increasing duration of use.[227] A French case-control study indicated a reduction of nonproliferative benign breast disease associated with low-dose COCs used before a first full-term pregnancy but no effect on proliferative disease or with use after a pregnancy.[228] A Canadian cohort study including use of modern low-dose COCs also showed reduction in risk of proliferative benign disease associated with increasing duration of use.[229] Because most benign breast disease is unrelated to breast cancer risk, the relevance of these benefits to breast cancer risk is probably limited. Further, an American case-control study did not find an increased risk of breast carcinoma in situ associated with oral contraceptive use.[230]

The Royal College of General Practitioners,[231] Oxford Family Planning Association,[232,233] the Nurses' Health Study,[234] and Walnut Creek[235] cohort studies indicated no significant differences in breast cancer rates between users and nonusers. However, these studies enrolled women at a time when COCs were used primarily by married couples spacing out their children. Beginning in the 1980s, oral contraception was primarily being used by women early in life, for longer durations, and to delay an initial pregnancy (remember, a full-term pregnancy before age 35 increases breast cancer risk for several years but protects against breast cancer later in life).[236,237]

Many studies have evaluated the relationships between COCs and breast cancer taking into account timing and duration of hormone use and also the recency of use relative to the diagnosis of breast cancer. The results of these individual studies have not been clear-cut.

A collaborative group reanalyzed data from 54 studies in 26 countries, studies that included 53,297 women with breast cancer and 100,239 women without breast cancer, in order to more precisely assess the relationship between the risk of breast cancer and COC use.[238,239] That overview grouped oral contraceptives into three categories: low, medium, and high dose (which correlated with EE doses <50, 50, and >50 μg). Those studies included relatively few women who had used COCs with EE doses less than 30 μg, so they were not analyzed separately. At the time of diagnosis, 9% of the women with breast cancer were under age 35, 25% were 35 to 44, 33% were 45 to 54, and 33% were age 55 and older. A similar percentage of women with breast cancer (41%) and women without breast cancer (40%) had used COCs at some time in their lives. Overall, the breast cancer RR in ever users of oral contraceptives was very slightly elevated and statistically significant: RR, 1.07; CI, 1.03 to 1.10.

The collaborative reanalysis found a stronger relationship with time since last use, with an elevated risk for current users (RR, 1.24; CI, 1.15 to 1.33) and in women who had stopped use 1 to 4 years before (recent use). Ten or more years after stopping use, there was no increased risk of breast cancer. The risk of metastatic disease was reduced (compared with localized tumors) among HC users compared to nonusers: RR, 0.88; CI, 0.81 to 0.95.

The investigators found these associations did not vary by family history of breast cancer, age of menarche, country of origin, ethnic groups, body weight, alcohol use, years of education, and study design. There was no variation according to specific type of estrogen or progestin in the various products. Importantly, there was no statistically significant effect of dose.

Overall, this massive analysis yielded good news. No major adverse impact of COCs emerged. Even though young women have higher RRs of breast cancer during current use and in the 5 years after stopping, this is a time when breast cancer is very rare, and the increase in the actual number of breast cancers would be modest. The difference between localized disease and metastatic disease was statistically greater and deserves further evaluation; however, more recent studies have not evaluated stage at diagnosis. Whether stage at diagnosis is a screening effect or a biologic effect is unknown.

The Norwegian-Swedish Women's Lifestyle and Health Cohort Study began in the early 1990s to follow over 100,000 women specifically to address the role of hormonal contraceptives on health.[240] Those results are compatible with the collaborative reanalysis.

A 2017 analysis using data from the nationwide Danish registries[241] included 11,517 breast cancers in women aged less than 49 years and reported an increase in breast cancer among current and recent HC users (HR 1.20; CI, 1.14 to 1.26), which was entirely compatible with earlier studies. Unfortunately, that analysis did not report separately about the lowest estrogen-dose HC, nor did it report on stage at diagnosis, so these questions remain unsettled.[242] Most data come from COC users, and lacking additional data, one must infer that using a contraceptive ring or patch would yield similar results.

What explanation could account for an increased risk associated only with current or recent use, no increase with duration of use, and a return to normal 10 years after exposure? A leading theory is that CHCs have a tumor promoter effect rather than an initiator effect. In essence, current and recent CHC use affects the growth of a preexisting malignancy, explaining the limitation of the association to current and recent use and the increase in localized disease. Detection/surveillance bias (more interaction with the health care system by oral contraceptive users) could also explain the slightly increased risk. Pregnancy and childbirth also transiently increase the risk of breast cancer for a period of several years, and this is followed by a lifetime reduction in risk.[236,237] And some have found that a concurrent or recent pregnancy adversely affects survival.[243,244] It is argued that breast cells that have already begun malignant transformation are adversely affected by the hormones of pregnancy, while normal stem cells become more resistant because of a pregnancy.

Among women with a breast cancer diagnosis in the years remote from CHC use, study results continue to be reassuring. In a case-control study of women aged 40 to 69 years in Toronto, Canada, those women who had used CHC for 5 or more years, 15 or more years previously, had a 50% reduced risk of breast cancer.[245] However, a case-control study from Sweden could detect neither a beneficial nor adverse effect of previous use of oral contraceptives (mainly EE 50 μg products) on the risk of breast cancer in women age 50 to 74 years.[246]

An American case-control study included 4,575 women diagnosed with breast cancer between aged 35 and 64 years.[247] The overall risk of breast cancer was not increased in CHC users (although the risk in current users was compatible with that identified in the studies cited above). There was no adverse effect of increasing duration of use or higher doses of estrogen. That study found no impact of CHC initiation at a younger age or among women with a family history of breast cancer. This large American study had consistently negative results. The next largest study, involving women from California, Canada, and Australia, focused on breast cancer diagnosed before age 40 and could not detect an increase in current or past users of oral contraceptives.[248] Furthermore, no increase in breast cancer mortality can be detected in women who have used oral contraceptives.[249,250]

Women with a family history of breast cancer or with BRCA1 and BRCA2 mutations have a higher baseline risk of breast cancer, and thus any additional risk conferred through CHC use would be magnified in such women. Several studies, mostly small, suggest that these women do have a further modest increase breast cancer risk with CHC use,[251–255] but in these studies, the risks were limited to varying subsets of women. Others studies have not identified any increased risk.[248,256,257] A meta-analysis of eight studies[258] suggests that CHC may increase breast cancer risk (OR, 1.21; CI, 0.93 to 1.58) in BRCA1/2 carriers. A second meta-analysis concludes that studies report heterogeneous and inconsistent breast cancer risks with CHC use among BRCA1/2 carriers, and thus the authors did not provide a pooled estimate.[259]

Several institutions in the United States collaborated on a case-control study of the association between CHC use and lobular and ductal breast cancer occurring in young women (under age 44).[260] Cases included 100 lobular cancers and 1,164 ductal cancers, and CHC use had no meaningful effects on breast cancer according to histologic subtype. Lobular cancer (15% of all breast cancers) has been increasing in the United States in recent years, prompting these investigators to ask whether this reflects exposure to exogenous hormones. According to their data, the answer is no. This is reassuring because lobular cancer is more hormonally sensitive than ductal breast cancer.

Nearly all of the hormonal contraception exposure data in these epidemiologic studies is on oral contraceptive use. Lacking extensive data about contraceptive ring and patch use, we must infer that the associations are likely to be similar for all types of CHCs.

Summary: Combined Hormonal Contraceptives and the Risk of Breast Cancer

- Studies consistently show that current and recent CHC use may be associated with about a 20% to 25% increased risk of early breast cancer, which may be limited to localized disease. This association has a limited effect on overall incidence because most breast cancer occurs among older women whose CHC use is usually far more than 5 years before.

- No study has shown any increase in breast cancer mortality among current or past CHC users.
- The increase in breast cancer in American women was greater in older women from 1973 to 1994, that is, among those who never had the opportunity to use oral contraception.[261] In women under 50 years of age, there was only a slight increase during this same time period.
- CHC use does not appear to further increase the risk of breast cancer in women with positive family histories of breast cancer or in women with proven benign breast disease.
- The clinician should take every opportunity to direct attention to other factors that affect breast cancer. Breast-feeding and control of alcohol intake are good examples and are also components of preventive health care. Especially important is this added motivation to encourage breast-feeding. Conversely, delayed fertility yields a major increase in breast cancer incidence, and current trends in age at first birth in the United States (and elsewhere) suggest that breast cancer rates will continue to increase.
- Given the hormone sensitivity of existing breast cancer, the MEC considers current breast cancer as an absolute contraindication (category 4) to CHC use and that recent breast cancer as category 3.[110]

Endometrial Cancer

Based on data from oral contraceptive exposure, CHC use protects against endometrial cancer. Use for at least 12 months reduces the risk of developing endometrial cancer by 50%; the protective effect increases with greater duration of CHC use.[262–267] This protection persists for 20 or more years after discontinuation (the actual length of duration of protection is unknown) and is greatest in women at highest risk: nulliparous and low-parity women and obese women.[267–269] This protection is similar for all three major histologic subtypes of endometrial cancer: adenocarcinoma, adenoacanthoma, and adenosquamous cancers. Finally, protection is seen with all monophasic formulations of oral contraceptives, including pills with EE dose less than 50 µg.[262,266,267,270] There are no data as yet with multiphasic preparations or the new progestin formulations, but because these products are still dominated by their progestational component, there is every reason to believe that they will be protective. One must also assume that contraceptive rings and patches will yield similar protection. Due to the obesity epidemic, endometrial cancer incidence is increasing, and thus the benefits of CHC use are increasingly important.[271]

Ovarian Cancer

Protection against ovarian cancer, the most lethal of female reproductive tract cancers, is one of the most important noncontraceptive benefits of using CHC. Because this cancer is often diagnosed at a late stage and mortality is high, the impact of this protection is enormous. CHC use may be particularly protective against the most aggressive ovarian cancers but is also protective against borderline cancers.[272,273] Several countries have observed a decline in mortality from ovarian cancer since the early 1970s, an effect attributable to CHC use.[274] Women with longer exposure to oral contraceptives have a marked decrease in ovarian cancer incidence.[275-278] The risk of developing epithelial ovarian cancer of all histologic subtypes in users of oral contraception is reduced by 40% compared with that of nonusers.[264,266,279-285] This protective effect increases with longer duration of use and continues for at least 20 years after stopping the medication.[269,286] This protection is detectable in women who use oral contraception for as little as 3 to 6 months (although at least 3 years of use are required for a notable impact), reaching an 80% reduction in risk with more than 10 years of use. This benefit has been associated with all monophasic formulations, including the low-dose products,[283-285,287] although one recent study does not fully agree.[288] As with other cancers, the data are mainly from oral contraceptive users, and we must infer that the protection will be similar for contraceptive ring and patch use. The protective effect of CHC is especially important for women at high risk of ovarian cancer (nulliparous women and women with a positive family history).[289,290] Continuous CHC use for 10 years by women with a positive family history for ovarian cancer can reduce the risk of epithelial ovarian cancer to a level equal to or less than that of women with a negative family history.[289] CHC use by women with BRCA1/2 mutations achieves similar ovarian cancer risk reduction and thus may be a risk-reducing strategy for women who are not ready for a risk-reducing surgery.[258,291-293] The benefits of ovarian cancer protection appear to outweigh the smaller and less certain increases in breast cancer risk.[259]

Cervical Cancer

Many studies show the risk for dysplasia and carcinoma in situ of the uterine cervix increases with CHC use for more than 1 year.[294-299] Invasive cervical cancer may be increased after 5 years of use, reaching a 2-fold increase after 10 years. More recent studies limited to women not vaccinated against human papillomavirus (HPV) have less consistent results.[300-302] Studies of this association in vaccinated populations are needed. The number of partners a woman has had and age at first coitus are important risk factors for cervical neoplasia that were not always accounted for in earlier analyses. Other confounding factors include exposure to HPV, barrier contraception use (protective), and smoking. Frequency of cervical screening in the study populations varied greatly, and CHC users may have more frequent cervical screening. These are difficult factors to control, and, therefore, the conclusions regarding cervical cancer are often difficult to interpret. The apparent increased risk of carcinoma in situ may be due to enhanced detection of disease (because oral contraceptive users have more frequent Pap testing).[297] Although the WHO identified a Pap test screening bias, their evidence still suggested an increased risk of cervical carcinoma in situ with long-term oral contraceptive use.[298]

The relationship between cervical adenocarcinoma and CHC use is clearer: a case-control study in Panama, Costa Rica, Colombia, and Mexico concluded that there was a significantly increased risk for invasive adeno-carcinoma.[303] Similar results were obtained in a case-control study in Los Angeles and in the WHO Collaborative Study.[304,305] In Los Angeles, the RR of adenocarcinoma of the cervix increased from 2.1 with ever use to 4.4 with 12 or more years of oral contraceptive use.[304] Because the incidence of adenocarcinoma of the cervix (10% of all cervical cancers) has increased in young women over the last 20 years, there is concern that this increase reflects the use of CHC.[306]

One meta-analysis concluded that the risk of cervical cancer increased with increasing duration of CHC use (for in situ and invasive cancer and both squamous cancer and adenocarcinoma).[307] A pooled analysis of case-control studies (including only HPV-positive women) concluded that the risk of cervical cancer in women with HPV increases about 3-fold but not until after 5 years of CHC use.[308]

A meta-analysis of 24 epidemiologic studies included 16,573 women with cervical cancer and 35,509 women without cervical cancer.[309] The risk of cervical cancer in situ and invasive cancer increased about 2-fold with increasing duration of use of oral contraceptives. After discontinuation of oral contraceptives, the risk steadily declined. There was no increase in risk with duration of use less than 5 years or after 10 or more years since last use. The same relationships were seen comparing women likely to have been screened and those likely not to have been screened. The results were similar among the HPV-positive women. A similar but smaller risk was associated with injectable progestin-only methods. Insufficient numbers were available to assess oral progestin-only contraceptives.

It has been well demonstrated that oral contraceptive users have more sexual partners, more HPV infections, and more Pap smears than do nonusers. The data in the meta-analyses confirm these associations, plus a greater incidence of smoking in oral contraceptive users. The analyses were not always able to adjust effectively for some of these factors. Adequate data are not available to allow case-control and cohort studies to control for Pap screening and for differences in condom use.

We currently know three important facts about cervical cancer. (1) HPV causes cervical cancer. (2) Cervical screening reduces cervical cancer incidence. (3) HPV vaccination can potentially eliminate most cases of cervical cancer. COC users, and presumably other CHC users, have behavior patterns that place them at greater risk of HPV infections. In addition, CHC could increase the ability of HPV to establish itself in the cervix. Once infected with HPV, CHC could influence the response of a woman to HPV, for example, suppressing the immune response. Therefore, we do not know for certain whether case-control and cohort data reflect an enhancing effect of CHC on cervical cancer development or whether the results are affected by the confounding problems of HPV infections and the prevalence of cervical screening. For cervical cancer (as for the other cancers), most of the epidemiologic data come from oral contraceptive users, and thus we can only make the reasonable assumption that contraceptive rings and patches will have similar effects. In addition, most of the data regarding cervical cancer came from unvaccinated populations using Pap testing rather than newer cervical screening modalities. Thus, the relationships described above may change in the future.

Cervical Cancer Summary

Squamous cell and particularly adenocarcinoma of the cervix have been repeatedly associated with longer duration CHC use. These studies reinforce the need to follow cervical screening algorithms for CHC users. Fortunately, steroid contraception does not mask abnormal cervical changes, and the necessity for prescription renewals offers the opportunity for consistent screening. Whether receiving CHC directly from a pharmacy or over-the-counter will decrease appropriate cervical screening among these women deserves examination. Whether there will be any association between cervical cancer and CHC among women who have received the HPV vaccine is also a question for future study. CHC use is appropriate for women with a history of cervical intraepithelial neoplasia (CIN), including those who have been surgically treated.

Colorectal Cancer

Numerous studies have reported on the little-known association between HC use and decreased colorectal cancer over the past 20 years. In 1997, the Nurses' Health Study (NHS) reported about a 40% reduced risk of colorectal cancer associated with 8 years of previous CHC use.[310] More recent analyses from NHS found no risk reduction with ever use, but a significantly decreased risk with 5 or more years duration of use.[311] Both case-control and cohort studies have reported reductions in the risk of colorectal cancer associated with the ever use of oral contraceptives.[312-314] As with the other cancers, we must assume that the associations measured among oral contraceptive users will apply to women who have used other forms of CHC. A 2001 meta-analysis concluded that CHC use is associated with an 18% colorectal cancer risk reduction, with a larger decrease in recent users.[315] Similarly, a 2009 meta-analysis reported a 19% risk reduction.[316] A larger 2015 meta-analysis including 15,790 cancer cases also reported an 18% risk reduction.[317] The similarity of these meta-analysis results is partly a result of including many of the same studies, but the results do support a risk reduction. That risk reduction is more modest than the endometrial cancer and ovarian cancer risk reductions but nonetheless highly meaningful for this far more common cancer.

Liver Cancer

Combination oral contraception has been linked to the development of hepatocellular carcinoma.[318,319] However, the very small number of cases in many studies, and, thus, the limited statistical power, requires great caution in interpretation. Due to the small size of the individual studies, a meta-analysis combined results from 14 case-control and 3 cohort studies, with 1,798 cases.[320] That analysis identified a modest, nonsignificant overall association between oral contraceptive use and liver cancer (RR, 1.23; CI, 0.93 to 1.63). Only a few studies provided enough information to evaluate a duration-response association, showing that the RR increased with longer duration of use; however, that trend was also not significant. Even case-control analysis of oral contraceptives containing CPA (known to be toxic to the liver in high doses) could detect no evidence of an increased risk of liver cancer.[321] As parenteral CHCs, such as the ring and patch, do not undergo a first pass through the liver, these methods might not have exactly the same association with hepatic cancer as oral contraceptives. In the United States, Japan, Sweden, England, and Wales, death rates from liver cancer did not change despite introduction and widespread CHC use.[322,323] More recently, liver cancer incidence and mortality has increased in the United States, but this is believed to be due to infection with hepatitis C and hepatitis B.[324]

Other Cancers

The Walnut Creek study suggested that melanoma was linked to combination oral contraception; however, the major risk factor for melanoma is exposure to sunlight. More accurate evaluation utilizing both the Royal College General Practitioners and the Oxford Family Planning Association prospective cohorts and accounting for exposure to sunlight did not indicate a significant difference in the risk of melanoma comparing users to nonusers.[325-327] A recent French cohort study reported an adjusted RR of 1.14 (CI, 0.95 to 1.38) for melanoma among ever users of CHC.[328] The Oxford-FPA prospective cohort study found no links between CHC use and kidney cancer, gallbladder cancer, or pituitary tumors.[329] Long-term oral contraceptive use may slightly increase the risk of molar pregnancy.[330-332] A Swedish cohort study found no association between HC use and pancreatic cancer.[333] A case-control study concluded that oral contraceptives reduce the risk of salivary gland cancer.[334] Two recent studies reported a reduced risk of lymphatic/hematopoietic cancers with HC use (RR, 0.79; CI, 0.64 to 0.97 and RR, 0.74; CI, 0.58 to 0.94, respectively).[335,336] All of those studies examined oral contraceptive exposures.

Overall Effects of Combined Hormonal Contraception on Cancer, Cancer Mortality, and Other Mortality

Many studies indicate that CHC use, particularly for more than 5 years, is associated with an increase in cervical cancer. The increased risk is greater for cervical adenocarcinoma. The importance of this association varies geographically according to baseline cervical cancer risks and the availability of cervical screening. Studies are also consistent in indicating an approximately 25% increase in breast cancer among current and recent users. Because current and recent CHC use mainly occurs among women aged 30 or younger when breast cancer incidence is quite low, the effect of this risk on the number of breast cancer cases is also low. For both breast cancer and cervical cancer, the increased risk wanes after discontinuation of CHC.

Consistent studies also show that CHC strongly and consistently protects against ovarian and endometrial cancers, with longer duration of use conferring greater risk reduction. The observed risk reduction persists for many years after discontinuing the CHC. CHC also confers risk reduction against colorectal cancer and possibly against hematopoietic cancers.

Taken together, the net cancer effects of CHC tend to be beneficial or neutral and even to outweigh the adverse cardiovascular effects of using CHC. In the Oxford-FPA cohort, long-term follow-up suggested that the beneficial effects of OC use on cancer incidence in that cohort outweighed the adverse effects.[337] Analyses from the RCGP cohort also found that the overall balance of cancer risks among past OC users was neutral with the increased risks entirely counterbalanced by benefits regarding endometrial, ovarian, and colorectal cancers that persisted at least 30 years.[336,337]

Other Risks and Benefits

Reproductive System

Effects of Combined Hormonal Contraceptives During Pregnancy

Safety of inadvertent COC use during early pregnancy has now been evaluated on large-scale population-level epidemiologic studies. In the 1970s, there was question of an association with cardiac anomalies.[338,339] Subsequent analyses by Simpson and Phillips, in a very thorough and critical review in 1990, concluded that there was no reliable evidence implicating COCs as cardiac teratogens.[340] Further, Simpson found no relationship between combined oral contraception during pregnancy and the following problems: hypospadias, limb reduction anomalies, neural tube defects, or mutagenic effects that would be responsible for chromosomally abnormal fetuses. Even virilization is not a practical consideration because the doses required (e.g., 20 to 40 mg NET per day) are in excess of anything currently used. These conclusions reflect use of COCs as well as progestins alone, but no data have emerged regarding nonoral CHCs.

In the past, there was also a concern regarding the VACTERL anomalies (vertebral, anal, cardiac, tracheoesophageal, renal, and limb). While initial case-control studies indicated a relationship with combined oral contraception, prospective studies have failed to observe any connection between sex steroids and the VACTERL complex.[341]

By 1990, meta-analyses of the risk of birth defects with COC ingestion during pregnancy included over 6,000 exposed and 83,000 unexposed patients. These meta-analyses concluded that there was no increase in risk for major malformations, congenital heart defects, or limb reduction defects.[342,343] Women who become pregnant while taking CHC or women who inadvertently take CHC during early pregnancy can receive advice that the risk of a significant congenital anomaly is no greater than the general rate of 2% to 3%.[344,345]

All of the data here assess effects of COCs. Although we lack specific data, because the hormones are the same, we can extrapolate the above findings to all CHC including the contraceptive ring and patch.

Reproduction After Discontinuing Combined Hormonal Contraception

FERTILITY. The early reports from the British prospective studies indicated that women who discontinued combined oral contraception for pregnancy had a slight delay in achieving pregnancy. In an analysis of the Oxford Family Planning Association cohort, recent COC users had a lower monthly fecundity rate of conception for the first 3 months and somewhat lower rate from 4 to 10 months. By the second year, 90% of previous COC users had become pregnant.[346] Another analysis of the Oxford-FPA study by Howe et al.[347] in 1985 showed that nulliparous women had a longer delay compared to women with proven fertility. There is no evidence of infertility following oral contraceptive use.[348,349] Furthermore, the studies indicating a delay in conception are influenced by pills with EE doses greater than 50 μg. In a prospective study from the United Kingdom reflecting modern, low-dose COCs, no delay to conception was found and long-term use was actually associated with greater fertility.[349] The EURAS Study on Oral Contraceptives was a prospective cohort study of 59,510 users of low-dose combined oral contraception. The early and 1-year pregnancy rates after discontinuation of oral contraceptives were not negatively affected, regardless of progestin type, duration of use, or parity.[350] After 2 years, the pregnancy rate was 88.3% and the average time to pregnancy was 5.5 cycles. The previous reports indicating a delay in achieving pregnancy may have been influenced not only by higher dose products but also by a failure to account for declining fertility with aging and the prescribing of COCs to women with anovulatory, irregular menstrual periods. It is unlikely that women discontinuing low-dose combined hormonal contraception experience any significant delay in achieving pregnancy compared with the experience in a general population. A recent systematic review and meta-analysis found no change in fertility with oral contraception use.[351]

These data reflect effects of COCs. Although we lack specific data, because the hormones are the same, we can extrapolate the above findings to all combined hormonal contraceptives including the contraceptive ring and patch.

SPONTANEOUS ABORTION. Incidence of spontaneous abortion is not increased after the cessation of COCs. The rate of spontaneous abortion and stillbirth is slightly lower in former pill users, 1% lower for spontaneous abortion and 0.3% lower for stillbirths.[352] Even in women who become pregnant after age 30, previous combined hormonal contraceptive use does not increase risk of spontaneous miscarriage.[353]

Similar to above, all of these data reflect effects of COCs. Although we lack specific data, because the hormones are the same, we can extrapolate the above findings to all combined hormonal contraceptives including the contraceptive ring and patch.

PREGNANCY OUTCOME. Combined hormonal contraceptives do not increase risk of aneuploidy or fetal malformation in future pregnancies nor do they change sex ratio. These observations are not altered when analyzed for duration of use.[340,352,354] These findings are consistent with spontaneous abortion data, which one would expect because chromosomal abnormalities are the principal cause of spontaneous miscarriage.

In a 3-year follow-up of children whose mothers had ever used COCs prior to conception, no differences were detected in weight, anemia, intelligence, or development.[355] Former pill users have no increased risks for the following: perinatal morbidity or mortality, prematurity, and low birth weight.[356,357] The only reason to recommend that women defer attempts to conceive after stopping the pill is to improve the accuracy of gestational dating to identify the last menstrual period. However, ubiquitous use of sonography confirms dating even with an unknown last menstrual period.

All of the data presented assess effects of COCs. Although we lack specific data, because the hormones are the same, we can extrapolate the above findings to all combined hormonal contraceptives including the contraceptive ring and patch.

Gynecologic Effects

HEAVY MENSTRUAL BLEEDING/ANEMIA. Combined hormonal contraceptive methods are effective in the treatment of heavy menstrual bleeding. In a placebo-controlled RCT of 120 women receiving an E2V/DNG COC, 29% of subjects had complete resolution of heavy menstrual bleeding compared to 3% in the placebo group ($p = 0.001$). The mean menstrual blood loss reduction over 90 days was 353 mL with treatment compared to 130 mL with placebo ($p < 0.001$).[358] This formulation received FDA approval for the indication of heavy menstrual bleeding in 2012. A systematic review concluded that, although data are limited and most studies are low quality, women using CHCs experienced 35% to 72% reductions in menstrual blood loss compared to placebo. Users of E2V/DNG also experienced a 5% to 16% increase in hemoglobin and 13% to 63% increase in hematocrit.[359] Reduction of heavy menstrual bleeding decreases iron deficiency anemia.[360,361] In anemic women, an increase in hemoglobin and ferritin levels accompanies COCs use.[362] A recent analysis of data from the Demographic and Health Surveys including 201,720 women across 12 low- and middle-income counties with anemia prevalence of 40% anemia showed that current combined oral contraception use was associated with decreased risk of anemia; the benefit increased with duration of use. Women were half as likely to have anemia after 2 years of use.[363]

DYSMENORRHEA/ENDOMETRIOSIS. Combined hormonal contraceptives provide dysmenorrhea relief even with low-dose formulations. In a prospective cohort study of 308 adolescents with 80% dysmenorrhea prevalence and 18% prevalence of severe dysmenorrhea, girls who had severe dysmenorrhea and a reduction of dysmenorrhea from oral contraceptives were eight times more likely to be consistent COC users.[364] A placebo-controlled double-blinded RCT of 76 adolescents with severe dysmenorrhea reported lower pain scores on a 10-point scale in the 20 µg COC group than the placebo group (3.1 vs. 5.8, $p = 0.004$). By the third COC cycle, participants reported less pain medication usage and decreased pain perception compared to placebo.[365] In a population-based study of Swedish women, those using COCs at baseline reported less dysmenorrhea than nonusers.[366] This was supported by a double-blind placebo-controlled RCT of 215 women with dysmenorrhea. Following treatment with 4 cycles of an EE 35 µg COC, women reported a 30-point decrease on the 100-point VAS compared to a 13-point decrease with placebo.[367] Continuous COC use versus cyclic use showed improvement in dysmenorrhea at 1 and 3 months but no difference at 6 months of usage.[368] A Cochrane review of 12 RCTs found that 11 showed reduced menstrual pain with continuous COC use compared to cyclic use.[369] Although the available data strongly support use of CHC to reduce dysmenorrhea, this is not a U.S. FDA-approved indication.

Combined hormonal contraceptives may reduce endometriosis-related pain although evidence is less robust.[370-372] Other studies have suggested that CHC can suppress and prevent recurrence of disease following conservative surgery for endometriosis[373,374]; however, this evidence is also limited. A 2018 Cochrane Review by Brown et al.[375] concluded that there is insufficient evidence to make a judgment on the effectiveness of combined hormonal contraception compared to placebo or compared to other medical treatments.

POLYCYSTIC OVARY SYNDROME
MENSTRUAL REGULATION
Combined oral contraception is an effective method for menstrual regulation in women with PCOS. In a Cochrane review conducted in 2007 by Costello et al.,[376] two trials found that EE 35 µg/CPA 2 mg COCs are more effective than metformin in improving menstrual pattern. Metformin was found to be inferior to COCs with OR 0.08 (95% CI, 0.01 to 0.45). This was found to be true among adolescents as well. A review of four RCTs of adolescents with polycystic ovary syndrome (PCOS) by Al Khalifah et al.[377] found that OCP treatment resulted in improvement in menstrual cycle frequency. Although these studies involved oral formulations, we can extrapolate the above findings to all combined hormonal contraceptives including the contraceptive ring and patch.

ANDROGENIC SYMPTOMS
All CHCs improve androgenic symptoms by increasing SHBG, by decreasing adrenal androgen production, and by decreasing conversion of testosterone to dihydrotestosterone (DHT). Although each contraceptive formulation has a progestin with varying degrees of antiandrogen activity, the overall combination with EE makes all formulations antiandrogenic. In a study by de Leo et al.[378] in 2010, 40 women with PCOS were randomized to one

of four treatment groups: EE 30 μg/DRSP 3 mg, EE 30 μg/CMA 2 mg, EE 30 μg/GSD 75 μg, and EE 30 μg/DSG 150 μg. Blood samples of androstenedione (A), total testosterone (T), free T, SHBG, and dehydroepiandrosterone sulfate (DHEAS) were obtained and showed mean concentrations of free T, total T and A dropped by 40% to 60%, and concentrations of DHEAS dropped by 20% to 50% ($p < 0.05$). Similarly, a meta-analysis by Amiri et al. in 2018 showed that COCs increase SHBG levels and decrease the Ferriman-Gallwey (FG) score, total T, free T, A, and DHEAS levels. Six to twelve months of COC use was more effective in improving hirsutism compared to short term. COCs containing CPA for 12 months had the strongest effect in improving hirsutism.[379] A review by de Medeiros in 2017[380] showed that the antiandrogenic benefits are similar among all COC preparations. Evidence suggests that these improvements in hirsutism and hyperandrogenemia apply to the combined contraceptive ring as well.[381]

Metabolic Changes

Women with PCOS can experience worsening lipid profiles with use of COCs. A meta-analysis by Amiri et al.[382] in 2018 showed that long-term COC use resulted in elevated LDL as well as HDL and triglycerides. No changes were noted with other metabolic outcomes, including BMI, fasting blood glucose, fasting insulin, or blood pressure. This held true for all COCs but with different timings.

Overall, CHCs have beneficial effects on symptoms of PCOS, including menstrual regulation and a reduction in acne, hirsutism, and endometrial cancer risk, but may result in a worsening lipid profile.

Benign Ovarian Tumors and Cysts. Functional ovarian cysts occur less frequently in women using higher dose combined oral contraception.[383] Current lower dose products have less of a protective effect.[384-388] Most cysts resolve without treatment within a few cycles, and persistent cysts tended to be endometriomas or paraovarian cysts versus physiologic cysts. Treatment with COCs does not hasten resolution of functional ovarian cysts.[389] COCs decrease the risk of benign ovarian tumors. In a case-control study evaluating 746 pathologically confirmed cases, 5 or more years of COC use decreased risk of a benign ovarian tumor (OR, 0.39) including serous adenomas, teratomas, endometriomas, and mucinous adenomas. The largest protective effect was toward endometriomas (OR, 0.15). Reduced risk persisted even 5 years after discontinuation (OR, 0.63).[390] Although the available data strongly support use of COC to treat endometriomas, this is not an FDA-approved indication in the United States. Overall, the findings in these studies using older and higher dose oral formulations can be extrapolated to all combined hormonal contraceptives including the contraceptive ring and patch, since all of our approved products undergo extensive pharmacodynamic studies that demonstrate a reduction in follicle growth.

Mental Health (Mood and Libido)

Mood and PMS

The evidence surrounding CHCs and mood changes is varied. A cross-sectional study by Keyes et al.[391] in 2013 showed that combined hormonal contraceptive users had lower reported depressive symptoms and less likely to report a suicide attempt compared to users of low-tier or non-contraceptive users. A critical review of 46 studies by Schaffir et al.[392] in 2016 showed that most CHC users have no effect or a beneficial effect on mood symptoms. A recent double-blind randomized placebo-controlled trial by Zethraeus et al.[393] in 2017 showed a decreased report of well-being with COC use compared to placebo although there were no differences in depressive symptoms. Another RCT with 202 women using an E2 1.5 mg/nomegestrol acetate 2.5 mg COC or placebo for three treatment cycles found small increases in anxiety, irritability, and mood swings in the inter-menstrual phase and improvement in the premenstrual phase by report of Daily Record of Severity of Problems.[394]

Among adolescents, a large Danish database analysis reported that hormonal contraception was associated with a first diagnosis of depression, initiation of antidepressants,[395] and with suicide attempts.[396] Database studies such as these offer ability to link prescriptions and diagnosis codes with a large number of subjects, but bias must be considered as confounders cannot be evaluated. A more recent survey study of 4,765 adolescents using COCs showed that there was no association between COCs use and lifetime depressive disorder (OR, 1.10; 95% CI, 0.88 to 1.37), nor current use of COCs and current depressive disorder.[397]

Two reviews of premenstrual syndrome (PMS) concluded that EE/DRSP COCs improve symptoms of premenstrual dysphoric disorder (PMDD). The evidence was limited and unclear for other COC formulations and for women with less severe symptoms.[398,399] The EE/DRSP 24-day formulation received FDA approval for treatment of PMDD in 2016.

Libido

Though infrequent, a reduction in libido may be a cause for seeking an alternative method of contraception.[400] Most women report an increase or no change in libido during COC use.[401,402] In a review in 2004, Davis and Castaño[400] found mixed results with women reporting positive effects, negative effects, as well as no effect on libido during COC use. This was again the conclusion in a 2012 review.[403] In a recent randomized, double-blind, placebo-controlled, crossover study with 74 women, both LNG and DRSP COCs reduced total and FT levels and increased SHBG concentrations.[404] There was no improvement in sexual function, mood, and quality of life indicators with the addition of DHEA.[405] More recent RCTs indicate that COCs may decrease libido. In a 2016 RCT by Ciaplinskiene et al.,[406] hormonal contraception with DRSP decreased desire (OR, 2.47; 95% CI, 1.22, 4.98; $p = 0.01$) and arousal (OR, 2.85; 95% CI, 1.34, 5.93; $p = 0.005$).

In another RCT, subjects reported decreased sexual desire and arousability after 5 cycles of either EE-LNG or EE-DRSP COC compared to baseline.[407]

Skin

Acne

Low-dose oral contraceptives improve acne regardless of which product is used. In a placebo-controlled RCT of 257 women with moderate acne, use of the COC (EE/NGM) compared with placebo significantly reduced patient perception of facial acne lesion counts by 62.0% versus 38.6% as well investigator's global assessment of improvement from 93.7% compared with 65.4% in the placebo group.[408] Another placebo-controlled RCT with 250 women with the same drugs and similar protocol resulted in fewer inflammatory lesions (mean reduction, 51.4% compared to 34.6%; $p = 0.01$) and improved investigator's global assessment (83.3% compared to 62.5%; $p = 0.001$) associated with COC use.[409] A placebo-controlled RCT with 350 women taking EE/LNG or placebo for six cycles showed significantly lower inflammatory, noninflammatory, and total lesion counts at cycle 6 with EE/LNG compared to placebo. Patients in the LNG/EE group also had significantly better clinician global and patient self-assessment scores than those in the placebo group at cycle 6.[410] A study of 41 patients with high-grade acne reported that after six cycles with triphasic low-dose EE/DL-norgestrel, the number of comedones had decreased by 79.6% (range, 50% to 100%) in 69.4% of the patients.[411] A RCT of 19 subjects comparing EE/GSD versus EE/DSG resulted in significant improvement in acne in both groups with 62% of cases in the EE/GTD group and 90% of those in the EE/DSG group had either minimal or no acne lesions.[412] An RCT with 34 women with acne comparing EE/DSG versus EE/LNG for 9 months, acne decreased by 52.8% in the EE/LNG group ($n = 9$) and by 58.5% in the EE/DSG group ($n = 7$) (between groups: P not significant).[413] A large placebo-controlled RCT with EE/DNG ($n = 525$), EE/CPA ($n = 537$), or placebo ($n = 264$) for six cycles showed that EE/DNG was superior to placebo and noninferior to EE/CPA ($p < 0.05$). Inflammatory lesions were reduced by 66% for EE/DNG, 65% EE/CPA, and 50% for placebo. Total lesions were reduced by 55% for EE/DNG, 54% for EE/CPA, and 39% for placebo. Percentage of patients with improvement in acne was 92% for EE/DNG, 90% for EE/CPA, and 76% for placebo.[414] A Cochrane review of 31 trials concluded that studies consistently showed that COCs reduced acne lesion counts, severity grades, and self-assessed acne.[415] A meta-analysis of 32 RCTs compared the efficacy of antibiotics to COCs in managing acne and concluded that COCs are equivalent to antibiotics at 6 months in reducing acne lesions and, thus, may be a better first-line alternative to systemic antibiotics. Total lesion reduction at 6 months was 52% with oral antibiotic treatment, 55% with COCs, and 29% with placebo.[416] Because all combined hormonal contraceptives work systemically, the findings related to acne may apply equally to the contraceptive ring and patch.

Chloasma

Chloasma, a patchy increase in facial pigment, was, at one time, found to occur in approximately 10% of oral contraceptive users. It is now a rare problem due to the decrease in estrogen dose. Once chloasma appears, it may fade gradually following CHC discontinuation and may never disappear completely.[417]

Gastrointestinal

Liver Adenomas

Prospective studies have not identified an increased incidence of liver adenomas.[418] In a collaborative study of 15 German liver centers, no increase in risk for liver adenomas in contemporary COC users could be detected.[419] This is reinforced by the rarity of the condition ever since low-dose oral contraception became available. If an enlarged liver is found, oral contraception should be stopped. Tumors and focal nodular hyperplasia regress when oral contraception is stopped.[420,421]

Gallbladder

Data from the Royal College of General Practitioners' prospective study in 1982 indicated an increase in gallstone incidence in the first years of oral contraceptive use.[422] In a 1994 analysis of the Nurses' Health Study, which included 96,211 female United States nurses with 425 cases of gallstones, researchers reported an increase in the symptomatic gallstone risk among current (RR, 1.6) and long-term COC users (RR, 1.5 for 10 to 14 years; RR, 1.6 for 15 or more years).[423] An Italian case-control study and a report from the Oxford-FPA cohort found no increase in gallbladder disease with oral contraceptive use even with adjustment for increasing age or body weight.[424,425] A UK database analysis also found no association between EE/DRSP or EE/LNG COC and gallbladder disease compared to unexposed women.[426] A secondary analysis of an RCT with women at University of Texas Southwestern Medical Center reported Mexican-American postpartum women initiating COC had a higher than expected rate of cholecystectomy in the next 6 months compared to the general population of women age 15 to 44 (25.3/1,000 woman-years vs. 4.2/1,000 woman-years).[427] While gallbladder disease is associated with high-dose pills, it is less common in more recent studies with lower dose pills. Women at higher risk for disease may experience symptoms when initiating COCs.

Other GI Problems

Follow-up analysis of the Oxford-FPA cohort identified 175 women with confirmed peptic ulcer disease and revealed similar rates of disease between previous COC users and nonusers (4/1,000 woman-years vs. 7/1,000 woman-years).[428] A 1990 case-control study of 46 women with ulcerative colitis failed to reveal association with CHC use.[429] Analysis in 1989 of Royal College of General Practitioners' study in which 42 women developed

Crohn's disease and 78 developed ulcerative colitis showed greater incidence of both conditions among oral contraceptive users compared to non-users (Crohn's RR, 1.7; ulcerative colitis RR, 1.3)[430] A 2017 meta-analysis of 20 cohort and case-control studies reported a 24% higher risk for developing Crohn's disease, a 30% higher risk for developing ulcerative colitis, and a 30% increased risk for the development of general inflammatory bowel disease in women with previous CHC exposure compared to no exposure.[431] All formulations of oral contraception are not recommended for patients with problems of gastrointestinal malabsorption, although transdermal or vaginal ring contraceptives may be an alternative. Similarly, combination hormonal injections, where available, may also be suitable for women with various GI problems.

Infectious Disease

Human Immunodeficiency Virus

Most studies have found no association between oral contraceptive use and HIV acquisition risk. A 1997 case-control study among Thai female commercial sex workers all using COCs with 118 HIV-1 positive cases and 258 HIV-1–negative controls revealed no significant association between CHCs and HIV-1 infection.[432] In a 2012 prospective cohort study of 1,314 couples in which the HIV-1–seronegative partner was female, there was no significant difference in rates of HIV-1 transmission between couples with oral contraception compared to no hormonal contraception.[433] A 2013 systematic review of 12 observational studies showed no association with HIV acquisition and CHCs.[434] In a 2015 cohort study of 1,393 serodiscordant Zambian couples, 252 incident infections occurred in women and there was no significant difference in rates of HIV transmission between couples with oral contraception compared to no hormonal contraception.[435] Meta-analysis of 18 studies, including 37,124 women and 1,830 incident HIV infections, found no evidence that COC increases women's risk of HIV.[436] A prospective cohort study using data from women enrolled in the HIV Prevention Trials Network in Malawi, South Africa, Zambia, and Zimbabwe with 2,830 participants, of whom 106 became HIV infected, showed no increased risk of HIV acquisition.[437]

CHCs use by HIV-positive women does not affect disease progression. In a subset analysis of data from the Women's Interagency HIV Study, no change in viral load was noted among the 73 women with HIV who reported COC use.[438] In a prospective cohort study of 273 Kenyan women all using COCs, HIV-1–RNA plasma viral loads or CD4 T-cell counts did not change during a 2-year period.[439] In a prospective study of 2,269 women with HIV-1 from seven countries in eastern and southern Africa with CD4 cell counts of at least 250 cells/μL, there was no evidence for accelerated disease progression compared to women with HIV not using hormonal contraception.[440]

Vaginitis (BV/Trichomonas/Candidiasis)

Oral contraception appears to protect against bacterial vaginosis and trichomonas infections and increase risk of candidiasis, although study outcomes are not always consistent. In a study of 818 women evaluated for trichomoniasis, candidiasis, and bacterial vaginosis monthly for 6 months, women using oral contraceptives experienced a nonsignificant lower rate of trichomoniasis (RR 0.83) and bacterial vaginosis (RR 0.86) as compared with placebo users. The rate of candidiasis was nearly identical to placebo users (RR 1.02).[441] However, in a Swedish cohort study with 131 women with clinical BV, there was a reduced risk of BV associated with oral contraceptive use (OR 0.4).[442] A prospective cohort study of 948 Kenyan prostitutes found that oral contraceptive users were at increased risk for acquisition of chlamydia (HR 1.8) and vaginal candidiasis (HR 1.5) and at decreased risk for bacterial vaginosis (HR 0.8).[443] In 133 women with BV diagnosed at a Baltimore clinic, use of combined hormonal contraception was associated with decreased risk of BV (OR 0.66).[444] Systematic review of 55 studies has shown that combined hormonal contraception reduces the risk of bacterial vaginosis infection BV (RR 0.68), including incident infection (RR 0.82) and recurrent infection (RR 0.69).[445] A systematic review of 36 studies and reanalysis of the Hormonal Contraception and HIV Acquisition study reports decrease in BV infection ranging from 10% to 20% and an increased risk of vaginal candidiasis although this evidence was less consistent.[446] A more recent retrospective study of vaginal sample data from a subset of participants from the Human Vaginal Microbiome Project with 682 women found that women using COCs were less likely to be colonized by BV-associated bacteria relative to women who used condoms. Women using COCs were more likely to be colonized by beneficial *Lactobacillus* species compared with women using condoms.[447]

The use of a contraceptive vaginal ring is not associated with vaginitis.[448–451] New evidence suggests the same findings with a 1-year ring. With 13-cycle use of the 1-year ring, infection detection rate remained stable with 3.3% of subjects clinically diagnosed with bacterial vaginosis, 15.0% with vulvovaginal candidiasis, and 0.8% with trichomoniasis. There were no significant changes in frequency or concentrations of other pathogens. High levels of agreement between vaginal and ring surface microbiota were observed.[452]

Cervicitis

Initial published studies reported a correlation of oral contraceptives with acquisition of chlamydial cervicitis.[238,453,454] A cross-sectional study conducted with colposcopic, cytologic, and microbiologic examination of 764 women with cervicitis compared to 819 controls reported an association between oral contraceptives and cervical ectropion suggesting that cervical ectropion may explain the increased detection of the chlamydial organism by culture.[455] More recent evidence conducted with PCR diagnosis suggests increased chlamydia infection and decreased gonorrhea infection. A study of 107 women with male partners diagnosed with gonorrhea infection found that 64% of participants had gonorrhea infection and women using CHC were less likely than nonusers to test positive for infection (32% vs. 76%) after adjusting for new partner, sexual frequency, and condom use.[456] In a 2015 study of 800 Rwandan female sex workers, oral contraceptive use was associated with increased chlamydial incidence found by PCR testing.[457]

Pelvic Inflammatory Disease

Despite the relationship between oral contraception and chlamydial cervicitis, there is no evidence of increased risk of tubal infertility or diagnosis of pelvic inflammatory disease (PID) with CHC use. In an evaluation of the Women's Health Study by the CDC, which included 648 women with PID, women using OCs in the prior 3 months had a decreased risk of PID.[458] A case-control study of 141 women with verified PID reported those with PID were less likely than control subjects to use oral contraceptives with stronger effect with chlamydial infection compared to gonorrheal infection.[459] A more recent study of 144 subjects with PID reported lower detection of chlamydial infection by IgA among previous or current oral contraceptive users compared to women who had never used birth control methods.[460] A case-control analysis of 2,761 cases with PID from the Women's health study showed no significant association between low-dose combination oral contraceptives and PID.[461]

To evaluate the effect of COCs on fertility, a study with 283 nulliparous infertile women with tubal adhesions or occlusion reported that past use of oral contraceptives had no effect on woman's risk of tubal infertility.[462] In a study of 546 women with salpingitis seen on laparoscopy, women using COCs had significantly milder degrees of inflammation of the fallopian tubes than women with other contraceptive methods.[463] A case-control study with 94 women with acute salpingitis due to chlamydial infection reported that women using OCs had significantly lower titer of antibodies to the organism than did nonusers.[464] This decreased inflammation may explain the improved fertility rate observed in previous users of oral contraception compared to nonusers.[348,349]

Hematologic Effects

Hematologic effects include an increased sedimentation rate, an increased total iron-binding capacity due to the increase in globulins, and a decrease in prothrombin time.

Prolactin-Secreting Adenomas

Because estrogen is known to stimulate prolactin secretion and to cause hypertrophy of the pituitary lactotrophs, it is appropriate to be concerned over a possible relationship between oral contraception and prolactin-secreting adenomas. Case-control studies have uniformly concluded that no such relationship exists.[465,466] Data from both the Royal College of General

Practitioners and the Oxford-FPA studies indicated no increase in the incidence of pituitary adenomas.[329,467] Previous use of oral contraceptives is not related to the size of prolactinomas at presentation and diagnosis.[467,468] Oral contraception can be prescribed for patients with pituitary microadenomas without fear of subsequent tumor growth.[469,470]

Eye/Ear Diseases

In the 1960s and 1970s, there were numerous anecdotal reports of eye disorders in women using oral contraception. An analysis of the two large British cohort studies (the Royal College of General Practitioners' Study and the Oxford FPA Study) could find no increase in risk for the following conditions: conjunctivitis, keratitis, iritis, lacrimal disease, strabismus, cataract, glaucoma, and retinal detachment.[471] Retinal vascular lesions were slightly more common in recent users of oral contraception, but this finding did not reach statistical significance. Contact lens may be less well tolerated, requiring more frequent use of wetting solutions. The Oxford Family Planning Association Study could detect no evidence of any adverse effects of oral contraception on ear disorders.[472]

Neurologic

Multiple Sclerosis

There is no evidence in three cohort studies (the Royal College of General Practitioners' Study, the Oxford FPA Study, and the Nurses' Health Study) of any effect of oral contraceptive use on the risk or course of multiple sclerosis.[473-476]

Choosing a CHC: Initiation and Management

Different pill types are numerous, and the number of brand names is far greater. Development of so many different pills has been motivated by a search for lower-risk and higher-benefit formulations, which would be good for individual and population health, and which would provide a commercial benefit for the developers. That said, the major noncontraceptive benefits (e.g., ovarian and endometrial cancer prevention, cycle regulation and reduced flow) as well as the risks appear to accrue to all pill types and are part of "class labeling." Many different pills are likely to share the other noncontraceptive benefits (e.g., acne reduction, dysmenorrhea reduction), but because carrying out clinical trials to demonstrate these benefits is costly, only a few brands have these benefits listed in their label, and many other pill labels are silent about what are quite likely to be the same benefits. Fewer options for nonoral methods exist.

Individual tolerability and preferences appear to vary. While on average most women will do well with any pill, idiosyncratic responses mean that some women will need to try several different formulations to find a pill that "feels right." Some women complain of mood dysregulation when using CHC,[69,477] but this has not been solidly associated with particular

271

formulations. CHC effectiveness is probably greater when using formulations with a shorter pill-free interval and using formulations in which the progestin component has a longer half-life[10]; while this evidence is limited, these results are plausible because such pills should minimize breakthrough ovulation, especially in face of imperfect pill use. Multiphasic pills are safe and effective but do not offer any special benefits. Continuous CHC use for several months or indefinitely provides effective menstrual suppression.

A woman's preferences are an excellent basis for choosing an initial pill (or ring or patch) from the many available—she may consider her own past experience, the good or bad experiences of her friends or family, and she may have preferences based on marketing messages. A product that a woman successfully used in the past is typically a good one to use again. Anecdotally, many women believe that the "lowest dose" will be safer or will have less effect on her weight, especially in regard to EE dose. While science does not support these particular prejudices regarding today's pill formulations, attending to a woman's preferences is reasonable and appropriate patient-centered care. Good practice also includes providing women with accurate information about contraceptive risks and benefits in order to assist her in making a contraceptive choice—certainly some women avoid combined hormonal contraception due to specific myths, and more accurate information may provide reassurance useful for them.[28] The clinician should be tactful in correcting misinformation.

A key basis for choosing a particular CHC brand is ease of access for that woman. Insurance coverage and required co-pays vary widely as do refill policies: frequent refills are a barrier to continuation, and we know that more affordable and readily available CHC supplies enhance continuation and reduce unintended pregnancy rates.[478,479] At this time, California and several other states permit dispensing an annual supply of pills; this is an encouraging trend. In contrast, in New York (and many other states), Medicaid will permit dispensing only three packs at a time, and most commercial insurances require going to the pharmacy for monthly refills. Many women with commercial insurance can receive three cycles at a time by mail order from their pharmacy-benefit manager. Clinicians should provide a maximal supply and not require women to return for unnecessary checkups; most state pharmacy regulations, however, will not permit prescriptions longer than 12 months. Any additional routine surveillance in a healthy woman with normal blood pressure is just a barrier to continuation. Online provision with refills is increasingly available.[480] The regulations around dispensing are state specific and rapidly changing; thus, clinicians need to be attentive to their local situation in order to minimize barriers.

Evaluating a woman for initiating CHC depends mainly on her detailed medical history and her family medical history of hormonally related cancers and cardiovascular disease. The many studies discussed earlier in this chapter give a good general idea of what are the most important contraindications. The most detailed compilation of contraindications related to medical conditions is available in the WHO or CDC medical eligibility criteria publications.[110,481] These evidence-based recommendations are formally updated every several years, are available through the CDC website, and are the most accurate information source about contraindications. Clinicians should use the MEC to evaluate whether a patient's medical history reveals conditions that are contraindications to using CHCs. In addition to providing a medical history, a woman considering CHC initiation should also have a blood pressure measurement. Finally, all the elements of a well woman visit might be appropriate for a woman seeking to initiate CHC[482]; however, these elements should not be a barrier to initiating hormonal contraception. Note in particular that a pelvic examination is not a prerequisite for initiating CHC.[483] Because initiating CHC depends mainly on medical history and not an examination or testing, an in-person assessment is generally unnecessary; in several states, women can now obtain CHC directly from a pharmacist and from many online vendors.[28,484] Several groups are working toward FDA approval for providing COCs over-the-counter, although the first products are likely to be progestin-only pills.

After deciding that a woman is medically eligible for CHC and choosing a specific formulation, one must decide when to begin. Pill (and patch and ring) product labels specify beginning the pill pack at the beginning of the woman's next menstrual cycle, often suggesting the first day of menses, the Sunday after initiating menses, or within 7 days. This guidance follows how phase 3 clinical trials generally initiate contraceptives. Contemporary guidance suggests that a woman can begin immediately or whenever it is "reasonably certain" that she is not pregnant. Since inadvertent hormonal exposure during early pregnancy is not teratogenic or otherwise harmful, many find the "reasonably certain" checklist to be too restrictive.[169,485,486] The benefit of an immediate start includes a quicker onset of contraceptive protection and may result in better continuation and fewer pregnancies, especially among ambivalent adolescents.[477,487] The worry about immediate initiation is the possibility of delaying the diagnosis of a very early pregnancy, but multiple studies have found that among women sexually active since their last menses, only about 2% will prove to have an early pregnancy only detected after initiating the method. As the potential harm to those 2% is minimal, withholding contraceptive initiation for the other 98% seems unwarranted.[486]

Ongoing surveillance during CHC use should fulfill several goals: first, avoid requiring extra visits that are a barrier to continuation by providing the maximum number of refills allowable by state regulations or insurance requirements. In a study of over 1,600 young OC initiators in the United States, the number one reason for discontinuation was difficulty in accessing refills; these results indicate the role that clinicians have in CHC discontinuation due to limiting easy refills.[69] However, it is important to see women often enough to update medical history and blood pressure and thus ensure that CHC remains a safe contraceptive. Most CHC users in the United States are healthy and below age 35 and need little surveillance; however, women 35 years and older and those with medical comorbidities

273

deserve follow-up at least once per year. Finally, offer a visit to reassess any woman who is dissatisfied with her current CHC for any reason and also to reassess those who have developed any new medical problem that might change the risk/benefit ratio for CHC use.

CHC "side effects"—including headache, weight gain, mood disorders, and sexual satisfaction changes—are often reported as a reason for discontinuing the contraceptive method.[488] However, these "side effects" may just be part of life, rather than an actual "side effect" of the method. In a 6-month double-blinded RCT of 507 women, Redmond and colleagues[70] found that women receiving COC or placebo reported types and numbers of "side effects" that were indistinguishable, and that a similar percentage of women discontinued over the study. A double-blinded, placebo-controlled trial among adolescents also found similar types and numbers of side effects in both groups of participants.[489] In the study of 1,600 young U.S. COC users, almost 50% reported at least one of these side effects, but half of the women attributed the new symptom to a cause other than the contraceptive. That said, the women who reported one of these symptoms, whether attributing it to the method or not, were more likely to discontinue the COC before 6 months.[69] In focus groups performed in preparation for that study, women did not cite concerns about initial breakthrough bleeding as a reason to discontinue the COC. Another analysis of the same young women showed that those who discontinued due to side effects during a past episode of COC use were more likely to discontinue again.[477] Placebo-controlled trials indicate that supposed oral contraceptive side effects are more myth than reality. The widespread beliefs in such side effects lead to a "nocebo effect" and may contribute to a disinclination to continue or even to start oral contraceptives.[28,490] For an individual patient, the clinician needs to be attentive to her unique symptoms and concerns, offer reassurance, and be willing to change to a different CHC or a different contraceptive altogether in order to increase patient satisfaction and to decrease pregnancy risk.

Postpartum and Postabortion Use

Initiating CHC postpartum merits a delay due to the elevated VTE risk that persists for at least 6 weeks.[491] Women should not begin CHC for at least 21 days postpartum (MEC category 4). From 21 to 42 days postpartum, if women have additional risk factors for VTE (beyond being postpartum), then the VTE risks may exceed the benefits of using CHC, and other contraceptive methods would be preferable (MEC category 3). For women without additional VTE risk factors, the benefits of starting CHC outweigh the risks (MEC category 2) from 21 to 42 days, and after 42 days, starting CHC is generally suitable (i.e., category 1). The exceptions are recommendations for lactating women due to additional concerns that CHC use may hinder successful lactation.[492] While the data to resolve this concern remain inconclusive, the MEC recommendations take a cautious approach of avoiding even theoretical risks to successful lactation. Thus, for lactating women, initiating CHC from 21 to 30 days postpartum (a finer category than used for nonlactating women), even without VTE risk factors, is still considered a category 3, and even after 42 days, initiating CHC remains a category 2. Some recommend waiting up to 6 months to begin CHC, both because of concerns that earlier CHC might inhibit lactation, and because of concerns about transferring hormones to the infant. Limited data support these precautionary concerns.[110] When starting CHC among postpartum women, 1 week of abstinence or backup contraception is suitable except for those women with lactational amenorrhea, who do not need backup.

Initiating CHC is appropriate immediately after a first-trimester or second-trimester abortion (MEC category 1). Because ovulation can follow abortion within weeks, prompt contraceptive initiation is wise for women who wish to delay the next pregnancy. Same-day initiation is safe and convenient and may obviate an unnecessary return visit. With same-day initiation, no backup method is necessary.

275

References

1. **Amador E, Zimmerman TS, Wacker WE,** FDA report on Enovid. Ad hoc advisory committee for the evaluation of a possible etiologic relation with thromboembolic conditions, JAMA 185:776, 1963.

2. **Vessey MP, Doll R,** Investigation of relation between use of oral contraceptives and thromboembolic disease, Br Med J 2:199–205, 1968.

3. **Gallo MF, Nanda K, Grimes DA, Lopez LM, Schulz KF,** 20 microg versus >20 microg estrogen combined oral contraceptives for contraception, Cochrane Database Syst Rev (8):CD003989, 2013.

4. **Van Vliet HA, Grimes DA, Lopez LM, Schulz KF, Helmerhorst FM,** Triphasic versus monophasic oral contraceptives for contraception, Cochrane Database Syst Rev (11):CD003553, 2011.

5. **Van Vliet HA, Raps M, Lopez LM, Helmerhorst FM,** Quadriphasic versus monophasic oral contraceptives for contraception, Cochrane Database Syst Rev (11):CD009038, 2011.

6. **Killick SR, Bancroft K, Oelbaum S, Morris J, Elstein M,** Extending the duration of the pill-free interval during combined oral contraception, Adv Contracept 6:33–40, 1990.

7. **van Heusden AM, Fauser BC,** Activity of the pituitary-ovarian axis in the pill-free interval during use of low-dose combined oral contraceptives, Contraception 59:237–243, 1999.

8. **Willis SA, Kuehl TJ, Spiekerman AM, Sulak PJ,** Greater inhibition of the pituitary–ovarian axis in oral contraceptive regimens with a shortened hormone-free interval, Contraception 74:100–103, 2006.

9. **Rible RD, Taylor D, Wilson ML, Stanczyk FZ, Mishell DR Jr,** Follicular development in a 7-day versus 4-day hormone-free interval with an oral contraceptive containing 20 mcg ethinyl estradiol and 1 mg norethindrone acetate, Contraception 79:182–188, 2009.

10. **Dinger J, Minh TD, Buttmann N, Bardenheuer K,** Effectiveness of oral contraceptive pills in a large U.S. cohort comparing progestogen and regimen, Obstet Gynecol 117:33–40, 2011.

11. **Kaunitz AM, Burkman RT, Fisher AC, Laguardia KD,** Cycle control with a 21-day compared with a 24-day oral contraceptive pill: a randomized controlled trial, Obstet Gynecol 114:1205–1212, 2009.

12. **Kaunitz AM, Portman DJ, Hait H, Reape KZ,** Adding low-dose estrogen to the hormone-free interval: impact on bleeding patterns in users of a 91-day extended regimen oral contraceptive, Contraception 79:350–355, 2009.

13. **Nakajima ST, Archer DF, Ellman H,** Efficacy and safety of a new 24-day oral contraceptive regimen of norethindrone acetate 1 mg/ethinyl estradiol 20 µg (Loestrin® 24 Fe), Contraception 75:16–22, 2007.

14. **Klipping C, Marr J, Korner P,** Ovulation inhibition effects of two low-dose oral contraceptive dosing regimens following intentional dosing errors (abstract), Obstet Gynecol 107:495, 2006.

15. **Creinin MD, Lippman JS, Eder SE, Godwin AJ, Olson W,** The effect of extending the pill-free interval on follicular activity: triphasic norgestimate/35 µg ethinyl estradiol versus monophasic levonorgestrel/20 µg ethinyl estradiol, Contraception 66:147–152, 2002.

16. **Baerwald AR, Olatunbosun OA, Pierson RA,** Effects of oral contraceptives administered at defined stages of ovarian follicular development, Fertil Steril 86:27–35, 2006.

17. **Westhoff CL, Torgal AH, Mayeda ER, Stanczyk FZ, Lerner JP, Benn EK, et al.,** Ovarian suppression in normal-weight and obese women during oral contraceptive use: a randomized controlled trial, Obstet Gynecol 116:275–283, 2010.

18. **Seidman L, Kroll R, Howard B, Ricciotti N, Hsieh J, Weiss H,** Ovulatory effects of three oral contraceptive regimens: a randomized, open-label, descriptive trial, Contraception 91:495–502, 2015.

19. **Reape KZ, DiLiberti CE, Hendy CH, Volpe EJ,** Effects on serum hormone levels of low-dose estrogen in place of placebo during the hormone-free interval of an oral contraceptive, Contraception 77:34–39, 2008.

20. **Archer DF, Jensen JT, Johnson JV, Borisute H, Grubb GS, Constantine GD,** Evaluation of a continuous regimen of levonorgestrel/ethinyl estradiol: phase 3 study results, Contraception 74:439–445, 2006.

21. **Kwiecien M, Edelman A, Nichols MD, Jensen JT,** Bleeding patterns and patient acceptability of standard or continuous dosing regimens of a low-dose oral contraceptive: a randomized trial, Contraception 67:9–13, 2003.

22. **Sulak PJ, Carl J, Gopalakrishnan I, Coffee A, Kuehl TJ,** Outcomes of extended oral contraceptive regimens with a shortened hormone-free interval to manage breakthrough bleeding, Contraception 70:281–287, 2004.

23. **Han L, Jensen JT,** Expert opinion on a flexible extended regimen of drospirenone/ethinyl estradiol contraceptive, Expert Opin Pharmacother 15:2071–2079, 2014.

24. **Jensen JT, Garie SG, Trummer D, Elliesen J,** Bleeding profile of a flexible extended regimen of ethinylestradiol/drospirenone in US women: an open-label, three-arm, active-controlled, multicenter study, Contraception 86:110–118, 2012.

25. **Edelman AB, Koontz SL, Nichols MD, Jensen JT,** Continuous oral contraceptives. Are bleeding patterns dependent on the hormones given? Obstet Gynecol 107:657–665, 2006.

26. **Archer DF, Kovalevsky G, Ballagh SA, Grubb GS,** Ovarian activity and safety of a novel levonorgestrel/ethinyl estradiol continuous oral contraceptive regimen, Contraception 80:245–253, 2009.

27. **Davis AR, Kroll R, Soltes B, Zhang N, Grubb GS, Constantine GD,** Occurrence of menses or pregnancy after cessation of a continuous oral contraceptive, Fertil Steril 89:1059–1063, 2008.

28. **Nelson AL, Cohen S, Galitsky A, Hathaway M, Kappus D, Kerolous M, et al.,** Women's perceptions and treatment patterns related to contraception: results of a survey of US women, Contraception 97:256–273, 2018.

29. **den Tonkelaar I, Oddens BJ,** Preferred frequency and characteristics of menstrual bleeding in relation to reproductive status, oral contraceptive use, and hormone replacement therapy use, Contraception 59:357–362, 1999.

30. **Shere M, Bapat P, Nickel C, Kapur B, Koren G,** The effectiveness of folate-fortified oral contraceptives in maintaining optimal folate levels to protect against neural tube defects: a systematic review, J Obstet Gynaecol Can 37:527–533, 2015.

31. **Lassi ZS, Salam RA, Haider BA, Bhutta ZA,** Folic acid supplementation during pregnancy for maternal health and

pregnancy outcomes, Cochrane Database Syst Rev (3):CD006896, 2013.

32. **Bakhru A, Stanwood N,** Performance of contraceptive patch compared with oral contraceptive pill in a high-risk population, Obstet Gynecol 108:378–386, 2006.

33. **Sonnenberg FA, Burkman RT, Speroff L, Westhoff C, Hagerty CG,** Cost-effectiveness and contraceptive effectiveness of the transdermal contraceptive patch, Am J Obstet Gynecol 192:1–9, 2005.

34. **Smallwood GH, Meador ML, Lenihan JP, Shangold GA, Fisher AC, Creasy GW, et al.,** Efficacy and safety of a transdermal contraceptive system, Obstet Gynecol 98:799–805, 2001.

35. **Zacur HA, Hedon B, Mansour D, Shangold GA, Fisher AC, Creasy GW,** Integrated summary of Ortho Evra™/Evra™ contraceptive patch adhesion in varied climates and conditions, Fertil Steril 77:S32–S35, 2002.

36. **Audet M-C, Moreau M, Koltun WD, Waldbaum AS, Shangold G, Fisher AC, et al.,** Evaluation of contraceptive efficacy and cycle control of a transdermal contraceptive patch vs an oral contraceptive. A randomized controlled trial, JAMA 285:2347–2354, 2001.

37. **Zieman M, Guillebaud J, Weisberg E, Shangold GA, Fisher AC, Creasy GW,** Contraceptive efficacy and cycle control with the Ortho Evra™/Evra™ transdermal system: the analysis of pooled data, Fertil Steril 77:S13–S18, 2002.

38. **Edelman A, Trussell J, Aiken ARA, Portman DJ, Chiodo JA III, Garner EIO,** The emerging role of obesity in short-acting hormonal contraceptive effectiveness, Contraception 97:371–377, 2018.

39. **Creinin MD, Meyn LA, Borgatta L, Barnhart K, Jensen J, Burke AE, et al.,** Multicenter comparison of the contraceptive ring and patch: a randomized controlled trial, Obstet Gynecol 111:267–277, 2008.

40. **van den Heuvel MW, van Bragt AJ, Alnabawy AK, Kaptein MC,** Comparison of ethinylestradiol pharmacokinetics in three hormonal contraceptive formulations: the vaginal ring, the transdermal patch and an oral contraceptive, Contraception 72:168–174, 2005.

41. **Jensen JT, Burke AE, Barnhart KT, Tillotson C, Messerle-Forbes M, Peters D,** Effects of switching from oral to transdermal or transvaginal contraception on markers of thrombosis, Contraception 78:451–458, 2008.

42. **Kaunitz AM, Portman D, Westhoff CL, Archer DF, Mishell DR Jr, Rubin A, et al.,** Low-dose levonorgestrel and ethinyl estradiol patch and pill: a randomized controlled trial, Obstet Gynecol 123:295–303, 2014.

43. **Kaunitz AM, Archer DF, Mishell DR Jr, Foegh M,** Safety and tolerability of a new low-dose contraceptive patch in obese and nonobese women, Am J Obstet Gynecol 212:318e1–318e8, 2015.

44. **Kaunitz AM, Portman D, Westhoff CL, Mishell DR Jr, Archer DF, Foegh M,** New contraceptive patch wearability assessed by investigators and participants in a randomized phase 3 study, Contraception 91:211–216, 2015.

45. **Trussell J, Portman D,** The creeping Pearl: why has the rate of contraceptive failure increased in clinical trials of combined hormonal contraceptive pills? Contraception 88:604–610, 2013.

46. **Hofmann B, Reinecke I, Schuett B, Merz M, Zurth C,** Pharmacokinetic overview of ethinyl estradiol dose and bioavailability using two transdermal contraceptive systems and a standard combined oral contraceptive, Int J Clin Pharmacol Ther 52:1059–1070, 2014.

47. **Westhoff CL, Reinecke I, Bangerter K, Merz M,** Impact of body mass index on suppression of follicular development and ovulation using a transdermal patch containing 0.55-mg ethinyl estradiol/2.1-mg gestodene: a multicenter, open-label, uncontrolled study over three treatment cycles, Contraception 90:272–279, 2014.

48. **Merz M, Kroll R, Lynen R, Bangerter K,** Bleeding pattern and cycle control of a low-dose transdermal contraceptive patch compared with a combined oral contraceptive: a randomized study, Contraception 91:113–120, 2015.

49. **Wiegratz I, Bassol S, Weisberg E, Mellinger U, Merz M,** Effect of a low-dose contraceptive patch on efficacy, bleeding pattern, and safety: a 1-year, multicenter, open-label, uncontrolled study, Reprod Sci 21:1518–1525, 2014.

277

50. **Dragoman M, Petrie K, Torgal A, Thomas T, Cremers S, Westhoff CL,** Contraceptive vaginal ring effectiveness is maintained during 6 weeks of use: a prospective study of normal BMI and obese women, Contraception 87:432–436, 2013.

51. **Shimoni N, Westhoff C,** Review of the vaginal contraceptive ring (NuvaRing), J Fam Plann Reprod Health Care 34:247–250, 2008.

52. **Petrie KA, Torgal AH, Westhoff CL,** Matched-pairs analysis of ovarian suppression during oral vs. vaginal hormonal contraceptive use, Contraception 84:e1–e4, 2011.

53. **Westhoff C, Osborne LM, Schafer JE, Morroni C,** Bleeding patterns after immediate initiation of an oral compared with a vaginal hormonal contraceptive, Obstet Gynecol 106:89–96, 2005.

54. **Gemzell-Danielsson K, Sitruk-Ware R, Creinin MD, Thomas M, Barnhart KT, Creasy G, et al.,** Segesterone acetate/ethinyl estradiol 12-month contraceptive vaginal system safety evaluation, Contraception 99:323–328, 2019.

55. **Archer DF, Merkatz R, Bahamondes L, Westhoff C, Darney P, Apter D, et al.,** Efficacy of the 1-year (13-cycle) segesterone acetate/ethinyl estradiol contraceptive vaginal system: results from phase 3 trials, Lancet Glob Health Published Online June 20, 2019. http://dx.doi.org/10.1016/ S2214-109X(19)30265

56. **Huang Y, Merkatz RB, Hillier SL, Roberts K, Blithe DL, Sitruk-Ware R, Creinin MD,** Effects of a one year reusable contraceptive vaginal ring on vaginal microflora and the risk of vaginal infection: an open-label prospective evaluation, PLoS One 10:e0134460, 2015.

57. **Duijkers I, Klipping C, Heger-Mahn D, Fayad GN, Frenkl TL, Cruz SM, et al.,** Phase II dose-finding study on ovulation inhibition and cycle control associated with the use of contraceptive vaginal rings containing 17beta-estradiol and the progestagens etonogestrel or nomegestrol acetate compared to NuvaRing, Eur J Contracept Reprod Health Care 23:245–254, 2018.

58. **Jensen JT, Edelman AB, Chen BA, Archer DF, Barnhart KT, Thomas MA, et al.,** Continuous dosing of a novel contraceptive vaginal ring releasing Nestorone(R) and estradiol: pharmacokinetics from a dose-finding study, Contraception 97:422–427, 2018.

59. **Miller L, Verhoeven CH, Hout J,** Extended regimens of the contraceptive vaginal ring: a randomized trial. Obstet Gynecol 106:473–482, 2005.

60. **Kaunitz AM, Garceau RJ, Cromie MA,** Comparative safety, efficacy, and cycle control of Lunelle monthly contraceptive injection (medroxyprogesterone acetate and estradiol cypionate injectable suspension) and Ortho-Novum 7/7/7 oral contraceptive (norethindrone/ethinyl estradiol triphasic). Lunelle Study Group, Contraception 60:179–187, 1999.

61. **Shulman LP, Oleen-Burkey M, Willke RJ,** Patient acceptability and satisfaction with Lunelle monthly contraceptive injection (medroxyprogesterone acetate and estradiol cypionate injectable suspension), Contraception 60:215–222, 1999.

62. **Rahimy MH, Ryan KK,** Lunelle monthly contraceptive injection (medroxyprogesterone acetate and estradiol cypionate injectable suspension): assessment of return of ovulation after three monthly injections in surgically sterile women, Contraception 60:189–200, 1999.

63. **Thurman A, Kimble T, Hall P, Schwartz JL, Archer DF,** Medroxyprogesterone acetate and estradiol cypionate injectable suspension (Cyclofem) monthly contraceptive injection: steady-state pharmacokinetics, Contraception 87:738–743, 2013.

64. **Sang GW, Shao QX, Ge RS, Ge JL, Chen JK, Song S, et al.,** A multicentred phase III comparative clinical trial of Mesigyna, Cyclofem and Injectable No. 1 given by intramuscular injection to Chinese women. II. The comparison of bleeding patterns, Contraception 51:185–192, 1995.

65. **Sang GW, Shao QX, Ge RS, Ge JL, Chen JK, Song S, et al.,** A multicentred phase III comparative clinical trial of Mesigyna, Cyclofem and Injectable No. 1 given monthly by intramuscular injection to Chinese women. I. Contraceptive efficacy and side effects, Contraception 51:167–183, 1995.

66. **Westhoff CL, Petrie KA, Cremers S,** Using changes in binding globulins to assess oral contraceptive compliance, Contraception 87:176–181, 2013.

67. **Nault AM, Peipert JF, Zhao Q, Madden T, Secura GM,** Validity of perceived weight gain in women using long-acting reversible contraception and depot medroxyprogesterone acetate, Am J Obstet Gynecol 208:48.e1–48.e8, 2013.

68. **Gaudet LM, Kives S, Hahn PM, Reid RL,** What women believe about oral contraceptives and the effect of counseling, Contraception 69:31–36, 2004.

69. **Westhoff CL, Heartwell S, Edwards S, Zieman M, Stuart G, Cwiak C, et al.,** Oral contraceptive discontinuation: do side effects matter? Am J Obstet Gynecol 196:412.e1–412.e6; discussion e6–e7, 2007.

70. **Redmond G, Godwin AJ, Olson W, Lippman JS,** Use of placebo controls in an oral contraceptive trial: methodological issues and adverse event incidence, Contraception 60:81–85, 1999.

71. **Carpenter S, Neinstein LS,** Weight gain in adolescent and young adult oral contraceptive users, J Adolesc Health Care 7:342, 1986.

72. **Reubinoff BE, Wurtman J, Rojansky N, Adler D, Stein P, Schenker JG, et al.,** Effects of hormone replacement therapy on weight, body composition, fat distribution, and food intake in early postmenopausal women: a prospective study, Fertil Steril 64:963–968, 1995.

73. **Moore LL, Valuck R, McDougall C, Fink W,** A comparative study of one-year weight gain among users of medroxyprogesterone acetate, levonorgestrel implants, and oral contraceptives, Contraception 52:215, 1995.

74. **Gupta S,** Weight gain on the combined pill—is it real? Hum Reprod Update 6:427–431, 2000.

75. **Coney P, Washenik K, Langley RGB, DiGiovanna JJ, Harrison DD,** Weight change and adverse event incidence with a low-dose oral contraceptive: two randomized, placebo-controlled trials, Contraception 63:297–302, 2001.

76. **Lindh I, Ellstrom AA, Milsom I,** The long-term influence of combined oral contraceptives on body weight, Hum Reprod 26:1917–1924, 2011.

77. **Gallo MF, Lopez LM, Grimes DA, Carayon F, Schulz KF, Helmerhorst FM,** Combination contraceptives: effects on weight, Cochrane Database Syst Rev (1):CD003987, 2014.

78. **Mayeda ER, Torgal AH, Westhoff CL,** Weight and body composition changes during oral contraceptive use in obese and normal weight women, J Womens Health (Larchmt) 23:38–43, 2014.

79. **Milsom I, Lete I, Bjertnaes A, Rokstad K, Lindh I, Gruber CJ, et al.,** Effects on cycle control and bodyweight of the combined contraceptive ring, NuvaRing, versus an oral contraceptive containing 30 microg ethinyl estradiol and 3 mg drospirenone, Hum Reprod 21:2304–2311, 2006.

80. **Burkman RT, Robinson JC, Kruszon-Moran D, Kimball AW, Kwiterovich P, Burford RG,** Lipid and lipoprotein changes associated with oral contraceptive use: a randomized clinical trial, Obstet Gynecol 71:33–38, 1988.

81. **Wahl P, Walden C, Knopp R, Hoover J, Wallace R, Heiss R, et al.,** Effect of estrogen/progestin potency on lipid/lipoprotein cholesterol, N Engl J Med 308:862, 1983.

82. **Tuppurainen M, Klimscheffskij R, Venhola M, Dieben TO,** The combined contraceptive vaginal ring (NuvaRing) and lipid metabolism: a comparative study, Contraception 69:389–394, 2004.

83. **Walsh BW, Sacks FM,** Effects of low dose oral contraceptives on very low density and low density lipoprotein metabolism, J Clin Invest 91:2126–2132, 1993.

84. **Adams MR, Clarkson TB, Koritnik DR, Nash HA,** Contraceptive steroids and coronary artery atherosclerosis in cynomolgus macaques, Fertil Steril 47:1010–1018, 1987.

85. **Clarkson TB, Adams MR, Kaplan JR, Shively CA, Koritnik DR,** From menarche to menopause: coronary artery atherosclerosis and protection in cynomolgus monkeys, Am J Obstet Gynecol 160:1280–1285, 1989.

86. **Clarkson TB, Shively CA, Morgan TM, Koritnik DR, Adams MR, Kaplan JR,** Oral contraceptives and coronary artery atherosclerosis of cynomolgus monkeys, Obstet Gynecol 75:217–222, 1990.

279

87. **Kushwaha R, Hazzard W,** Exogenous estrogens attenuate dietary hypercholesterolemia and atherosclerosis in the rabbit, Metabolism 30:57–66, 1981.

88. **Hough JL, Zilversmit DB,** Effect of 17 beta estradiol on aortic cholesterol content and metabolism in cholesterol-fed rabbits, Arteriosclerosis 6:57–63, 1986.

89. **Henriksson P, Stamberger M, Eriksson M, Rudling M, Diczfalusy U, Berglund L, et al.,** Oestrogen-induced changes in lipoprotein metabolism: role in prevention of atherosclerosis in the cholesterol-fed rabbit, Eur J Clin Invest 19:395–403, 1989.

90. **Croft P, Hannaford PC,** Risk factors for acute myocardial infarction in women: evidence from the Royal College of General Practitioners' oral contraception study, Br Med J 298:165–168, 1989.

91. **Colditz GA; the Nurses' Health Study Research Group,** Oral contraceptive use and mortality during 12 years of follow-up: the Nurses' Health Study, Ann Intern Med 120:821–826, 1994.

92. **Beasley A, Estes C, Guerrero J, Westhoff C,** The effect of obesity and low-dose oral contraceptives on carbohydrate and lipid metabolism, Contraception 85:446–452, 2012.

93. **Stampfer MJ, Willett WC, Colditz GA, Speizer FE, Hennekens CH,** Past use of oral contraceptives and cardiovascular disease: a meta-analysis in the context of the Nurses' Health Study, Am J Obstet Gynecol 163:285–291, 1990.

94. **Godsland IF, Crook D, Simpson R, Proudler T, Gelton C, Lees B, et al.,** The effects of different formulations of oral contraceptive agents on lipid and carbohydrate metabolism, N Engl J Med 323:1375–1381, 1990.

95. **Wynn V, Godsland I,** Effects of oral contraceptives on carbohydrate metabolism, J Reprod Med 31:892–897, 1986.

96. **Berenson AB, van den Berg P, Williams KJ, Rahman M,** Effect of injectable and oral contraceptives on glucose and insulin levels, Obstet Gynecol 117:41–47, 2011.

97. **Kim C, Siscovick DS, Sidney S, Lewis CE, Kiefe CI, Koepsell TD,** Oral contraceptive use and association with glucose, insulin, and diabetes in young adult women: the CARDIA Study. Coronary Artery Risk Development in Young Adults, Diabetes Care 25:1027–1032, 2002.

98. **Kjos SL, Peters RK, Xiang A, Thomas D, Schaefer U, Buchanan TA,** Contraception and the risk of type 2 diabetes mellitus in Latina women with prior gestational diabetes mellitus, JAMA 280:533–538, 1998.

99. **Korytkowski MT, Mokan M, Horwitz MJ, Berga SL,** Metabolic effects of oral contraceptives in women with polycystic ovary syndrome, J Clin Endocrinol Metab 80:3327–3334, 1995.

100. **Brady WA, Kritz-Silverstein D, Barrett-Connor E, Morales AJ,** Prior oral contraceptive use is associated with higher blood pressure in older women, J Womens Health 7:221–227, 1998.

101. **Hannaford PC, Kay CR,** Oral contraceptives and diabetes mellitus, Br Med J 299:315, 1989.

102. **Rimm EB, Manson JE, Stampfer MJ, Colditz GA, Willett WC, Rosner B, et al.,** Oral contraceptive use and the risk of type 2 (non-insulin-dependent) diabetes mellitus in a large prospective study of women, Diabetologia 35:967–972, 1992.

103. **Duffy TJ, Ray R,** Oral contraceptive use: prospective follow-up of women with suspected glucose intolerance, Contraception 30:197, 1984.

104. **Chasan-Taber L, Colditz GA, Willett WC, Stampfer MJ, Hunter DJ, Colditz GA, et al.,** A prospective study of oral contraceptives and NIDDM among U.S. women, Diabetes Care 20:330–335, 1997.

105. **Kjos SL, Shoupe D, Douyan S, Friedman RL, Bernstein GS, Mestman JH, et al.,** Effect of low-dose oral contraceptives on carbohydrate and lipid metabolism in women with recent gestational diabetes: results of a controlled, randomized, prospective study, Am J Obstet Gynecol 163:1822, 1990.

106. **Skouby SO, Malsted-Pedersen L, Kuhl C, Bennet P,** Oral contraceptives in diabetic women: metabolic effects of compounds with different estrogen/progestogen profiles, Fertil Steril 46:858–864, 1986.

107. **Petersen KR, Skouby SO, Sidelmann J, Mølsted-Petersen L, Jespersen J,** Effects of contraceptive steroids on

cardiovascular risk factors in women with insulin-dependent diabetes mellitus, Am J Obstet Gynecol 171:400, 1994.

108. **Garg SK, Chase HP, Marshall G, Hoops SL, Holmes DL, Jackson WE,** Oral contraceptives and renal and retinal complications in young women with insulin-dependent diabetes mellitus, JAMA 271:1099, 1994.

109. **Klein BE, Klein R, Moss SE,** Mortality and hormone-related exposures in women with diabetes, Diabetes Care 22:248–252, 1999.

110. **Curtis KM, Tepper NK, Jatlaoui TC, Berry-Bibee E, Horton LG, Zapata LB, et al.,** U.S. Medical Eligibility Criteria for contraceptive use, 2016, MMWR Recomm Rep 65:1–103, 2016.

111. **Meade TW,** Oral contraceptives, clotting factors, and thrombosis, Am J Obstet Gynecol 142:758–761, 1982.

112. **The Oral Contraceptive and Hemostasis Study Group,** The effect of seven monophasic oral contraceptive regimens on hemostatic variables: conclusions from a large randomized multicenter study, Contraception 67:173–185, 2003.

113. **Westhoff CL, Pike MC, Cremers S, Eisenberger A, Thomassen S, Rosing J,** Endogenous thrombin potential changes during the first cycle of oral contraceptive use, Contraception 95:456–463, 2017.

114. **Jespersen J, Petersen KR, Skouby SO,** Effects of newer oral contraceptives on the inhibition of coagulation and fibrinolysis in relation to dosage and type of steroid, Am J Obstet Gynecol 163:396–403, 1990.

115. **Notelovitz M, Kitchens CS, Khan FY,** Changes in coagulation and anticoagulation in women taking low-dose triphasic oral contraceptives: a controlled comparative 12-month clinical trial, Am J Obstet Gynecol 167:1255–1261, 1992.

116. **Schlit AF, Grandjean P, Donnez J, Lavenne E,** Large increase in plasmatic 11-dehydro-TXB$_2$ levels due to oral contraceptives, Contraception 51:53–58, 1995.

117. **Wiegratz I, Stahlberg S, Mantehy T, Sänger N, Mittmann K, Lange E, et al.,** Effects of conventional or extended-cycle regimen of an oral contraceptive containing 30 mcg ethinylestradiol and 2 mg dienogest on various hemostasis parameters, Contraception 78:384–391, 2008.

118. **van Vliet HA, Bertina RM, Dahm AE, Rosendaal FR, Rosing J, Sandset PM, et al.,** Different effects of oral contraceptives containing different progestogens on protein S and tissue factor pathway inhibitor, J Thromb Haemost 6:346–351, 2008.

119. **Farris M, Bastianelli C, Rosato E, Brosens I, Benagiano G,** Pharmacodynamics of combined estrogen-progestin oral contraceptives: 2. Effects on hemostasis, Expert Rev Clin Pharmacol 10:1129–1144, 2017.

120. **Fruzzetti F, Cagnacci A,** Venous thrombosis and hormonal contraception: what's new with estradiol-based hormonal contraceptives? Open Access J Contracept 9:75–79, 2018.

121. An open label, randomized study to evaluate the effects of seven monophasic oral contraceptive regimens on hemostatic variables. Outline of the protocol. Oral Contraceptive and Hemostasis Study Group, Contraception 59:345–355, 1999.

122. **Stanczyk FZ, Mathews BW, Cortessis VK,** Does the type of progestin influence the production of clotting factors? Contraception 95:113–116, 2017.

123. **Rosing J, Tans G, Nicolaes GA, Thomassen MC, van Oerle R, van der Ploeg PM, et al.,** Oral contraceptives and venous thrombosis: different sensitivities to activated protein C in women using second- and third-generation oral contraceptives, Br J Haematol 97:233–238, 1997.

124. **Segers O, van Oerle R, ten Cate H, Rosing J, Castoldi E,** Thrombin generation as an intermediate phenotype for venous thrombosis, Thromb Haemost 103:114–122, 2010.

125. **Tans G, van Hylckama Vlieg A, Thomassen MC, Curvers J, Bertina RM, Rosing J, et al.,** Activated protein C resistance determined with a thrombin generation-based test predicts for venous thrombosis in men and women, Br J Haematol 122:465–470, 2003.

126. **Kluft C, Zimmerman Y, Mawet M, Klipping C, Duijkers IJ, Neuteboom J,**

et al., Reduced hemostatic effects with drospirenone-based oral contraceptives containing estetrol vs. ethinyl estradiol, Contraception 95:140–147, 2017.

127. Fleischer K, van Vliet HA, Rosendaal FR, Rosing J, Tchaikovski S, Helmerhorst FM, Effects of the contraceptive patch, the vaginal ring and an oral contraceptive on APC resistance and SHBG: a cross-over study, Thromb Res 123:429–435, 2009.

128. Johnson JV, Lowell J, Badger GJ, Rosing J, Tchaikovski S, Cushman M, Effects of oral and transdermal hormonal contraception on vascular risk markers: a randomized controlled trial, Obstet Gynecol 111:278–284, 2008.

129. United Nations Development Programme/United Nations Population Fund/World Health Organization/World Bank Special Programme of Research, Development, Research Training in Human Reproduction, Task Force on Long-acting Systemic Agents for Fertility Regulation, Comparative study of the effects of two once-a-month injectable contraceptives (Cyclofem and Mesigyna) and one oral contraceptive (Ortho-Novum 1/35) on coagulation and fibrinolysis, Contraception 68:159–176, 2003.

130. Böttiger LE, Boman G, Eklund G, Westerholm B, Oral contraceptives and thromboembolic disease: effects of lowering oestrogen content, Lancet i:1097–1101, 1980.

131. Gerstman BB, Piper JM, Tomita DK, Ferguson WJ, Stadel BV, Lundin FE, Oral contraceptive estrogen dose and the risk of deep venous thromboembolic disease, Am J Epidemiol 133:32–37, 1991.

132. Vessey M, Mant D, Smith A, Yeates D, Oral contraceptives and venous thromboembolism: findings in a large prospective study, Br Med J 292:526, 1986.

133. Helmrich SP, Rosenberg L, Kaufman DW, Strom B, Shapiro S, Venous thromboembolism in relation to oral contraceptive use, Obstet Gynecol 69:91–95, 1987.

134. Thorogood M, Mann J, Murphy M, Vessey M, Risk factors for fatal venous thromboembolism in young women: a case-control study, Int J Epidemiol 21:48–52, 1992.

135. Oral contraceptives, venous thrombosis, and varicose veins. Royal College of General Practitioners' Oral Contraception Study, J R Coll Gen Pract 28:393–399, 1978.

136. Rosenberg L, Hennekens CH, Rosner B, Belanger C, Rothman KH, Speizer FE, Oral contraceptive use in relation to nonfatal myocardial infarction, Am J Epidemiol 11:59–66, 1980.

137. Incidence of arterial disease among oral contraceptive users. Royal College of General Practitioners' Oral Contraceptive Study, J R Coll Gen Pract 33:75–82, 1983.

138. Lidegaard Ø, Oral contraception and risk of a cerebral thromboembolic attack: results of a case-control study, Br Med J 306:956–963, 1993.

139. Lawson DH, Davidson JF, Jick H, Oral contraceptive use and venous thromboembolism: absence of an effect of smoking, Br Med J 2:729–730, 1977.

140. Petitti DB, Wingerd J, Pellegrin F, Ramcharan S, Oral contraceptives, smoking, and other factors in relation to risk of venous thromboembolic disease, Am J Epidemiol 108:480–485, 1978.

141. Porter JB, Hershel J, Walker AM, Mortality among oral contraceptive users, Obstet Gynecol 70:29–32, 1987.

142. Jick H, Jick SS, Gurewich V, Myers MW, Vasilakis C, Risk of idiopathic cardiovascular death and nonfatal venous thromboembolism in women using oral contraceptives with differing progestagen components, Lancet 348:1589–1593, 1995.

143. Lidegaard Ø, Lokkegaard E, Svendsen AL, Agger C, Hormonal contraception and risk of venous thromboembolism: national follow-up study, Br Med J 339:b2890, 2009. doi:10.1136/bmj.b2890.

144. Lidegaard Ø, Nielsen LH, Skovlund CW, Skjeldestad FE, Lokkegaard E, Risk of venous thromboembolism from use of oral contraceptives containing different progestogens and oestrogen doses: Danish cohort study, 2001–9, BMJ 343:d6423, 2011.

145. WHO Collaborative Study of Cardiovascular Disease and Steroid Hormone Contraception, Venous thromboembolic disease and combined oral contraceptives: results of

international multicentre case-control study, Lancet 346:1575–1582, 1995.

146. **Spitzer WO, Lewis MA, Heinemann LAJ, Thorogood M, MacRae KD; on behalf of the Transnational Research Group on Oral Contraceptives and the Health of Young Women,** Third generation oral contraceptives and risk of venous thromboembolic disorders: an international case-control study, Br Med J 312:83–88, 1996.

147. **van Hylckama Vlieg A, Helmerhorst FM, Vandenbroucke JP, Doggen CJ, Rosendaal FR,** The venous thrombotic risk of oral contraceptives, effects of oestrogen dose and progestogen type: results of the MEGA case-control study, BMJ 339:b2921, 2009.

148. **Dinger J, Do Minh T, Heinemann K,** Impact of estrogen type on cardiovascular safety of combined oral contraceptives, Contraception 94:328–339, 2016.

149. **WHO Collaborative Study of Cardiovascular Disease and Steroid Hormone Contraception,** Effect of different progestagens in low oestrogen oral contraceptives on venous thromboembolic disease, Lancet 346:1582–1588, 1995.

150. **Lidegaard Ø, Edström B, Kreiner S,** Oral contraceptives and venous thromboembolism. A case-control study, Contraception 5:291–301, 1998.

151. **Lidegaard O, Edstrom B, Kreiner S,** Oral contraceptives and venous thromboembolism: a five-year national case-control study, Contraception 65:187–196, 2002.

152. **Farmer RDT, Lawrenson RA, Thompson CR, Kennedy JG, Hambleton IR,** Population-based study of risk of venous thromboembolism associated with various oral contraceptives, Lancet 349:83–88, 1997.

153. **Farmer RDT, Lawrenson RA, Todd JC, Williams TJ, MacRae KD, Tyrer F, et al.,** A comparison of the risks of venous thromboembolic disease in association with different combined oral contraceptives, Br J Clin Pharmacol 49:580–590, 2000.

154. **Farmer RDT, Todd J-C, Lewis MA, MacRae KD, Williams TJ,** The risks of venous thromboembolic disease among German women using oral contraceptives: a database study, Contraception 57:67–70, 1998.

155. **Farmer RDT, Williams TJ, Simpson EL, Nightingale AL,** Effect of 1995 pill scare on rates of venous thromboembolism among women taking combined oral contraceptives: analysis of General Practice Research Database, Br Med J 321:477–478, 2000.

156. **Suissa S, Blais L, Spitzer WO, Cusson J, Lewis M, Heinemann L,** First-time use of newer oral contraceptives and the risk of venous thromboembolism, Contraception 56:141–146, 1997.

157. **Todd J, Lawrenson R, Farmer RD, Williams TJ, Leydon GM,** Venous thromboembolic disease and combined oral contraceptives: a re-analysis of the MediPlus database, Hum Reprod 14:1500–1505, 1999.

158. **Heinemann LAJ, Lewis MA, Assmann A, Thiel C,** Case-control studies on venous thromboembolism: bias due to design? A methodological study on venous thromboembolism and steroid hormone use, Contraception 65:207–214, 2002.

159. **Heinemann LAJ, Lewis MA, Assman A, Gravens L, Guggenmoos-Holzmann I,** Could preferential prescribing and referral behaviour of physicians explain the elevated thrombosis risk found to be associated with third generation oral contraceptives?, Pharmacoepidemiol Drug Saf 5:285–294, 1996.

160. **Jamin C, de Mouzon J,** Selective prescribing of third generation oral contraceptives (OCs), Contraception 54:55–56, 1996.

161. **Van Lunsen WH,** Recent oral contraceptive use patterns in four European countries: evidence for selective prescribing of oral contraceptives containing third generation progestogens, Eur J Contracept Reprod Health 1:39–45, 1996.

162. **Lewis MA, Heinemann LAJ, MacRae KD, Bruppacher R, Spitzer WO,** The increased risk of venous thromboembolism and the use of third generation progestagens: role of bias in observational research, Contraception 54:5–13, 1996.

163. **Sheldon T,** Dutch GPs warned against new contraceptive pill, Br Med J 324:869, 2002.

283

164. **Pearce HM, Layton D, Wilton LV, Shakir SA,** Deep vein thrombosis and pulmonary embolism reported in the Prescription Event Monitoring Study of Yasmin, Br J Clin Pharmacol 60:98–102, 2005.

165. **Dinger JC, Heinemann LA, Kuhl-Habich D,** The safety of a drospirenone-containing oral contraceptive: final results from the European Active Surveillance Study on oral contraceptives based on 142,475 women-years of observation, Contraception 75:344–354, 2007.

166. **Seeger JD, Loughlin J, Eng PM, Clifford CR, Cutone J, Walker AM,** Risk of thromboembolism in women taking ethinylestradiol/drospirenone and other oral contraceptives, Obstet Gynecol 110:587–593, 2007.

167. **Dinger J, Bardenheuer K, Heinemann K,** Cardiovascular and general safety of a 24-day regimen of drospirenone-containing combined oral contraceptives: final results from the International Active Surveillance Study of Women Taking Oral Contraceptives, Contraception 89:253–263, 2014.

168. **Dinger J, Mohner S, Heinemann K,** Cardiovascular risk associated with the use of an etonogestrel-containing vaginal ring, Obstet Gynecol 122:800–808, 2013.

169. **Tepper NK, Curtis KM, Jatlaoui TC, Whiteman MK,** Removing barriers to contraception through use of criteria to assess pregnancy risk, Contraception 95:323–325, 2017.

170. **Heinemann LA, Dinger JC,** Range of published estimates of venous thromboembolism incidence in young women, Contraception 75:328–336, 2007.

171. **Pomp ER, le Cessie S, Rosendaal FR, Doggen CJ,** Risk of venous thrombosis: obesity and its joint effect with oral contraceptive use and prothrombotic mutations, Br J Haematol 139:289–296, 2007.

172. **Ridker PM, Miletich JP, Hennekens CH, Buring JE,** Ethnic distribution of factor V Leiden in 4047 men and women: implications for venous thromboembolism screening, JAMA 277:1305–1307, 1997.

173. **Hajjar KA,** Factor V Leiden: an unselfish gene?, N Engl J Med 331:1585–1587, 1994.

174. **Vensson PJ, Dahlbäck B,** Resistance to activated protein C as a basis for venous thrombosis, N Engl J Med 330:517–522, 1994.

175. **Hellgren M, Svensson PJ, Dahlbäck B,** Resistance to activated protein C as a basis for venous thromboembolism associated with pregnancy and oral contraceptives, Am J Obstet Gynecol 173:210–213, 1995.

176. **Vandenbroucke JP, Koster T, Briet E, Reitsma PH, Bertina RM, Rosendaal FR,** Increased risk of venous thrombosis in oral-contraceptive users who are carriers of factor V Leiden mutation, Lancet 344:1453–1457, 1994.

177. **Spannagl M, Heinemann AJ, Schramm W,** Are factor V Leiden carriers who use oral contraceptives at extreme risk for venous thromboembolism?, Eur J Contracept Reprod Health Care 5:105–112, 2000.

178. **Bloemenkamp KW, Rosendaal FR, Helmerhorst FM, Vandenbroucke JP,** Higher risk of venous thrombosis during early use of oral contraceptives in women with inherited clotting defects, Arch Intern Med 160:49–52, 2000.

179. **Reich LM, Bower M, Key NS,** Role of the geneticist in testing and counseling for inherited thrombophilia, Genet Med 5:133–143, 2003.

180. **Kovacs L, Bartfai G, Apro G, Annus J, Bulpitt C, Belsey E, et al.,** The effect of the contraceptive pill on blood pressure: a randomized controlled trial of three progestogen-oestrogen combinations in Szeged, Hungary, Contraception 33:69–77, 1986.

181. **Nichols M, Robinson G, Bounds W, Newman B, Guillebaud J,** Effect of four combined oral contraceptives on blood pressure in the pill-free interval, Contraception 47:367, 1993.

182. **Qifang S, Deliang L, Ziurong J, Haifang L, Zhongshu Z,** Blood pressure changes and hormonal contraceptives, Contraception 50:131, 1994.

183. **Darney P,** Safety and efficacy of a triphasic oral contraceptive containing desogestrel: results of three multicenter trials, Contraception 48:323, 1993.

184. Chasan-Taber L, Willett WC, Manson JE, Spiegelman D, Hunter DJ, Curhan G, et al., Prospective study of oral contraceptives and hypertension among women in the United States, Circulation 94:483–489, 1996.

185. WHO Collaborative Study of Cardiovascular Disease and Steroid Hormone Contraception, Acute myocardial infarction and combined oral contraceptives: results of an international multicentre case-control study, Lancet 349:1202–1209, 1997.

186. WHO Collaborative Study of Cardiovascular Disease and Steroid Hormone Contraception, Ischaemic stroke and combined oral contraceptives: results of an international, multicentre case-control study, Lancet 348:498–505, 1996.

187. WHO Collaborative Study of Cardiovascular Disease and Steroid Hormone Contraception, Haemorrhagic stroke, overall stroke risk, and combined oral contraceptives: results of an international, multicentre, case-control study, Lancet 348:505–510, 1996.

188. Lubianca JN, Faccin CS, Fuchs FD, Oral contraceptives: a risk factor for uncontrolled blood pressure among hypertensive women, Contraception 67:19–24, 2003.

189. Lidegaard Ø, Kreiner S, Cerebral thrombosis and oral contraceptives. A case-control study, Contraception 57:303–314, 1998.

190. Lidegaard Ø, Edström B, Oral contraceptives and myocardial infarction. A case-control study (abstract), Eur J Contracept Reprod Health Care 1:72–73, 1996.

191. Petitti DB, Sidney S, Quesenberry CP Jr, Bernstein A, Incidence of stroke and myocardial infarction in women of reproductive age, Stroke 28:280–283, 1997.

192. Sidney S, Petitti DB, Quesenberry CP, Klatsky AL, Ziel HK, Wolf S, Myocardial infarction in users of low-dose oral contraceptives, Obstet Gynecol 88:939–944, 1996.

193. Lewis MA, Heinemann LAJ, Spitzer WO, MacRae KD, Bruppacher R; for the Transnational Research Group on Oral Contraceptives and the Health of Young Women, The use of oral contraceptives and the occurrence of acute myocardial infarction in young women. Results from the Transnational Study on Oral Contraceptives and the Health of Young Women, Contraception 56:129–140, 1997.

194. Lewis MA, Spitzer WO, Heinemann LAJ, MacRae KD, Bruppacher R, Lowered risk of dying of heart attack with third generation pill may offset risk of dying of thromboembolism, Br Med J 315:679–680, 1997.

195. Dunn N, Thorogood M, Garagher B, de Caestecker L, MacDonald TM, McCollum C, et al., Oral contraceptives and myocardial infarction: results of the MICA case-control study, Br Med J 318:1579–1583, 1999.

196. Rosenberg L, Palmer JR, Rao RS, Shapiro S, Low-dose contraceptive use and the risk of myocardial infarction, Arch Intern Med 161:1065–1070, 2001.

197. Tanis BC, van den Bosch MA, Kemmeren JM, Cats VM, Helmerhorst FM, Algra A, et al., Oral contraceptives and the risk of myocardial infarction, N Engl J Med 345:1787–1793, 2001.

198. Edgren RA, Progestagens, In: Givens J, ed. Clinical Uses of Steroids, Yearbook, Chicago, 1980, pp 1–29.

199. Basdevant A, Conard J, Pelissier C, Guyene T-T, Lapousterle C, Mayer M, et al., Hemostatic and metabolic effects of lowering the ethinyl-estradiol dose from 30 mcg to 20 mcg in oral contraceptives containing desogestrel, Contraception 48:193–204, 1993.

200. Winkler UH, Schindler AE, Endrikat J, Düsterberg B, A comparative study of the effects of the hemostatic system of two monophasic gestodene oral contraceptives containing 20 mg and 30 mg ethinylestradiol, Contraception 53:75–84, 1996.

201. Jick H, Porter J, Rothman KJ, Oral contraceptives and nonfatal stroke in healthy young women, Ann Intern Med 89:58–60, 1978.

202. Vessey MP, Lawless M, Yeates D, Oral contraceptives and stroke: findings in a large prospective study, Br Med J 289:530, 1984.

203. Hannaford PC, Croft PR, Kay CR, Oral contraception and stroke: evidence

from the Royal College of General Practitioners' Oral Contraception Study, Stroke 25:935–942, 1994.

204. **Petitti DB, Sidney S, Bernstein A, Wolf S, Quesenberry C, Ziel HK,** Stroke in users of low-dose oral contraceptives, N Engl J Med 335:8–15, 1996.

205. **Schwartz SM, Siscovick DS, Longstreth WT Jr, Psaty BM, Beverly RK, Raghunathan TE, et al.,** Use of low-dose oral contraceptives and stroke in young women, Ann Intern Med 127:596–603, 1997.

206. **Schwartz SM, Petitti DB, Siscovick DS, Longstreth NT Jr, Sidney S, Raghunathan TE, et al.,** Stroke and use of low-dose oral contraceptives in young women: a pooled analysis of two US studies, Stroke 29:2277–2284, 1998.

207. **Heinemann LAJ, Lewis MA, Spitzer WO, Thorogood M, Guggenmoos-Holzmann I, Bruppacher R, et al.,** Thromboembolic stroke in young women. A European case-control study on oral contraceptives, Contraception 57:29–37, 1998.

208. **Lidegaard Ø, Kreiner S,** Contraceptives and cerebral thrombosis: a five-year national case-control study, Contraception 65:197–205, 2002.

209. **Lipton RB, Vigal ME, Diamond MP, Freitag F, Reed ML, Stewart WF,** Migraine prevalence, disease burden, and the need for preventive therapy, Neurology 68:343–349, 2007.

210. **Tietjen GE,** The relationship of migraine and stroke, Neuroepidemiology 19:13–19, 2000.

211. **Chang CL, Donaghy M, Poulter N,** Migraine and stroke in young women: case-control study, Br Med J 318:13, 1999.

212. **Donaghy M, Chang CL, Poulter N,** Duration, frequency, recency, and type of migraine and the risk of ischaemic stroke in women of childbearing age, J Neurol Neurosurg Psychiatry 73:747–750, 2002.

213. **Tzourio C, Tehindrazanarierelo A, Iglésias S, Alpérovitch A, Chgedru F, d'Anglejan-Chatillon J, et al.,** Case-control study of migraine and risk of ischaemic stroke in young women, Br Med J 310:830, 1995.

214. **Lidegaard Ø,** Oral contraceptives, pregnancy and the risk of cerebral thromboembolism: the influence of diabetes, hypertension, migraine and previous thrombotic disease, Br J Obstet Gynaecol 102:153, 1995.

215. **Curtis KM, Chrisman CE, Peterson HB,** Contraception for women in selected circumstances, Obstet Gynecol 99:1100–1112, 2002.

216. **MacClellan LR, Giles W, Cole J, Wozniak M, Stern B, Mitchell BD, et al.,** Probable migraine with visual aura and risk of ischemic strone: the stroke prevention in young women study, Stroke 38:2438–2445, 2007.

217. **Vessey M, Painter R, Yeates D,** Mortality in relation to oral contraceptive use and cigarette smoking, Lancet 362:185–191, 2003.

218. **Martinelli I, Sacchi E, Landi G, Taioli E, Duca F, Mannucci PM,** High risk of cerebral-vein thrombosis in carriers of a prothrombin-gene mutation and in users of oral contraceptives, N Engl J Med 338:1793–1797, 1998.

219. **de Bruijn SFTM, Stam J, Koopman MMW, Vandenbroucke JP; for the Cerebral Venous Sinus Thrombosis Study Group,** Case-control study of risk of cerebral sinus thrombosis in oral contraceptive users who are carriers of hereditary prothrombotic conditions, Br Med J 316:589–592, 1998.

220. **Cosmi B, Legnani C, Bernardi F, Coccheri S, Palareti G,** Role of family history in identifying women with thrombophilia and higher risk of venous thromboembolism during oral contraception, Arch Intern Med 163:1105–1109, 2003.

221. **Baglin T, Luddington R, Brown K, Baglin C,** Incidence of recurrent venous thromboembolism in relation to clinical and thrombophilic risk factors: prospective cohort study, Lancet 362:523–526, 2003.

222. **Pabinger I, Schneider B; for the GTH Study Group,** Thrombotic risk of women with hereditary antithrombin III, protein C, and protein S deficiency taking oral contraceptive medication, Thromb Haemost 5:548–552, 1994.

223. **Beral V, Hermon C, Kay C, Hannaford P, Darby S, Reeves G,** Mortality associated with oral contraceptive use: 25-year follow-up of cohort of 46,000

women from Royal College of General Practitioners' oral contraception study, Br Med J 318:96–100, 1999.

224. **Brinton LA, Vessey MP, Flavel R, Yeates D,** Risk factors for benign breast disease, Am J Epidemiol 113:203–214, 1981.

225. **Franceschi S, La Vecchia C, Parazzini F, Fasoli M, Regallo M, Decarli A, et al.,** Oral contraceptives and benign breast disease: a case-control study, Am J Obstet Gynecol 1984;149:602–606.

226. **Rohan TE, L'Abbe KA, Cook MG,** Oral contraceptives and risk of benign proliferative epithelial disorders of the breast, Int J Cancer 50:891–894, 1992.

227. **Vessey M, Yeates D,** Oral contraceptives and benign breast disease: an update of findings in a large cohort study, Contraception 76:418–424, 2007.

228. **Charreau I, Plu-Bureau G, Bachelot A, Contesso G, Guinebretiere JM, L'e MG,** Oral contraceptive use and risk of benign breast disease in a French case-control study of young women, Eur J Cancer Prev 2:147–154, 1993.

229. **Rohan TE, Miller AB,** A cohort study of oral contraceptive use and risk of benign breast disease, Int J Cancer 82:191–196, 1999.

230. **Gill JK, Press MF, Patel AV, Bernstein L,** Oral contraceptive use and risk of breast carcinoma in situ (United States), Cancer Causes Control 17:1155–1162, 2006.

231. Further analyses of mortality in oral contraceptive users. Royal College of General Practitioners' Oral Contraceptive Study, Lancet 1:541, 1981.

232. **Vessey M, McPherson K, Villard-Mackintosh L, Yeates D,** Oral contraceptives and breast cancer: latest findings in a large cohort study, Br J Cancer 59:613, 1989.

233. **Vessey M, Baron J, Doll R, McPherson K, Yeates D,** Oral contraceptives and breast cancer: final report of an epidemiological study, Br J Cancer 47:455, 1982.

234. **Romieu I, Willett WC, Colditz GA, Stampfer MJ, Rosner B, Hennekens CH, et al.,** Prospective study of oral contraceptive use and risk of breast cancer in women, J Natl Cancer Inst 81:1313, 1989.

235. **Ramcharan S, Pellegrin FA, Ray RM, Hsu J-P,** The Walnut Creek Contraceptive Drug Study. A prospective study of the side effects of oral contraceptives, J Reprod Med 25:360, 1980.

236. **Nichols HB, Schoemaker MJ, Cai J, Xu J, Wright LB, Brook MN, et al.,** Breast cancer risk after recent childbirth: a pooled analysis of 15 prospective studies, Ann Intern Med 170:22–30, 2019.

237. **Lambe M, Hsieh C, Trichopoulos D, Ekbom A, Pavia M, Adami H-O,** Transient increase in the risk of breast cancer after giving birth, N Engl J Med 331:5–9, 1994.

238. **Collaborative Group on Hormonal Factors in Breast Cancer,** Breast cancer and hormonal contraceptives: collaborative reanalysis of individual data on 53,297 women with breast cancer and 100,239 women without breast cancer from 54 epidemiological studies, Lancet 347:1713–1727, 1996.

239. Breast cancer and hormonal contraceptives: further results. Collaborative Group on Hormonal Factors in Breast Cancer, Contraception 54:1S–106S, 1996.

240. **Kumle M, Weiderpass B, Braaten T, Persson I, Adami H-O, Lund E,** Use of oral contraceptives and breast cancer risk: the Norwegian-Swedish Women's Lifestyle and Health Cohort Study, Cancer Epidemiol Biomarkers Prev 11:1375–1381, 2002.

241. **Morch LS, Skovlund CW, Hannaford PC, Iversen L, Fielding S, Lidegaard O,** Contemporary hormonal contraception and the risk of breast cancer, N Engl J Med 377:2228–2239, 2017.

242. **Westhoff CL, Pike MC,** Hormonal contraception and breast cancer, Contraception 98:171–173, 2018.

243. **Guinee VF, Olsson H, Moller T, Hess KR, Taylor SH, Fahey T, et al.,** Effect of pregnancy on prognosis for young women with breast cancer, Lancet 343:1587, 1994.

244. **Kroman N, Wohlfart J, Andersen KW, Mouriudsen HT, Westergaard U, Melbye M,** Time since childbirth and prognosis in primary breast cancer: population based study, Br Med J 315:851–855, 1997.

245. **Rosenberg L, Palmer JR, Clarke EA, Shapiro S,** A case-control study of the

risk of breast cancer in relation to oral contraceptive use, Am J Epidemiol 136:1437–1444, 1992.

246. **Magnusson CM, Persson IR, Baron JA, Ekbom A, Bergström R, Adami H-O,** The role of reproductive factors and use of oral contraceptives in the aetiology of breast cancer in women aged 50 to 74 years, Int J Cancer 80:231–236, 1999.

247. **Marchbanks PA, McDonald JA, Wilson HG, Folger SG, Mandel MG, Daling JR, et al.,** Oral contraceptives and the risk of breast cancer, N Engl J Med 346:2025–2032, 2002.

248. **Milne RL, Knight JA, John EM, Dite GS, Balbuena R, Ziogas A, et al.,** Oral contraceptive use and risk of early-onset breast cancer in carriers and noncarriers of BRCA1 and BRCA2 mutations, Cancer Epidemiol Biomarkers Prev 14:350–356, 2005.

249. **Wingo PA, Austin H, Marchbanks PA, Whiteman MK, Hsia J, Mandel MG, et al.,** Oral contraceptives and the risk of death from breast cancer, Obstet Gynecol 110:793–800, 2007.

250. **Trivers KF, Gammon MD, Abrahamson PE, Lund MJ, Flagg EW, Moorman PG, et al.,** Oral contraceptives and survival in breast cancer patients aged 20 to 54 years, Cancer Epidemiol Biomarkers Prev 16:1822–1827, 2007.

251. **Grabrick DM, Hartmann LC, Cerhan JR, Vierkant RA, Therneau TM, Vachon CM, et al.,** Risk of breast cancer with oral contraceptive use in women with a family history of breast cancer, JAMA 284:1791–1798, 2000.

252. **Ursin G, Henderson BE, Haile RW, Pike MC, Zhou N, Diep A, et al.,** Does oral contraceptive use increase the risk of breast cancer in women with *BRCA1/ BRCA2* mutations more than in other women?, Cancer Res 57:3678–3681, 1997.

253. **Narod S, Dube MP, Klijn J, Lubinski J, Lynch HT, Ghadirian P, et al.,** Oral contraceptives and the risk of breast cancer in BRCA1 and BRCA2 mutation carriers, J Natl Cancer Inst 94:1773–1779, 2002.

254. **Haile RW, Thomas DC, McGuire V, Felberg A, John EM, Milne R, et al.,** BRCA1 and BRCA2 mutation carriers, oral contraceptive use, and breast

cancer before age 50, Cancer Epidemiol Biomarkers Prev 15:1863–1870, 2006.

255. **Brohet RM, Goldgar DE, Easton DF, Antonious AC, Andrieu N, Chang-Claude J, et al.,** Oral contraceptives and breast cancer risk in the international BRCA1/2 carrier cohort study: a report from EMBRACE, GENEPSO, GEO-HEBON, and the IBCCS Collaborating Group, J Clin Oncol 25:3831–3836, 2007.

256. **Lee E, Ma H, McKean-Cowdin R, Van Den Berg D, Bernstein L, Henderson BE, et al.,** Effect of reproductive factors and oral contraceptives on breast cancer risk in BRCA1/2 mutation carriers and noncarriers: results from a population based study, Cancer Epidemiol Biomarkers Prev 17:3170–3178, 2008.

257. **Figueiredo JC, Haile RW, Bernstein L, Malone KE, Largent J, Langholz B, et al.,** Oral contraceptives and postmenopausal hormones and risk of contralateral breast cancer among BRCA1 and BRCA2 mutation carriers and noncarriers: the WECARE Study, Breast Cancer Res Treat 120:175–183, 2010.

258. **Moorman PG, Havrilesky LJ, Gierisch JM, Coeytaux RR, Lowery WJ, Peragallo Urrutia R, et al.,** Oral contraceptives and risk of ovarian cancer and breast cancer among high-risk women: a systematic review and meta-analysis, J Clin Oncol 31:4188–4198, 2013.

259. **Cibula D, Zikan M, Dusek L, Majek O,** Oral contraceptives and risk of ovarian and breast cancers in BRCA mutation carriers: a meta-analysis, Expert Rev Anticancer Ther 11:1197–1207, 2011.

260. **Nyante SJ, Gammon MD, Malone KE, Daling JR, Brinton LA,** The association between oral contraceptive use and lobular and ductal breast cancer in young women, Int J Cancer 122:936–941, 2007.

261. **American Cancer Society,** Cancer Reference Information. http://www-cancerorg/docroot/CRI/content/CRI_2_4_2X_What_are_the_risk_factors_for_breast_cancer_5asp, 2009.

262. Combination oral contraceptive use and the risk of endometrial cancer. The Cancer and Steroid Hormone Study of the Centers for Disease Control and the National Institute of Child Health and Human Development, JAMA 257:796, 1987.

263. **Schlesselman JJ,** Risk of endometrial cancer in relation to use of combined oral contraceptives. A practitioner's guide to meta-analysis, Hum Reprod 12:1851–1863, 1997.

264. **Salazar-Martinez E, Lazcano-Ponce EC, Gonzalez Lira-Lira G, Escudero-De los Rios P, Salmeron-Castro J, Hernandez-Avila M,** Reproductive factors of ovarian and endometrial cancer risk in a high fertility population in Mexico, Cancer Res 59:3658–3662, 1999.

265. **Schlesselman JJ,** Oral contraceptives and neoplasia of the uterine corpus, Contraception 43:557, 1991.

266. **Vessey MP, Painte R,** Endometrial and ovarian cancer and oral contraceptives—findings in a large cohort study, Br J Cancer 71:1340, 1995.

267. **Weiderpass E, Adami HO, Baron JA, Magnusson C, Lindgren A, Persson I,** Use of oral contraceptives and endometrial cancer risk (Sweden), Cancer Causes Control 10:277–284, 1999.

268. **Jick SS, Walker AM, Jick H,** Oral contraceptives and endometrial cancer, Obstet Gynecol 82:931–935, 1993.

269. **Michels KA, Pfeiffer RM, Brinton LA, Trabert B,** Modification of the associations between duration of oral contraceptive use and ovarian, endometrial, breast, and colorectal cancers, JAMA Oncol 4:516–521, 2018.

270. **Sherman ME, Sturgeon S, Brinton LA, Potischman N, Kurman RJ, Berman ML, et al.,** Risk factors and hormone levels in patients with serous and endometrioid uterine carcinomas, Mod Pathol 10:963–968, 1997.

271. **Jamison PM, Noone AM, Ries LA, Lee NC, Edwards BK,** Trends in endometrial cancer incidence by race and histology with a correction for the prevalence of hysterectomy, SEER 1992 to 2008, Cancer Epidemiol Biomarkers Prev 22:233–241, 2013.

272. **Poole EM, Merritt MA, Jordan SJ, Yang HP, Hankinson SE, Park Y, et al.,** Hormonal and reproductive risk factors for epithelial ovarian cancer by tumor aggressiveness, Cancer Epidemiol Biomarkers Prev 22:429–437, 2013.

273. **Rasmussen ELK, Hannibal CG, Dehlendorff C, Baandrup L, Junge J, Vang R, et al.,** Parity, infertility, oral contraceptives, and hormone replacement therapy and the risk of ovarian serous borderline tumors: a nationwide case-control study, Gynecol Oncol 144:571–576, 2017.

274. **Mant JWF, Vessey MP,** Ovarian and endometrial cancers, Cancer Surv 19:287, 1994.

275. **Adami HO, Bergstrom R, Persson I, Sparen P,** The incidence of cancer in Sweden, 1960–1984, Am J Epidemiol 132:446–452, 1990.

276. **Silva IS, Swerdlow AJ,** Recent trends in incidence of and mortality from breast, ovarian and endometrial cancer in England and Wales and their relation to changing fertility and oral contraceptive use, Br J Cancer 72:485–492, 1995.

277. **Oriel KA, Hartenbach EM, Remington PL,** Trends in United States ovarian cancer mortality, 1979–1995, Obstet Gynecol 93:30–33, 1999.

278. **Lurie G, Thompson P, McDuffie KE, Carney ME, Terada KY, Goodman MT,** Association of estrogen and progestin potency of oral contraceptives with ovarian carcinoma risk, Obstet Gynecol 109:597–607, 2007.

279. **The Cancer and Steroid Hormone Study of the CDC and NICHD,** The reduction in risk of ovarian cancer associated with oral-contraceptive use, N Engl J Med 316:650, 1987.

280. **Hankinson SE, Colditz GA, Hunter DJ, Spencer TL, Rosner B, Stampfer MJ,** A quantitative assessment of oral contraceptive use and risk of ovarian cancer, Obstet Gynecol 80:708–714, 1992.

281. **Whittemore AS, Harris R, Itnyre J; the Collaborative Ovarian Cancer Group,** Characteristics relating to ovarian cancer risk: collaborative analysis of 12 US case-control studies. II: Invasive epithelial ovarian cancers in white women, Am J Epidemiol 136:1184–1203, 1992.

282. **Wittenberg L, Cook LS, Rossing MA, Weiss NS,** Reproductive risk factors for mucinous and non-mucinous epithelial ovarian cancer, Epidemiology 10:761–763, 1999.

283. **Ness RB, Grisso JA, Klapper J, Schlesselman JJ, Silberzweig S, Vergona R, et al.,** Risk of ovarian cancer in relation to estrogen and progestin dose and use characteristics of oral contraceptives, Am J Epidemiol 152:233–241, 2000.

289

284. **Royar J, Becher H, Chang-Claude J,** Low-dose oral contraceptives: protective effect on ovarian cancer risk, Int J Cancer 95:370–374, 2001.

285. **Collaborative Group on Epidemiological Studies of Ovarian Cancer; Beral V, Doll R, Hermon C, Peto R, Reeves G,** Ovarian cancer and oral contraceptives: collaborative reanalysis of data from 45 epidemiological studies including 23,257 women with ovarian cancer and 87,303 controls, Lancet 371:303–314, 2008.

286. **Tworoger SS, Fairfield KM, Colditz GA, Rosner BA, Hankinson SE,** Association of oral contraceptive use, other contraceptive methods, and infertility with ovarian cancer risk, Am J Epidemiol 166:894–901, 2007.

287. **Rosenberg L, Palmer JR, Zauber AG, Warshauer ME, Lewis JL Jr, Strom BL, et al.,** A case-control study of oral contraceptive use and invasive epithelial ovarian cancer, Am J Epidemiol 139:654–661, 1994.

288. **Shafrir AL, Schock H, Poole EM, Terry KL, Tamimi RM, Hankinson SE, et al.,** A prospective cohort study of oral contraceptive use and ovarian cancer among women in the United States born from 1947 to 1964, Cancer Causes Control 28:371–383, 2017.

289. **Gross TP, Schlesselman JJ,** The estimated effect of oral contraceptive use on the cumulative risk of epithelial ovarian cancer, Obstet Gynecol 83:419–424, 1994.

290. **Walker GR, Schlesselman J, Ness RB,** Family history of cancer, oral contraceptive use, and ovarian cancer risk, Am J Obstet Gynecol 186:8–14, 2002.

291. **Narod SA, Risch H, Moslehi R, Dørum A, Neuhausen S, Olsson H, et al.,** Oral contraceptives and the risk of hereditary ovarian cancer, N Engl J Med 339:424–428, 1998.

292. **Whittemore AS, Balise RR, Pharoah PD, Dicioccio RA, Oakley-Girvan I, Ramus SJ, et al.,** Oral contraceptive use and ovarian cancer risk among carriers of BRCA1 or BRCA2 mutations, Br J Cancer 91:1911–1915, 2004.

293. **McLaughlin JR, Risch HA, Lubinski J, Moller P, Ghadirian P, Lynch H, et al.,** Reproductive risk factors for ovarian cancer in carriers of BRCA1 or BRCA2 mutations: a case-control study, Lancet Oncol 8:26–34, 2007.

294. **Brinton LA,** Oral contraceptives and cervical neoplasia, Contraception 43:581–595, 1991.

295. **Delgado-Rodriguez M, Sillero-Arenas M, Martin-Moreno JM, Galvez-Vargas R,** Oral contraceptives and cancer of the cervix uteri. A meta-analysis, Acta Obstet Gynecol Scand 71:368–376, 1992.

296. **Gram IT, Macaluso M, Stalsberg H,** Oral contraceptive use and the incidence of cervical intraepithelial neoplasia, Am J Obstet Gynecol 167:40, 1992.

297. **Irwin KL, Rosero-Bixby L, Oberle MW, Lee NC, Whatley AS, Fortney JA, et al.,** Oral contraceptives and cervical cancer risk in Costa Rica: detection bias or causal association?, JAMA 259:59, 1988.

298. **Ye Z, Thomas DB, Ray RM; the WHO Collaborative Study of Neoplasia and Steroid Contraceptives,** Combined oral contraceptives and risk of cervical carcinoma in situ, Int J Epidemiol 24:19, 1995.

299. **Ylitalo N, Sorensen P, Josefsson A, Frisch M, Sparen P, Ponten J, et al.,** Smoking and oral contraceptives as risk factors for cervical carcinoma in situ, Int J Cancer 81:357–365, 1999.

300. **Adhikari I, Eriksson T, Luostarinen T, Lehtinen M, Apter D,** The risk of cervical atypia in oral contraceptive users, Eur J Contracept Reprod Health Care 23:12–17, 2018.

301. **Roura E, Travier N, Waterboer T, de Sanjose S, Bosch FX, Pawlita M, et al.,** The influence of hormonal factors on the risk of developing cervical cancer and pre-cancer: results from the EPIC Cohort. PLoS One 11:e0147029, 2016.

302. **Longatto-Filho A, Hammes LS, Sarian LO, Roteli-Martins C, Derchain SF, Erzen M, et al.,** Hormonal contraceptives and the length of their use are not independent risk factors for high-risk HPV infections or high-grade CIN, Gynecol Obstet Investig 71:93–103, 2011.

303. **Brinton LA, Reeves WC, Brenes MM, Herrero R, de Britton RC, Gaitan E, et al.,** Oral contraceptive use and risk of invasive cervical cancer, Int J Epidemiol 19:4–11, 1990.

290

304. Ursin G, Peters RK, Hendeson BE, d'Ablaing G III, Monroe KR, Pike MC, Oral contraceptive use and adenocarcinoma of cervix, Lancet 344:1390–1394, 1994.

305. Thomas DB, Ray RM; the World Health Organization Collaborative Study of Neoplasia and Steroid Contraceptives, Oral contraceptives and invasive adenocarcinomas and adenosquamous carcinomas of the uterine cervix, Am J Epidemiol 144:281–289, 1996.

306. Schwartz SM, Weiss NS, Increased incidence of adenocarcinoma of the cervix in young women in the United States, Am J Epidemiol 124:1045–1047, 1986.

307. Smith JS, Green J, de Gonzalez AB, Appleby P, Peto J, Plummer M, et al., Cervical cancer and use of hormonal contraceptives: a systematic review, Lancet 361:1159–1167, 2003.

308. Moreno V, Bosch FX, Muñoz N, Meijer CJLM, Shah KV, Walboomers JMM, et al., Effect of oral contraceptives on risk of cervical cancer in women with human papillomavirus infection: the IARC multicentric case-control study, Lancet 359:1085–1192, 2002.

309. International Collaboration of Epidemiological Studies of Cervical Cancer, Cervical cancer and hormonal contraceptives: collaborative reanalysis of individual data for 16,573 women with cervical cancer and 35,509 women without cervical cancer from 24 epidemiological studies, Lancet 370:1609–1621, 2007.

310. Martinez ME, Grodstein F, Giovannucci E, Colditz GA, Speizer FE, Hennekens C, et al., A prospective study of reproductive factors, oral contraceptive use, and risk of colorectal cancer, Cancer Epidemiol Biomarkers Prev 6:1–5, 1997.

311. Charlton BM, Wu K, Zhang X, Giovannucci EL, Fuchs CS, Missmer SA, et al., Oral contraceptive use and colorectal cancer in the Nurses' Health Study I and II, Cancer Epidemiol Biomarkers Prev 24:1214–1221, 2015.

312. Levi F, Pasche C, Lucchini F, La Vecchia C, Oral contraceptives and colorectal cancer, Dig Liver Dis 35:85–87, 2003.

313. Nichols HB, Trentham-Dietz A, Hampton JM, Newcomb PA, Oral contraceptive use, reproductive factors, and colorectal cancer risk: findings from Wisconsin, Cancer Epidemiol Biomarkers Prev 14:1212–1218, 2005.

314. Hannaford P, Elliott A, Use of exogenous hormones by women and colorectal cancer: evidence from the Royal College of General Practitioners' Oral Contraception Study, Contraception 71:95–98, 2005.

315. Fernandez E, La Vecchia C, Balducci A, Chatenoud L, Franceschi S, Negri E, Oral contraceptives and colorectal cancer risk: a meta-analysis, Br J Cancer 84:722–727, 2001.

316. Bosetti C, Bravi F, Negri E, La Vecchia C, Oral contraceptives and colorectal cancer risk: a systematic review and meta-analysis, Hum Reprod Update 15:489–498, 2009.

317. Luan NN, Wu L, Gong TT, Wang YL, Lin B, Wu QJ, Nonlinear reduction in risk for colorectal cancer by oral contraceptive use: a meta-analysis of epidemiological studies, Cancer Causes Control 26:65–78, 2015.

318. Neuberger J, Forman D, Doll R, Williams R, Oral contraceptives and hepatocellular carcinoma, Br Med J 292:1355, 1986.

319. Palmer JR, Rosenberg L, Kaufman DW, Warshauer ME, Stolley P, Shapiro S, Oral contraceptive use and liver cancer, Am J Epidemiol 130:878, 1989.

320. An N, Oral contraceptives use and liver cancer risk: a dose-response meta-analysis of observational studies, Medicine (Baltimore) 94:e1619, 2015.

321. Oral contraceptives and liver cancer. Results of the Multicentre International Liver Tumor Study (MILTS), Contraception 56:275–284, 1997.

322. Mant JWF, Vessey MP, Trends in mortality from primary liver cancer in England and Wales 1975–92: influence of oral contraceptives, Br J Cancer 72:800–803, 1995.

323. Waetjen LE, Grimes DA, Oral contraceptives and primary liver cancer: temporal trends in three countries, Obstet Gynecol 88:945–949, 1996.

324. El-Serag HB, Mason AC, Rising incidence of hepatocellular carcinoma in the

United States, N Engl J Med 340:745–750, 1999.

325. **Green A,** Oral contraceptives and skin neoplasia, Contraception 43:653–666, 1991.

326. **Hannaford PC, Villard-Mackintosh L, Vessey MP, Kay CR,** Oral contraceptives and malignant melanoma, Br J Cancer 63:430–433, 1991.

327. **Vessey MP, Painter R, Powell J,** Skin disorders in relation to oral contraception and other factors, including age, social class, smoking and body mass index. Findings in a large cohort study, Br J Dermatol 143:815–820, 2000.

328. **Cervenka I, Mahamat-Saleh Y, Savoye I, Dartois L, Boutron-Ruault MC, Fournier A, et al.,** Oral contraceptive use and cutaneous melanoma risk: a French prospective cohort study, Int J Cancer 143:2390–2399, 2018.

329. **Milne R, Vessey M,** The association of oral contraception with kidney cancer, colon cancer, gallbladder cancer (including extrahepatic bile duct cancer) and pituitary tumors, Contraception 43:667, 1991.

330. **Berkowitz RS, Bernstein MR, Harlow BL, Rice LW, Lage JM, Goldstein DP, et al.,** Case-control study of risk factors for partial molar pregnancy, Am J Obstet Gynecol 173:788, 1995.

331. **Palmer JR, Driscoll SG, Rosenberg L, Berkowitz RS, Lurain JR, Soper J, et al.,** Oral contraceptive use and risk of gestational trophoblastic tumors, J Natl Cancer Inst 91:635–640, 1999.

332. **Parazzini F, Cipriani S, Mangili G, Garavaglia E, Guarnerio P, Ricci E, et al.,** Oral contraceptives and risk of gestational trophoblastic disease, Contraception 65:425–427, 2002.

333. **Andersson G, Borgquist S, Jirstrom K,** Hormonal factors and pancreatic cancer risk in women: the Malmo Diet and Cancer Study, Int J Cancer 143:52–62, 2018.

334. **Horn-Ross PL, Morrow M, Ljung BM,** Menstrual and reproductive factors for salivary gland cancer risk in women, Epidemiology 10:528–530, 1999.

335. **Michels KA, Brinton LA, Pfeiffer RM, Trabert B,** Oral contraceptive use and risks of cancer in the NIH-AARP diet and health study, Am J Epidemiol 187:1630–1641, 2018.

336. **Iversen L, Sivasubramaniam S, Lee AJ, Fielding S, Hannaford PC,** Lifetime cancer risk and combined oral contraceptives: the Royal College of General Practitioners' Oral Contraception Study, Am J Obstet Gynecol 216:580.e1–580.e9, 2017.

337. **Vessey M, Yeates D,** Oral contraceptive use and cancer: final report from the Oxford-Family Planning Association contraceptive study, Contraception 88:678–683, 2013.

338. **Janerich DT, Dugan JM, Standfast SJ, Strite L,** Congenital heart disease and prenatal exposure to exogenous sex hormones, Br Med J 1:1058, 1977.

339. **Nora JJ, Nora AH, Blu J, Ingram J, Foster D,** Exogenous progestogen and estrogen implicated in birth defects, JAMA 240:837, 1978.

340. **Simpson JL, Phillips OP,** Spermicides, hormonal contraception and congenital malformations, Adv Contracept 6:141–167, 1990.

341. **Michaelis J, Michaelis H, Gluck E, Koller S,** Prospective study of suspected associations between certain drugs administered during early pregnancy and congenital malformations, Teratology 27:57, 1983.

342. **Bracken MB,** Oral contraception and congenital malformations in offspring: a review and meta-analysis of the prospective studies, Obstet Gynecol 76:552–557, 1990.

343. **Raman-Wilms L, Tseng AL, Wighardt S, Einarson TR, Koren G,** Fetal genital effects of first trimester sex hormone exposure: a meta-analysis, Obstet Gynecol 85:141–149, 1995.

344. **Ressequie LJ, Hick JF, Bruen JA, Noller KL, O'Fallon WM, Kurland LT,** Congenital malformations among offspring exposed in utero to progestins, Olsted County, Minnesota, 1936–1974, Fertil Steril 43:514, 1985.

345. **Katz Z, Lancet M, Skornik J, Chemke J, Mogilemer B, Klinberg M,** Teratogenicity of progestogens given during the first trimester of pregnancy, Obstet Gynecol 65:775, 1985.

346. **Vessey MP, Wright NH, McPherson K, Wiggins P,** Fertility after stopping different methods of contraception, Br Med J 1:265, 1978.

347. **Howe G, Westhoff C, Vessey M, Yeates D,** Effects of age, cigarette smoking, and other factors on fertility: findings in a large prospective study, Br Med J (Clin Res Ed) 290:1697–1700, 1985.

348. **Bagwell MA, Coker AL, Thompson SJ, Baker ER, Addy CL,** Primary infertility and oral contraceptive steroid use, Fertil Steril 63:1161, 1995.

349. **Farrow A, Hull MGR, Northstone K, Taylor H, Ford WCL, Golding J,** Prolonged use of oral contraception before a planned pregnancy is associated with a decreased risk of delayed conception, Hum Reprod 17:2754–2761, 2002.

350. **Cronin M, Schellschmidt I, Dinger J,** Rate of pregnancy after using drospirenone and other progestin-containing oral contraceptives, Obstet Gynecol 114:616–622, 2009.

351. **Girum T, Wasie A,** Return of fertility after discontinuation of contraception: a systematic review and meta-analysis, Contracept Reprod Med 3:9, 2018.

352. **Rothman KJ,** Fetal loss, twinning, and birth weight after oral-contraceptive use, N Engl J Med 297:468, 1977.

353. **Ford JH, MacCormac L,** Pregnancy and lifestyle study: the long-term use of the contraceptive pill and the risk of age-related miscarriage, Hum Reprod 10:1397–1402, 1995.

354. **Rothman KJ, Liess J,** Gender of offspring after oral-contraceptive use, N Engl J Med 295:859, 1976.

355. **Magidor S, Poalti H, Harlap S, Baras M,** Long-term follow-up of children whose mothers used oral contraceptives prior to contraception, Contraception 29:203, 1984.

356. **Vessey M, Doll R, Peto R, Johnson B, Wiggins P,** A long-term follow-up study of women using different methods of contraception—an interim report, J Biosoc Sci 8:373, 1976.

357. The outcome of pregnancy in former oral contraceptive users, Br J Obstet Gynaecol 83:608, 1976.

358. **Jensen JT, Parke S, Mellinger U, Machlitt A, Fraser IS,** Effective treatment of heavy menstrual bleeding with estradiol valerate and dienogest: a randomized controlled trial, Obstet Gynecol 117:777–787, 2011.

359. **Uhm S, Perriera L,** Hormonal contraception as treatment for heavy menstrual bleeding: a systematic review, Clin Obstet Gynecol 57:694–717, 2014.

360. **Milman N, Kirchhoff M, Jorgensen T,** Iron status markers, serum ferritin and hemoglobin in 1359 Danish women in relation to menstruation, hormonal contraception, parity, and postmenopausal hormone treatment, Ann Hematol 65:96–102, 1992.

361. **Galan P, Yoon HC, Preziosi P, Viteri P, Fieux B, Briancon S, et al.,** Determining factors in the iron status of adult women in the SU.VI.MAX study. SUpplementation en VItamines et Minéraux AntioXydants, Eur J Clin Nutr 52:383–388, 1998.

362. Effects of contraceptives on hemoglobin and ferritin. Task Force for Epidemiological Research on Reproductive Health, United Nations Development Programme/United Nations Population Fund/World Health Organization/World Bank Special Programme of Research, Development and Research Training in Human Reproduction, World Health Organization, Geneva, Switzerland, Contraception 58:261–273, 1998.

363. **Bellizzi S, Ali MM,** Effect of oral contraception on anemia in 12 low- and middle-income countries, Contraception 97:236–242, 2018.

364. **Robinson JC, Plichter S, Weisman CS, Nathanson CA, Ensminger M,** Dysmenorrhea and use of oral contraceptives in adolescent women attending a family planning clinic, Am J Obstet Gynecol 166:578–583, 1992.

365. **Davis AR, Westhoff C, O'Connell K, Gallagher N,** Oral contraceptives for dysmenorrhea in adolescent girls: a randomized trial, Obstet Gynecol 106:97–104, 2005.

366. **Lindh I, Ellstrom AA, Milsom I,** The effect of combined oral contraceptives and age on dysmenorrhoea: an epidemiological study, Hum Reprod 27:676–682, 2012.

367. **Harada T, Momoeda M,** Evaluation of an ultra-low-dose oral contraceptive for dysmenorrhea: a placebo-controlled, double-blind, randomized trial, Fertil Steril 106:1807–1814, 2016.

293

368. **Dmitrovic R, Kunselman AR, Legro RS,** Continuous compared with cyclic oral contraceptives for the treatment of primary dysmenorrhea: a randomized controlled trial, Obstet Gynecol 119:1143–1150, 2012.

369. **Edelman A, Micks E, Gallo MF, Jensen JT, Grimes DA,** Continuous or extended cycle vs. cyclic use of combined hormonal contraceptives for contraception, Cochrane Database Syst Rev (7):CD004695, 2014.

370. **Vercellini P, Frontino G, De Giorgi O, Pietropaolo G, Pasin R, Crosignani PG,** Continuous use of an oral contraceptive for endometriosis-associated recurrent dysmenorrhea that does not respond to a cyclic pill regimen, Fertil Steril 80:560–563, 2003.

371. **Harada T, Momoeda M, Taketani Y, Hoshiai H, Terakawa N,** Low-dose oral contraceptive pill for dysmenorrhea associated with endometriosis: a placebo-controlled, double-blind, randomized trial, Fertil Steril 90:1583–1588, 2008.

372. **Seracchioli R, Mabrouk M, Frascà C, Manuzzi L, Montanari G, Keramyda A, et al.,** Long-term cyclic and continuous oral contraceptive therapy and endometrioma recurrence: a randomized controlled trial, Fertil Steril 93:52–56, 2010.

373. **Mabrouk M, Frasca C, Geraci E, Montanari G, Ferrini G, Raimondo D, et al.,** Combined oral contraceptive therapy in women with posterior deep infiltrating endometriosis, J Minim Invasive Gynecol 18:470–474, 2011.

374. **Seracchioli R, Mabrouk M, Manuzzi L, Vicenzi C, Frasca C, Elmakky A, et al.,** Post-operative use of oral contraceptive pills for prevention of anatomical relapse or symptom-recurrence after conservative surgery for endometriosis, Hum Reprod 24:2729–2735, 2009.

375. **Brown J, Crawford TJ, Datta S, Prentice A,** Oral contraceptives for pain associated with endometriosis, Cochrane Database Syst Rev 5:Cd001019, 2018.

376. **Costello M, Shrestha B, Eden J, Sjoblom P, Johnson N,** Insulin-sensitising drugs versus the combined oral contraceptive pill for hirsutism, acne and risk of diabetes, cardiovascular disease, and endometrial cancer in polycystic ovary syndrome, Cochrane Database Syst Rev (1):CD005552, 2007.

377. **Al Khalifah RA, Florez ID, Dennis B, Thabane L, Bassilious E,** Metformin or oral contraceptives for adolescents with polycystic ovarian syndrome: a meta-analysis, Pediatrics 137, 2016.

378. **De Leo V, Di Sabatino A, Musacchio MC, Morgante G, Scolaro V, Cianci A, et al.,** Effect of oral contraceptives on markers of hyperandrogenism and SHBG in women with polycystic ovary syndrome, Contraception 82:276–280, 2010.

379. **Amiri M, Kabir A, Nahidi F, Shekofteh M, Ramezani Tehrani F,** Effects of combined oral contraceptives on the clinical and biochemical parameters of hyperandrogenism in patients with polycystic ovary syndrome: a systematic review and meta-analysis, Eur J Contracept Reprod Health Care 23:64–77, 2018.

380. **de Medeiros SF,** Risks, benefits size and clinical implications of combined oral contraceptive use in women with polycystic ovary syndrome, Reprod Biol Endocrinol 15:93, 2017.

381. **Battaglia C, Mancini F, Fabbri R, Persico N, Busacchi P, Facchinetti F, et al.,** Polycystic ovary syndrome and cardiovascular risk in young patients treated with drospirenone-ethinylestradiol or contraceptive vaginal ring. A prospective, randomized, pilot study, Fertil Steril 94:1417–1425, 2010.

382. **Amiri M, Ramezani Tehrani F, Nahidi F, Kabir A, Azizi F, Carmina E,** Effects of oral contraceptives on metabolic profile in women with polycystic ovary syndrome: a meta-analysis comparing products containing cyproterone acetate with third generation progestins, Metabolism 73:22–35, 2017.

383. **Vessey M, Metcalfe A, Wells C, McPherson K, Westhoff C, Yeates D,** Ovarian neoplasms, functional ovarian cysts, and oral contraceptives, Br Med J (Clin Res Ed) 294:1518–1520, 1987.

384. **Holt VL, Cushing-Haugen KL, Daling JR,** Oral contraceptives, tubal sterilization, and functional ovarian cyst risk, Obstet Gynecol 102:252–258, 2003.

385. **Lanes SF, Birmann B, Walker AM, Singer S,** Oral contraceptive type and functional ovarian cysts, Am J Obstet Gynecol 166:956–961, 1992.

386. **Holt VL, Daling JR, McKnight B, Moore D, Stergachis A, Weiss NS,** Functional ovarian cysts in relation to the use of monophasic and triphasic oral contraceptives, Obstet Gynecol 79:529–533, 1992.

387. **Young RL, Snabes MC, Frank ML, Reilly M,** A randomized, double-blind, placebo-controlled comparison of the impact of low-dose and triphasic oral contaceptives on follicular development, Am J Obstet Gynecol 167:678–682, 1992.

388. **Grimes DA, Godwin AJ, Rubin A, Smith JA, Lacarra M,** Ovulation and follicular development associated with three low-dose oral contraceptives: a randomized controlled trial, Obstet Gynecol 83:29–34, 1994.

389. **Grimes DA, Jones LB, Lopez LM, Schulz KF,** Oral contraceptives for functional ovarian cysts, Cochrane Database Syst Rev (4):CD006134, 2014.

390. **Westhoff C, Britton JA, Gammon MD, Wright T, Kelsey JL,** Oral contraceptive and benign ovarian tumors, Am J Epidemiol 152:242–246, 2000.

391. **Keyes KM, Cheslack-Postava K, Westhoff C, Heim CM, Haloossim M, Walsh K, et al.,** Association of hormonal contraceptive use with reduced levels of depressive symptoms: a national study of sexually active women in the United States, Am J Epidemiol 178:1378–1388, 2013.

392. **Schaffir J, Worly BL, Gur TL,** Combined hormonal contraception and its effects on mood: a critical review, Eur J Contracept Reprod Health Care 21:347–355, 2016.

393. **Zethraeus N, Dreber A, Ranehill E, Blomberg L, Labrie F, von Schoultz B, et al.,** A first-choice combined oral contraceptive influences general well-being in healthy women: a double-blind, randomized, placebo-controlled trial, Fertil Steril 107:1238–1245, 2017.

394. **Lundin C, Danielsson KG, Bixo M, Moby L, Bengtsdotter H, Jawad I, et al.,** Combined oral contraceptive use is associated with both improvement and worsening of mood in the different phases of the treatment cycle—a double-blind, placebo-controlled randomized trial, Psychoneuroendocrinology 76:135–143, 2017.

395. **Skovlund CW, Morch LS, Kessing LV, Lidegaard O,** Association of hormonal contraception with depression. JAMA Psychiatry 73:1154–1162, 2016.

396. **Skovlund CW, Morch LS, Kessing LV, Lange T, Lidegaard O,** Association of hormonal contraception with suicide attempts and suicides, Am J Psychiatry 175:336–342, 2018.

397. **McKetta S, Keyes KM,** Oral contraceptive use and depression among adolescents, Ann Epidemiol 29:46–51, 2019.

398. **Freeman EW, Halbreich U, Grubb GS, Rapkin AJ, Skouby SO, Smith L, et al.,** An overview of four studies of a continuous oral contraceptive (levonorgestrel 90 mcg/ethinyl estradiol 20 mcg) on premenstrual dysphoric disorder and premenstrual syndrome, Contraception 85:437–445, 2012.

399. **Lopez LM, Kaptein AA, Helmerhorst FM,** Oral contraceptives containing drospirenone for premenstrual syndrome, Cochrane Database Syst Rev (2):CD006586, 2012.

400. **Davis AR, Castaño PM,** Oral contraceptives and libido in women, Annu Rev Sex Res 15:297–320, 2004.

401. **Oranratanaphan S, Taneepanichskul S,** A double blind randomized control trial, comparing effect of drospirenone and gestodene to sexual desire and libido, J Med Assoc Thai 89:S17–S22, 2006.

402. **Greco T, Graham CA, Bancroft J, Tanner A, Doll HA,** The effects of oral contraceptives on androgen levels and their relevance to premenstrual mood and sexual interest: a comparison of two triphasic formulations containing norgestimate and either 35 or 25 ug of ethinyl estradiol, Contraception 76:8–17, 2007.

403. **Burrows LJ, Basha M, Goldstein AT,** The effects of hormonal contraceptives on female sexuality: a review, J Sex Med 9:2213–2223, 2012.

404. **Coelingh Bennink HJT, Zimmerman Y, Laan E, Termeer HMM, Appels N, Albert A, et al.,** Maintaining physiological testosterone levels by adding dehydroepiandrosterone to combined oral contraceptives: I. Endocrine effects, Contraception 96:322–329, 2017.

405. **Zimmerman Y, Foidart JM, Pintiaux A, Minon JM, Fauser BC, Cobey K,**

et al., Restoring testosterone levels by adding dehydroepiandrosterone to a drospirenone containing combined oral contraceptive: II. Clinical effects, Contraception 91:134–142, 2015.

406. **Ciaplinskiene L, Zilaitiene B, Verkauskiene R, Zalinkevicius R, Bumbuliene Z, Vanagiene V, et al.,** The effect of a drospirenone-containing combined oral contraceptive on female sexual function: a prospective randomised study, Eur J Contracept Reprod Health Care 21:395–400, 2016.

407. **van Lunsen RHW, Zimmerman Y, Coelingh Bennink HJT, Termeer HMM, Appels N, Fauser B, et al.,** Maintaining physiologic testosterone levels during combined oral contraceptives by adding dehydroepiandrosterone: II. Effects on sexual function. A phase II randomized, double-blind, placebo-controlled study, Contraception 98:56–62, 2018.

408. **Lucky AW, Henderson TA, Olson WH, Robisch DM, Lebwohl M, Swinyer LJ,** Effectiveness of norgestimate and ethinyl estradiol in treating moderate acne vulgaris, J Am Acad Dermatol 37:746–754, 1997.

409. **Redmond GP, Olson WH, Lippman JS, Kafrissen ME, Jones TM, Jorizzo JL,** Norgestimate and ethinyl estradiol in the treatment of acne vulgaris: a randomized, placebo-controlled trial, Obstet Gynecol 89:615–622, 1997.

410. **Thiboutot D, Archer DF, Lemay A, Washenik K, Roberts J, Harrison DD,** A randomized, controlled trial of a low-dose contraceptive containing 20 µg of ethinyl estradiol and 100 µg of levonorgestrel for acne treatment, Fertil Steril 76:461–468, 2001.

411. **Lemay A, Dewailly SD, Grenier R, Huard J,** Attenuation of mild hyperandrogenic activity in postpubertal acne by a triphasic oral contraceptive containing low doses of ethynyl estradiol and D,L-norgestrel, J Clin Endocrinol Metab 71:8, 1990.

412. **Mango D, Ricci S, Manna P, Miggiano GAD, Serra GB,** Clinical and hormonal effects of ethinyl estradiol combined with gestodene and desogestrel in young women with acne vulgaris, Contraception 53:163–170, 1996.

413. **Rosen MP, Breitkopf DM, Nagamani M,** A randomized controlled trial of second- versus third-generation oral contraceptives in the treatment of acne vulgaris, Am J Obstet Gynecol 188:1158–1160, 2003.

414. **Palombo-Kinne E, Schellschmidt I, Schumacher U, Gräser T,** Efficacy of a combined oral contraceptive containing 0.030 mg ethinylestradiol/2 mg dienogest for the treatment of papulopustular acne in comparison with placebo and 0.035 mg ethinylestradiol/2 mg cyproterone acetate, Contraception 79:282–289, 2009.

415. **Arowojolu AO, Gallo MF, Lopez LM, Grimes DA,** Combined oral contraceptive pills for treatment of acne, Cochrane Database Syst Rev (7), 2012.

416. **Koo EB, Petersen TD, Kimball AB,** Meta-analysis comparing efficacy of antibiotics versus oral contraceptives in acne vulgaris, J Am Acad Dermatol 71:450–459, 2014.

417. **Torok HM,** A comprehensive review of the long-term and short-term treatment of melasma with a triple combination cream, Am J Clin Dermatol 7:223–230, 2006.

418. **Hannaford PC, Kay CR, Vessey MP, Painter R, Mant J,** Combined oral contraceptives and liver disease, Contraception 55:145–151, 1997.

419. **Heinemann LA, Weimann A, Gerken G, Thiel C, Schlaud M, Do Minh T,** Modern oral contraceptive use and benign liver tumors: the German Benign Liver Tumor Case-Control Study, Eur J Contracept Reprod Health Care 3:194–200, 1998.

420. **Cherqui D, Rahmouni A, Charlotte F, Boulahdour H, Metreau JM, Meignan M, et al.,** Management of focal nodular hyperplasia and hepatocellular adenoma in young women: a series of 41 patients with clinical radiological and pathological correlations, Hepatology 22:1674–1681, 1995.

421. **Côté C,** Regression of focal nodular hyperplasia of the liver after oral contraceptive discontinuation, Clin Nucl Med 9:587–590, 1997.

422. Oral contraceptives and gallbladder disease. Royal College of General Practitioners' Oral Contraception Study, Lancet 2:957, 1982.

423. Grodstein F, Colditz GA, Hunter DJ, Manson JE, Willett WC, Stampfer MJ, A prospective study of symptomatic gallstones in women: relation with oral contraceptives and other risk factors, Obstet Gynecol 84:207, 1994.

424. La Vecchia C, Negri E, D'Avanzo B, Parazzini F, Genitle A, Franceschi S, Oral contraceptives and noncontraceptive oestrogens in the risk of gallstone disease requiring surgery, J Epidemiol Community Health 46:234–236, 1992.

425. Vessey M, Painter R, Oral contraceptive use and benign gallbladder disease; revisited, Contraception 50:167, 1994.

426. Jick S, Pennap D, Drospirenone- and levonorgestrel-containing oral contraceptives and the risk of gallbladder disease, Contraception 86:220–223, 2012.

427. Stuart GS, Tang JH, Heartwell SF, Westhoff CL, A high cholecystectomy rate in a cohort of Mexican American women who are postpartum at the time of oral contraceptive pill initiation, Contraception 76:357–359, 2007.

428. Vessey MP, Villard-Mackintosh L, Painter R, Oral contraceptives and pregnancy in relation to peptic ulcer, Contraception 46:349, 1992.

429. Lashner BA, Kane SV, Hanauer SB, Lack of association between oral contraceptive use and ulcerative colitis, Gastroenterology 99:1032, 1990.

430. Logan RF, Kay CR, Oral contraception, smoking and inflammatory bowel disease—findings in the Royal College of General Practitioners Oral Contraception Study, Int J Epidemiol 18:105–107, 1989.

431. Ortizo R, Lee SY, Nguyen ET, Jamal MM, Bechtold MM, Nguyen DL, Exposure to oral contraceptives increases the risk for development of inflammatory bowel disease: a meta-analysis of case-controlled and cohort studies, Eur J Gastroenterol Hepatol 29:1064–1070, 2017.

432. Taneepanichskul S, Phuapradit W, Chaturachinda K, Association of contraceptives and HIV-1 infection in Thai female commercial sex workers, Aust N Z J Obstet Gynaecol 37:86–88, 1997.

433. Heffron R, Donnell D, Rees H, Celum C, Mugo N, Were E, et al., Use of hormonal contraceptives and risk of HIV-1 transmission: a prospective cohort study, Lancet Infect Dis 12:19–26, 2012.

434. Polis CB, Phillips SJ, Curtis KM, Hormonal contraceptive use and female-to-male HIV transmission: a systematic review of the epidemiologic evidence, AIDS 27:493–505, 2013.

435. Wall KM, Kilembe W, Vwalika B, Htee Khu N, Brill I, Chomba E, et al., Hormonal contraception does not increase women's HIV acquisition risk in Zambian discordant couples, 1994–2012, Contraception 91:480–487, 2015.

436. Morrison CS, Chen PL, Kwok C, Baeten JM, Brown J, Crook AM, et al., Hormonal contraception and the risk of HIV acquisition: an individual participant data meta-analysis, PLoS Med 12:e1001778, 2015.

437. Balkus JE, Brown ER, Hillier SL, Coletti A, Ramjee G, Mgodi N, et al., Oral and injectable contraceptive use and HIV acquisition risk among women in four African countries: a secondary analysis of data from a microbicide trial, Contraception 93:25–31, 2016.

438. Cejtin HE, Jacobson L, Springer G, Watts DH, Levine AJ, Greenblatt R, et al., Effect of hormonal contraceptive use on plasma HIV-1-RNA levels among HIV-infected women, AIDS 17:1702–1704, 2003.

439. Richardson BA, Otieno PA, Mbori-Ngacha D, Overbaugh J, Farquhar C, John-Stewart GC, Hormonal contraception and HIV-1 disease progression among postpartum Kenyan women, AIDS 21:749–753, 2007.

440. Heffron R, Mugo N, Ngure K, Celum C, Donnell D, Were E, et al., Hormonal contraceptive use and risk of HIV-1 disease progression, AIDS 27:261–267, 2013.

441. Barbone F, Austin H, Louv WC, Alexander WJ, A follow-up study of methods of contraception, sexual activity, and rates of trichomoniasis, candidiasis, and bacterial vaginosis, Am J Obstet Gynecol 163:510, 1990.

442. Shoubnikova M, Hellberg D, Nilsson S, Mårdh P-A, Contraceptive use in women with bacterial vaginosis, Contraception 55:355–358, 1997.

443. Baeten JM, Nyange PM, Richardson BA, Lavreys L, Chohan B, Martin HL

297

Jr, et al., Hormonal contraception and risk of sexually transmitted disease acquisition: results from a prospective study, Am J Obstet Gynecol 185:380–385, 2001.

444. **Rifkin SB, Smith MR, Brotman RM, Gindi RM, Erbelding EJ,** Hormonal contraception and risk of bacterial vaginosis diagnosis in an observational study of women attending STD clinics in Baltimore, MD, Contraception 80:63–67, 2009.

445. **Vodstrcil LA, Hocking JS, Law M, Walker S, Tabrizi SN, Fairley CK, et al.,** Hormonal contraception is associated with a reduced risk of bacterial vaginosis: a systematic review and meta-analysis, PLoS One 8:e73055, 2013.

446. **van de Wijgert JH, Verwijs MC, Turner AN, Morrison CS,** Hormonal contraception decreases bacterial vaginosis but oral contraception may increase candidiasis: implications for HIV transmission, AIDS 27:2141–2153, 2013.

447. **Brooks JP, Edwards DJ, Blithe DL, Fettweis JM, Serrano MG, Sheth NU, et al.,** Effects of combined oral contraceptives, depot medroxyprogesterone acetate and the levonorgestrel-releasing intrauterine system on the vaginal microbiome, Contraception 95:405–413, 2017.

448. **Roy S, Wilkins J, Mishell DR Jr,** The effect of a contraceptive vaginal ring and oral contraceptives on the vaginal flora, Contraception 24:481–491, 1981.

449. **Schwan A, Ahren T, Victor A,** Effects of contraceptive vaginal ring treatment on vaginal bacteriology and cytology, Contraception 28:341–347, 1983.

450. **Roumen FJME, Boon ME, van Velzen D, Dieben TOM, Coelingh Bennink HJT,** The cervico-vaginal epithelium during 20 cycles' use of a combined contraceptive vaginal ring, Hum Reprod 11:2443–2448, 1996.

451. **Lete I, Cuesta MC, Marin JM, Guerra S,** Vaginal health in contraceptive vaginal ring users—a review. Eur J Contracept Reprod Health Care 18:234–241, 2013.

452. **Huang Y, Merkatz RB, Hillier SL, Roberts K, Blithe DL, Sitruk-Ware R, et al.,** Effects of a one year reusable contraceptive vaginal ring on vaginal microflora and the risk of vaginal infection: an open-label prospective evaluation, PLoS One 2015;10:e0134460.

453. **Cates W Jr, Washington AE, Rubin GL, Peterson HB,** The pill, chlamydia and PID, Fam Plann Perspect 17:175, 1985.

454. **Cottingham J, Hunter D,** *Chlamydia trachomatis* and oral contraceptive use: a quantitative review, Genitourin Med 68:209–216, 1992.

455. **Critchlow CW, Wölner-Hanssen P, Eschenbach DA, Kiviat NB, Koutsky LA, Stevens CE, et al.,** Determinants of cervical ectopia and of cervicitis: age, oral contraception, specific cervical infection, smoking, and douching, Am J Obstet Gynecol 173:534, 1995.

456. **Gursahaney PR, Meyn LA, Hillier SL, Sweet RL, Wiesenfeld HC,** Combined hormonal contraception may be protective against *Neisseria gonorrhoeae* infection, Sex Transm Dis 37:356–360, 2010.

457. **Borgdorff H, Verwijs MC, Wit FW, Tsivtsivadze E, Ndayisaba GF, Verhelst R, et al.,** The impact of hormonal contraception and pregnancy on sexually transmitted infections and on cervicovaginal microbiota in African sex workers, Sex Transm Dis 42:143–152, 2015.

458. **Rubin GL, Ory WH, Layde PM,** Oral contraceptives and pelvic inflammatory disease, Am J Obstet Gynecol 140:630, 1980.

459. **Wolner-Hanssen P, Eschenbach DA, Paavonen J, Kiviat N, Stevens CE, Critchlow C, et al.,** Decreased risk of symptomatic chlamydial pelvic inflammatory disease associated with oral contraceptive use, JAMA 263:54, 1990.

460. **Spinillo A, Gorini G, Piazzi G, Balataro F, Monaco A, Zara F,** The impact of oral contraception on chlamydial infection among patients with pelivic inflammatory disease, Contraception 54:163–168, 1996.

461. **Panser LA, Phipps WR,** Type of oral contraceptive in relation to acute, initial episodes of pelvic inflammatory disease, Contraception 43:91, 1991.

462. **Cramer DW, Goldman MB, Schiff I, Belisla S, Albrecht B, Stadel B, et al.,** The relationship of tubal infertility to barrier method and oral contraceptive use, JAMA 257:2446, 1987.

463. Svensson L, Westrom L, Mardh P, Contraceptives and acute salpingitis, JAMA 251:2553, 1984.

464. Wolner-Hanssen P, Oral contraceptive use modifies the manifestations of pelvic inflammatory disease, Br J Obstet Gynaecol 93:619–624, 1986.

465. Pituitary Adenoma Study Group, Pituitary adenomas and oral contraceptives: a multicenter case-control study, Fertil Steril 39:753, 1983.

466. Shy FKK, McTiernan AM, Daling JR, Weiss NS, Oral contraceptive use and the occurrence of pituitary prolactinomas, JAMA 249:2204, 1983.

467. Wingrave SJ, Kay CR, Vessey MP, Oral contraceptives and pituitary adenomas, Br Med J 280:685, 1980.

468. Hulting A-L, Werner S, Hagenfeldt K, Oral contraceptives do not promote the development or growth of prolactinomas, Contraception 27:69, 1983.

469. Corenblum B, Donovan L, The safety of physiological estrogen plus progestin replacement therapy and oral contraceptive therapy in women with pathological hyperprolactinemia, Fertil Steril 59:671, 1993.

470. Testa G, Vegetti W, Motta T, Alagna F, Bianchedi D, Carlucci C, et al., Two-year treatment with oral contraceptives in hyperprolactinemic patients, Contraception 58:69–73, 1998.

471. Vessey MP, Hannaford P, Mant J, Painter R, Frith P, Chappel D, Oral contraception and eye disease: findings in two large cohort studies, Br Med J 82:538–542, 1998.

472. Vessey M, Painter R, Oral contraception and ear disease: findings in a large cohort study, Contraception 63:61–63, 2001.

473. Villard-Mackintosh L, Vessey MP, Oral contraceptives and reproductive factors in multiple sclerosis incidence, Contraception 47:161–168, 1993.

474. Thorogood M, Hannaford PC, The influence of oral contraceptives on the risk of multiple sclerosis, Br J Obstet Gynaecol 105:1296–1299, 1998.

475. Hernan MA, Hohol MJ, Olek MJ, Spiegelman D, Ascherio A, Oral contraceptives and the incidence of multiple sclerosis, Neurology 55:848–854, 2000.

476. Zapata LB, Oduyebo T, Whiteman MK, Houtchens MK, Marchbanks PA, Curtis KM, Contraceptive use among women with multiple sclerosis: a systematic review, Contraception 94:612–620, 2016.

477. Kalmuss D, Koenemann S, Westhoff C, Heartwell S, Edwards S, Zieman M, et al., Prior pill experiences and current continuation among pill restarters, Perspect Sex Reprod Health 40:138–143, 2008.

478. White KO, Westhoff C, The effect of pack supply on oral contraceptive pill continuation: a randomized controlled trial, Obstet Gynecol 118:615–622, 2011.

479. Foster DG, Hulett D, Bradsberry M, Darney P, Policar M, Number of oral contraceptive pill packages dispensed and subsequent unintended pregnancies, Obstet Gynecol 117:566–572, 2011.

480. Zuniga C, Grossman D, Harrell S, Blanchard K, Grindlay K, Breaking down barriers to birth control access: an assessment of online platforms prescribing birth control in the USA, J Telemed Telecare 2019. doi: 10.1177/1357633X18824828.

481. Gaffield ML, Kiarie J, WHO medical eligibility criteria update, Contraception 94:193–194, 2016.

482. American College of Obstetrics and Gynecology, Well-Woman Recommendations 2018. https://www.acog.org/About-ACOG/ACOG-Departments/Annual-Womens-Health-Care/Well-Woman-Recommendations

483. Westhoff CL, Jones HE, Guiahi M, Do new guidelines and technology make the routine pelvic examination obsolete? J Womens Health (Larchmt) 20:5–10, 2011.

484. Lu S, Rafie S, Hamper J, Strauss R, Kroon L, Characterizing pharmacist-prescribed hormonal contraception services and users in California and Oregon pharmacies, Contraception 99:239–243, 2018.

485. Stanback J, Yacobson I, Harber L, Proposed clinical guidance for excluding pregnancy prior to contraceptive initiation, Contraception 95:326–330, 2017.

486. **Morroni C, Findley M, Westhoff C,** Does using the "pregnancy checklist" delay safe initiation of contraception? Contraception 95:331–334, 2017.

487. **Westhoff C, Heartwell S, Edwards S, Zieman M, Cushman L, Robilotto C, et al.,** Initiation of oral contraceptives using a quick start compared with a conventional start: a randomized controlled trial, Obstet Gynecol 109:1270–1276, 2007.

488. **Rosenberg MJ, Waugh MS,** Oral contraceptive discontinuation: a prospective evaluation of frequency and reasons, Am J Obstet Gynecol 179:577–582, 1998.

489. **O'Connell K, Davis AR, Kerns J,** Oral contraceptives: side effects and depression in adolescent girls, Contraception 75:299–304, 2007.

490. **Grimes DA, Schulz KF,** Nonspecific side effects of oral contraceptives: nocebo or noise? Contraception 83:5–9, 2011.

491. **Kamel H, Navi BB, Sriram N, Hovsepian DA, Devereux RB, Elkind MS,** Risk of a thrombotic event after the 6-week postpartum period, N Engl J Med 370:1307–1315, 2014.

492. **Tepper NK, Phillips SJ, Kapp N, Gaffield ME, Curtis KM,** Combined hormonal contraceptive use among breastfeeding women: an updated systematic review, Contraception 94:262–274, 2016.

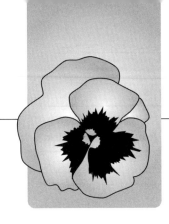

8

Injectable Contraception

Laneta Dorflinger, PhD
and Sharon L. Achilles, MD, PhD

njectable contraceptives are widely available, moderately effective, medium-acting (1 to 3 months) reversible methods that can be used discretely and do not require daily action by the user. More than 50 million women worldwide use injectable methods for contraception, which is an estimated 7% of all contraceptive use among married or in-union women.[1,2] In the United States, injectable contraceptive use constitutes approximately 4.5% of overall contraceptive use, with use being highest among younger women, women of black race, and never-married women.[3]

A single injection delivers a depot of active drug, resulting in a serum drug concentration that peaks and then gradually declines to provide a nondaily hormonal contraceptive option that lasts up to several months, with duration dependent on specific formulation. Although users who adhere to the recommended injection schedule enjoy highly effective protection, noncompliance often leads to typical-use effectiveness for this method that is similar to other short-acting reversible hormonal methods. Depot-medroxyprogesterone acetate (DMPA) delivered by intramuscular (IM) or subcutaneous (SC) injection every 3 months is the most widely used injectable contraceptive worldwide and is currently the only FDA-approved injectable contraceptive used clinically in the United States. Other injectable contraceptives available globally include a formulation of the progestin norethindrone enanthate (NET-EN) as well as combined injectable formulations that contain a progestin (typically medroxyprogesterone acetate [MPA] or NET-EN) combined with an estrogen (typically estradiol cypionate or estradiol valerate) (Table 8.1).

DMPA became available in the 1960s with initial indications as treatment for threatened and habitual abortion, as well as gonadal suppression for treatment of endometriosis.[4] Investigators soon recognized that DMPA had potential as a potent contraceptive and initiated studies to explore the impact of various doses on effectiveness, side effects, and duration. Ultimately, a dose of 150 mg delivered intramuscularly in the deltoid or gluteus was marketed for 3 months of contraceptive protection. The method became widely available and used worldwide, but remained off-label in the United States for many years due to concerns about breast cancer risk based on data from Beagle dogs, which metabolize MPA differently than do humans.[5,6] Following publication of large trials by the World Health Organization

Table 8.1 Injectable Contraceptive Methods

Injectable	Brand Name*	Dose	Dosing Frequency	Route	Formulation
Progestin-only					
MPA	Depo-Provera® Triclofem® Triclovera® OSKB 1® Depogen™	150 mg	3 months	IM	Suspension of aqueous microcrystals
MPA	depo-subQ provera 104® Sayana® Sayana Press®	104 mg	3 months	SC	Suspension of aqueous microcrystals
NET-EN	Noristerat® Syngestal® Norigest® Doryxas®	200 mg	2 months	IM	Oily solution
Combination					
MPA/E2C	Cyclofem® Cyclofemina® Novafem® Cyclogeston®	25 mg/ 5 mg	monthly	IM	Aqueous suspension
NET-EN/E2V	Mesigyna® Norigynon®	50 mg/ 5 mg	monthly	IM	Oily solution
DHPA/E2E	Perlutan® Perlutal® Topasel® Deladroxate®	150 mg/ 10 mg	monthly	IM	Oily solution
DHPA/E2E	Anafertin®	75 mg/ 5 mg	monthly	IM	Oily solution

*Listed brand names are not exhaustive.
Abbreviations: MPA, medroxyprogesterone acetate; NET-EN, norethindrone (also known as norethisterone) enanthate; E2C, estradiol cypionate; E2V, estradiol valerate; DHPA, dihydroxyprogesterone acetophenide; E2E, estradiol enanthate; IM, intramuscular; SC, subcutaneous.

demonstrating no impact of DMPA on human breast cancer, the U.S. FDA granted approval in 1992 for DMPA as a contraceptive. An SC formulation (104 mg/0.65 mL) of MPA was approved by the FDA in 2004 that offered a lower dose option with added potential for self-administration.[7,8] Studies on self-injection of DMPA SC have shown substantial improvement in continuation when compared with clinic-based provision, and women cite important benefits of saving time and money when not having monthly clinic visits.[9,10] The SC formulation is provided in prefilled syringes, while the IM formulation is provided in vials or prefilled syringes. Following injection, micronized drug is slowly released from the IM or SC depot. As currently labeled, both products are to be administered every 12 to 14 weeks.

Extensive research, largely led by the World Health Organization's Special Programme on Human Reproduction, was carried out throughout the 1980s and 1990s to evaluate lower doses of DMPA and non–DMPA-based alternative progestin-only injectables aimed at minimizing side effects and developing shorter-acting injectable options containing estrogen to improve bleeding profiles.[5,11] Arising largely from the work led by the World Health Organization, NET-EN as well as estrogen/progestin combination injectables became widely available as alternative injectables. NET-EN is a long-chain ester of norethindrone formulated as an oily solution containing 200 mg/mL for IM administration bimonthly. Several clinical trials defined the clinical characteristics and duration of action of NET-EN and compared effectiveness to that of DMPA IM.[5,12–14] In a large comparative trial of DMPA 150 mg every 3 months and NET-EN 200 mg every 2 months, the 24-month pregnancy rate was the same for both regimens (0.4 per 100 women).[14] Although the duration of bleeding and spotting was similar, women using DMPA were 21% more likely to develop amenorrhea compared to women using NET-EN.[15] Return to ovulation may be somewhat more rapid following NET-EN use compared to DMPA IM use.[16] Mean time to return of fertility is variable with both of these injectables and, on average, is shorter in NET-EN users compared to DMPA users.[11,17] Today, NET-EN is registered in a number of countries although global use appears to be modest when compared with DMPA. The highest prevalence of use is in South Africa where 12% of modern contraceptive users, constituting nearly one third of all injectable contraceptive users, are using NET-EN.[18]

Bleeding irregularities are an important reason that women discontinue progestin-only injectable contraceptives, hence the desire to develop alternatives such as combined injectable methods aimed to improve bleeding patterns.[5,19] Studies spanned more than a decade and ultimately advanced the broader availability of the combination of MPA 25 mg plus estradiol cypionate 5 mg (DMPA 25 mg plus E2C 5 mg) and the combination of NET-EN 50 mg plus estradiol valerate 5 mg (NET-EN 50 mg plus E2V 10 mg), the two most widely available combination products today.[5,19] Other combination injectables are available, particularly in Latin America, and are listed in **Table 8.1**, but use is low compared with the DMPA/E2C and NET-EN/E2V products. When combination products (DMPA 25 mg plus

E2C 5 mg or NET-EN 50 mg plus E2V 10 mg) were compared with relevant progestin-only formulations (DMPA or NET-EN, respectively), the combination injectables showed more regular bleeding patterns, less amenorrhea, and less discontinuation for reasons related to bleeding changes. Nevertheless, discontinuation for reasons other than changes in bleeding patterns, including the burden of monthly clinic visits, as well as discontinuation overall were greater for the combination monthly products.[20] In the United States, DMPA 25 mg plus E2C 5 mg was marketed between 2000 and 2002 as Lunelle®; however, this product was ultimately withdrawn from the market due to limited market demand and production issues.

Pharmacokinetics

Injectable contraceptives deliver a relatively large bolus of active drug compared to either short-acting contraceptives (pills, patch, and ring) or long-acting reversible contraceptives (intrauterine devices [IUDs] and subdermal implants) to maintain a serum drug concentration adequate for contraceptive efficacy for several weeks or months. The pharmacokinetic profiles for injectable contraceptives reflect these differences. **Figure 8.1** illustrates pharmacokinetic curve approximations extrapolated to 1 year using publicly available data for the first injection cycle of IM and SC

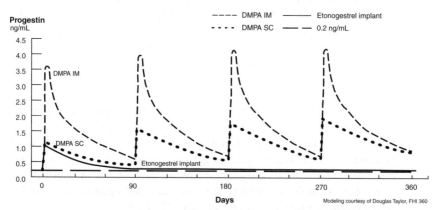

Figure 8.1 Mean serum concentration-time profile of DMPA IM, DMPA SC, and etonogestrel implant over 12 months. DMPA curves reflect actual data for the first 90-day injection interval and modeled data for injection intervals 2 to 4. *Circles* represent trough values at 6 and 12 months reported during long-term use of DMPA IM (*dashed line*) and DMPA SC (*dotted line*).[21] The implant (*solid line*) has the lowest peak. The *dashed line* at 0.2 ng/mL indicates the estimated threshold needed for a contraceptive effect. (Data sources: etonogestrel implant, physician prescribing information.[22]; DMPA IM, FDA label and review of a generic formulation.[23,24]; DMPA SC, blended from PK studies at three injection sites [abdomen, thigh, and upper arm].[25–27])

formulations of DMPA. The data are compared with a "sustained-release" etonogestrel implant that maintains serum progestin concentrations just above the theoretical threshold concentration for ovulation inhibition for 3 years or longer.[21]

Following DMPA IM or SC injection, serum MPA levels increase for 1 to 3 weeks to peak levels (C_{max}). Minimum levels of MPA necessary to ensure contraceptive effectiveness (approximately 0.2 ng/mL) are achieved within the first 24 hours following either IM or SC injection of DMPA.[6,24,28] Peak levels decline to mean trough concentrations of approximately 0.4 to 1 ng/mL by 90 days.[6,8,24,25,27,29] While no currently published studies directly compare the pharmacokinetics of DMPA administered IM versus SC, SC administration may have lower average C_{max} and serum MPA concentrations compared to IM administration in the first 30 days after injection. MPA accumulates with continued IM or SC administration such that trough serum concentrations increase over several injection intervals until a steady state is reached **(Figure 8.1)**. At 12 months, 90-day trough concentrations (C_{91}) for both IM and SC products are similar, about 0.8 ng/mL, which is twice the average trough value reported for the SC product during the first cycle of administration (about 0.4 ng/mL).[25] Specifically with regard to the SC product, this small amount of accumulation may explain the reported longer time to ovulation following multiple injections (10 months) compared to single injection (7 months).[25,30]

As with other hormonal contraceptives, studies of women using DMPA have reported wide interindividual and interstudy variability in pharmacokinetic profiles.[30–33] Interindividual variability in drug concentrations may be related to drug metabolism differences and may contribute to different individual experiences with bleeding and other side effects although no studies have yet carefully explored this. Two ongoing studies are aimed at partially addressing this question by carefully evaluating pharmacokinetic parameters using varying and repeated SC doses in individual women (Clinicaltrials.gov NCT02456584 and NCT02732418). Published C_{max} values following DMPA IM administration range from 2.2 to 24 ng/mL,[34–46] and those following DMPA SC administration range from 0.95 to 1.56 ng/mL.[8,24–26,29] Some data suggest there may be ethnic differences in drug absorption and clearance for IM injectable contraceptives between Asian and Latin American women.[47] Interestingly, no pharmacokinetic differences have been observed in Asian and U.S. women using DMPA SC.[25,26] Explanations for the wide range of reported C_{max} levels following DMPA IM administration include different sampling times (some studies have less frequent sampling such that a true average C_{max} cannot be calculated), pharmacokinetic properties related to varying sites of IM injection, injection techniques (including massage or rubbing the injection site), intrinsic participant factors (including BMI, ethnic and metabolic differences), small sample sizes in some studies, and different MPA assays. Further complicating our understanding of the relationship of MPA pharmacokinetics and side effects is that assays for progestins, including MPA, have evolved over time from radioimmunoassay (RIA) to gas chromatography–mass spectrometry (GC-MS) to high-performance liquid chromatography or ultra-high-performance liquid chromatography with tandem mass spectrometry (HPLC- or UPLC-MS/MS).[25,48,49] RIA may overestimate serum levels due to cross-reactivity of antibodies with metabolites or other circulating hormones.[50-52] Results using GC, LC-, or HPLC-/UPLC-based approaches as opposed to RIA show less interstudy variation and have consistently reported lower average C_{max} levels for DMPA IM, ranging from 2 to 4.5 ng/mL.[7,22,25,34,35] All three pharmacokinetic studies of DMPA SC[24-26] measured serum drug concentrations with liquid chromatography, so the differences in the literature are not as varied as those seen with DMPA IM.

Mechanism of Action/Pharmacodynamics

The primary mechanism of action for injectable contraceptives (IM and SC formulations) is suppression of ovulation.[16,25,53-56] Following DMPA administration, the circulating level of the MPA effectively blocks the luteinizing hormone (LH) surge, preventing ovulation even though follicle-stimulating hormone (FSH) is not necessarily suppressed.[57] FSH levels similar to the midfollicular stage of cycling women can occur across the 3-month injection cycle in DMPA users such that follicular growth is maintained sufficiently to stimulate endogenous estrogen secretion comparable to the early follicular phase of a normal menstrual cycle with use of either IM or SC DMPA.[6,25,58] FSH can also be suppressed in some users of DMPA IM.[59,60] The reasons for these differences are not well understood, but may be related to the age of women studied,[61,62] the timing and frequency of sampling, and pharmacogenetic variations in cytochrome P-450 enzymes, which metabolize contraceptive steroids and have been shown to influence pharmacokinetics and responses.[63] In addition to ovulation suppression, thickening of cervical mucus and changes in the endometrium also occur following administration of DMPA,[6,64] yet the potential contribution of these effects, if any, to the mechanism of action is unclear given the dominant role of ovulation suppression.

Return to ovulation and fertility is commonly delayed after stopping injectable contraceptives **(Figure 8.2)**. Unlike drugs in short-acting contraceptives (pills, patch, and ring) and LARC methods (IUDs and implants), all of which are quickly metabolized following cessation of use, injectables are formulated as drug depots, intentionally designed to be long-lasting following dosing. The benefit of drug depots is less frequent dosing, which is convenient for the user. The drawbacks include unpredictable delay in return to fertility and inability to stop the drug quickly in the event of allergy or anaphylaxis. Significant allergy to contraceptive steroid hormones is rare as are instances of significant reaction to inactive ingredients in injectable contraceptives (parabens, polyethylene glycols, and polysorbates).[65,66]

Approximately half of women who discontinue DMPA can expect normal menses to return by 6 months after the last injection, but approximately 25% will not resume a normal menstrual pattern for at least 1 year.[25,67] Among 15 women who received multiple doses of DMPA SC, the median time to

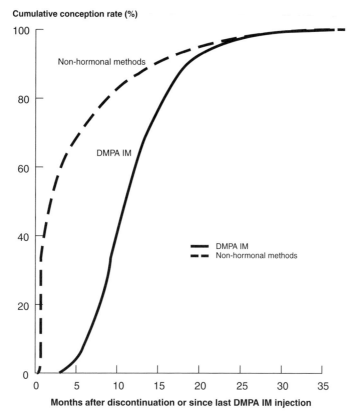

Figure 8.2 Return to fertility after stopping DMPA. Cumulative conception rate (%) among women seeking pregnancy following discontinuation of a nonhormonal method or following last injection of DMPA IM. (Adapted from **Schwallie PC, Assenzo JR,** The effect of depomedroxyprogesterone acetate on pituitary and ovarian function, and the return of fertility following its discontinuation: a review, Contraception 10:181–202, 1974.)

ovulation was 10 months after the last injection; earliest return to ovulation was 6 months after the last injection; and 12 women (80%) ovulated within 1 year of the last injection.[30] Subcutaneous administration of DMPA may be associated with a slightly greater delay in return to ovulation compared to the IM route. In a comparative study, median time to return of ovulation after a single IM injection of DMPA IM and a single injection of DMPA SC was 183 and 212 days, respectively, although this was not statistically different.[25] In this study, the 12-month rates of return to ovulation for DMPA IM users and DMPA SC users were 95% and 97%, respectively.[25] Return to fertility following DMPA use is also delayed when compared to other methods, and the delay may be slightly greater with DMPA SC than DMPA IM.[4,30]

Approximately two thirds of women conceived within 12 months, over 80% conceived within 15 months, and over 90% conceived within 18 months from the last injection of DMPA IM.[4] Among 28 women using DMPA SC who stopped treatment to become pregnant, only 1 became pregnant within a year of the last injection, and a second became pregnant 443 days after the last injection (7 women were lost to follow-up).[30] Clinician counseling for initiation of DMPA must include details regarding this potential for delay in return to fertility. Women who strongly wish to become pregnant within a year should not initiate or continue use of DMPA.

Efficacy

Approximately 6 out of 100 women will become pregnant in the first year of DMPA use with typical use. Injectable contraceptives have perfect-use contraceptive efficacy similar to that observed with typical use of LARC methods, greater than 99%.[68] However, similar to short-acting contraceptive methods, the end-user–dependent need for timely and consistent dosing results in typical-use contraceptive effectiveness that diverges from perfect-use efficacy (see Table 1.2).

In a large multicenter international clinical trial conducted by the WHO, no pregnancies occurred during 5,429 woman-months of experience among women receiving IM DMPA 150 mg every 3 months.[69] Similarly, no pregnancies occurred in two large multinational clinical trials of DMPA SC, with over 16,000 women-months of use, which specifically included large numbers of overweight and obese women.[70] The collective data suggest that contraceptive efficacy for DMPA is not significantly impacted by weight[71] or by use of medications that stimulate hepatic enzymes,[34,72-74] which may be related to both high potency and relatively high serum concentrations of MPA following administration. Like other progestin-only methods, DMPA protects against ectopic pregnancy; a systematic review identified only four ectopic pregnancies in the published literature over almost 50 years.[75]

The first contraceptive injection can be given at any time if it is reasonably certain that the woman is not pregnant.[76] To optimize effective contraception, the first injection should ideally be administered within the first 7 days of the menstrual cycle (before a dominant follicle emerges), or a backup method is recommended for 7 days.[76,77] The quick-start, same-day start can be used with injectable contraceptives, and quick-starting contraception has been shown to result in better contraceptive initiation rates and similar contraceptive continuation compared with traditional contraceptive initiation protocols that direct clinicians to restrict initiation to the first 7 days of the menstrual cycle.[78-82] In situations when the health care provider cannot be reasonably certain that the woman is not pregnant, the benefits of initiating injectable contraception likely exceed any risk and therefore quick-start initiation is reasonable.[76] As is true for most pharmacologic drugs, the limited available data on risks associated with exposure to DMPA in pregnancy are retrospective and significantly confounded limiting their interpretability.[83] However, no indication of significant fetal harm or patterns of serious congenital anomaly exist to support termination of an otherwise desired pregnancy in the setting of DMPA exposure.

There is currently a small study under way designed to evaluate pharmacodynamic effects of DMPA used shortly after unprotected intercourse for emergency contraception (Clinicaltrials.gov NCT03395756). In common clinical practice, DMPA can be quick-started anytime provided the urine pregnancy test is negative with a recommendation to perform a pregnancy test in 2 weeks if she has had any potential unprotected sex in the 2 weeks preceding injection.

The duration of action of DMPA IM can be iatrogenically shortened if attention is not paid to proper IM administration, which is ideally given deeply into the muscle using the Z-track technique to minimize drug leakage.[84] Additionally, the injection should be given in a protected anatomic location, and the site should not be massaged following administration to protect the drug depot from disruption of the microcrystals, which could accelerate drug release and impact duration of efficacy.

When given properly, there is an effective 2-week grace period that allows for late reinjections of DMPA. For many women, there may be a longer grace period as several studies, including a meta-analysis, have concluded that reinjection up to 4 weeks late continued to provide equivalent protection against pregnancy based on return to ovulation and pregnancy occurrence.[85,86] Nevertheless, given wide interindividual variations in metabolism and potential for harm (unplanned pregnancy) in those who may metabolize drug more rapidly, the recommended dosing interval continues to be 12 to 14 weeks. Notably, the package inserts for both DMPA IM and SC recommend only a 1-week grace period.[23,30] Thus, women who are more than 2 weeks late for reinjection should be tested for pregnancy and quickly restarted if the test is negative. An ongoing clinical trial is evaluating the effectiveness, pharmacokinetics, safety, and acceptability of DMPA SC when given every 4 months, essentially equivalent to maximizing a 4-week grace period; results will inform future guidance with regard to a safe reinjection interval (Clinicaltrials.gov NCT03154125). Notably, no minimal time limits exist for early injections, so repeat injection can be given early when necessary, for instance, if the patient will be traveling or otherwise unable to return at the routine dosing interval.[76]

Contraceptive continuation rates in users of injectable contraceptives tend to be lower than continuation rates for LARC users,[87] and in a recent study in which some participants self-selected and others were randomized to contraception, self-selection did not appear to impact continuation for participants using injectables.[88] The observed unintended pregnancy rates for injectable users are comparable to unintended pregnancy rates in short-acting contraceptive users, further suggesting that discontinuation is likely frequent in injectable contraceptive users.[89] Recent data strongly suggest that continuation rates are significantly increased with use of SC injections that can be self-administered as compared to clinician-administered IM injections.[9,90,91] One nonrandomized study in Ugandan women[90] and two randomized studies in Malawian[9] and American women[91] all demonstrate significantly increased method continuation rates at 12 months (81% vs. 65%, $p < 0.05$; 73% vs. 45%, $p < 0.001$; and 69% vs. 54%, $p = 0.005$, respectively) in women using self-administered SC injections compared to health worker–administered IM injections. As has been observed with other short-acting contraceptives, decreasing barriers to continued use, such as eliminating the need for clinician administration, should improve patient satisfaction and continuation of injectable contraceptives.[92]

Bleeding Profile

Use of injectable progestins generally causes reduced menstrual bleeding and many users will stop having monthly menses. Bleeding and spotting typically decrease progressively with each reinjection so that after 12 months, 60% of users experience amenorrhea (compared with 20% of women using a levonorgestrel [LNG] IUS).[93-96] Women using DMPA SC report similar bleeding patterns compared to those using DMPA IM,[70,97] with 63% versus 64% achieving amenorrhea at the end of the first year of treatment and 71% versus 80% after 2 years, respectively, in a direct comparison.[27]

Some women experience prolonged and/or irregular bleeding with injectable progestins. Irregular bleeding can be disturbing and annoying, and up to 25% of patients discontinue in the first year because of irregular bleeding.[15,98,99] The bleeding is rarely heavy; in fact, hemoglobin values typically rise in DMPA users.[100] With honest, open, patient-centered contraceptive counseling, including setting realistic expectations of anticipated bleeding patterns, discontinuation of contraception due to irregular bleeding or other common side effects can be minimized.[101,102] Unscheduled bleeding is most common in the first year of DMPA use compared to after greater than 12 months of use.[103] Therefore, encouraging patients to continue use, if they otherwise like the method, with reassurance that unscheduled bleeding commonly resolves is a reasonable approach. Endometrial biopsy data from women using DMPA demonstrate that glandular atrophy commonly occurs both in women experiencing and not experiencing unscheduled bleeding, so these findings alone do not explain bleeding patterns.[104] In the largest therapeutic trial of treatment of presumed atrophy in DMPA users with unscheduled bleeding, 278 DMPA users with unscheduled bleeding were assigned to receive ethinyl estradiol (EE) 50 µg, estrone sulfate 2.5 mg, or placebo for 14 days.[105] Although EE was significantly more effective than placebo in stopping bleeding during treatment (bleeding stopped in 93%, 76%, and 74%, respectively), bleeding tended to recur after discontinuation of EE. Besides treatment with supplemental estrogen, other commonly discussed treatment modalities include nonsteroidal anti-inflammatory drugs (NSAIDs), mefenamic acid, tranexamic acid, and doxycycline. The U.S. SPR for Contraceptive Use (2016) suggests 5 to 7 days of NSAIDs to treat unscheduled spotting or light bleeding,[76] although data supporting efficacy are limited. Mefenamic acid (500 mg twice per day for 5 days) may have limited utility in short-term control of bleeding associated with DMPA use; however, it was not statistically more effective than placebo by week 4 of use.[106] A randomized placebo-controlled trial of 100 DMPA users with unscheduled bleeding found that tranexamic acid 250 mg orally four times per day for 5 days was significantly more effective in halting bleeding compared to placebo with 88% versus 8% stopping, respectively ($p < 0.001$).[107] The women who received tranexamic acid also experienced significantly fewer bleeding/spotting days over 4 weeks (mean of 5.7 vs. 17.5 days, $p < 0.05$). Finally, a double-blind placebo-controlled randomized trial of 68 DMPA users experiencing unscheduled bleeding demonstrated doxycycline 100 mg twice daily for 5 days was not more effective than placebo for stopping bleeding or for improving bleeding in the 3 months following treatment.[108] Hence, therapeutic approaches to normalize bleeding for injectable contraceptive users have not consistently been effective and have largely not altered patient discontinuation rates.[109]

Metabolic Effects

Bone

The FDA-approved label for DMPA (IM and SC) contains a "black box" warning regarding bone loss with long-term use.[23,27,30] No data are available to inform whether use during adolescence or early adulthood, a critical period of bone accretion, leads to reduced peak bone mass and alteration of risk for osteoporotic fracture in later life. Given the absence of evidence and the theoretical concern, the FDA label takes a conservative position and indicates that DMPA should not be used longer than 2 years unless other contraceptive methods are considered inadequate. In contrast to the FDA product label, Kaunitz and Grimes[110,111] reviewed existing evidence and concluded that the changes in bone mineral density are largely reversible and comparable to changes associated with naturally occurring hypoestrogenism with pregnancy and lactation, which most women experience for periods of their lives, suggesting use should not be restricted.[110,111] The observed bone loss and reversibility appear comparable for IM and SC administration of DMPA in a relatively small comparative study.[27] In a study of postmenopausal women who were former long-term users of either DMPA or copper IUD, there was no difference in forearm bone densities providing additional evidence that bone density changes are reversible and do not adversely impact long-term bone density measurements.[112] Furthermore, there is no evidence of change in fracture risk, the clinically relevant outcome, associated with short- or long-term use.[110,111] There are, however, no data on clinical fracture risk among postmenopausal women who previously used DMPA. While the current evidence does not justify restricting use of DMPA, additional research is needed to address questions of whether specific populations at risk of low bone density, for example, underweight women, women with eating disorders, women who are immobilized or wheelchair bound, as well as adolescents who have not reached peak bone mass, may be at potential increased risk for fracture during or after long-term use.

Cardiovascular

Although the absolute safety with regard to thrombosis has not been proven in a controlled study, clinically, there have not been apparent trends for increased thromboembolic events when progestin-only injectables are used, including during use by high-risk women with a personal history of venous thromboembolism (VTE). The U.S. Medical Eligibility for Criteria for Contraceptive Use lists injectable progestin-only contraceptives as a category 2 for women at highest risk for thrombosis, including women with an acute deep vein thrombosis or pulmonary embolus.[113] A recent systematic review and meta-analysis (8 studies met inclusion criteria: 3 retrospective cohort and 5 case-control) of thromboembolic events in users of progestin-only contraception showed a modestly increased relative risk of thromboembolic events in injectable progestin users compared to nonhormonal contraceptive users (2.67, 95% CI 1.29 to 5.53).[114] However, studies of this type do not have the ability to adjust for important baseline medical conditions that affect both thrombosis risk and the decision to prescribe DMPA. The authors acknowledged the limited available published data including the potential confounding if medically higher-risk women are in the progestin-only contraceptive user group.[114]

Additional data supporting an absence of any important effect on thrombosis risk with progestin-only injectables come from a small prospective cohort study of healthy reproductive age women initiating DMPA or copper IUD. This study evaluated biomarkers related to coagulation pathways at baseline and 12 months after initiation of the contraceptive and found that women using DMPA had changes in biomarkers that would predict lower risk of VTE compared to women using copper IUD.[115] Clinically, given these overall reassuring data, we recommend routinely offering injectable progestin-only methods as an option for women with cardiovascular risk factors, including personal or family history of cardiovascular events following the MEC guidelines.

General Metabolism/Weight Gain

Weight gain is commonly reported by many DMPA users. Although several studies have found no weight increase in DMPA users,[116–118] the preponderance of studies demonstrates moderate increases in weight.[35,119–128] A retrospective cohort study of women continuously using IM DMPA, LNG IUS, or copper IUD for 10 years reported mean weight gains of 6.6 kg, 4.0 kg, and 4.9 kg, respectively ($p < 0.05$ for comparison to either IUD group).[120] In a prospective study that followed weight-matched new users of DMPA and copper IUDs during 1 year of use, DMPA users had a 1.9-kg increase in weight of which 1.6 kg was increased fat mass compared to no change in weight in IUD users.[121] With the SC method, an average weight gain of

1.5 kg was observed after 1 year and 4.5 kg after 3 years, changes that are comparable to the IM formulation.[70,129]

Specific individuals and certain ethnic groups may be more susceptible to weight gain. For example, significant weight gain has been reported in Navajo women using DMPA[122] and in black adolescents compared with white adolescents and obese adolescents compared to nonobese adolescents.[123,130] In a cohort comparison study of obese adolescents initiating use of DMPA, oral contraceptives, or no hormonal contraception, only those initiating DMPA gained significant weight (9.4 kg after 18 months).[130] In two prospective cohort studies, about 25% of adult women and 21% of adolescents initiating DMPA use experienced significant weight gain within 6 months, and these women and adolescents continued having significant weight gain with continued DMPA use.[124,125]

Since the available data suggest that women and adolescents who are susceptible to significant weight gain with DMPA can be identified soon after initiation, we recommend that patients initiating DMPA monitor their weight at home and contact the office or return for a visit if significant change is noticed. Clinics providing DMPA should use the first and second reinjection visits as an opportunity to evaluate weight changes objectively. One study found that women who gain excessive weight experience a 5% increase within 6 months.[124]

In addition to weight gain, some women initiating and using MPA-based injectables undergo significant metabolic changes, including increases in all parameters of serum lipids (total cholesterol, LDL, HDL, and triglycerides), Castelli index (I and II), and serum glucose.[131,132] With these metabolic changes, there is some evidence of increased risk of adverse health outcomes, including development of diabetes.[133,134] The impact of DMPA-induced weight gain on cardiovascular outcomes is less clear and warrants further study.[131,135,136]

Special Considerations

Unique Features

Injectable contraceptives are globally available. Largely due to relatively low commodity cost, no requirement for cold-chain storage, and limited clinical skills necessary for safe administration, injectable contraceptives have been among the most commonly available and widely used methods in resource-poor settings.

Injectable contraceptives do not require daily compliance from the user enabling ease of use and discretion, features that are amplified by needing no further action at the time of coitus and being undetectable by the sexual partner. Injectable contraceptives and LARC methods may be particularly appealing to women who prefer not to adhere to a frequent dosing schedule as is required by short-acting methods to maintain contraceptive efficacy. Despite widespread popularity of injectable contraceptives, difficulty in complying with clinic-based reinjection schedules presents challenges for users and contributes to high discontinuation.[137]

Cancer Risk

Overall, studies over several decades have not identified a substantial risk of cancer with DMPA use, and there may be a reduction in endometrial and ovarian cancer risk.[28,138] The WHO Collaborative Study of Neoplasia and Steroid Contraceptives was a large hospital-based case-control study that has provided extensive data about the impact of DMPA on risk of cancer, including breast, uterine, cervical, ovarian, and liver cancers.[138] DMPA use was associated with a protective effect against endometrial cancer, which was as strong as or stronger than that seen with oral contraceptives.[139] While the WHO found no association between DMPA use and risk of epithelial ovarian cancer,[140] another large case-control study found a significant, nearly 40% reduction in risk of epithelial ovarian cancer with DMPA use,[141] as did a study from South Africa.[142] Evidence of an association of DMPA use with invasive cervical cancer is mixed as the WHO found an association between DMPA use and risk of in situ cervical cancer,[143] but no evidence for an increased risk of invasive cervical cancer.[144,145] Independently, a separate study from South Africa reported an increased risk among current and recent users, but not among women who had discontinued use more than 10 years previously.[142] These mixed data suggest either confounding or a weak association. Studies evaluating DMPA use and risk of breast cancer are also not consistent, but generally suggest no overall increased risk.[28,146–150] Some studies suggest that current or recent users and longer-term users of DMPA may have an increased risk of breast cancer.[142,147–150] However, the Women's Contraceptive and Reproductive Experiences (CARE), a large study conducted by the Centers for Disease Control and Prevention, found no evidence of increased risk, including no evidence of increased risk in current or recent users, long-term users, or women who began use at a young age.[149] A recent systematic review of progestin use and breast cancer risk also found no association.[151] No associations were identified between DMPA use and liver cancer in a case-controlled study conducted by the World Health Organization.[152]

Sexually Transmitted Infection and HIV Risk

Use of injectable progestin-only contraceptives may be associated with an increased risk of sexually transmitted infections. Several prospective studies have reported an increased risk of cervical infection, particularly with chlamydia, in women using DMPA compared to women using combined oral contraceptive pills or women using nonhormonal contraception,[153,154] although other studies have not demonstrated any difference in risk.[155] A published systematic review concluded that the evidence linking hormonal contraception to increased risk of sexually transmitted infection remains limited with inadequate adjustment for confounding, lack of appropriate controls, and small sample sizes.[156] Historically, many studies aiming to link hormonal contraception and genital tract infections have relied heavily on self-reported sexual behavior and contraceptive use, and this has likely contributed to the mixed data available in the published literature.[157–159]

The published literature on use of injectable progestin-only contraceptives and HIV acquisition risk is also mixed. The most recent systematic review published in 2016 concluded that the preponderance of data suggest an increased risk of HIV, particularly in women using DMPA.[160] This review of the highest-quality available data prompted both the World Health Organization[161] and the Centers for Disease Control and Prevention[162] to update their respective Medical Eligibility Criteria (MEC) for use of injectable progestins by women at high risk of HIV, changing the risk category from 1 (no risk) to category 2 (benefits generally outweigh risks). This highlighted the concern of a possible increased risk for HIV acquisition among women using progestin-only injectable contraceptives, though it remained unclear whether this reflected a true biologic effect or was due to methodologic issues with the studies. The committee emphasized that women should not be denied DMPA because of concerns about this possible increased risk and that women considering DMPA should be advised about the possible risk and about available HIV prevention measures.[162]

To address methodologic concerns associated with available prior studies, a randomized clinical trial was conducted. The Evidence for Contraceptive Options and HIV Outcomes (ECHO) study enrolled over 7,800 women at 12 sites in Eswatini, Kenya, South Africa, and Zambia, and compared the relative risk of HIV acquisition among women randomized to use DMPA-IM, copper intrauterine device (Cu-IUD), or levonorgestrel (LNG) implant as contraception.[163,164]. The study was carefully conducted, had excellent retention and follow-up, and found no substantial difference in HIV risk among the three methods. The HIV seroconversion rates were high enough across all groups (4.19, 3.94, and 3.31/100 person-years in DMPA-IM, Cu-IUD, and LNG implant users, respectively) that the study had ample power to detect at least a 30% difference in incidence between methods.

While there are biologically plausible mechanisms and supporting in vitro data[165] by which DMPA use may increase HIV acquisition, such as alteration in mucosal architecture, HIV target cell densities/susceptibilities, or innate immune responses, the ECHO trial results do not support an increased risk.[163] More research is needed on understanding biologic and physiologic impacts of specific progestins[166] and mode of progestin administration[29,167] particularly for future development of safe and effective multipurpose prevention modalities[168] and for better integration of HIV and family planning services.[169]

Use in Special Populations

When is it safe to discontinue use of injectable contraception in perimenopausal women without risking pregnancy? Injectable progestin use in the later reproductive years can cause uncertainty in determining when menopause occurs given that amenorrhea is common, particularly in long-term users. While menopause can be assumed in the majority of women by age 55, it is possible that some women with a family history of late menopause and women with an absence of associated menopausal symptoms, such as hot flashes and sleep disturbances, may not have reached menopause by this age. Ultimately, stopping contraception when fertility is low (after age 50) is a personal decision, and the role of the clinician is to provide accurate information to support an informed choice. Measuring FSH levels is typically not helpful in this determination given the wide FSH fluctuations in perimenopause and the wide interindividual variation in FSH values with clinical menopause, with approximately 7% of women maintaining low FSH levels well into clinical menopause.[170] Two recent studies that evaluated FSH levels in perimenopausal women using DMPA IM suggest measuring FSH levels without interrupting DMPA use may enable diagnosis of probable menopause when at least two samples taken late in the injection cycle and at different times are evaluated.[61,62] Neither study sampled FSH at a time point later than the normal redosing period, which is greater than 3 months from last DMPA injection. Doing so would be a reasonable approach given suppression of ovulation continues beyond the labeled duration and the likelihood of diagnosing menopause would be enhanced since FSH should rise in a menopausal woman as DMPA levels fall. Given the wide fluctuations in FSH, we do not recommend routinely measuring FSH to diagnose menopause.

Medical Eligibility Criteria for Contraceptive Use Considerations

Progestin-only injectable contraceptive methods are appropriate for most women including those over age 35 who smoke and those with common or significant medical problems. Injectables are also appropriate for women with obesity, hypertension, depression, diabetes, HIV, headache disorders, uterine structural abnormalities, sickle cell anemia, structural heart disease, history of thromboembolism, and history of organ transplantation.[71,113,171] Indeed, DMPA use may be beneficial to women with some medical conditions, reducing frequency and intensity of sickle cell crises,[172–174] effectively treating pain associated with endometriosis,[175] and possibly reducing or eliminating menstrual migraines, though there is currently a lack of primary research evidence to support this frequently mentioned claim.

New Formulations

Substantial research over several decades has focused on developing new progestin-only injectables. These studies aim primarily to increase the duration of action to enable longer injection intervals, and to minimize the dose to decrease side effects as compared to DMPA and NET-EN.[176] Increasing the interval between injections has been shown to enhance adherence and continuation when compared to shorter injection intervals, improving the acceptability of the method.[176] Recent research on user preferences for new technologies reported that interest was highest for a longer-acting injectable among six new methods presented.[176,177] In the mid-1970s, a major initiative supported the synthesis and screening of hundreds of long-acting esters of norethindrone and LNG that could be formulated as 3- to 6-month injections.[5] Two LNG esters were evaluated in women (butanoate and cyclobutylcarboxylate) and LNG butanoate was selected to advance to further clinical testing.[47] Initial pharmacokinetic/pharmacodynamic studies showed a promising dose-dependent response and duration; however, this research was subsequently stalled for many years due to issues with formulation stability.[5] A recently completed phase I trial with a new LNG butanoate formulation also failed to achieve the desired pharmacokinetic profile prompting additional reformulation work.[178] Two current strategies under investigation will adapt existing DMPA formulations to extend the duration of action in order to achieve 6 months of contraceptive protection when given subcutaneously (Clinicaltrials.gov NCT02456584 and NCT02817464).

New Research on Alternative Delivery Formulations for Injectables

A variety of formulation change approaches are currently being explored that have potential to extend duration, including biodegradable polymers formulated as microspheres, porous silicon microparticles, biodegradable gels, and new suspension formulations of LNG, etonogestrel, and segesterone acetate (formally known as Nestorone®). All research activities are currently in preclinical and proof-of-concept stages, far from being commercially available.[176] The earlier formulations of microsphere-based products that advanced to clinical trials, including microspheres containing norethindrone,[179-181] were ultimately abandoned due to problems with scaling up the products.

Postpartum and Postabortion Use

Injectable progestin-only contraceptives can be safely used by breastfeeding women in the immediate postpartum period. The WHO Medical Eligibility Criteria rates injectable progestin-only method use in breastfeeding women less than 1 month postpartum as category 2, meaning that the benefits generally outweigh the risks.[113] There is no evidence that administration of injectable progestin-only contraception prior to hospital discharge following delivery impacts milk production or initiation or continuation of breastfeeding.[182,183] DMPA levels are similar in breast milk and serum,[184] yet no effects on infant growth and development have been observed in breastfed infants of women using progestin-only injectables.[182,185,186] Furthermore, in a careful study of male infants being breastfed by women treated with DMPA, no MPA metabolites could be detected in the infant's urine and no alterations could be observed in the infant levels of FSH, LH, testosterone, and cortisol.[45]

Injectable progestin-only contraceptives can also be safely used immediately following a complete spontaneous or induced abortion, including medical or surgical abortion.[187] The MEC lists injectable progestin-only contraception as category 1 (no risk) following abortion regardless of trimester and also in the setting of septic abortion.[113] In the interest of minimizing or eliminating the need for in-person follow-up following medical abortion, researchers have investigated the possibility of administering DMPA at the time of mifepristone and found an increased risk of medical abortion failure. In a pilot study of 20 women electing medical abortion and DMPA administration within 15 minutes of mifepristone administration, 15% had medical abortion failure at follow-up.[188] Furthermore, in a multinational randomized controlled trial of quick-start versus after-start, in which DMPA was administered with mifepristone or after medical abortion completion, respectively, ongoing pregnancy was 3.6% in the quick-start group compared with less than 1% in the after-start group.[189] Given these findings, we do not recommend routinely offering DMPA administration on the day of mifepristone administration; however, it can be administered as soon as 24 to 48 hours after mifepristone[190] without impacting medical abortion success, which may be beneficial for some women, including women who opt for self-administration of DMPA SC.

References

1. **United Nations, Department of Economic and Social Affairs, Population Division,** Estimates and Projections of Women of Reproductive Age Who Are Married or in a Union: 2018 Revision, 2018.

2. **United Nations, Department of Economic and Social Affairs, Population Division,** Trends in Contraceptive Use Worldwide 2015 (ST/ESA/SER.A/349), 2015.

3. **Daniels K, Daugherty J, Jones J, et al.,** Current contraceptive use and variation by selected characteristics among women aged 15-44: United States, 2011-2013, Natl Health Stat Report (86):1–14, 2015.

4. **Schwallie PC, Assenzo JR,** The effect of depo-medroxyprogesterone acetate on pituitary and ovarian function, and the return of fertility following its discontinuation: a review, Contraception 10:181–202, 1974.

5. **Benagiano G, d'Arcangues C, Harris Requejo J, et al.,** The special programme of research in human reproduction: forty years of activities to achieve reproductive health for all, Gynecol Obstet Invest 74:190–217, 2012.

6. **Mishell DR,** Pharmacokinetics of depot medroxyprogesterone acetate contraception, J Reprod Med 41:381–390, 1996.

7. **U.S. Food and Drug Administration (FDA),** New Drug Application No.: 020246.

8. **U.S. Food and Drug Administration (FDA),** Depo-SubQ Provera 104 (Medroxyprogesterone Acetate) Injectable Suspension New Drug Application No.: 021583, 2014.

9. **Burke HM, Chen M, Buluzi M, et al.,** Effect of self-administration versus provider-administered injection of subcutaneous depot medroxyprogesterone acetate on continuation rates in Malawi: a randomised controlled trial, Lancet Glob Health 6:e568–e578, 2018.

10. **Burke HM, Packer C, Buluzi M, et al.,** Client and provider experiences with self-administration of subcutaneous depot medroxyprogesterone acetate (DMPA-SC) in Malawi, Contraception 98:405–410, 2018.

11. **d'Arcangues C, Snow R,** Injectable contraceptives, In: Runnebaum B, Rabe T, eds. Fertility Control-Update and Trends, Springer-Verlag, Berlin, 1999, pp 121–149.

12. **Benagiano G, Diczfalusy E, Goldzieher JW, et al.,** Multinational comparative clinical evaluation of two long-acting injectable contraceptive steroids: norethisterone oenanthate and medroxyprogesterone acetate. 1. Use-effectiveness, Contraception 15:513–533, 1977.

13. **Benagiano G, Diczfalusy E, Diethelm P, et al.,** Multinational comparative clinical evaluation of two long-acting injectable contraceptive steroids: norethisterone oenanthate and medroxyprogesterone acetate: 2. Bleeding patterns and side effects, Contraception 17:395–406, 1978.

14. **Toppozada HK, Koetsawang S, Aimakhu VE, et al.,** Multinational comparative clinical trial of long-acting injectable contraceptives: norethisterone enanthate given in two dosage regimens and depot-medroxyprogesterone acetate. Final report, Contraception 28:1–20, 1983.

15. **Draper BH, Morroni C, Hoffman M, et al.,** Depot medroxyprogesterone

versus norethisterone oenanthate for long-acting progestogenic contraception, Cochrane Database Syst Rev (3):CD005214, 2006.

16. **Garza-Flores J, Cardenas S, Rodríguez V, et al.,** Return to ovulation following the use of long-acting injectable contraceptives: a comparative study, Contraception 31:361–366, 1985.

17. **ICMR National Programme of Research in Human Reproduction: Task Force on Hormonal Contraception,** Return of fertility following discontinuation of an injectable contraceptive–Norethisterone oenanthate (NET EN) 200 mg dose, Contraception 34:573–582, 1986.

18. **South Africa, Department of Health, Statistics South Africa,** South Africa demographic and health survey, 2016: key indicators report, 2017.

19. **World Health Organization,** Facts about once-a-month injectable contraceptives: memorandum from a WHO meeting, Bull World Health Organ 71:677–689, 1993.

20. **Gallo MF, Grimes DA, Lopez LM, et al.,** Combination injectable contraceptives for contraception, Cochrane Database Syst Rev (3):CD004568, 2013.

21. **Kaunitz AM, Darney PD, Ross D, et al.,** Subcutaneous DMPA vs. intramuscular DMPA: a 2-year randomized study of contraceptive efficacy and bone mineral density, Contraception 80:7–17, 2009.

22. **Food and Drug Administration (FDA),** Package insert Nexplanon (etonogestrel implant), 2017.

23. **U.S. Food and Drug Administration (FDA),** Abbreviated New Drug Application No.: 76-533.

24. **Food and Drug Administration (FDA),** Package insert for DEPO-PROVERA CI (medroxyprogesterone acetate) injectable suspension, for intramuscular use, 2016.

25. **Halpern V, Combes SL, Dorflinger LJ, et al.,** Pharmacokinetics of subcutaneous depot medroxyprogesterone acetate injected in the upper arm, Contraception 89:31–35, 2014.

26. **Jain J, Dutton C, Nicosia A, et al.,** Pharmacokinetics, ovulation suppression and return to ovulation following a lower dose subcutaneous formulation of Depo-Provera, Contraception 70:11–18, 2004.

27. **Toh YC, Jain J, Rahimy MH, et al.,** Suppression of ovulation by a new subcutaneous depot medroxyprogesterone acetate (104 mg/0.65 mL) contraceptive formulation in Asian women, Clin Ther 26:1845–1854, 2004.

28. **Kaunitz AM,** Depot medroxyprogesterone acetate for contraception, UpToDate, 2018. https://www.uptodate.com/contents/depot-medroxyprogesterone-acetate-for-contraception

29. **Polis CB, Achilles SL, Hel Z, et al.,** Is a lower-dose, subcutaneous contraceptive injectable containing depot medroxy-progesterone acetate likely to impact women's risk of HIV? Contraception 97:191–197, 2018.

30. **Food and Drug Administration (FDA),** Package Insert for depo-subQ provera 104™ medroxyprogesterone acetate injectable suspension 104 mg/0.65 mL, 2017.

31. **Shelton JD, Halpern V,** Subcutaneous DMPA: a better lower dose approach, Contraception 89:341–343, 2014.

32. **Mathrubutham M, Fotherby K,** Medroxyprogesterone acetate in human serum, J Steroid Biochem 14:783–786, 1981.

33. **Smit J, Botha J, McFadyen L, et al.,** Serum medroxyprogesterone acetate levels in new and repeat users of depot medroxyprogesterone acetate at the end of the dosing interval, Contraception 69:3–7, 2004.

34. **Nanda K, Amaral E, Hays M, et al.,** Pharmacokinetic interactions between depot medroxyprogesterone acetate and combination antiretroviral therapy, Fertil Steril 90:965–971, 2008.

35. **Bonny AE, Lange HL, Rogers LK, et al.,** A pilot study of depot medroxy-progesterone acetate pharmacokinetics and weight gain in adolescent females, Contraception 89:357–360, 2014.

36. **Ortiz A, Hirol M, Stanczyk FZ, et al.,** Serum medroxyprogesterone acetate (MPA) concentrations and ovarian function following intramuscular injection of depo-MPA, J Clin Endocrinol Metab 44:32–38, 1977.

37. **Jeppsson S, Gershagen S, Johansson ED, et al.,** Plasma levels of medroxyprogesterone acetate (MPA), sex-hormone binding globulin, gonadal steroids, gonadotrophins and prolactin in women during long-term use of depo-MPA (Depo-Provera) as a contraceptive agent,

Acta Endocrinol (Copenh) 99:339–343, 1982.

38. **Fotherby K, Saxena BN, Shrimanker K, et al.,** A preliminary pharmacokinetic and pharmacodynamic evaluation of depot-medroxyprogesterone acetate and norethisterone oenanthate, Fertil Steril 34:131–139, 1980.

39. **Kirton KT, Cornette JC,** Return of ovulatory cyclicity following an intramuscular injection of medroxyprogesterone acetate (Provera), Contraception 10:39–45, 1974.

40. **Koetsawang S,** Injected long—acting medroxyprogesterone acetate. Effect on human lactation and concentrations in milk, J Med Assoc Thai 60:57–60, 1977.

41. **Shrimanker K, Saxena BN, Fotherby K,** A radioimmunoassay for serum medroxyprogesterone acetate, J Steroid Biochem 9:359–363, 1978.

42. **Fotherby K, Koetsawang S, Mathrubutham M,** Pharmacokinetic study of different doses of Depo Provera, Contraception 22:527–536, 1980.

43. **Fotherby K, Koetsawang S,** Metabolism of injectable formulations of contraceptive steroids in obese and thin women, Contraception 26:51–58, 1982.

44. **Fang S, Sun D, Jiang H, et al.,** Concentration changes of medroxyprogesterone acetate in serum and milk in lactating woman who used Depo Geston®, J Reprod Contracept 15:157–162, 2004.

45. **Virutamasen P, Leepipatpaiboon S, Kriengsinyot R, et al.,** Pharmacodynamic effects of depot-medroxyprogesterone acetate (DMPA) administered to lactating women on their male infants, Contraception 54:153–157, 1996.

46. **Jeppsson S, Johansson JS,** Medroxyprogesterone acetate, estradiol, FSH and LH in peripheral blood after intramuscular administration of Depo-ProveraR to women, Contraception 14:461–469, 1976.

47. **Garza-Flores J, Hall PE, Perez-Palacios G,** Long-acting hormonal contraceptives for women, J Steroid Biochem Mol Biol 40:697–704, 1991.

48. **Augustine MS, Bonny AE, Rogers LK,** Medroxyprogesterone acetate and progesterone measurement in human serum: assessments of contraceptive efficacy, J Anal Bioanal Tech S5:005, 2014. doi: 10.4172/2155-9872.S5-005.

49. **Blue SW, Winchell AJ, Kaucher AV, et al.,** Simultaneous quantitation of multiple contraceptive hormones in human serum by LC–MS/MS, Contraception 97:363–369, 2018.

50. **Callahan R, Stanczyk F, Taylor D, et al.,** Measuring total plasma Levonorgestrel (LNG) levels among users of contraceptive implants: a comparison of radioimmunoassay and mass spectrometry methods, Fertility Control Club, Barcelona, Spain, 2015. http://www.comtecmed.com/FCC/2015/Uploads/Editor/PDF/2.pdf.

51. **Rahimy MH, Ryan KK, Hopkins NK,** Lunelle monthly contraceptive injection (medroxyprogesterone acetate and estradiol cypionate injectable suspension): steady-state pharmacokinetics of MPA and E2 in surgically sterile women, Contraception 60:209–214, 1999.

52. **Wang Y, Zhang T, Zhao H, et al.,** Measurement of serum progesterone by isotope dilution liquid chromatography tandem mass spectrometry: a candidate reference method and its application to evaluating immunoassays, Anal Bioanal Chem 411:2363–2371, 2019. doi: 10.1007/s00216-019-01676-7.

53. **Thurman A, Kimble T, Hall P, et al.,** Medroxyprogesterone acetate and estradiol cypionate injectable suspension (Cyclofem) monthly contraceptive injection: steady-state pharmacokinetics, Contraception 87:738–743, 2013.

54. **Recio R, Garza-Flores J, Schiavon R, et al.,** Pharmacodynamic assessment of dihydroxyprogesterone acetophenide plus estradiol enanthate as a monthly injectable contraceptive, Contraception 33:579–589, 1986.

55. **Schiavon R, Benavides S, Oropeza G, et al.,** Serum estrogens and ovulation return in chronic users of a once-a-month injectable contraceptive, Contraception 37:591–598, 1988.

56. **Bassol S, Garza-Flores J,** Review of ovulation return upon discontinuation of once-a-month injectable contraceptives, Contraception 49:441–453, 1994.

57. **Mishell DR,** Effect of 6-alpha-methyl-17-alpha-hydroxyprogesterone on urinary excretion of luteinizing hormone, Am J Obstet Gynecol 99:86–90, 1967.

58. **Fraser IS, Weisberg E,** A comprehensive review of injectable contraception with special emphasis on depot medroxyprogesterone acetate, Med J Aust 1:3–19, 1981.

59. **Mishell DR, Kharma KM, Thorneycroft IH, et al.,** Estrogenic activity in women receiving an injectable progestogen for contraception, Am J Obstet Gynecol 113:372–376, 1972.

60. **Miller L, Patton DL, Meier A, et al.,** Depomedroxyprogesterone-induced hypoestrogenism and changes in vaginal flora and epithelium, Obstet Gynecol 96:431–439, 2000.

61. **Beksinska ME, Smit JA, Kleinschmidt I, et al.,** Detection of raised FSH levels among older women using depomedroxyprogesterone acetate and norethisterone enanthate, Contraception 68:339–343, 2003.

62. **Juliato CT, Fernandes A, Marchi NM, et al.,** Usefulness of FSH measurements for determining menopause in long-term users of depot medroxyprogesterone acetate over 40 years of age, Contraception 76:282–286, 2007.

63. **Neary M, Lamorde M, Olagunju A, et al.,** The effect of gene variants on levonorgestrel pharmacokinetics when combined with antiretroviral therapy containing efavirenz or nevirapine, Clin Pharmacol Ther 102:529–536, 2017.

64. **Kapp N, Gaffield ME,** Initiation of progestogen-only injectables on different days of the menstrual cycle and its effect on contraceptive effectiveness and compliance: a systematic review, Contraception 87:576–582, 2013.

65. **Lestishock L, Pariseau C, Rooholamini S, et al.,** Anaphylaxis from depot medroxyprogesterone acetate in an adolescent girl, Obstet Gynecol 118:443–445, 2011.

66. **Selo-Ojeme DO, Tillisi A, Welch CC,** Anaphylaxis from medroxyprogesterone acetate, Obstet Gynecol 103:1045–1046, 2004.

67. **Gardner JM, Mishell DR,** Analysis of bleeding patterns and resumption of fertility following discontinuation of a long acting injectable contraceptive, Fertil Steril 21:286–291, 1970.

68. **Winner B, Peipert JF, Zhao Q, et al.,** Effectiveness of long-acting reversible contraception, N Engl J Med 366:1998–2007, 2012.

69. **Said S, Omar K, Koetsawang S, et al.,** A multicentred phase III comparative clinical trial of depot-medroxyprogesterone acetate given three-monthly at doses of 100 mg or 150 mg: 1. Contraceptive efficacy and side effects. World Health Organization Task Force on Long-Acting Systemic Agents for Fertility Regulation. Special Programme of Research, Development and Research Training in Human Reproduction, Contraception 34:223–235, 1986.

70. **Jain J, Jakimiuk AJ, Bode FR, et al.,** Contraceptive efficacy and safety of DMPA-SC, Contraception 70:269–275, 2004.

71. **Lopez LM, Bernholc A, Chen M, et al.,** Hormonal contraceptives for contraception in overweight or obese women, Cochrane Database Syst Rev (8):CD008452, 2016.

72. **Robinson JA, Jamshidi R, Burke AE,** Contraception for the HIV-positive woman: a review of interactions between hormonal contraception and antiretroviral therapy, Infect Dis Obstet Gynecol 2012:890160, 2012.

73. **Dutton C, Foldvary-Schaefer N,** Contraception in women with epilepsy: pharmacokinetic interactions, contraceptive options, and management, Int Rev Neurobiol 83:113–134, 2008.

74. **Nanda K, Stuart GS, Robinson J, et al.,** Drug interactions between hormonal contraceptives and antiretrovirals, AIDS 31:917–952, 2017.

75. **Callahan R, Yacobson I, Halpern V, et al.,** Ectopic pregnancy with use of progestin-only injectables and contraceptive implants: a systematic review, Contraception 92:514–522, 2015.

76. **Curtis KM,** U.S. selected practice recommendations for contraceptive use, 2016, MMWR Recomm Rep 65:1–66, 2016.

77. **Petta CA, Faúndes A, Dunson TR, et al.,** Timing of onset of contraceptive effectiveness in Depo-Provera users. II. Effects on ovarian function, Fertil Steril 70:817–820, 1998.

321

78. **Steinauer JE, Sokoloff A, Roberts EM, et al.,** Immediate versus delayed initiation of the contraceptive patch after abortion: a randomized trial, Contraception 89:42–47, 2014.

79. **Nelson AL, Katz T,** Initiation and continuation rates seen in 2-year experience with same day injections of DMPA, Contraception 75:84–87, 2007.

80. **Edwards SM, Zieman M, Jones K, et al.,** Initiation of oral contraceptives—start now! J Adolesc Health 43:432–436, 2008.

81. **Stechna S, Mravcak S, Schultz P, et al.,** The Quick Start Contraception Initiation Method during the 6-week postpartum visit: an efficacious way to improve contraception in Federally Qualified Health Centers, Contraception 88:160–163, 2013.

82. **Balkus J, Miller L,** Same-day administration of depot-medroxyprogesterone acetate injection: a retrospective chart review, Contraception 71:395–398, 2005.

83. **Pardthaisong T, Gray RH,** In utero exposure to steroid contraceptives and outcome of pregnancy, Am J Epidemiol 134:795–803, 1991.

84. **Yilmaz D, Khorshid L, Dedeoğlu Y,** The effect of the Z-Track technique on pain and drug leakage in intramuscular injections, Clin Nurse Spec 30:E7–E12, 2016.

85. **Paulen ME, Curtis KM,** When can a woman have repeat progestogen-only injectables—depot medroxyprogesterone acetate or norethisterone enanthate? Contraception 80:391–408, 2009.

86. **Steiner MJ, Kwok C, Stanback J, et al.,** Injectable contraception: what should the longest interval be for reinjections? Contraception 77:410–414, 2008.

87. **O'Neil-Callahan M, Peipert JF, Zhao Q, et al.,** Twenty-four-month continuation of reversible contraception, Obstet Gynecol 122:1083–1091, 2013.

88. **Hubacher D, Spector H, Monteith C, et al.,** Long-acting reversible contraceptive acceptability and unintended pregnancy among women presenting for short-acting methods: a randomized patient preference trial, Am J Obstet Gynecol 216:101–109, 2017.

89. **Reeves MF, Zhao Q, Secura GM, et al.,** Risk of unintended pregnancy based on intended compared to actual contraceptive use, Am J Obstet Gynecol 215:71.e1–71.e6, 2016.

90. **Cover J, Namagembe A, Tumusiime J, et al.,** Continuation of injectable contraception when self-injected v. administered by a facility-based health worker: a non-randomized, prospective cohort study in Uganda, Contraception 98:383–388, 2018.

91. **Kohn JE, Simons HR, Della Badia L, et al.,** Increased 1-year continuation of DMPA among women randomized to self-administration: results from a randomized controlled trial at Planned Parenthood, Contraception 97:198–204, 2018.

92. **Nelson AL, Westhoff C, Schnare SM,** Real-world patterns of prescription refills for branded hormonal contraceptives: a reflection of contraceptive discontinuation, Obstet Gynecol 112:782–787, 2008.

93. **Polaneczky M, Guarnaccia M, Alon J, et al.,** Early experience with the contraceptive use of depot medroxyprogesterone acetate in an inner-city clinic population, Fam Plann Perspect 28:174–178, 1996.

94. **Adeyemi AS, Adekanle DA,** Progestogen-only injectable contraceptive: experience of women in Osogbo, southwestern Nigeria, Ann Afr Med 11:27–31, 2012.

95. **Schreiber CA, Teal SB, Blumenthal PD, et al.,** Bleeding patterns for the Liletta® levonorgestrel 52 mg intrauterine system, Eur J Contracept Reprod Health Care 23:116–120, 2018.

96. **Food and Drug Administration (FDA),** Package insert for Mirena® (levonorgestrel-releasing intrauterine system), 2017.

97. **Arias RD, Jain JK, Brucker C, et al.,** Changes in bleeding patterns with depot medroxyprogesterone acetate subcutaneous injection 104 mg, Contraception 74:234–238, 2006.

98. **Aktun H, Moroy P, Cakmak P, et al.,** Depo-Provera: use of a long-acting progestin injectable contraceptive in Turkish women, Contraception 72:24–27, 2005.

99. **Nanda K, Morrison CS, Kwok C, et al.,** Discontinuation of oral contraceptives and depot medroxyprogesterone acetate among women with and without HIV in Uganda, Zimbabwe and Thailand, Contraception 83:542–548, 2011.

100. **World Health Organization, Reproductive Health and Research, K4Health,** Family Planning: A Global Handbook For Providers: Evidence-Based Guidance Developed Through Worldwide Collaboration, World Health Organization, Department of Reproductive Health and Research; John Hopkins Bloomberg School of Public Health, Center for Communication programs, Knowledge for Health Project, Geneva, 2018.

101. **Dehlendorf C, Henderson JT, Vittinghoff E, et al.,** Association of the quality of interpersonal care during family planning counseling with contraceptive use, Am J Obstet Gynecol 215:78. e1–78.e9, 2016.

102. **Nelson AL,** Counseling issues and management of side effects for women using depot medroxyprogesterone acetate contraception, J Reprod Med 41:391–400, 1996.

103. **Hubacher D, Lopez L, Steiner MJ, et al.,** Menstrual pattern changes from levonorgestrel subdermal implants and DMPA: systematic review and evidence-based comparisons, Contraception 80:113–118, 2009.

104. **Sereepapong W, Chotnopparatpattara P, Taneepanichskul S, et al.,** Endometrial progesterone and estrogen receptors and bleeding disturbances in depot medroxyprogesterone acetate users, Hum Reprod 19:547–552, 2004.

105. **Said S, Sadek W, Rocca M, et al.,** Clinical evaluation of the therapeutic effectiveness of ethinyl oestradiol and oestrone sulphate on prolonged bleeding in women using depot medroxyprogesterone acetate for contraception. World Health Organization, Special Programme of Research, Development and Research Training in Human Reproduction, Task Force on Long-acting Systemic Agents for Fertility Regulation, Hum Reprod 11:1–13, 1996.

106. **Tantiwattanakul P, Taneepanichskul S,** Effect of mefenamic acid on controlling irregular uterine bleeding in DMPA users, Contraception 70:277–279, 2004.

107. **Senthong A-J, Taneepanichskul S,** The effect of tranexamic acid for treatment irregular uterine bleeding secondary to DMPA use, J Med Assoc Thai 92: 461–465, 2009.

108. **Abdel-Aleem H, Shaaban OM, Abdel-Aleem MA, et al.,** Doxycycline in the treatment of bleeding with DMPA: a double-blinded randomized controlled trial, Contraception 86:224–230, 2012.

109. **Abdel-Aleem H, d'Arcangues C, Vogelsong KM, et al.,** Treatment of vaginal bleeding irregularities induced by progestin only contraceptives, Cochrane Database Syst Rev (7):CD003449, 2013.

110. **Kaunitz AM, Grimes DA,** Removing the black box warning for depot medroxyprogesterone acetate, Contraception 84:212–213, 2011.

111. **Kaunitz AM, Arias R, McClung M,** Bone density recovery after depot medroxyprogesterone acetate injectable contraception use, Contraception 77:67–76, 2008.

112. **Viola AS, Castro S, Marchi NM, et al.,** Long-term assessment of forearm bone mineral density in postmenopausal former users of depot medroxyprogesterone acetate, Contraception 84:122–127, 2011.

113. **Centers for Disease Control and Prevention,** U.S. medical eligibility criteria for contraceptive use, 2016, MMWR Morb Mortal Wkly Rep 65:1–104, 2016.

114. **Mantha S, Karp R, Raghavan V, et al.,** Assessing the risk of venous thromboembolic events in women taking progestin-only contraception: a meta-analysis, BMJ 345:e4944, 2012.

115. **Melhado-Kimura V, Bizzacchi JMA, Quaino SKP, et al.,** Effect of the injectable contraceptive depot-medroxyprogesterone acetate on coagulation parameters in new users, J Obstet Gynaecol Res 43:1054–1060, 2017.

116. **Mainwaring R, Hales HA, Stevenson K, et al.,** Metabolic parameter, bleeding, and weight changes in U.S. women using progestin only contraceptives, Contraception 51:149–153, 1995.

117. **Taneepanichskul S, Reinprayoon D, Jaisamrarn U,** Effects of DMPA on weight and blood pressure in long-term acceptors, Contraception 59:301–303, 1999.

118. **Silva Dos Santos PN, de Souza AL, Batista GA, et al.,** Binge eating and biochemical markers of appetite in new users of the contraceptive depot medroxyprogesterone acetate, Arch Gynecol Obstet 294:1331–1336, 2016.

119. **Vickery Z, Madden T, Zhao Q, et al.,** Weight change at 12 months in users of three progestin-only contraceptive methods, Contraception 88:503–508, 2013.

120. **Modesto W, de Nazaré Silva dos Santos P, Correia VM, et al.,** Weight variation in users of depot-medroxyprogesterone acetate, the levonorgestrel-releasing intrauterine system and a copper intrauterine device for up to ten years of use, Eur J Contracept Reprod Health Care 20:57–63, 2015.

121. **Dal'Ava N, Bahamondes L, Bahamondes MV, et al.,** Body weight and body composition of depot medroxyprogesterone acetate users, Contraception 90:182–187, 2014.

122. **Espey E, Steinhart J, Ogburn T, et al.,** Depo-provera associated with weight gain in Navajo women, Contraception 62:55–58, 2000.

123. **Bonny AE, Britto MT, Huang B, et al.,** Weight gain, adiposity, and eating behaviors among adolescent females on depot medroxyprogesterone acetate (DMPA), J Pediatr Adolesc Gynecol 17:109–115, 2004.

124. **Le Y-CL, Rahman M, Berenson AB,** Early weight gain predicting later weight gain among depot medroxyprogesterone acetate users, Obstet Gynecol 114:279–284, 2009.

125. **Bonny AE, Secic M, Cromer B,** Early weight gain related to later weight gain in adolescents on depot medroxyprogesterone acetate, Obstet Gynecol 117:793–797, 2011.

126. **Moore LL, Valuck R, McDougall C, et al.,** A comparative study of one-year weight gain among users of medroxyprogesterone acetate, levonorgestrel implants, and oral contraceptives, Contraception 52:215–219, 1995.

127. **Lange HLH, Belury MA, Secic M, et al.,** Dietary intake and weight gain among adolescents on depot medroxyprogesterone acetate, J Pediatr Adolesc Gynecol 28:139–143, 2015.

128. **Silva P, Qadir S, Fernandes A, et al.,** Dietary intake and eating behavior in depot medroxyprogesterone acetate users: a systematic review, Braz J Med Biol Res 51:e7575, 2018.

129. **Westhoff C, Jain JK, Milsom I, et al.,** Changes in weight with depot medroxyprogesterone acetate subcutaneous injection 104 mg/0.65 mL, Contraception 75:261–267, 2007.

130. **Bonny AE, Ziegler J, Harvey R, et al.,** Weight gain in obese and nonobese adolescent girls initiating depot medroxyprogesterone, oral contraceptive pills, or no hormonal contraceptive method, Arch Pediatr Adolesc Med 160:40–45, 2006.

131. **Dilshad H, Yousuf RI, Shoaib MH, et al.,** Cardiovascular disease risk associated with the long-term use of depot medroxyprogesterone acetate, Am J Med Sci 352:487–492, 2016.

132. **Dilshad H, Ismail R, Naveed S, et al.,** Effect of hormonal contraceptives on serum lipids: a prospective study, Pak J Pharm Sci 29:1379–1382, 2016.

133. **Kim C, Seidel KW, Begier EA, et al.,** Diabetes and depot medroxyprogesterone contraception in Navajo women, Arch Intern Med 161:1766–1771, 2001.

134. **Xiang AH, Kawakubo M, Buchanan TA, et al.,** A longitudinal study of lipids and blood pressure in relation to method of contraception in Latino women with prior gestational diabetes mellitus, Diabetes Care 30:1952–1958, 2007.

135. **Cursino K, de Lima GA, de Nazaré Silva Dos Santos P, et al.,** Subclinical cardiovascular disease parameters after one year in new users of depot medroxyprogesterone acetate compared to copper-IUD, Eur J Contracept Reprod Health Care 23:1–6, 2018.

136. **Batista GA, Souza AL Marin DM, et al.,** Body composition, resting energy expenditure and inflammatory markers: impact in users of depot medroxyprogesterone acetate after 12 months follow-up, Arch Endocrinol Metab 61:70–75, 2017.

137. **Baumgartner JN, Morroni C, Mlobeli RD, et al.,** Timeliness of contraceptive reinjections in South Africa and its relation to unintentional discontinuation, Int Fam Plan Perspect 33:66–74, 2007.

138. **Skegg DC,** Safety and efficacy of fertility-regulating methods: a decade of research, Bull World Health Organ 77:713–721, 1999.

139. **The WHO Collaborative Study of Neoplasia and Steroid Contraceptives,** Depot-medroxyprogesterone acetate (DMPA) and risk of endometrial cancer, Int J Cancer 49:186–190, 1991.

140. The WHO Collaborative Study of Neoplasia and Steroid Contraceptives, Depot-medroxyprogesterone acetate (DMPA) and risk of epithelial ovarian cancer, Int J Cancer 49:191–195, 1991.
141. Wilailak S, Vipupinyo C, Suraseranivong V, et al., Depot medroxyprogesterone acetate and epithelial ovarian cancer: a multicentre case-control study, BJOG 119:672–677, 2012.
142. Urban M, Banks E, Egger S, et al., Injectable and oral contraceptive use and cancers of the breast, cervix, ovary, and endometrium in black South African women: case-control study, PLoS Med 9:e1001182, 2012.
143. Thomas DB, Ye Z, Ray RM, Cervical carcinoma in situ and use of depot-medroxyprogesterone acetate (DMPA). WHO Collaborative Study of Neoplasia and Steroid Contraceptives, Contraception 51:25–31, 1995.
144. Thomas DB, Ray RM, Depot-medroxyprogesterone acetate (DMPA) and risk of invasive adenocarcinomas and adenosquamous carcinomas of the uterine cervix. WHO Collaborative Study of Neoplasia and Steroid Contraceptives, Contraception 52:307–312, 1995.
145. The WHO Collaborative Study of Neoplasia and Steroid Contraceptives, Depot-medroxyprogesterone acetate (DMPA) and risk of invasive squamous cell cervical cancer, Contraception 45:299–312, 1992.
146. WHO Collaborative Study of Neoplasia and Steroid Contraceptives, Breast cancer and depot-medroxyprogesterone acetate: a multinational study, Lancet 338:833–838, 1991.
147. Paul C, Skegg DC, Spears GF, Depot medroxyprogesterone (Depo-Provera) and risk of breast cancer, BMJ 299:759–762, 1989.
148. Shapiro S, Rosenberg L, Hoffman M, et al., Risk of breast cancer in relation to the use of injectable progestogen contraceptives and combined estrogen/progestogen contraceptives, Am J Epidemiol 151:396–403, 2000.
149. Strom BL, Berlin JA, Weber AL, et al., Absence of an effect of injectable and implantable progestin-only contraceptives on subsequent risk of breast cancer, Contraception 69:353–360, 2004.
150. Li CI, Beaber EF, Tang MTC, et al., Effect of depo-medroxyprogesterone acetate on breast cancer risk among women 20 to 44 years of age, Cancer Res 72:2028–2035, 2012.
151. Samson M, Porter N, Orekoya O, et al., Progestin and breast cancer risk: a systematic review, Breast Cancer Res Treat 155:3–12, 2016.
152. Mati JG, Kenya P, Kungu A, et al., Depot-medroxyprogesterone acetate (DMPA) and risk of liver cancer. The WHO Collaborative Study of Neoplasia and Steroid Contraceptives, Int J Cancer 49:182–185, 1991.
153. Morrison CS, Bright P, Wong EL, et al., Hormonal contraceptive use, cervical ectopy, and the acquisition of cervical infections, Sex Transm Dis 31:561–567, 2004.
154. Baeten JM, Nyange PM, Richardson BA, et al., Hormonal contraception and risk of sexually transmitted disease acquisition: results from a prospective study, Am J Obstet Gynecol 185:380–385, 2001.
155. Romer A, Shew ML, Ofner S, et al., Depot medroxyprogesterone acetate use is not associated with risk of incident sexually transmitted infections among adolescent women, J Adolesc Health 52:83–88, 2013.
156. Mohllajee AP, Curtis KM, Martins SL, et al., Hormonal contraceptive use and risk of sexually transmitted infections: a systematic review, Contraception 73:154–165, 2006.
157. Achilles SL, Mhlanga FG, Musara P, et al., Misreporting of contraceptive hormone use in clinical research participants, Contraception 97:346–353, 2018.
158. Pyra M, Lingappa JR, Heffron R, et al., Concordance of self-reported hormonal contraceptive use and presence of exogenous hormones in serum among African women, Contraception 97:357–362, 2018.
159. Bartz D, Maurer R, Kremen J, et al., High-risk sexual behaviors while on depot medroxyprogesterone acetate as compared to oral contraception, Contracept Reprod Med 2:8, 2017.
160. Polis CB, Curtis KM, Hannaford PC, et al., An updated systematic review of epidemiological evidence on hormonal contraceptive methods and HIV

325

acquisition in women, AIDS 30: 2665–2683, 2016.

161. **World Health Organization,** Hormonal contraceptive eligibility for women at high risk of HIV. Guidance Statement: Recommendations concerning the use of hormonal contraceptive methods by women at high risk of HIV, 2017.

162. **Tepper NK, Krashin JW, Curtis KM, et al.,** Update to CDC's U.S. Medical eligibility criteria for contraceptive use, 2016: revised recommendations for the use of hormonal contraception among women at high risk for HIV infection, MMWR Morb Mortal Wkly Rep 66:990–994, 2017.

163. **Ahmed K, Baeten JM, Beksinska M, Bekker LG, Bukusi EA, Donnell D, Gichangi PB, et al.,** HIV incidence among women using intramuscular depot medroxyprogesterone acetate, a copper intrauterine device, or a levonorgestrel implant for contraception: a randomised, multicentre, open-label trial. Lancet, 2019. doi: 10.1016/S0140-6736(19)31288-7.

164. **Hofmeyr GJ, Morrison CS, Baeten JM, et al.,** Rationale and design of a multicenter, open-label, randomised clinical trial comparing HIV incidence and contraceptive benefits in women using three commonly-used contraceptive methods (the ECHO study), Gates Open Res 1:17, 2017.

165. **Hapgood JP, Kaushic C, Hel Z,** Hormonal contraception and HIV-1 acquisition: biological mechanisms, Endocr Rev 39:36–78, 2018.

166. **Achilles SL, Hillier SL,** The complexity of contraceptives: understanding their impact on genital immune cells and vaginal microbiota, AIDS 27:S5–S15, 2013.

167. **Schivone G, Dorflinger L, Halpern V,** Injectable contraception: updates and innovation, Curr Opin Obstet Gynecol 28:504–509, 2016.

168. **Polis CB, Phillips SJ, Hillier SL, et al.,** Levonorgestrel in contraceptives and multipurpose prevention technologies: does this progestin increase HIV risk or interact with antiretrovirals? AIDS 30:2571–2576, 2016.

169. **Riley HEM, Steyn PS, Achilles SL, et al.,** Hormonal contraceptive methods and HIV: research gaps and programmatic priorities, Contraception 96:67–71, 2017.

170. **El Khoudary SR, Santoro N, Chen H-Y, et al.,** Trajectories of estradiol and follicle-stimulating hormone over the menopause transition and early markers of atherosclerosis after menopause, Eur J Prev Cardiol 23:694–703, 2016.

171. **Worly BL, Gur TL, Schaffir J,** The relationship between progestin hormonal contraception and depression: a systematic review, Contraception 97:478–489, 2018.

172. **de Abood M, de Castillo Z, Guerrero F, et al.,** Effect of Depo-Provera or Microgynon on the painful crises of sickle cell anemia patients, Contraception 56:313–316, 1997.

173. **De Ceulaer K, Gruber C, Hayes R, et al.,** Medroxyprogesterone acetate and homozygous sickle-cell disease, Lancet 2:229–231, 1982.

174. **Bahamondes L, Valeria Bahamondes M, Shulman LP,** Non-contraceptive benefits of hormonal and intrauterine reversible contraceptive methods, Hum Reprod Update 21:640–651, 2015.

175. **Barra F, Scala C, Ferrero S,** Current understanding on pharmacokinetics, clinical efficacy and safety of progestins for treating pain associated with endometriosis, Expert Opin Drug Metab Toxicol 14:399–415, 2018.

176. **Halpern V, Stalter RM, Owen DH, et al.,** Towards the development of a longer-acting injectable contraceptive: past research and current trends, Contraception 92:3–9, 2015.

177. **Callahan R, Mackenzie A, Brunie A,** User preferences for new long-acting contraceptive technologies, Contraception 96:295–296, 2017.

178. **Edelman AB, Cherala G, Li H, et al.,** Levonorgestrel butanoate intramuscular injection does not reliably suppress ovulation for 90 days in obese and normal-BMI women: a pilot study, Contraception 95:55–58, 2017.

179. **Rivera R, Alvarado G, Flores C, et al.,** Norethisterone contraceptive microspheres, J Steroid Biochem 27:1003–1007, 1987.

180. **Grubb GS, Welch JD, Cole L, et al.,** A comparative evaluation of the safety and

contraceptive effectiveness of 65 mg and 100 mg of 90-day norethindrone (NET) injectable microspheres: a multicenter study, Fertil Steril 51:803–810, 1989.

181. Singh M, Saxena BB, Singh R, et al., Contraceptive efficacy of norethindrone encapsulated in injectable biodegradable poly-dl-lactide-co-glycolide microspheres (NET-90): phase III clinical study, Adv Contracept 13:1–11, 1997.

182. Phillips SJ, Tepper NK, Kapp N, et al., Progestogen-only contraceptive use among breastfeeding women: a systematic review, Contraception 94:226–252, 2016.

183. Chen BA, Haddad LB, Achilles SL, et al., Effect of timing of postpartum depot medroxyprogesterone acetate initiation on breastfeeding continuation and contraceptive use: a randomized trial, Contraception 96:278–279, 2017.

184. Saxena BN, Shrimanker K, Grudzinskas JG, Levels of contraceptive steroids in breast milk and plasma of lactating women, Contraception 16:605–613, 1977.

185. Jimenez J, Ochoa M, Soler MP, et al., Long-term follow-up of children breast-fed by mothers receiving depot-medroxyprogesterone acetate, Contraception 30:523–533, 1984.

186. Pardthaisong T, Yenchit C, Gray R, The long-term growth and development of children exposed to Depo-Provera during pregnancy or lactation, Contraception 45:313–324, 1992.

187. Roe AH, Bartz D, Society of Family Planning clinical recommendations: contraception after surgical abortion, Contraception 99:2–9, 2019.

188. Sonalkar S, McClusky J, Hou MY, et al., Administration of depot medroxyprogesterone acetate on the day of mifepristone for medical abortion: a pilot study, Contraception 91:174–177, 2015.

189. Raymond EG, Weaver MA, Louie KS, et al., Effects of depot medroxyprogesterone acetate injection timing on medical abortion efficacy and repeat pregnancy: a randomized controlled trial, Obstet Gynecol 128:739–745, 2016.

190. Lang C, Chen ZE, Johnstone A, et al., Initiating intramuscular depot medroxyprogesterone acetate 24-48 hours after mifepristone administration does not affect success of early medical abortion, BMJ Sex Reprod Health 44:242–247, 2018.

327

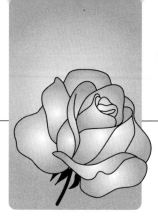

9

Shorter-Acting Progestin-Only Contraception

Elizabeth Micks, MD, MPH and
Sarah Prager, MD, MAS

Contraceptives containing only progestins are available in intrauterine devices (IUDs), subdermal implants, injectable contraceptives, and shorter-acting progestin-only pills (POPs), patches, and vaginal rings. This chapter will address the shorter-acting progestin-only methods.

The Progestin-Only Pill

The POP contains a small dose of a progestational agent and must be taken daily, in a continuous fashion.[1,2] The first oral contraceptives were initially designed to be POPs; only through an accident did the combined estrogen-progestin pill evolve. The first POPs were marketed after combined pills with the intention to reduce the side effects and thromboembolic risks associated with estrogen-containing pills.[3] Continuous dosing was expected to improve compliance. The first POP, containing chlormadinone acetate 0.5 mg, was approved in France in 1968. Several other POPs became available in the United States and Europe in the early 1970s, including norgestrel, norethindrone (also known as norethisterone), and levonorgestrel (the levo enantiomer of norgestrel).[4]

The only POP currently available in the United States is norethindrone 0.35 mg, used by approximately 0.4% of contracepting women.[5] The brand-name products initially marketed were Micronor and Nor-QD; today, numerous therapeutic equivalent products are also available including Camila and Jolivette. Other formulations commercially available around the globe include pills containing 0.03 mg levonorgestrel, 0.5 mg ethynodiol diacetate, and 0.075 mg desogestrel (**Table 9.1**).[6] Of these, only the levonorgestrel, norethindrone, and desogestrel pills are in common use. Levonorgestrel and norethindrone POPs have been available for decades, and desogestrel POPs have been available since 2003.

Two more POPs are currently under development. A norgestrel 0.075 mg pill, which was previously marketed as Ovrette, is being developed with the intention of over-the-counter sales in the United States (Clinicaltrials.gov NCT03585712). A novel 24/4 cyclic regimen POP containing drospirenone 4.0 mg daily for 24 days followed by a 4-day hormone-free interval has been studied over the last decade.[7,8] The product was approved in the United States in June 2019 (brand-name Slynd) with plans for marketing in late 2019.

Table 9.1 Progestin-Only Pills

Drug	Dose	Brand-Name Products	Therapeutic Equivalent Products	U.S. Availability
Norethindrone (norethisterone)	0.35 mg	Micronor, Nor-QD	Camila, Jolivette, Heather, Errin, Nora-Be, Noriday	Yes
Norgestrel	0.075 mg	Ovrette	Cryselle, Minicon, Neogest	No*
Levonorgestrel	0.03 mg	Norgeston, Microlut, Microval		No
Lynestrenol	0.5 mg	Exluton	Minikare	No
Ethynodiol diacetate	0.5 mg	Femulen		No
Desogestrel	0.075 mg	Cerazette		No
Drospirenone	4 mg	Slynd		Yes

*Approved but not currently available.

Mechanism of Action

POPs historically have about 25% of the amount of circulating progestin as combined oral contraceptives (COCs); hence, they are commonly referred to as the "minipill."[6] For POPs containing levonorgestrel, norgestrel, and norethindrone, this low dose of progestin results in predominantly cervical and endometrial effects, though the precise mechanism of action is based on very limited clinical evidence.[9] POPs appear to cause the cervical mucus to become thick and impermeable, likely the major contraceptive effect.[2] These progestins have less of an effect on ovulatory function, as the gonadotropins are not consistently suppressed. Hence, approximately 40% of patients using these POPs ovulate normally.[10–12] Tubal physiology may also be affected, but this is speculative.

However, POPs containing desogestrel and drospirenone provide more inhibition of ovulation. The desogestrel POP suppresses ovulation comparable to that of COCs.[13,14] The drospirenone POP also suppresses ovulation; this suppression is maintained over a 4-day hormone-free interval and is comparable to desogestrel POPs dosed daily.[7,8,15]

Because of the low dose, and lack of ovulation inhibition, norethindrone norgestrel, levonorgestrel, ethynodiol diacetate, and lynestrenol POPs must be taken every day at about the same time of day. Based on limited data, the changes in cervical mucus associated with the POP appear to develop quickly and diminish quickly.[9] Thickened cervical mucus reportedly occurs within 2 to 4 hours of dosing, with impermeability to sperm declining 22 hours after administration, and by 24 hours, some sperm penetration occurs.[16] While the available data support the need for consistent "on-time" dosing of POPs, and use of a backup method in the event of a late pill, the quality of this evidence is weak.[9] The requirement for maintaining this rigorous schedule may present a barrier to some potential users. In contrast, users of desogestrel POPs can miss a pill by up to 12 hours, and drospirenone POP users can delay taking a pill for 24 hours without impacting the contraceptive efficacy.[8,17]

Efficacy

Perfect-use failure rates have been documented to be as low as 1.1 per 100 women in the first year of use.[18,19] The actual use failure rate for all contraceptive pills (COCs and POPs) reported from the National Survey of Family Growth 2006 to 2010 is 7.2 per 100 women in the first year of use.[20] In this cohort, failure rates differ by age (10.4 per 100 women aged 25 to 29 vs. 4.1 per 100 women aged 30 to 44) and by race/ethnicity (13.1 per 100 black women and 6.1 per 100 white women). A systematic review of POPs for contraception did not find statistically significant differences in efficacy between POP types, though the analyses favored desogestrel over levonorgestrel and norethindrone over desogestrel.[6] Higher rates of discontinuation were seen with desogestrel due to bleeding irregularities, which likely limited its overall efficacy. There are no published efficacy data comparing drospirenone POPs with any other formulations. When women are able to adhere to recommended timing of POP administration, the failure rate may be comparable to the rate (<1 per 100 woman-years) with COCs.[18] However, use of population data to compare effectiveness of POPs and COCs is limited by selection bias, as users of POPs may have lower fertility risk for a variety of reasons (e.g., age, breastfeeding).

Who Might Use Progestin-Only Pills

POPs can be an effective, well-tolerated contraceptive method for many women. This method is frequently used by individuals who prefer an oral contraceptive and have an intolerance to, a personal preference to avoid, or a medical contraindication to estrogen-containing contraceptives. According to the U.S. Medical Eligibility Criteria (MEC) for Contraceptive Use, POPs are category 1 (no restrictions) or category 2 (advantages generally outweigh theoretical or proven risks) for women over the age of 35 who smoke or for those who have migraines with aura, history of venous or arterial thrombosis, hypertension, diabetes with vascular disease, or cardiovascular disease.[21] In general, women with liver tumors, cirrhosis, or breast cancer should not use the POP or other methods of hormonal contraception. Individuals with certain forms of bariatric surgery (malabsorptive procedures) that impair drug absorption should not use oral contraceptives.

All potential POP users must be counseled regarding the need for consistent timing to maximize efficacy, using a patient-centered approach. Theoretically, POPs may be associated with decreased efficacy in certain populations, such as adolescents and obese women. Use of POPs in adolescent women is poorly studied and less common, so precise estimates of failure rates are not available. However, clinicians may avoid the use of POPs in adolescents due to concerns about their compliance with the dosing regimen. Studies of obese women using COCs demonstrate they may require a longer period of time to reach full contraceptive efficacy, though the data do not suggest higher doses of hormones are necessary.[22] Based on very limited epidemiologic data, obese women who use POPs are not at higher risk of pregnancy than nonobese women.[23]

Pill Taking

The POP may be safely initiated at any point in the menstrual cycle.[24] Though cervical mucus changes are noted within 2 to 4 hours, reliable contraceptive protection may not be fully established for 48 hours.[2,10,24] Unless a person is within 5 days since the start of menstrual bleeding or within 7 days of abortion or pregnancy loss, a backup method should be used for 2 days after POP initiation.

Pill taking can be keyed to a daily event to ensure regular administration at the same time of the day. Use of a smart phone alarm may be useful.[25] If pills are forgotten or gastrointestinal illness impairs absorption, the POP should be resumed as soon as possible, and a backup method should be used immediately and until the pills have been resumed for at least 2 days.[24] If two or more pills are missed in a row and there is no menstrual bleeding in 4 to 6 weeks, a pregnancy test should be obtained. *If more than 3 hours late in taking a POP (except desogestrel or drospirenone), a backup method should be used for 48 hours.*[24] *The desogestrel POP allows a 12-hour late time period. Drospirenone POPs may allow at least a 24-hour late time period.*[7]

Side Effects

Due to the unpredictable effect on ovulation, irregular bleeding is a common side effect. The daily progestational impact on the endometrium also contributes to this problem. Patients can expect to have normal, ovulatory cycles (40% to 50%), short, irregular cycles (40%), or a total lack of cycles ranging from irregular bleeding to spotting and amenorrhea (10%).[2] This irregularity is the major reason why women discontinue the POP method of contraception.[19] Compared to levonorgestrel and norethindrone, desogestrel POPs are associated with more unpredictable bleeding with initial use and decreased bleeding over time, most likely due to stronger inhibition of ovulation.[6,13] Irregular bleeding is also seen with drospirenone-only pills, though this decreases over time (72.2% in cycle 1 and 22.8% in cycle 13).[15]

Women on progestin-only contraception can develop functional, ovarian follicular cysts,[26] primarily because follicular development is not suppressed. Nearly all cysts regress and do not generally cause a clinical problem of any significance. However, women who experience frequent, symptomatic ovarian cysts on a POP should consider switching to a combined method (if not contraindicated) or longer-acting progestins such as injectables or implants that more effectively suppress both follicle development and ovulation.

Few studies have assessed the effect of POPs on weight, but based on limited evidence, they are not known to cause weight gain.[27] Progestin-only methods of contraception including the POP may increase acne for some women, and this side effect may differ by progestin type.[28] The androgenic activity of levonorgestrel, for instance, decreases the circulating levels of sex hormone–binding globulin (SHBG).[29] Therefore, free steroid levels (levonorgestrel and testosterone) will be increased despite the low dose. This action is in contrast to the action of COCs in which the effect of the progestin is countered by the estrogen-induced increase in SHBG and reduced testosterone. The incidence of other minor side effects is very low, possibly at the same rate that would be encountered with a placebo.

Risks and Benefits

Unlike with COCs, triglyceride and lipid levels, carbohydrate metabolism, and coagulation factors remain unchanged with POPs.[30–33] A prospective, noncomparative study of the drospirenone POP conducted at 41 European sites reported no changes in laboratory parameters.[15] There is no evidence that POPs increase the risk of cardiovascular disease or thrombosis, though data are limited because relatively small numbers have chosen to use this method of contraception compared to COCs.[34,35] Both the World Health Organization case-control study and the transnational case-control study found no increased risks of stroke, myocardial infarction, or venous thromboembolism with POPs.[36,37] A more recent meta-analysis that included six studies of POPs found no increased risk of venous thromboembolism.[38]

The POP does not appear to be associated with an increased risk of developing new cancers. While some studies have shown that hormonal contraceptives are specifically associated with an increased risk of breast cancer, there is no evidence that this is the case for POPs.[39,40]

As with other methods of hormonal contraception, the overall incidence of ectopic pregnancy is reduced with POPs, but when pregnancy occurs, it is more likely to be ectopic.[41] A previous ectopic pregnancy should not be regarded as a contraindication to the POP.[21]

Studies are unable to help us understand if some of the noncontraceptive benefits associated with COCs apply to the POP because of the relatively small numbers of POP users. However, the progestin impact on the cervical mucus and endometrium would imply some of the benefits may be similar (e.g., reduced risks of pelvic infection and endometrial cancer). Although limited by small numbers, one case-control study indicated that protection against endometrial cancer was even greater with POPs than with COCs.[42]

Drug Interactions

Orally administered progestins are metabolized in the liver by the cytochrome P450 CYP3A4 isoenzyme in addition to other isoenzymes. Because of the relatively low doses of progestin administered, patients using medications that induce CYP3A4 should avoid this method of contraception due to the potential for decreased efficacy, unless other methods of contraception are unavailable or unacceptable.[21] For this reason, the MEC considers use of the following medications to be category 3 (the theoretical or proven risks usually outweigh the advantages of using the method) for POPs:

1. Anticonvulsants: phenytoin, carbamazepine, barbiturates, primidone, topiramate, and oxcarbazepine
2. Antimicrobials: rifampin and rifabutin

Other medications may also reduce efficacy, but to a lesser degree. The MEC considers use of the following medications to be category 2 (the advantages of using the method generally outweigh the theoretical or proven risks) for POPs:

1. Nonnucleoside reverse transcriptase inhibitor (NNRTI): efavirenz
2. Ritonavir-boosted protease inhibitors: atazanavir, darunavir, fosamprenavir, saquinavir, and tipranavir
3. Protease inhibitors without ritonavir: fosamprenavir, and nelfinavir
4. St. John's wort

Vaginal and Transdermal Progestin-Only Contraception

Transdermal and vaginal progestin-only contraceptives are not currently available in the United States. The progesterone vaginal ring (PVR) is approved in several Latin American countries and has only demonstrated efficacy in women who are breastfeeding at least four times daily. The PVR releases natural progesterone and can be used continuously for 3 months. Rings can be used successively for up to 1 year if breastfeeding continues. Among breastfeeding women, the PVR has been shown to be as effective as the copper IUD.[43,44]

As with POPs, the PVR appears to reliably suppress ovulation in breastfeeding women.[45] In earlier studies of a progesterone-releasing vaginal ring, the serum progesterone level needed to suppress ovulation was found to be approximately half that of normal luteal phase levels, much lower than that required to suppress ovulation in nonlactating women.[46] Progesterone has poor oral bioavailability and minimal drug is passed to the infant, making this an optimal method for breastfeeding women.

A transdermal levonorgestrel contraceptive patch has been evaluated in early phase clinical trials.[47]

Considerations for Postpartum and Postabortion Use

In the United States, the POP is commonly used during the postpartum period, primarily due to concerns about thrombosis risk. Unfortunately, providers still commonly recommend POPs for breastfeeding women due to concerns about decreased breast milk supply with estrogen-containing methods. A recent systematic review found an inconsistent impact of COCs on breastfeeding duration and success.[48] The body of evidence is limited by poor methodologic quality, consisting primarily of older studies using different formulations and doses of estrogen. The investigators recommend that, given the significant limitations of this body of evidence, the importance of contraception for postpartum women, and the theoretical concerns that have been raised about the use of combined hormonal contraception by women who are breastfeeding, rigorous studies examining these issues are needed.

Among postpartum women who are breastfeeding, the contraceptive effect of the POP is combined with prolactin-induced suppression of ovulation.[49] The mechanism of action of POPs in breastfeeding women is similar to that of prolonged lactational amenorrhea.[50] Furthermore, the major side effect of irregular bleeding may be minimized in this population.

The POP can be initiated immediately postpartum or postabortion.[21] For postpartum women whose menses have not returned, a backup method does not need to be used after initiation if they are within 21 days postpartum and not breastfeeding or within 6 months postpartum if exclusively breastfeeding (or the vast majority [≥85%] of feeds are breastfeeds). If menstrual cycles have resumed and it has been more than 5 days since bleeding started, they also need to use backup for 2 days. Women more than 7 days postabortion should use a backup method of contraception for 2 days after POP initiation.[24]

There is no evidence that POPs have an adverse effect on breastfeeding as measured by milk volume and infant growth and development.[51-54] In fact, there may be a modest positive impact; in one study, women using the levonorgestrel POP breastfed longer and added supplementary feeding at a later time.[55] A study investigating the impact of early initiation found no adverse effects on breastfeeding.[56]

The public health impact of limiting oral contraceptive use in breastfeeding women to POPs should be considered. A recent retrospective study suggests negative impact of limiting oral contraceptive choice to POPs for breastfeeding women.[57] Among 745 women, 203 (27%) experienced a repeat pregnancy within 18 months; those prescribed a POP were significantly more likely to experience a rapid repeat pregnancy compared to women choosing any other reversible method or no method (aOR = 5.1, 95% CI 2.2 to 12.1). POP users accounted for 50% of the rapid repeat pregnancies in this population. The investigators did not have information on breastfeeding rates in the population. This information, combined with the limitations of research related to combined pills in breastfeeding women, can inform women and patients that POPs may not be the best choice for women needing contraception in the postpartum period.

References

1. **Chi I,** The safety and efficacy issues of progestin-only oral contraceptives—an epidemiologic perspective, Contraception 47:1–21, 1993.
2. **McCann MF, Potter LS,** Progestin-only oral contraception: a comprehensive review, Contraception 50:S1–S195, 1994.
3. **Rudel HW, Martinez Manautou J, Maqueo Topete M,** The role of progestogens in the hormonal control of fertility, Fertil Steril 16:158–169, 1965.
4. **Bennett JP,** The second generation of hormonal contraceptives, In: Bennett JP, ed., Chemical Contraception, Palgrave, London, 1974.
5. **Hall KS, Trussell J, Schwarz EB,** Progestin-only contraceptive pill use among women in the United States, Contraception 86:653–658, 2012.
6. **Grimes DA, Lopez LM, O'Brien PA, Raymond EG,** Progestin-only pills for contraception, Cochrane Database Syst Rev (11):CD007541, 2013.
7. **Duijkers IJ, Heger-Mahn D, Drouin D, Skouby S,** A randomised study comparing the effect on ovarian activity of a progestogen-only pill (POP) containing desogestrel and a new POP containing drospirenone in a 24/4 regimen, Eur J Contracept Reprod Health Care 20:419–427, 2015.
8. **Duijkers IJM, Heger-Mahn D, Drouin D, Colli E, Skouby S,** Maintenance of ovulation inhibition with a new progestogen-only pill containing drospirenone after scheduled 24-h delays in pill intake, Contraception 93:303–309, 2016.
9. **Han L, Taub R, Jensen JT,** Cervical mucus and contraception: what we know and what we don't, Contraception 96:310–321, 2017.
10. **Moghissi KS, Marks C,** Effects of microdose norgestrel on endogenous gonadotropic and steroid hormones, cervical mucus properties, vaginal cytology, and endometrium, Fertil Steril 22:424–434, 1971.

11. **Moghissi KS, Syner FN, McBride LC,** Contraceptive mechanism of microdose norethindrone, Obstet Gynecol 41:585–594, 1973.

12. **Landgren BM, Diczfalusy E,** Hormonal effects of the 300 microgram norethisterone (NET) minipill. I. Daily steroid levels in 43 subjects during a pretreatment cycle and during the second month of NET administration, Contraception 21:87–113, 1980.

13. A double-blind study comparing the contraceptive efficacy, acceptability and safety of two progestogen-only pills containing desogestrel 75 micrograms/ day or levonorgestrel 30 micrograms/ day. Collaborative Study Group on the Desogestrel-containing Progestogen-only Pill, Eur J Contracept Reprod Health Care 3:169–178, 1998.

14. **Milsom I, Korver T,** Ovulation incidence with oral contraceptives: a literature review, J Fam Plann Reprod Health Care 34:237–246, 2008.

15. **Archer DF, Ahrendt HJ, Drouin D,** Drospirenone-only oral contraceptive: results from a multicenter noncomparative trial of efficacy, safety and tolerability, Contraception 92:439–444, 2015.

16. **Cox H,** The precoital use of mini-dosage progestogens, J Reprod Fertil (Suppl 5):167–172, 1968.

17. **Korver T, Klipping C, Heger-Mahn D, Duijkers I, van Osta G, Dieben T,** Maintenance of ovulation inhibition with the 75-microg desogestrel-only contraceptive pill (Cerazette) after scheduled 12-h delays in tablet intake, Contraception 71:8–13, 2005.

18. **Trussell J,** Contraceptive failure in the United States, Contraception 83:397–404, 2011.

19. **Broome M, Fotherby K,** Clinical experience with the progestogen-only pill, Contraception 42:489–495, 1990.

20. **Sundaram A, Vaughan B, Kost K, Bankole A, Finer L, Singh S, Trussell J,** Contraceptive failure in the United States: estimates from the 2006–2010 National Survey of Family Growth, Perspect Sex Reprod Health 49:7–16, 2017.

21. **Curtis KM, Tepper NK, Jatlaoui TC, Berry-Bibee E, Horton LG, Zapata LB,** **Simmons KB, Pagano HP, Jamieson DJ, Whiteman MK,** U.S. Medical Eligibility Criteria for contraceptive use, 2016, MMWR Recomm Rep 65:1–103, 2016.

22. **Edelman AB, Cherala G, Munar MY, Dubois B, McInnis M, Stanczyk FZ, Jensen JT,** Prolonged monitoring of ethinyl estradiol and levonorgestrel levels confirms an altered pharmacokinetic profile in obese oral contraceptives users, Contraception 87:220–226, 2013.

23. **Vessey M,** Oral contraceptive failures and body weight: findings in a large cohort study, J Fam Plann Reprod Health Care 27:90–91, 2001.

24. **Curtis KM, Jatlaoui TC, Tepper NK, Zapata LB, Horton LG, Jamieson DJ, Whiteman MK,** U.S. Selected Practice Recommendations for contraceptive use, 2016, MMWR Recomm Rep 65:1–66, 2016.

25. **Smith C, Gold J, Ngo TD, Sumpter C, Free C,** Mobile phone-based interventions for improving contraception use, Cochrane Database Syst Rev (6):CD011159, 2015.

26. **Tayob Y, Adams J, Jacobs HS, Guillebaud J,** Ultrasound demonstration of increased frequency of functional ovarian cysts in women using progestogen-only oral contraception, Br J Obstet Gynaecol 92:1003–1009, 1985.

27. **Lopez LM, Ramesh S, Chen M, Edelman A, Otterness C, Trussell J, Helmerhorst FM,** Progestin-only contraceptives: effects on weight, Cochrane Database Syst Rev (8):CD008815, 2016.

28. **Lortscher D, Admani S, Satur N, Eichenfield LF,** Hormonal contraceptives and acne: a retrospective analysis of 2147 patients, J Drugs Dermatol 15:670–674, 2016.

29. **Pakarinen P, Lahteenmaki P, Rutanen EM,** The effect of intrauterine and oral levonorgestrel administration on serum concentrations of sex hormone-binding globulin, insulin and insulin-like growth factor binding protein-1, Acta Obstet Gynecol Scand 78:423–428, 1999.

30. **Godsland IF, Crook D, Simpson R, Proudler T, Felton C, Lees B, Anyaoku V, Devenport M, Wynn V,** The effects of different formulations of oral contra-

337

ceptive agents on lipid and carbohydrate metabolism, N Engl J Med 323:1375–1381, 1990.

31. **Ball MJ, Ashwell E, Gillmer MD,** Progestagen-only oral contraceptives: comparison of the metabolic effects of levonorgestrel and norethisterone, Contraception 44:223–233, 1991.

32. **Winkler UH,** Blood coagulation and oral contraceptives. A critical review, Contraception 57:203–209, 1998.

33. **Winkler UH, Howie H, Buhler K, Korver T, Geurts TB, Coelingh Bennink HJ,** A randomized controlled double-blind study of the effects on hemostasis of two progestogen-only pills containing 75 microgram desogestrel or 30 microgram levonorgestrel, Contraception 57:385–392, 1998.

34. **Lidegaard O, Edstrom B, Kreiner S,** Oral contraceptives and venous thromboembolism: a five-year national case-control study, Contraception 65:187–196, 2002.

35. **Lidegaard O, Lokkegaard E, Svendsen AL, Agger C,** Hormonal contraception and risk of venous thromboembolism: national follow-up study, BMJ 339:b2890, 2009.

36. Cardiovascular disease and use of oral and injectable progestogen-only contraceptives and combined injectable contraceptives. Results of an international, multicenter, case-control study. World Health Organization Collaborative Study of Cardiovascular Disease and Steroid Hormone Contraception, Contraception 57:315–324, 1998.

37. **Heinemann LA, Assmann A, DoMinh T, Garbe E,** Oral progestogen-only contraceptives and cardiovascular risk: results from the Transnational Study on Oral Contraceptives and the Health of Young Women, Eur J Contracept Reprod Health Care 4:67–73, 1999.

38. **Mantha S, Karp R, Raghavan V, Terrin N, Bauer KA, Zwicker JI,** Assessing the risk of venous thromboembolic events in women taking progestin-only contraception: a meta-analysis, BMJ 345:e4944, 2012.

39. **Morch LS, Skovlund CW, Hannaford PC, Iversen L, Fielding S, Lidegaard O,** Contemporary hormonal contraception and the risk of breast cancer, N Engl J Med 377:2228–2239, 2017.

40. **Samson M, Porter N, Orekoya O, Hebert JR, Adams SA, Bennett CL, Steck SE,** Progestin and breast cancer risk: a systematic review, Breast Cancer Res Treat 155:3–12, 2016.

41. **Furlong LA,** Ectopic pregnancy risk when contraception fails. A review, J Reprod Med 47:881–885, 2002.

42. **Weiderpass E, Adami HO, Baron JA, Magnusson C, Bergström R, Lindgren A, Correia N, Persson I,** Risk of endometrial cancer following estrogen replacement with and without progestins, J Natl Cancer Inst 91:1131–1137, 1999.

43. **Sivin I, Diaz S, Croxatto HB, Miranda P, Shaaban M, Sayed EH, Xiao B, Wu SC, Du M, Alvarez F, Brache V, Basnayake S, McCarthy T, Lacarra M, Mishell DR Jr, Koetsawang S, Stern J, Jackanicz T,** Contraceptives for lactating women: a comparative trial of a progesterone-releasing vaginal ring and the copper T 380A IUD, Contraception 55:225–232, 1997.

44. **RamaRao S, Clark H, Merkatz R, Sussman H, Sitruk-Ware R,** Progesterone vaginal ring: introducing a contraceptive to meet the needs of breastfeeding women, Contraception 88:591–598, 2013.

45. **Nath A, Sitruk-Ware R,** Progesterone vaginal ring for contraceptive use during lactation, Contraception 82:428–434, 2010.

46. **Croxatto HB, Diaz S,** The place of progesterone in human contraception, J Steroid Biochem 27:991–994, 1987.

47. **Westhoff CL, Chen BA, Jensen JT, Barnhart K, Thomas M, Teal S, Blithe D,** Phase I/II pharmacokinetic and pharmacodynamic evaluation of two levonorgestrel-only contraceptive patches in a multicenter randomized trial, Contraception 98:151–157, 2018.

48. **Tepper NK, Phillips SJ, Kapp N, Gaffield ME, Curtis KM,** Combined hormonal contraceptive use among breastfeeding women: an updated systematic review, Contraception 94:262–274, 2016.

49. **Dunson TR, McLaurin VL, Grubb GS, Rosman AW,** A multicenter clinical trial of a progestin-only oral contraceptive in lactating women, Contraception 47:23–35, 1993.

50. **Diaz S, Miranda P, Brandeis A, Cardenas H, Croxatto HB,** Mechanism of action of progesterone as contraceptive for lactating women, Ann N Y Acad Sci 626:11–21, 1991.

51. **Tankeyoon M, Dusitsin N, Chalapati S, Koetsawang S, Saibiang S, Sas M, Gellen JJ, Ayeni O, Gray R, Pinol A, Zegers L,** Effects of hormonal contraceptives on milk volume and infant growth. WHO Special Programme of Research, Development and Research Training in Human Reproduction Task force on oral contraceptives, Contraception 30:505–522, 1984.

52. Progestogen-only contraceptives during lactation: I. Infant growth. World Health Organization Task force for Epidemiological Research on Reproductive Health; Special Programme of Research, Development and Research Training in Human Reproduction, Contraception 50:35–53, 1994.

53. Progestogen-only contraceptives during lactation: II. Infant development. World Health Organization, Task Force for Epidemiological Research on Reproductive Health; Special Programme of Research, Development, and Research Training in Human Reproduction, Contraception 50:55–68, 1994.

54. **Lopez LM, Grey TW, Stuebe AM, Chen M, Truitt ST, Gallo MF,** Combined hormonal versus nonhormonal versus progestin-only contraception in lactation, Cochrane Database Syst Rev (3):CD003988, 2015.

55. **McCann MF, Moggia AV, Higgins JE, Potts M, Becker C,** The effects of a progestin-only oral contraceptive (levonorgestrel 0.03 mg) on breast-feeding, Contraception 40:635–648, 1989.

56. **Halderman LD, Nelson AL,** Impact of early postpartum administration of progestin-only hormonal contraceptives compared with nonhormonal contraceptives on short-term breast-feeding patterns, Am J Obstet Gynecol 186:1250–1256, 2002; discussion 1256–1258.

57. **Sackeim MG, Gurney EP, Koelper N, Sammel MD, Schreiber CA,** Effect of contraceptive choice on rapid repeat pregnancy, Contraception 99:184–186, 2019.

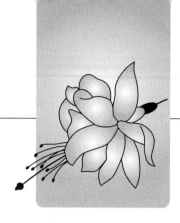

10

Barrier Methods of Contraception

Jill Schwartz, MD, MPH

Barrier methods of contraception have been the most widely used contraceptive techniques throughout recorded history. Although barriers represent the oldest of contraceptive methods, our response to the personal and social impact of sexually transmitted infections (STIs) has placed new importance on these approaches for dual prevention of pregnancy and human immunodeficiency virus (HIV) and other STIs. Male and female condoms represent the first line of defense, and other multipurpose prevention technologies (MPT) strategies are now in development.

Physical barrier methods (e.g., condoms, diaphragm, and cervical cap) and chemical barriers (e.g., spermicides) have higher and more variable perfect-use failure (2% to 20%) than do other modern methods, and also show the largest difference between perfect use and typical use.[1,2] For this reason, we classify these as the "least effective" contraceptive methods, along with withdrawal and fertility awareness–based methods (see Chapter 1, Figure 1.4). However, for many couples, a barrier may represent an appropriate choice despite higher perfect-use failure. The coital-dependent timing of use likely contributes to typical-use failure. For this reason, clinicians counseling women on use of barrier methods should stress correct and consistent use to bring users closer to perfect-use efficacy.

The importance of this counseling cannot be overemphasized. Many clinicians seem to give up on women who do not accept moderately or highly effective methods. Correct and consistent use of a less effective method will generally result in better outcomes than incorrect and inconsistent use of a more effective method. Obviously, long-acting reversible contraceptive (LARC) methods do not meet the needs of all couples, and women and their partners have differing tolerance for a contraceptive failure. For example, some women may prioritize a method that they control, and accept a higher risk of failure with a barrier method. In contrast, barrier methods represent a poor choice for women unable to accept the risk of contraceptive failure. The role of the clinician is to guide this discussion. In the past, primary care providers frequently recommended barrier methods to women with medical comorbidities that increase the risk of both pregnancy and hormonal contraception. For women with contraindications to pregnancy, best practice would involve directed counseling for medically appropriate LARC methods or permanent contraception.

Modern History of Barrier Methods

> Barrier methods likely existed even in ancient times. Barrier methods have always represented an important risk reduction strategy for prevention of STIs. See the *History of Contraception* online chapter in the eBook for details of this interesting story.

Modern physical barrier methods include male and female condoms, vaginal diaphragms, cervical caps, and vaginal sponges. Some of these methods are used in combination with a chemical barrier or spermicide. Early methods like the latex All-Flex diaphragm and the original cervical cap ("Prentif") are no longer available. While a silicone diaphragm similar to the original diaphragm is still marketed, novel diaphragms and caps have been introduced to increase availability. The "one size fits most" diaphragm (Caya®) was introduced in the United States in 2014, and the FemCap™ cervical cap became available in Europe in 1999 and the United States in 2003. In addition, new designs of the male and female condoms have also emerged. Alternatives to nonoxynol-9 (N-9), the only spermicide currently approved by the FDA, have been under development for decades or available in countries other than the United States. In the past decade, early testing of MPT products that combine a barrier method and HIV prevention strategies, such as a single-sized diaphragm delivering an antiretroviral drug, has been initiated.

Protection from Sexually Transmitted Infections

Barrier methods (condoms and diaphragms) provide protection against STIs and pelvic infection,[3-7] including infections due to chlamydia, gonorrhea, *Trichomonas*, herpes simplex, cytomegalovirus, and HIV. Couples should be counseled that consistent and correct use of the male latex condom reduces the risk for transmission of HIV and other STIs. Use of female condoms can provide protection from STIs, although data are limited. STI protection has a beneficial impact on the risk of tubal infertility and ectopic pregnancy.[5,8] Women who have never used barrier methods of contraception are almost twice as likely to develop cervical cancer.[8,9]

Nonspermicidal male and FC2 female condom are indicated for preventing pregnancy, as well as HIV and other STIs. Condoms lubricated with N-9 and other barrier methods bear the label that they reduce the risk of pregnancy but do not protect against HIV/STIs.

The risk of toxic shock syndrome is increased with female barrier methods, but the actual incidence is so rare that this is not a significant clinical consideration.[10] However, guidelines do indicate that the risks of diaphragm/spermicide use outweigh the advantages in women with a history of toxic shock syndrome (Medical Eligibility Criteria [MEC] category 3).[11]

The Diaphragm

The first effective contraceptive method under a woman's control was the vaginal diaphragm. Distribution of diaphragms led to Margaret Sanger's arrest in New York City in 1918. By 1940, one third of contracepting U.S. couples were using the diaphragm. Contraceptive provision was still a contentious issue in 1965 when the Supreme Court's decision in *Griswold v. Connecticut* ended the ban on contraception in that state. By this time, diaphragm use had decreased to 10% of contraceptors following the introduction of oral methods and intrauterine devices (IUDs). By 1995, this rate fell to about 1.9%; today, less than 1% of U.S. women[12] are diaphragm users. The Ortho All-Flex® diaphragm was the predominant diaphragm but the manufacturer opted to cease distribution in December 2013, leaving, at the time, only the Milex fitted silicone diaphragm in the United States (https://www.coopersurgical.com). Lower utilization led to decreased availability of vaginal diaphragms; today, most pharmacies no longer stock them routinely. A next-generation single-size method known as Caya (formerly SILCS) was developed by PATH and tested by CONRAD in an iterative process using clinician and end-user feedback to design a product that would be easier to use, more comfortable, more anatomically accurate, and easier to access. Caya **(Figure 10.1)** requires a prescription in the United States but is available over the counter or through Internet sales in many countries. Use of a contraceptive gel is recommended with both standard fitted diaphragms and Caya.

Efficacy

According to the most recent data from the National Survey of Family Growth, 12% of women using diaphragms experience pregnancy with typical use and 6% with perfect use.[1,2] These numbers may underestimate both the risk of failure and success as the current group of users may not reflect historic patterns. Randomized comparator studies completed in the 1980s and 1990s reported typical-use failure as high as 29% and perfect-use failure as low as 2% among parous diaphragm users.[13] While older married women with longer use achieve the highest efficacy, motivated young women

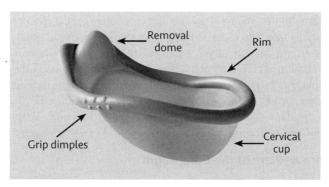

Figure 10.1 Caya Diaphragm.

can use diaphragms very successfully if they are properly encouraged and counseled. There have been no adequate studies to determine whether efficacy is different with and without spermicides.[14] A retrospective review of use patterns in Brazil found a lower rate of pregnancy (0.6% perfect, 2.8% typical use) in women who used the diaphragm continuously (removing only for bathing and then immediately reinserting) than in women following the traditional recommendations for pericoital use (6.5% perfect, 9.8% typical).[15]

Side Effects

The diaphragm is a safe method of contraception that rarely causes even minor side effects. Although irritation from latex was occasionally reported in the past, latex products are no longer available. Still, some women experience vaginal irritation due to the gel used with the diaphragm or, less commonly, complain of discomfort from the diaphragm itself. Fewer than 1% discontinue diaphragm use for these reasons. Urinary tract infections are two to threefold more common among standard diaphragm users than among women using oral contraception.[16,17] Possibly, the rim of the diaphragm presses against the urethra and causes irritation that is perceived as infectious in origin, or true infection may result from touching the perineal area or from incomplete emptying of the bladder. It is also possible that spermicides used with the diaphragm increase the risk of bacteriuria with *E. coli*, perhaps due to an alteration in the normal vaginal flora.[18] Clinical experience suggests that voiding after sexual intercourse may help. In persistent cases, a single postcoital dose of a prophylactic antibiotic may prevent the development of infection. The single-size Caya diaphragm has an anterior notch designed to minimize urethral pressure and causes fewer urinary symptoms than does the standard diaphragm.[19]

Improper fitting or prolonged retention (beyond 24 hours) can cause vaginal abrasion or mucosal irritation. There is no link between the normal use of diaphragms and the development of toxic shock syndrome.[20] It makes sense, however, to minimize the risk of toxic shock by not keeping the diaphragm in the vagina for more than 24 hours.

Benefits

Diaphragm use reduces the incidence of gonorrhea, *Trichomonas*, and chlamydia infection,[21] pelvic inflammatory disease,[5,22] and tubal infertility.[3,8] There are no data, as of yet, regarding the effect of diaphragm use on the transmission of HIV, but because the vagina remains exposed, the diaphragm is unlikely to fully protect against HIV. Indeed, a clinical trial demonstrated no added benefit against HIV with a diaphragm when used with condoms.[23] An important advantage of the diaphragm is low cost. Diaphragms are durable and with proper care can be used for 2 years or longer.

Choice and Use of the Diaphragm

Caya is a silicone barrier used with a contraceptive gel.[19,24] It comes in one size that fits most women, and, therefore, interaction with a clinician and the requirement for fitting can be avoided, simplifying provision and access.

The Milex® Wide-Seal diaphragm is also made of silicone and comes in eight sizes (60 to 95 mm) that require fitting.

Fitting

A pelvic exam or traditional diaphragm fitting is not required for the single-sized contoured device, yet an initial fitting by the provider can help determine if the method is appropriate for the user. Caya is correctly placed when it completely covers the cervix.

During fitting of a standard diaphragm, the clinician must have available aseptic fitting rings or diaphragms in all diameters. Fitting kits are available through the manufacturer. The Milex Wide-Seal fitting devices should be scrubbed after each use with mild soap and autoclaved according to the fitting kit instructions. To measure the distance from the inside of the pubic symphysis to the posterior fornix, the index finger and middle finger are brought together and inserted into the vagina until the posterior fornix is reached. The examining hand is lifted so that the index finger makes contact with the pubic arch, and the point directly below the inferior margin of the pubic bone is noted with the tip of the thumb (**Figure 10.2**).

If the chosen diaphragm based on this measured distance is too tightly pressed against the pubic symphysis or is uncomfortable, a smaller size should be tried. If the diaphragm is too loose (comes out with a cough or bearing down), the next larger size should be tested. After a good fit is obtained, the diaphragm is removed by hooking the index finger under the rim behind the symphysis and pulling. It is important to instruct the patient in these procedures during and after the fitting. The patient should then insert the diaphragm (**Figure 10.3A, B**), practice checking for proper placement (**Figure 10.3C**), and attempt removal (**Figure 10.3D**) before leaving the office.

Timing

Diaphragm users need instruction about the timing of diaphragm use in relation to sexual intercourse and the use of spermicide. None of this advice has been rigorously assessed in clinical studies; therefore, these recommendations represent product instructions and the consensus of clinical experience.

About a tablespoonful of spermicide should be placed in the dome of the diaphragm prior to insertion, and some of the spermicide should be spread around the rim. The diaphragm should be left in place for at least 6 hours (but no more than 24 hours) after coitus. In the event of repeated intercourse, or if the diaphragm was inserted 2 or more hours before intercourse, additional spermicide should be placed in the vagina while the diaphragm is in place.

Reassessment

Weight loss or gain, vaginal delivery, and even sexual intercourse can change vaginal caliber. The fit of a standard diaphragm should be assessed during routine pelvic examinations or whenever the woman is concerned that the fit doesn't seem correct.

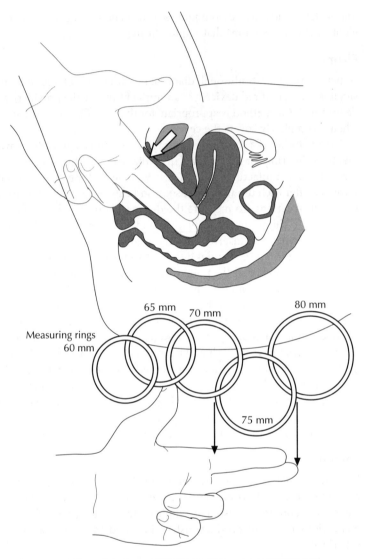

65 mm

70 mm

80 mm

Measuring rings
60 mm

75 mm

After S. Koperski from **Jackson, Berger, Keith**, *Vaginal Contraception*, G.K. Hall Publishers.

Figure 10.2 Standard diaphragm fitting set.

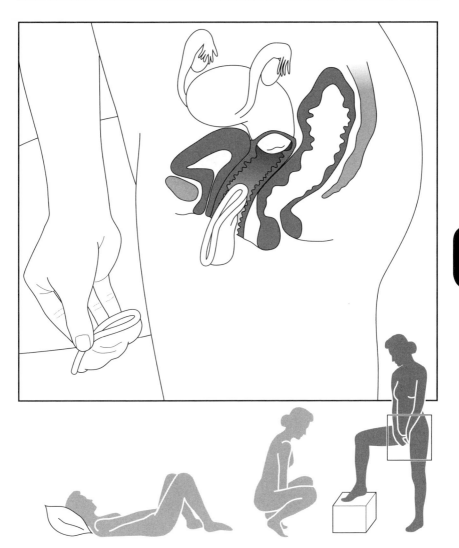

A   After S. Koperski from **Jackson, Berger, Keith**, *Vaginal Contraception*, G.K. Hall Publishers.

Figure 10.3 A: Starting self-insertion of the standard diaphragm.

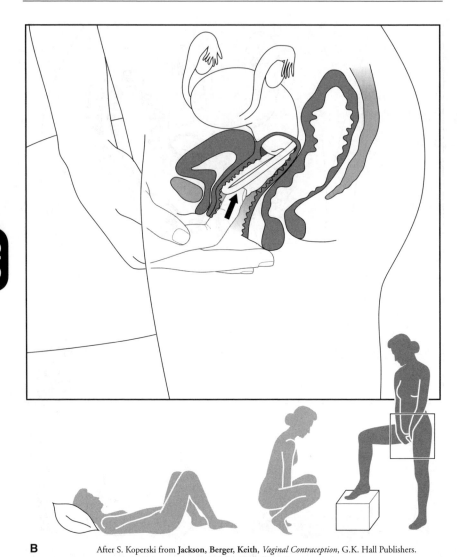

B   After S. Koperski from **Jackson, Berger, Keith**, *Vaginal Contraception*, G.K. Hall Publishers.

Figure 10.3 B: Completing self-insertion of the standard diaphragm.

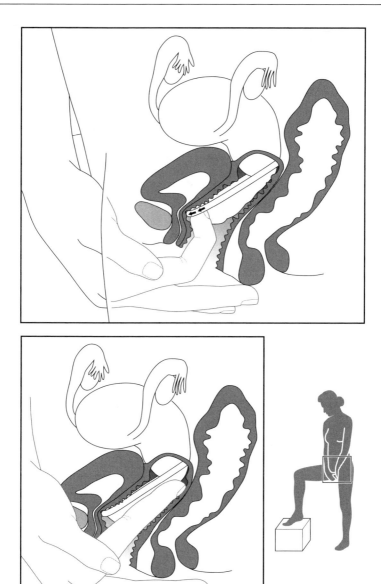

C After S. Koperski from **Jackson, Berger, Keith,** *Vaginal Contraception,* G.K. Hall Publishers.

Figure 10.3 C: Confirmation of correct position of the standard diaphragm behind the pubic bone (upper panel) and over the cervix (lower panel).

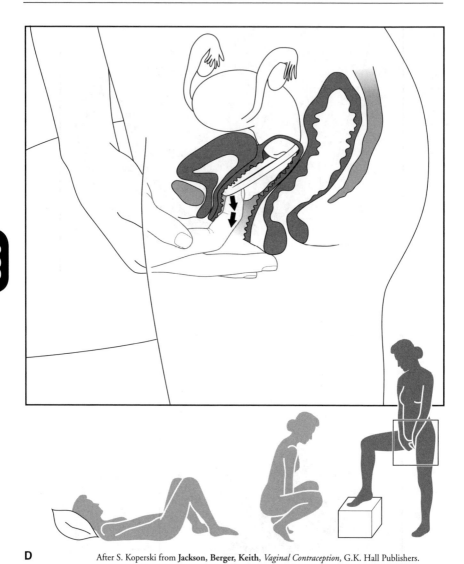

D   After S. Koperski from **Jackson, Berger, Keith**, *Vaginal Contraception*, G.K. Hall Publishers.

Figure 10.3 D: Technique for self-removal of the standard diaphragm.

Care of the Diaphragm

After removal, the diaphragm should be washed with soap and water, rinsed, and dried. It is wise to check for holes and tears before use and to use water to periodically check for leaks. Diaphragms should be stored within the supplied case in a cool and dark location. With proper care, the device should last at least 2 years.

The Cervical Cap

The only cervical cap that is currently widely available is the FemCap (FemCap, Inc. Del Mar, CA, www.femcap.com); the method requires a prescription in the United States but can be ordered without one elsewhere.[25-27] FemCap is made of nonallergenic, durable silicone rubber, with a dome to cover the cervix, a rim that fits into the vaginal fornices, and an uneven brim that flares out and conforms to the vaginal walls around the cervix. These features trap sperm in the groove and minimize dislodgement.[28] There are three inner rim diameter sizes, one for nulliparous women (22 mm), one for women who have been pregnant but not had a vaginal delivery (26 mm), and one for women who have had a vaginal delivery (30 mm). In a randomized trial, the pregnancy rate with FemCap was nearly twofold higher than a diaphragm, with 6-month cumulative typical-use pregnancy probabilities of 13.5% compared to 7.9%.[29] The pregnancy rate was noticeably higher in women with previous vaginal deliveries.

Spermicide is placed in the bowl prior to placement over the cervix. It must remain inserted for at least 6 hours after intercourse and should not be left in the vagina for more than 48 hours. FemCap has a strap over the dome to aid in removal **(Figure 10.4)**.

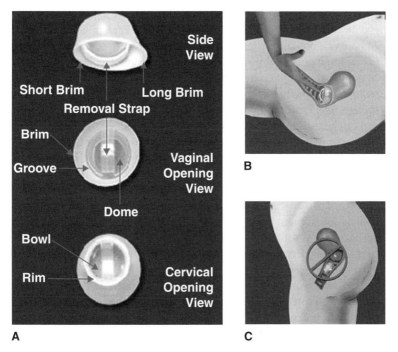

Figure 10.4   FemCap. A: FemCap features. **B:** The FemCap should cover the cervix completely. **C:** Example of incorrect FemCap placement. (Courtesy of FemCap Inc.)

The Contraceptive Sponge

Vaginal contraceptive sponges are soft, porous, single-size nonprescription devices designed for sustained spermicide release. Basically, the sponge is a spermicide product in a carrier that will block the entrance to the cervical canal and absorb semen, exposing the semen to concentrated spermicide.

The Today® sponge is a dimpled polyurethane disc impregnated with N-9 1 g and designed for use up to 24 hours including multiple acts of intercourse. Similar to other physical barriers, the device should remain in place for at least 6 hours after the last act of intercourse. Approximately 20% of the N-9 is released over the 24 hours that the sponge is left in the vagina.

Protectaid® is a polyurethane sponge not currently available in the United States that contains three spermicides and a dispersing gel.[30] The spermicidal agents are sodium cholate, N-9, and benzalkonium chloride (BZK). This combination exerts antiviral actions in vitro.[31] The dispersing agent, polydimethylsiloxane, forms a protective coating over the entire vagina, providing sustained protection. The Pharmatex sponge is a foam cylinder impregnated with 60 mg of the spermicide BZK that is also unavailable in the United States. The U.S. FDA requires efficacy data prior to marketing a contraceptive device, and only the Today sponge has complied with this requirement.

Prior to insertion in the vagina, the Today sponge is moistened with water (squeezing out the excess) and then placed firmly against the cervix. It can be inserted immediately before sexual intercourse or up to 24 hours beforehand. There should always be a lapse of at least 6 hours after sexual intercourse before removal, even if the sponge has been in place for 24 hours before intercourse (maximal wear time, therefore, is 30 hours). It is removed by hooking a finger through the ribbon attached to the back of the sponge. The Protectaid and Pharmatex sponges do not require moistening and can be inserted up to 12 hours before intercourse. Some reports suggest that these may be easier to remove than the Today sponge. Obviously, the sponge is not a good choice for women with anatomic changes that make proper insertion and placement difficult.

The effectiveness of the sponge is similar to that of spermicide with a typical failure rate during the first year of 27% and 14% in parous and nulliparous women, respectively.[1,2,32,33] This disparity in efficacy suggests that one size may not fit all users and the sponge may not adequately cover the larger parous cervix.[34] In comparator studies, the sponge is also inferior to the diaphragm.[13]

For some women, however, the sponge is preferred because it provides continuous protection for 24 hours regardless of the frequency of coitus. In addition, it is easier to use, available without prescription, and less messy as compared to spermicide.

Side effects associated with the sponge include allergic reactions in about 4% of users. Another 8% complain of vaginal dryness, soreness, or itching. Some women find removal difficult. There has been some concern that the sponge may damage the vaginal epithelium and enhance HIV transmission.[35] Women using the sponge have lower rates of infection with gonorrhea, *Trichomonas*, and chlamydia compared to a control group of women using no or surgical contraception.[5]

Spermicides

Jellies, creams, foams, melting suppositories, foaming tablets, foaming suppositories, and soluble films are used as vehicles for chemical agents that inactivate sperm in the vagina before they can move into the upper genital tract. Some are used together with diaphragms, caps, and condoms, but even used alone, they can provide modest protection against pregnancy.

Various chemicals and a wide array of vehicles have been used vaginally as contraceptives for centuries. The first commercially available spermicidal pessaries were made in England in 1885 of cocoa butter and quinine sulfite. These or similar materials were used until the 1920s when effervescent tablets that released carbon dioxide and phenyl mercuric acetate were marketed. Modern spermicides, introduced in the 1950s, contain surface active agents (surfactants) that damage the sperm cell membranes. The most common and only currently available active ingredient of spermicides sold in the United States is N-9. Most preparations contain N-9 100 to 150 mg in each vaginal application, with concentrations ranging from 3% to 12.5% in gels and foams and up to 28% in vaginal films. Other spermicides available outside the United States include the cationic surfactant BZK and phenol derivative menfegol, but use appears limited. All of these agents have been associated with vaginal irritation in some users due to the nonspecific action of membrane disruption.

Acid-buffering gels, including BufferGel, Amphora™ (previously Acidform), Contragel® (also known as Caya gel), RepHresh™, and Replens™, represent promising alternatives to N-9. These products are composed of several different agents with varying buffering capacities and tend to be hyperosmolar. Amphora and Contragel both show promise as contraceptive gels for use in conjunction with the Caya diaphragm. There are substantial clinical data from Amphora[36] and over 35 years of use of Contragel in Europe, with recent data demonstrating contraceptive activity when used in conjunction with Caya.[37] The regulatory pathway in the United States requires safety and efficacy studies, and these are in progress for Amphora including a comparator study with N-9 (Clinicaltrials.gov NCT01306331) and an additional open-label study (Clinicaltrials.gov NCT03243305).

Spermicides have different instructions, but, for the most part, the product is simply inserted with an applicator or finger. N-9 gels such as Gynol II® are effective upon insertion but only remain effective for about an hour. Vaginal contraceptive films require application not less than 15 minutes and not more than 3 hours prior to sexual intercourse. If ejaculation does not occur within the period of effectiveness, the spermicide should be reapplied. Reapplication should take place for each coital episode.

Although in vitro studies have demonstrated that spermicides kill or inactivate most STI pathogens, including HIV, clinical studies do not support protection against STIs. Spermicides have been reported to prevent

HIV seroconversion as well as to have no effect; therefore, spermicides by themselves cannot be counted on for protection against HIV.[38-42] In a controlled, clinical trial in female sex workers, N-9 failed to protect against HIV transmission, and an increased risk of infection was observed with frequent use.[43] Clinical studies have indicated reductions in the risk of gonorrhea,[44-46] pelvic infections,[22] and chlamydial infection.[44,46] However, these studies probably reflected condom use. In trials with a placebo, N-9 provided no protection against gonorrhea or chlamydia.[43,47-50] *N-9 spermicides should not be used alone for protection from STIs or use at all in high-risk individuals.*

Efficacy

Only periodic abstinence demonstrates as wide a range of efficacy in different studies as do the studies of spermicides. Efficacy seems to depend more on the population studied, including frequency of intercourse, than the agent used. The typical-use failure rate of spermicides during the first year of use is 21%.[1,2] Failure rates of approximately 20% to 25% during a year's use are most typical.[2,51] A randomized trial comparing vaginal contraceptive film (N-9 72 mg) with foaming tablets (N-9 100 mg) recorded similar 6-month pregnancy rates (24.9% and 28.0%, respectively).[51] A randomized assessment of various products concluded that a N-9 dose of 52.5 mg was less effective (22% in 6 months) than those containing 100 or 150 mg (about 15% in 6 months; intermediate doses were not tested).[52] These are very high failure rates, amounting to approximately 30% to 40% for 1 year of use. **Although better than no method, spermicides alone should not be recommended for contraception unless method failure and pregnancy are acceptable. The limited available data support inferiority for spermicides used alone compared with condoms used alone.**[53]

Vaginal postcoital douches are ineffective contraceptives even if they contain spermicidal agents. Postcoital douching is too late to prevent the rapid ascent of sperm (within seconds) to the fallopian tubes.

Advantages

Spermicides are relatively inexpensive and widely available in many retail outlets without prescription. These features may make spermicides more accessible to women of all ages with limited access to health care providers and appealing to others who have infrequent or unpredictable sexual intercourse. In addition, spermicides are simple to use.

Side Effects

Spermicides have been used for many decades and are generally regarded as safe. One serious past concern was a possible association between spermicide use and congenital abnormalities or spontaneous miscarriages. Epidemiologic analysis, including a meta-analysis, concluded that there is insufficient evidence to support these associations.[54-56] Spermicides are not absorbed through the vaginal mucosa in concentrations high enough to have systemic effects.[57] Vaginal and cervical mucosal damage (de-epithelialization without inflammation) has been observed with N-9,[58,59] and frequent use in high-risk women may increase HIV transmission.[43] Based on these findings, the FDA mandated that labeling for N-9 products carry a warning saying they do not protect against STIs/HIV, and current U.S. Medical Eligibility Criteria advises that women with a high risk of HIV face an unacceptable health risk with the use of spermicides (MEC 4).[11]

The principal side effect is allergy, which occurs in 1% to 5% of users, is most commonly minor, and is related to either the vehicle or the spermicidal agent. Using a different product often solves the problem. Spermicide users also have an altered vaginal flora promoting the colonization of *E. coli*, leading to a greater susceptibility to urinary tract infections as noted with diaphragm/spermicide users.[17,60]

The Search for Contraceptives to Prevent STIs: Multipurpose Prevention Technologies

For the last several decades, extensive research has been devoted to the development of contraceptive microbicides to prevent STIs, especially HIV. The ideal agent would be a topical microbicide that would prevent infection and destroy or immobilize sperm. Any new agent must match the latex condom, which is highly effective in blocking bacteria and viruses. The road is long, extending from in vitro work to clinical application. An acceptable agent must avoid damage to vaginal epithelial cells and disruption of vaginal flora, and the delivery system must be user-friendly. Carraguard, a microbicide that contains carrageenan, a substance derived from seaweed, is a good example. After extensive development by the Population Council, a large, long-term phase 3 clinical trial in South Africa concluded that Carraguard did not prevent vaginal transmission of HIV.[61] Similarly, C31G and cellulose sulfate gels have both been shown to be vaginal contraceptives but were not demonstrated to prevent HIV, so development was halted.[62,63] Acid-buffering agents have been evaluated in phase 1 clinical trials, when loaded in a diaphragm-like device,[64,65] and Amphora, in addition to being evaluated for contraception (Clinicaltrials.gov NCT03107377), is in testing for the prevention of urogenital chlamydia and gonorrhea and recurrent bacterial vaginosis. However, safety should be well established before recommending use in high–HIV risk individuals or countries.

With the introduction of new technologies comes the risk of behavioral changes. Those involved in the field debate the potential for risk compensation with use of oral pre-exposure prophylaxis (PrEP) for HIV prevention, noting the concern that reduction in condom use could lead to an increase in other STIs and potentially unplanned pregnancy in women. A South African study showed that condom use may increase in adolescents using PrEP due to increased awareness of personal HIV risk.[66] Conversely, use of PrEP in men who have sex with men (MSM) was associated with increased diagnoses of rectal chlamydia and any STIs.[67] Oral PrEP is a critical HIV prevention method, but with increasing availability and use, emergent trends in risk perception and consequent behavior in specific populations should be observed to assess the potential impact on reproductive health.

Male Condoms

Although male condoms are an effective contraceptive method as well as a protector against STIs, a great deal remains to be accomplished to reach the optimal level of use. With the recognition that condoms are not right for everyone and for every situation, this centuries-old method remains an effective strategy to prevent pregnancy and the only contraceptive method to prevent HIV. In survey data from 2011 to 2015, 97.4% of sexually experienced females aged 15 to 19 had ever used condoms, indicating that nearly all sexually active women will use condoms at some point in their life.[68]

There are three specific goals to effectively use condoms: correct use, consistent use, and affordable, easy availability. If these goals are met, the 21st century will see the annual manufacture of 20 billion condoms per year.

When used correctly and consistently, male condoms are approximately 90% effective in reducing HIV transmission and 98% effective in preventing pregnancy during 1 year of use.[69] Condoms must be used consistently and correctly to achieve the high levels of protection against HIV.

Various types of condoms are available. Although most are made of latex, polyurethane condoms are also now manufactured. "Natural skin" (lamb's intestine) condoms are not approved for prevention of STIs and represent a very small proportion of sales. Latex condoms are 0.3 to 0.8 mm thick. Sperm are 0.003 mm in diameter and cannot penetrate condoms. The organisms that cause STIs also do not penetrate latex or polyurethane condoms, but they can penetrate condoms made from intestine.[70,71] Evidence indicates that condom use also prevents transmission of human papillomavirus (HPV).[72] Consistent use of condoms when one partner is HIV seropositive is highly effective in preventing HIV transmission, with one study showing no seroconversion in 124 serodiscordant heterosexual couples who used condoms consistently compared with 12.7% conversion after 24 months in couples with inconsistent use.[73,74] Women who are partners of condom users are less likely to be HIV positive.[75] An extensive literature review concluded that consistent use of condoms provides protection against HIV to a degree comparable to condom efficacy in preventing pregnancy (reflecting some inconsistent use and other routes of transmission).[74] In addition, condoms protect against transmission of the herpes simplex virus from infected men to women.[76]

Polyurethane condoms are expected to protect against STIs and HIV, based on in vitro efficacy as a barrier to bacteria and viruses. They are odorless, may have greater sensitivity, and are resistant to deterioration from storage and oil-based lubricants. Those individuals who have the infrequent problem of latex allergy can use polyurethane condoms. Breakage and slippage have been reported to be comparable with latex condoms.[77] However, in a randomized, well-designed study, the polyurethane condom had a sixfold higher breakage rate, and another study comparing latex and polyurethane condoms found a higher pregnancy rate with the polyurethane condom.[78,79]

Condoms can be straight or tapered, smooth or ribbed, colored or clear, and lubricated or nonlubricated. These are all marketing ventures aimed at attracting individual notions of pleasure and enjoyment.[80] An often-repeated concern is the alleged reduction in penile glans sensitivity that accompanies condom use,[80] although this claim has never been objectively studied and may be more of a perception than reality. A clinician can overcome this objection by advocating the use of thinner, more novel condoms. To encourage use in clinical practice, health care providers should remind women that while many men will choose the alternative of sex without a condom to sex with a condom, they will generally prefer sex with a condom to no sex. Setting expectations regarding the rules of conduct in a sexual relationship to focus on pregnancy and disease prevention benefits women and men.

Prospective users need instructions if they are to avoid pregnancy and STIs. A condom must be placed on the penis before it touches a partner. Uncircumcised men must pull the foreskin back prior to placement. Before unrolling the condom to the base of the penis, air should be squeezed out of the reservoir tip with a thumb and forefinger **(Figure 10.5)**. The tip of the condom should extend beyond the end of the penis to provide a reservoir to collect the ejaculate (a half inch of pinched tip). If lubricants are used, they must be water or silicone based. Oil-based lubricants (such as Vaseline) will weaken the latex. Couples should be concerned that any vaginal medication can compromise condom integrity. After intercourse, the condom should be held at the base as the penis is withdrawn. Semen must not be allowed to spill or leak. The condom should be handled gently because fingernails

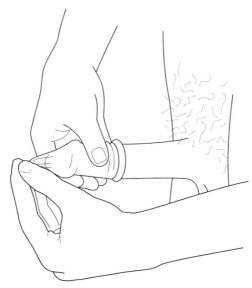

Figure 10.5 Proper placement of condom to leave reservoir at tip.

and rings can penetrate the material and cause leakage. If there is evidence of condom failure (spill, leakage, or breakage), emergency contraception is recommended (see Chapter 12).

Summary: Key Steps for Maximal Condom Efficacy

1. Use condoms for every act of coitus.
2. The best HIV/STI barrier is a condom without N-9.
3. Place the condom before vaginal contact.
4. Create a reservoir at the tip.
5. Withdraw while the penis is still erect.
6. Hold the base of the condom during withdrawal.

Clinicians should provide instructions on proper use of condoms when discussing their use for contraception or STI prevention. Condoms are available without a prescription and are used without medical supervision. Therefore, clinicians should use every opportunity to inform patients about their proper use.

Inconsistent or incorrect use explains most condom failures. Condoms sometimes break or slip during use. Breakage rates range from 1 to 8 per 100 episodes of vaginal intercourse (somewhat higher for anal intercourse). Slippage rates range from 1% to 5%.[81,82] These failures decrease over time; breakage and slippage (sufficient to increase the risk of pregnancy or STIs) occur at a rate of about 1% among experienced users.[83] In a U.S. survey, one pregnancy resulted for every three condom breakages.[84] In addition, even when slippage or breakage occurs, the condom may provide some protection against pregnancy and STIs due to an overall reduction in exposure to semen.[85]

Breakage represents a greater problem for couples at risk for STIs. An infected man transmits gonorrhea to a susceptible woman approximately two thirds of the time.[86] If the woman is infected, transmission to the man occurs one third of the time.[87] The chances of HIV infection after a single sexual exposure range from 1 in 1,000 to 1 in 10.[88,89]

Condom breakage rates depend on sexual behavior and practices, experience with condom use, the condition of the condoms, and manufacturing quality. Condoms can remain in good condition for up to 5 years unless exposed to ultraviolet light, excessive heat or humidity, ozone, or oils. Condom manufacturers regularly check samples of their products to make sure they meet national standards. These procedures limit the proportion of defects to less than 0.1% of all condoms distributed. Contraceptive failure is more likely to be due to nonuse or incorrect use. While carrying a condom in a wallet may demonstrate willingness and preparedness on the part of a man, clinicians should stress checking expiration date in the event of nonuse. Policies that make condoms available to both young men and women should improve outcomes.

For women using a condom to prevent pregnancy, emergency contraception (EC) is indicated when a condom breaks or if there is reason to believe spillage or leakage occurred. See Chapter 12 for a detailed discussion of EC. As efficacy of EC is directly related to timing of administration following unprotected sex, clinicians should provide educations and advanced prescription of EC to couples who rely on condoms for contraception and encourage them to keep an appropriate method available for self-medication.

For the immediate future, prevention of STIs and control of the HIV epidemic will require a great increase in the use of male condoms. Clinician involvement in the effort to educate regarding condom use may help increase uptake and provide empowering information to encourage cooperation of a reluctant partner. Emphasizing that prevention of STIs will also preserve future fertility may motivate some patients. *We recommend that any women not in a stable, monogamous relationship use a dual approach combining the contraceptive efficacy offered by LARC methods, hormonal contraception, or permanent contraception with the use of a condom for prevention of STIs.*

359

The Female Condom

The FC1® was the first female condom to receive approval from the U.S. FDA.[90] The design is a polyurethane pouch, which lines the vagina; an internal ring in the closed end of the pouch covers the cervix, and an external ring remains outside the vagina, partially covering the perineum. The FC2® (fc2.us.com) is the second-generation female condom from the Female Health Company. It addressed the issues of cost and noise with the FC1 by replacing the polyurethane with a less expensive nitrile material and is also reportedly less noisy than its predecessor. The female condom is prelubricated with silicone, contains no spermicide, and can be used with oil- or water-based lubricants. The FC2 condom is inserted by squeezing the inner ring and pushing it and the pouch up into the vagina typically 2 to 20 minutes before sex. It is for one-time use and should be removed after sex by twisting the outer ring and pulling out gently. The FC2 is indicated for preventing pregnancy, HIV/AIDS, and other STIs, and perfect-use 1-year pregnancy rates are 5%.[1] The female condom is impervious in vitro to cytomegalovirus and HIV.[91] The integrity of the female condom is maintained with up to eight multiple uses with washing, drying, and relubricating.[92] The devices are more cumbersome than condoms, and studies have indicated relatively high rates of problems such as slippage.[93] Women who have successfully used barrier methods and who are strongly motivated to avoid STIs are more likely to choose the female condom. With careful use, the efficacy rate should be similar to that of the diaphragm and the cervical cap.[94,95]

Other female condoms available outside the United States include the Woman's Condom developed by PATH (Shanghai Dahua Medical Apparatus Company) featuring a polyurethane pouch, dissolving capsule for insertion, and foam shapes for stability;[96] the VA w.o.w.® (Medtech Health Products Ltd., India), which has a pouch attached to a rounded triangular outer ring and a sponge to aid insertion; and the Cupid female condom (Cupid Limited, India) with an octagonal outer ring at the open end of the sheath.[97]

In September 2018, the FDA released a final rule to down-classify (class III to II) and rename the female condom as the single-use internal condom. This new classification expands the use of these devices to anal intercourse, consistent with how they are being used in practice.[98] This rule will also reduce the regulatory burden and allow for a similar approval process as the male condom, potentially leading to the emergence of more commercial varieties.

Postpartum/Postabortion

If no contraceptive method is used, it is possible to become pregnant soon after having a baby or after a spontaneous or induced abortion. Barrier methods have the benefit that they are effective immediately and can be used when intercourse resumes. The recommended time interval for resumption of intercourse can be 1 week or less after abortion but can vary based on individual circumstances. The cervical cap, diaphragm, and sponge can be used starting 6 weeks after childbirth; fit of the diaphragm or cervical cap should be confirmed, as the same device used prior to pregnancy may no longer fit correctly.

References

1. **Trussell J,** Contraceptive efficacy, In: Hatcher RA, Nelson AL, Trussell J, Cwaik C, Cason P, Policar, M, Aiken, A, Marrazzo J, Policar M, eds., Contraceptive Technology, 21st Revised ed., Arent Media, New York, 2018.

2. **Sundaram A, Vaughan B, Kost K, Bankole A, Finer L, Singh S, Trussell J,** Contraceptive failure in the United States: estimates from the 2006–2010 National Survey of Family Growth, Perspect Sex Reprod Health 49:7–16, 2017.

3. **Grimes DA, Cates W Jr,** Family planning and sexually transmitted diseases, In: Holmes KK, Mardh P-A, Sparling PF, eds. Sexually Transmitted Diseases, 2nd ed., McGraw-Hill, New York, 1990, p 1087.

4. **Cramer DW, Goldman MB, Schiff I, Belisla S, Albrecht B, Stadel B, Gibson M, Wilson E, Stillman R, Thompson I,** The relationship of tubal infertility to barrier method and oral contraceptive use, JAMA 257:2446, 1987.

5. **Rosenberg MJ, Davidson AJ, Chen J-H, Judson FN, Douglas JM,** Barrier contraceptives and sexually transmitted diseases in women: a comparison of female-dependent methods and condoms, Am J Public Health 82:669, 1992.

6. **Rowe PJ,** You win some and you lose some—contraception and infections, Aust N Z J Obstet Gynaecol 34:299, 1994.

7. **Cates W Jr, Stone K,** Family planning, sexually transmitted diseases and contraceptive choice: a literature update: part I, Fam Plann Perspect 24:75, 1992.

8. **Kost K, Forrest JD, Harlap S,** Comparing the health risks and benefits of contraceptive choices, Fam Plann Perspect 23:54, 1991.

9. **Coker AL, Hulka BS, McCann MF, Walton LA,** Barrier methods of contraception and cervical intraepithelial neoplasia, Contraception 45:1, 1992.

10. **Schwartz B, Gaventa S, Broome CV, Reingold AL, Hightower AW, Perlman JA, Wolf PH,** Nonmenstrual toxic shock syndrome associated with barrier contraceptives: report of a case-control study, Rev Infect Dis 11:S43, 1989.

11. **Curtis KM, Tepper NK, Jatlaoui TC, et al.,** U.S. medical eligibility criteria for contraceptive use, 2016, MMWR Recomm Rep 65:1–104, 2016. doi:http://dx.doi.org/10.15585/mmwr.rr6503a1.

12. **Daniels K, Daugherty J, Jones J, Mosher W,** Current contraceptive use and variation by selected characteristics among women aged 15-44: United States, 2011-2013, Natl Health Stat Report (86):1–14, 2015.

13. **Trussell J, Sturgen K, Strickler J, Dominik R,** Comparative contraceptive efficacy of the female condom and other barrier methods, Fam Plann Perspect 26:66, 1994.

14. **Cook L, Nanda K, Grimes D,** The diaphragm with and without spermicide for contraception: a Cochrane review, Hum Reprod 17:867, 2002.

15. **Ferreira, AE, et al.,** Effectiveness of the diaphragm, used continuously, without spermicide, Contraception 48:29–35, 1993.

16. **Fihn SD, Latham RH, Roberts P, Running K, Stamm WE,** Association between diaphragm use and urinary tract infection, JAMA 254:240, 1985.

17. **Hooton TM, Scholes D, Hughes JP, Winter C, Roberts PL, Stapleton AE, Stergachis A, Stamm WE,** A prospective study of risk factors for symptomatic urinary tract infection in young women, N Engl J Med 335:468, 1996.

18. **Hooton TM, Hillier S, Johnson C, Roberts P, Stamm WE,** Escherichia coli bacteriuria and contraceptive method, JAMA 265:64, 1991.

19. **Schwartz JL, Weiner DH, Lai JJ, Frezieres RG, Creinin MD, Archer DF, Bradley L, Barnhart KT, Poindexter A, Kilbourne-Brook M, Callahan MM, Mauck CK,** Contraceptive efficacy, safety, fit, and acceptability of a single-size diaphragm developed with end-user input, Obstet Gynecol (4):895–903, 2015.

20. **Centers for Disease Control and Prevention,** Toxic shock syndrome, United States, 1970–1982, MMWR Morb Mortal Wkly Rep 31:201, 1982.

21. **Keith L, Berger G, Moss W,** Prevalence of gonorrhea among women using various methods of contraception, Br J Vener Dis 51:307, 1975.

22. **Kelaghan J, Rubin GL, Ory HW, Layde PM,** Barrier method contraceptives and pelvic inflammatory disease, JAMA 248:184, 1982.

23. **Padian NS, van der Straten A, Ramjee G, Chipato T, de Bruyn G, Blanchard K, Shiboski S, Montgomery ET, Fancher H, Cheng H, Rosenblum M, van der Laan M, Jewell N, McIntyre J; MIRA Team,** Diaphragm and lubricant gel for prevention of HIV acquisition in southern African women: a randomized controlled trial, Lancet 370:251, 2007.

24. **Coffey PS, Kilbourne-Brook M, Brache V, Cochón L,** Comparative acceptability of the SILCS and Ortho ALL-FLEX diaphragms among couples in the Dominican Republic, Contraception 78:418, 2008.

25. **Bernstein G, Kilzer LH, Coulson AH, Nakamara RM, Smith GC, Bernstein R, Frezieres R, Clark VA, Coan C,** Studies of cervical caps, Contraception 26:443, 1982.

26. **Richwald GA, Greenland S, Gerber MM, Potik R, Kersey L, Comas MA,** Effectiveness of the cavity-rim cervical cap: results of a large clinical study, Obstet Gynecol 74:143, 1989.

27. **Gollub EL, Sivin I,** The Prentif cervical cap and pap smear results: a critical appraisal, Contraception 40:343, 1989.

28. **Shihata AA,** The FemCap: a new contraceptive choice, Eur J Contracept Reprod Health Care 3:160, 1998.

29. **Mauck C, Callahan M, Weiner DH, Dominik R; and the FemCap® Investigators Group,** A comparative study of the safety and efficacy of FemCap®, a new vaginal barrier contraceptive, and the Ortho All-Flex® diaphragm, Contraception 60:71, 1999.

30. **Courtot AM, Nikas G, Gravanis A, Psychoyos A,** Effects of cholic acid and "Protectaid" formulations on human sperm motility and ultrastructure, Hum Reprod 9:1999, 1994.

31. **Psychoyos A, Creatsas G, Hassan E,** Spermicidal and antiviral properties of cholic acid: contraceptive efficacy of a new vaginal sponge (Protectaid®) containing sodium cholate, Hum Reprod 8:866, 1993.

32. **Edelman DA, McIntyre SL, Harper J,** A comparative trial of the Today

contraceptive sponge and diaphragm: a preliminary report, Am J Obstet Gynecol 150:869, 1984.

33. **Creatsas G, Guerrero E, Guilbert E, Drouin J, Serfaty D, Lemieux L, Suissa S, Colin P,** A multinational evaluation of the efficacy, safety and acceptability of the Protectaid contraceptive sponge, Eur J Contracept Reprod Health Care 6:172, 2001.

34. **McIntyre SL, Higgins JE,** Parity and use-effectiveness with the contraceptive sponge, Am J Obstet Gynecol 155:796, 1986.

35. **Costello Daly C, Helling-Giese GE, Mati JK, Hunter DJ,** Contraceptive methods and the transmission of HIV: implications for family planning, Genitourin Med 70:110, 1994.

36. **Bayer LL, Jensen JT,** ACIDFORM: a review of the evidence, Contraception 90:11–18, 2014.

37. **Mauck C, Brache V, Kimble T, Doncel GF, Schwartz JL,** A phase I randomized postcoital testing and safety study of the Caya diaphragm used with 3% Nonoxynol-9 gel, ContraGel, or no gel, Contraception 96:124–130, 2017.

38. **Hicks DR, Martin LS, Getchell JP, Health JL, Francis DP, McDougal JS, Curran JW, Voeller B,** Inactivation of HTLV-III/LAV-infected cultures of normal human lymphocytes by nonoxynol-9 in vitro, Lancet 2:1422, 1985.

39. **Kreiss J, Ngugi E, Holmes K, Ndinya-Achola J, Waiyaki P, Roberts PL, Ruminjo I, Sajabi R, Kimata J, Fleming TR, Anzala A, Holton D, Plummer F,** Efficacy of nonoxynol-9 contraceptive sponge use in preventing heterosexual acquisition of HIV in Nairobi prostitutes, JAMA 268:477, 1992.

40. **Zekeng L, Feldblum PJ, Oliver RM, Kaptue L,** Barrier contraceptive use and HIV infection among high risk women in Cameroon, AIDS 7:725, 1993.

41. **Wittkowski KM, Susser E, Kietz K,** The protective effect of condoms and nonoxynol-9 against HIV infection, Am J Public Health 88:590, 1998.

42. **Centers for Disease Control and Prevention,** Nonoxynol-9 spermicide contraception use—United States, 1999, MMWR Morb Mortal Wkly Rep 51:389, 2002.

43. **Van Damme L, Ramjee G, Alary M, Vuylsteke B, Chandeying V, Rees H, Sirivongrangson P, Mukenge-Tshibaka L, Ettiegne-Traore V, Uaheowitchai C, Karim SS, Masee B, Perriens J, Laga M; for the COL-1492 Study Group,** Effectiveness of COL-1492, a nonoxynol-9 vaginal gel, on HIV-1 transmission in female sex workers: a randomised controlled trial, Lancet 360:971, 2002.

44. **Louv WC, Austin H, Alexander WJ, Stagno S, Cheeks J,** A clinical trial of nonoxynol-9 as a prophylaxis for cervical Neisseria gonorrhoeae and Chlamydia trachomatis infections, J Infect Dis 158:518, 1988.

45. **Austin H, Louv WC, Alexander WJ,** A case-control study of spermicides and gonorrhea, JAMA 251:2822, 1984.

46. **Niruthisard S, Roddy RE, Chutivongse S,** Use of nonoxynol-9 and reduction in rate of gonococcal and chlamydial cervical infections, Lancet 339:1371, 1992.

47. **Roddy RE, Zekeng L, Ryan KA, Tamoufém U, Weir SS, Wong EL,** A controlled trial of nonoxynol 9 film to reduce male-to-female transmission of sexually transmitted diseases, N Engl J Med 339:504, 1998.

48. **Roddy RE, Zekeng L, Ryan KA, Tamoufe U, Tweedy KG,** Effect of nonoxynol-9 gel on urogenital gonorrhea and chlamydial infection: a randomized controlled trial, JAMA 287:1117, 2002.

49. **Richardson BA, Lavreys L, Martin HL Jr, Stevens CE, Ngugi E, Mandaliya K, Bwayo J, Ndinya-Achola J, Kreiss JK,** Evaluation of a low-dose nonoxynol-9 gel for the prevention of sexually transmitted diseases: a randomized clinical trial, Sex Transm Dis 28:394, 2001.

50. **Barbone F, Austin H, Louv WC, Alexander WJ,** A follow-up study of methods of contraception, sexual activity, and rates of trichomoniasis, candidiasis, and bacterial vaginosis, Am J Obstet Gynecol 163:510, 1990.

51. **Raymond E, Dominik R; and the Spermicide Trial Group,** Contraceptive effectiveness of two spermicides: a randomized trial, Obstet Gynecol 93:896, 1999.

52. **Raymond EG, Chen PL, Luoto J; for the Spermicide Trial Group,** Contraceptive

effectiveness and safety of five nonoxynol-9 spermicides: a randomized trial, Obstet Gynecol 103:430, 2004.

53. **Steiner MJ, Hertz-Picciotto I, Schulz KF, Sangi-Haghpeykar H, Earle BB, Trussell J,** Measuring true contraceptive efficacy. A randomized approach—condom vs. spermicide vs. no method, Contraception 58:375–378, 1998.

54. **Louik C, Mitchell AA, Werler MM, Hanson JW, Shapiro S,** Maternal exposure to spermicides in relation to certain birth defects, N Engl J Med 317:474, 1987.

55. **Bracken MB, Vita K,** Frequency of non-hormonal contraception around conception and association with congenital malformations in offspring, Am J Epidemiol 117:281, 1983.

56. **Einarson TR, Koren G, Mattice D, Schechter-Tsafiri O,** Maternal spermicide use and adverse reproductive outcome: a meta-analysis, Am J Obstet Gynecol 162:655, 1990.

57. **Malyk B,** Preliminary results: serum chemistry values before and after the intravaginal administration of 5% nonoxynol-9 cream, Fertil Steril 35:647, 1981.

58. **Niruthisard S, Roddy RE, Chutivonge S,** The effects of frequent nonoxynol-9 use on vaginal and cervical mucosa, Sex Transm Dis 268:521, 1991.

59. **Roddy RE, Cordero M, Cordero C, Fortney JA,** A dosing study of nonoxynol-9 and genital irritation, AIDS 4:165, 1993.

60. **Hooton TM, Fennell CL, Clark AM, Stamm WE,** Nonoxynol-9: differential antibacterial activity and enhancement of bacterial adherence to vaginal epithelial cells, J Infect Dis 164:1216, 1991.

61. **Skoler-Karpoff S, Ramjee G, Ahmed K, Altini L, Plagianos MG, Friedland B, Govender S, De Kock A, Cassim N, Palanee T, Dozier G, Maguire R, Lahteenmaki P,** Efficacy of Carraguard for prevention of HIV infection in women in South Africa: a randomised, double-blind, placebo-controlled trial, Lancet 372:1977, 2008.

62. **Burke AE, Barnhart K, Jensen JT, Creinin MD, Walsh TL, Wan LS, et al.,** Contraceptive efficacy, acceptability, and safety of C31G and nonoxynol-9 spermicidal gels: a randomized controlled trial, Obstet Gynecol 116:1265–1273, 2010.

63. **Mauck CK, Freziers RG, Walsh TL, Peacock K, Schwartz JL, Callahan MM,** Noncomparative contraceptive efficacy of cellulose sulfate gel, Obstet Gynecol 111:739–746, 2008. doi:10.1097/AOG.0b013e3181644598.

64. **Williams DL, Newman DR, Ballagh SA, Creinin MD, Barnhart K, Weiner DH, Bell AJ, Jamieson DJ,** Phase I safety trial of two vaginal microbicide gels (Acidform or BufferGel) used with a diaphragm compared to KY jelly used with a diaphragm, Sex Transm Dis 34:977, 2007.

65. **Ballagh SA, Brache V, Mauck C, Callahan MM, Cochon L, Wheeless A, Moench TR,** A phase I study of the functional performance, safety and acceptability of the BufferGel® Duet™, Contraception 77:130, 2008.

66. **Maljaars LP, Gill K, Smith PJ, et al.,** Condom migration after introduction of pre-exposure prophylaxis among HIV-uninfected adolescents in South Africa: a cohort analysis, South Afr J HIV Med 18:712, 2017. doi:10.4102/sajhivmed.v18i1.712.

67. **Traeger MW, Schroeder SE, Wright EJ, Hellard ME, Cornelisse VJ, Doyle JS, Stoové MA,** Effects of pre-exposure prophylaxis for the prevention of human immunodeficiency virus infection on sexual risk behavior in men who have sex with men: a systematic review and meta-analysis, Clin Infect Dis 67:676–686, 2018. doi:10.1093/cid/ciy182.

68. **Abma J, Martinez GM,** Sexual activity and contraceptive use among teenagers in the United States, 2011–2015, Natl Health Stat Report (104):1, 2017.

69. **Weller S, Davis K,** Condom effectiveness in reducing heterosexual HIV transmission, Cochrane Database Syst Rev (1):CD003255, 2002.

70. **Stone KM, Grimes DA, Magder LS,** Primary prevention of sexually transmitted diseases: a primer for clinicians, JAMA 255:1763, 1986.

71. **Van de Perre P, Jacobs D, Sprecher-Goldberger S,** The latex condom, an efficient barrier against sexual transmission of AIDS-related viruses, AIDS 1:49, 1987.

72. **Winer RL, Hughes JP, Feng Q, O'Reilly S, Kiviat NB, Holmes KK, Koutsky LA,** Condom use and the risk of genital human papillomavirus infection in young women, N Engl J Med 354:2645, 2006.

73. **DeVincenzi I; for the European Study Group on Heterosexual Transmission of HIV,** A longitudinal study of human immunodeficiency virus transmission by heterosexual partners, N Engl J Med 331:341, 1994.

74. **Davis KR, Weller SC,** The effectiveness of condoms in reducing heterosexual transmission of HIV, Fam Plann Perspect 31:272, 1999.

75. **Diaz T, Schable B, Chu SY; and the Supplement to HIV and AIDS Surveillance Project Group,** Relationship between use of condoms and other forms of contraception among human immunodeficiency virus-infected women, Obstet Gynecol 86:277, 1995.

76. **Wald A, Langenberg AG, Link K, Izu AE, Ashley R, Warren T, Tyring S, Douglas JM Jr, Corey L,** Effect of condoms on reducing the transmission of herpes simplex virus type 2 from men to women, JAMA 285:3100, 2001.

77. **Rosenberg MJ, Waugh MS, Solomon HM, Lyszkowski ADL,** The male polyurethane condom: a review of current knowledge, Contraception 53:141, 1996.

78. **Frezieres RG, Walsh TL, Nelson AL, Clark VA, Coulson AH,** Breakage and acceptability of a polyurethane condom: a randomized, controlled study, Fam Plann Perspect 30:73, 1998.

79. **Steiner MJ, Dominik R, Rountree RW, Nanda K, Dorflinger L,** Contraceptive effectiveness of a polyurethane condom and a latex condom: a randomized controlled trial, Obstet Gynecol 101:539, 2003.

80. **Grady WR, Klepinger DH, Billy JOG, Tanfer K,** Condom characteristics: the perceptions and preferences of men in the United States, Fam Plann Perspect 25:67, 1993.

81. **Trussell J, Warner DL, Hatcher RA,** Condom slippage and breakage rates, Fam Plann Perspect 24:20, 1992.

82. **Sparrow MJ, Lavill K,** Breakage and slippage of condoms in family planning clients, Contraception 50:117, 1994.

83. **Rosenberg MJ, Waugh MS,** Latex condom breakage and slippage in a controlled clinical trial, Contraception 56:17, 1997.

84. **Liskin L, Wharton C, Blackburn RD, Kestelman P,** Condoms—now more than ever, Population Reports Series H: Barrier Methods:1–36, 1990.

85. **Walsh TL, Frezieres RG, Peacock K, Nelson AL, Clark VA, Bernstein L, Wraxall BGD,** Use of prostate-specific antigen (PSA) to measure semen exposure resulting from male condom failures: implications for contraceptive efficacy and the prevention of sexually transmitted disease, Contraception 67:139, 2003.

86. **Platt R, Rice PA, McCormack WM,** Risk of acquiring gonorrhea and prevalence of abnormal adnexal findings among women recently exposed to gonorrhea, JAMA 250:3205, 1983.

87. **Hooper RR, Reynolds GM, Jones OG, Zaidi A, Wiesner RJ, Latimer KP, Lester A, Campbell AF, Harrison WO, Karney WW, Holmes KK,** Cohort study of venereal disease. I. The risk of gonorrhea transmission from infected women to men, Am J Epidemiol 108:136, 1978.

88. **Anderson RM, Medley GF,** Epidemiology of HIV infection and AIDS: incubation and infectious periods, survival and vertical transmissions, AIDS 2:557, 1988.

89. **Cameron DW, Simonsen JN, D'Costa LJ, Ronald AR, Maitha GM, Gakinya MN, Cheang M, et al.,** Female to male transmission of human immunodeficiency virus type 1: risk factors for seroconversion in men, Lancet 2:403, 1989.

90. **Soper DE, Brockwell NJ, Dalton JP,** Evaluation of the effects of a female condom on the female lower genital tract, Contraception 44:21, 1991.

91. **Drew WL, Blair M, Miner RC, Conant M,** Evaluation of the virus permeability of a new condom for women, Sex Transm Dis 17:110, 1990.

92. **Beksinska M, Rees HV, Dickson-Tetteh KE, Mqoqi N, Kleinschmidt I, McIntyre JA,** Structural integrity of the female condom after multiple uses, washing, drying, and re-lubrication, Contraception 63:33, 2001.

93. **Bounds W, Guillebaud J, Newman GB,** Female condom (Femidom): a clinical study of its use-effectiveness and patient acceptability, Br J Fam Plann 18:36, 1992.

94. **Farr G, Gabelnick H, Sturgen K, Dorflinger L,** Contraceptive efficacy and acceptability of the female condom, Am J Public Health 84:1960, 1994.

95. **Trussell J,** Contraceptive efficacy of the Reality® female condom, Contraception 58:147–148, 1998.

96. **Chen BA, Blithe DL, Muraguri GR, Lance AA, Carr BR, Jensen JT, et al.,** Acceptability of the Woman's Condom in a phase III multicenter open-label study, Contraception 99:357–362, 2019.

97. **Beksinska ME, Piaggio G, Smit JA, Wu J, Zhang Y, Pienaar J, Greener R, Zhou Y, Joanis C,** Performance and safety of the second-generation female condom (FC2) versus the Woman's, the VA worn-of-women, and the Cupid female condoms: a randomised controlled non-inferiority crossover trial, Lancet Glob Health 1:e146–e152, 2013.

98. **Kelvin EA, Mantell JE, Candelario N, et al.,** Off-Label use of the female condom for anal intercourse among men in New York City, Am J Public Health 101:2241–2244, 2011. doi:10.2105/AJPH.2011.300260.

11

Behavioral Methods of Contraception

Anita L. Nelson, MD and
Diana Crabtree Sokol, MD, MSc

Introduction

Behavioral methods of contraception, such as fertility awareness–based methods (FABMs), coitus interruptus (withdrawal), and a range of other sexual practices, appeal to couples who might, for religious, personal, or medical reasons, wish to avoid contraceptive methods that require medication or devices. Behavioral methods also appeal to those couples who, at least temporarily, lack access to modern methods. Compared to other contraceptives, these methods are associated with the largest gaps between failure rates with correct and consistent use and those with typical use. Patient education and motivation are particularly critical to success with these methods.[1]

However, when considering behavioral methods, we often forget to include the lactational amenorrhea method (LAM), which is more effective than FABM and withdrawal and is specific to the postpartum woman. LAM is vitally important for short-term and long-term maternal and child health. In this chapter, we devote an entire section to postpartum breast physiology and LAM.

FABMs utilize various techniques to detect at-risk days in the woman's cycle when unprotected intercourse is most likely to result in pregnancy. During those identified at-risk days, couples can choose to abstain from intercourse altogether (periodic abstinence) or to use other contraceptive methods of birth control, usually barriers or withdrawal.

However, we stress that abstinence alone is not a behavioral method of contraception. Abstinence is a behavior—a lifestyle choice. Conspicuously, women, men, or couples who choose abstinence are not sexually active and, therefore, do not need contraception. It is important to note that people that choose abstinence may use the method intermittently and not continually; thus, these persons may still need education about contraceptive options. Data from the National Survey of Family Growth (NSFG) reveal that over 7% of reproductive age women report having had sexually intercourse in the last 3 months without using a method of contraception.[2] We need to improve the use of effective contraceptive strategies for women and men who consider themselves abstinent, but engage in occasional sex.

Globally, FABM, withdrawal, LAM, and other behavioral approaches are classified as "nonmodern" or "traditional methods."[3] Utilization of the different methods in this category varies greatly across the world. As of 2016, 3.0% of reproductive age contracepting women worldwide report using periodic abstinence, but in some areas, that number can be up to 20%.[4] In the United States, estimates of FABM use are complicated by assignment rules. The percent of sexually active women who relied on FABM use was estimated to be 2.2% in the 2013 to 2015 NSFG, but rose to 3.2% if couples who used condoms, withdrawal, or EC during at-risk days were included.[5] Withdrawal by itself is used by many more couples; most people have used withdrawal at some time in their lives.[6] In 2008 to 2012, 15.8% of women reported consistently relying on withdrawal and intermittent or episodic use was even more common.[7] In a 2012 survey of 4,634 U.S. women aged 18 to 39, 13% reported that withdrawal was the most effective method they had used in the last 30 days; 12% relied on it exclusively, but another 21% had used it in combination with some other more effective method.[8]

Behavioral methods other than LAM are associated with higher failure rates than barrier, hormonal, intrauterine, and permanent contraceptive methods. Women who participate in clinical trials of FABM may be highly motivated to use the method but differ from women in clinical trials of more effective options in their willingness to accept a higher pregnancy risk. Collectively, FABMs are estimated to have a 15% first-year failure rate in typical use.[9] With correct and consistent use, FABM techniques have first-year failure rates that range from 2% to 23%.[9] Withdrawal has a 4% first-year pregnancy rate with correct and consistent use, but a 20% first-year failure rate in typical use.[9] A systematic review concluded that effectiveness studies of each FABM in typical use are few and only of low to moderate quality; variability in the studies precludes any comparisons between individual FABM techniques.[10,11] Most studies show high first-year discontinuation rates for FABM.[12]

FABM, withdrawal, and other behavioral methods require clear communication between sexual partners, agreement about their reproductive plans, and a commitment from both partners to make their method work. The success of FABM assumes the woman has the ability to say no to unprotected intercourse, but the 35% of women who suffer sexual/physical violence and coercion worldwide may well lack that ability.[13]

Many clinicians consider behavioral methods to be poor options for most women.[14,15] In some circles, withdrawal is not even considered a legitimate contraceptive method, even though its contributions to fertility control have been well documented for over a century. For sexually active women, health care providers tend to discourage use of these behavioral methods, especially FABM, because of the relatively high failure rates and, perhaps, their personal lack of familiarity with FABM, their lack of time to provide adequate counseling, or their underestimation of the potential these methods offer for contraception.[16] Obstetricians often do not routinely discuss LAM as a contraceptive, especially in developed countries where breastfeeding rates are low to moderate and breastfeeding for a full 6 months is uncommon.[17] Depriving a patient access to expert guidance about these methods forces her to seek out information from less reliable sources, which perpetuates the cycle of suboptimal usage and higher failure rates.

There are definite advantages to behavioral methods. These methods have no or minimal direct costs. No drugs or medical system interactions are required for most techniques. Withdrawal is always available; it can be used with any coital act at any time in the cycle. It is one of the only methods available to men. There are no medical contraindications to any behavioral method although cycle variability in women with irregular menstrual cycles precludes use of most FABM and the onset of menstrual-like bleeding provides notice that LAM should no longer be used.

Fertility Awareness–Based Methods

FABMs utilize various techniques to detect at-risk days in the woman's cycle when unprotected intercourse is most likely to result in pregnancy. During those identified at-risk days, couples can choose to abstain from intercourse altogether (periodic abstinence) or to use other contraceptive methods of birth control, usually barriers or withdrawal. FABMs help couples gain understanding about their reproductive functioning and potential. This understanding can facilitate achieving pregnancy when it is desired and can help women recognize and anticipate symptoms of premenstrual syndrome or other catamenial problems.[18] FABMs also provide an opportunity for anovulatory women to detect their reduced fertility.

The various FABMs differ in the techniques used to calculate at-risk days and what methods to use during those days. There are three approaches used to calculate at-risk days (**Box 11.1**).

Each technique has traditional tools for women to use, but most also utilize more modern apps. In older parlance, these methods were collectively referred to as "natural family planning." This unfortunate phrase should be avoided, not only because it implies that all other methods are "unnatural" but also because it is technically incorrect. Libido in women is known to increase around the time of ovulation.[19–21] To call a method "natural" that asks couples

---

Box 11.1 Fertility Awareness Approaches

Method	Approach
Cycle length–based	Estimating the timing of ovulation in relation to menses
Sign/symptom-based ovulation detection	Rely on physical signs and symptoms to detect ovulation
Mixed methods	Combine information from the woman's history, physical changes, and laboratory tests

to abstain at the time in the woman's cycle when she is most "receptive" to sexual advances seems to be a cruel perversion of terminology.[10]

Each FABM technique relies on assumptions about the biology of ovulatory cycles and fertilization. Although there have been modern refinements in the estimates of fertility potential by cycle day,[22] most FABMs still rely on earlier observations of the timing of ovulation[23] and assume the following about ovulation and sperm.

Ovulation occurs at the following median times:

- 35 to 44 hours after the initial rise of luteinizing hormone (LH)
- 16 hours after the LH peak (range 8 to 40 hours)
- 24 hours after the estradiol peak (range 17 to 32 hours)
- 8 hours after the rise in progesterone (range 12.5 hours before to 10 hours after)
- 12 to 16 days before the onset of next menses, depending on cycle length

In addition, the following observations about ovulation and sperm are assumed to be true:

- No more than one ovulation occurs each cycle.
- Ova can only be fertilized during the 12 to 24 hours following ovulation.
- Sperm have the capacity to fertilize ova 3 days after they have been deposited in the vagina (however, this is really 5 days—see below).

Taken together, these estimates lead to the conclusion that there are only 6 days in a cycle when fertilization is possible—the 5 days preceding ovulation and the day of ovulation. However, variability in cycle-to-cycle lengths means that the time during a cycle when those 6 days occur may fluctuate, and even more days must be considered to be at risk when prospective assessments of fertility potential are being made. In addition, the fact that sperm can fertilize an egg for up to 5 days (not just 3 days as assumed in early FABM models) insures some built-in failure rate but makes the cycle length–based methods more acceptable by reducing the number of at-risk days.

Cycle Length–Based Methods

"Calendar Method" and "Rhythm Method"

Success with these cycle length methods requires that the woman has relatively minor variability in her cycle-to-cycle lengths. To determine if a woman can rely on these methods to identify the at-risk days, she must first record her menstrual cycles for 6 to 12 months. Classically, women collected this information during the year of engagement that preceded their wedding at a time when it was assumed the couple needed no contraception. Once enough information has been collected to determine the woman's shortest and the longest cycles, her at-risk days are identified using the following formulas:

- First at-risk (fertile) day each cycle = number of days in shortest cycle minus 18
- Last at-risk (fertile) day each cycle = number of days in longest cycle minus 11

Recent studies have shown that 20% of women studied for just four cycles had cycle lengths that varied by at least 14 days, making this method almost unfeasible. Another 26% had cycles that varied by 7 days or more, which would mean that they would be at risk for pregnancy at least 15 days per cycle.[24]

To use this technique, the woman indicates the at-risk days for the cycle on a calendar (paper or electronic) as soon as she starts her menses (hence the name "calendar method"). Women must be aware of cycles that are outliers (extra-long or short cycles) to see if they need to recalculate their at-risk days. Clinicians should be aware that women often report using the "rhythm method" without gathering the needed baseline information or doing any calculations; they only abstain for a few days when they sense (often incorrectly) that they are fertile.[25-27]

An older meta-analysis reported first-year failure rates for the calendar/rhythm method ranged from 15% to 19%.[28] An international study of women who used periodic abstinence based on the calendar method reported a typical use failure rate of 14%.[29] The unpredictable nature of a late ovulation, even in women who typically have regular cycles, likely contributes to these failure rates.[30] If couples use barrier methods during at-risk days, the failure rates may be lower because of higher compliance.[27]

Standard Days Method ("CycleBeads")

More recently, props, such as "CycleBeads," have been introduced to help women (couples) track at-risk days. The Standard Days Method relies on the observation that 78% of cycles range between 26 and 32 days, meaning that fertility is most likely to occur on days 8 to 21.[31] The beads **(Figure 11.1)** are color coded to alert users to at-risk days and to let them know if the cycle length is outside the appropriate range for the method.

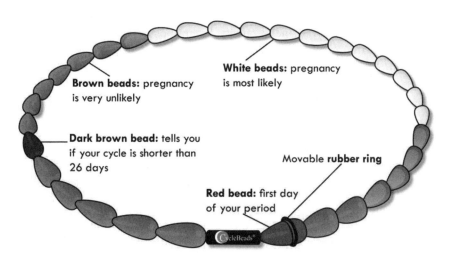

Figure 11.1 CycleBeads. An elastic band is advanced over a new bead each day to inform the user (and her partner) where she is in her cycle. CycleBeads are available at https://www.cyclebeads.com/shop.

Color-coded beads are assembled in a circle; an elastic band is advanced over one colored bead a day. The red bead represents the first day of bleeding and is followed by 7 brown (safe day) beads. CycleBeads 8 to 19, which represent the at-risk days, are colored white; in some versions, these beads glow in the dark. Beads 20 to 25 are brown. Bead 26 is brown-black and is used to remind women that if their menses start before this day, their cycles are too short, and this is not an appropriate method for them to use. Beads 27 to 31 are brown again. The 32nd bead is a black cylinder with an arrow arm showing the direction to advance the elastic band; this color reminds the woman that if she has not started her menses by then, she should consider pregnancy testing, or that her cycles are too long for her to rely on these beads.

First-year failure rates from the Standard Days Method clinical trial were 4.8% with correct and consistent use and 12% for the whole study population.[32] A meta-analysis of studies from 14 countries where the Standard Days Method was provided as a routine option showed a 14% failure rate,[33] consistent with a recent systematic review finding of 12%.[29] Interestingly, in one clinical trial, 23% of women had unprotected intercourse during at least one identified fertile day during one or more of the 13-cycle trials.[34] Based on these failure rates, WHO has classified Standard Days Method as a "modern method," a classification that has been openly challenged.[35,36]

"Apps" Based on Cycle Length Alone

Approximately 80% of 18- to 49-year-olds in the United States own a smart phone. Each of the technology giants, like Apple® and Google®, provides health applications for free to their users. Over 1,100 applications (apps) for tracking the menstrual cycles have come on the market, some requiring payment and others available for free.[37] These applications are highly variable in quality. Some apps provide digital platforms for existing cycle length–based methods, such as the calendar method and the Standard Days Method (available at https://www.cyclebeads.com/online). The data collected by some apps have been used to develop algorithms to predict fertility. For example, using the data of over 7,000 women with reliable menstrual and ovulation records, investigators fitted linear functions to the length of the cycle and timing of ovulation and concluded that the middle day of a mean menstrual cycle was the best estimate of the next ovulation.[38] A dynamic optimal timing (DOT) model was developed based on data from two cohort studies with over 10,000 women with cycles of 20 to 40 days. These identified between 11 and 13 at-risk days per cycle.[39,40] When women first start to use this method, many days are identified as high risk, but as information about the woman's cycle becomes more robust with time, the algorithm can more accurately recognize fewer at-risk days.[41] The first 6-month failure rate was 3.5%; the researchers reported that all those pregnancies resulted from incorrect use.[42]

In general, smart phone applications based on menstrual cycle data alone have been disappointing. Fewer than 20% of apps correctly predict the at-risk dates.[37,43] Because of this high error rate, it is important the clinicians guide their patients to accurate apps. Generally, apps discussed later in this chapter that utilize additional clues about ovulation timing are better options. Some observers have raised questions about the social, cultural, ethical, political, and privacy issues raised by these apps.[44]

Sign/Symptom-Based Ovulation Detection

Another approach to identify fertile days relies on biologic changes that can be detected around the time of ovulation. Persistently elevated estradiol levels (>200 pg/mL for 50 hours) that trigger the LH surge prior to ovulation induce several changes in cervical mucus, vaginal secretions, and saliva. Other physical changes, such as basal body temperature (BBT) and alterations in cervical mucus texture and composition, generally follow in short order. Together, these effects can help detect impending ovulation; their resolution can suggest the end of the at-risk days. These methods can be used by regularly cycling women as well as those with less predictable menstrual patterns, including women transitioning from breastfeeding or hormonal contraceptive use and women with irregular or infrequent menstrual cycles.[45,46]

For most of the cycle, the mucus secreted by the cervix is composed of poorly hydrated mucin. The resulting mucus is thick, scant, and viscous, forming a barrier to sperm and microorganisms. High estrogen levels at midcycle induce a number of changes to the composition and hydration of mucus that result in an increase in volume and a highly fluid low-viscosity consistency favorable to sperm penetration.[47,48]

Billings Ovulation Method

The Billings technique uses cervical mucus changes to monitor potential fertility throughout the woman's cycle. This method was approved by the Vatican and tested and promoted by the World Health Organization (WHO).[10,49] The woman evaluates the characteristics of her cervical mucus sampled at the introitus at least twice daily after her menses. Some experts advise that the woman assess her cervical mucus before and after each episode of urination by wiping front to back with toilet tissue to obtain a specimen. The woman assesses mucus presence or absence, quantity, color, fluidity, glossiness, transparency, and stretchiness (elasticity), charting the most fertile characteristics of the mucus over the entire day on a color-coded chart each night. She should evaluate the mucus for one to three cycles to familiarize herself with her patterns before attempting to rely on the method. Couples committed to this method need to avoid actions that complicate mucus evaluation including douching and intercourse on consecutive days; the day off permits mucus evaluation without any contamination by the ejaculate.

Early phase cervical mucus is scant and sticky. The volume of cervical mucus increases 2 to 9 days before ultrasound-detected ovulation.[50]

The Billings method assumes that cervical mucus can be detected on the vulva near the introitus by most women 4 to 7 days ahead of ovulation.[51] As ovulation approaches, the mucus becomes more abundant, clearer in color, and elastic. The last day with clear (transparent like a raw egg white), slippery, and elastic (it can be stretched for several centimeters before it breaks) mucus is called the "peak day." This day, of course, can only be retrospectively diagnosed. In the Billings method, the peak day mucus is assumed to occur at the time of ovulation. However, more recent studies show that ovulation actually occurs with a mean of 0.9 days following that peak day but ranges from 2 days before peak mucus to 3 days after.[50]

Classically, women using the Billings method were told to follow four rules to utilize their cervical mucus findings as effectively as possible to prevent pregnancy:[52,53]

- There must be no intercourse if the woman has any bleeding or spotting.
- Early in her cycle, when there is no cervical mucus or the secretions are consistently scant, cloudy, and sticky, intercourse can occur but no more frequently than every other day (although multiple acts are permitted on any 1 allowable day).
- Coitus is to be avoided once mucus becomes abundant and clear.
- Abstinence must be maintained or a backup method used until 4 days following the peak day mucus (assumed ovulation day). If the earlier cervical mucus changes resolve without signs of ovulation, intercourse may resume after 4 days of dryness.

Under the Billing method, 95% of all women will have 4 to 12 days of observable secretions, so many days of abstinence or other method use may be required. Since sperm can survive for up to 5 days, some experts now advise that women who rely on the Billings method classify all days when secretions can be detected as "at-risk days."[54] Older studies estimate first-year failure rates with classical Billings method to be 3% and 23% in more generalized use.[52,54,55] Cervical or vaginal infections and vaginally administered medications interfere with interpretations of cervical mucus.

A modification of the Billings method, the Creighton model NaPro Education Technology, uses picture and a more precise, standardized way to describe the cervical secretions.[56]

TwoDay Method

This method greatly simplifies the Billings method by decreasing the number of cervical mucus analyses. The TwoDay Method is a real-time, focused method in which the patient touches her introitus (with finger or tissue) at least once daily or as frequently as each time she urinates to determine by sensation or observation if there is *any* moisture present. The woman asks, "Am I dry today?" If she is dry, she then asks "Was I dry yesterday?" Unprotected coitus is allowed only if she has been dry for 2 consecutive days. Although multiple acts of coitus may be allowed on any one day, the next permissible day for coitus would be 3 days later because the moisture from that day's ejaculate will be detected as wetness the following day. This method is portable, allows for cycle-to-cycle variability (including infrequent menses), and is easy to teach. One multicountry study found that first-year failure rate with correct and consistent use was 3.5%; the total first-year failure rate in the study was 14%.[57] Typical use failure rates are not available.

Basal Body Temperature Method

This method is based on the fact that progesterone is thermogenic. In the follicular phase, BBT generally ranges from 97.0°F to 98.0°F. One day before ovulation, the BBT drops to its nadir. With the formation of the corpus luteum following ovulation, progesterone production increases and the BBT rises 0.5°F to 1.5°F. The higher temperature is maintained until the progesterone levels fall in late in the luteal phase, usually within 1 to 2 days before or at the onset of menstruation.[47]

To detect changes in temperature, a special BBT thermometer is required. Whereas a standard thermometer is accurate to 0.2°F, a BBT thermometer is accurate to 0.1°F. Women are asked to plot, on paper or on an electronic chart, their BBT taken at rest at the *same* time each day using the digital thermometers applied to the same site (e.g., oral, axillary, etc.) without arising for the preceding 3 to 6 hours. These conditions can be challenging. Illness, sleep disturbances, getting out of bed to urinate, or answer a baby's call can render the measured temperature invalid. Sleeping in late on weekends is not permissible. Even if the woman can collect accurate measurements, only 80% of cycles may have interpretable patterns.

To interpret the results, ovulation can be detected by using the "coverline method" or the "three-over-six rule." In the former, a horizontal threshold line is drawn at a level 0.15°F above the highest temperature recorded in the first 10 days of the cycle; ovulation is documented when temperatures taken later in the cycle cross that line. For the second, three consecutive temperatures must be 0.2°F higher than the highest point of the previous six temperature measurements, with at least a 0.4°F difference between the lowest and highest measurements.[47] BBT measurements are most effective as a postovulatory method that allows unprotected intercourse to start only after BBTs have been elevated for at least 3 days. Abstinence or other methods must be used at all other times earlier in the cycle—usually 16 days a cycle.[18]

Hormonal Testing

Most hormone monitors are designed to detect rising estradiol levels, which portends the onset of fertility and LH levels to indicate impending ovulation. Ovulation does not occur *before* the urinary LH peak day or the serum LH surge day.[50,58] Over-the-counter kits to detect the presence of urinary LH are best used once or twice a day starting from idealized cycle day 10 or 11 to detect the initial LH increase.[58] Interestingly, in 75% of cases, the onset of the LH surge starts between midnight and 08:00 hours.[47,59] Once LH is detected by these tests, ovulation generally follows in 20 ± 3 hours.[47] But since these tests may detect LH well before the peak, ovulation may occur as late as 3 days after a positive test.[47]

Urinary LH detection kits may be helpful for timing intercourse when couples seek pregnancy, but by *themselves* may have limited value in preventing pregnancy unless they are used in algorithms that permit unprotected intercourse only in the postovulatory period (4 days after LH surge). This limitation is because the LH surge occurs too close to the time of ovulation and cannot alert couples of impending risk 3 to 5 days before ovulation. LH detection may also be useful as a component in mixed methods.

Other body fluids have also been tested for their ability to predict ovulation. In 88% of cycles, at-risk days correspond to times when ferning is seen in saliva samples, a sign of impending ovulation. This test is used in some family planning products such as Ovate 1 Ovulation Monitor and Maybe Baby Saliva Ovulation Tester. On average, the onset of ferning precedes ovulation by 6 days. Electric resistance of saliva and vaginal secretions also changes about 6 days prior to ovulation.

Mixed Methods

Symptothermal Methods

This category includes a wide range of method combinations. When BBT measurements are paired with cervical mucus monitoring, unprotected intercourse *before* ovulation that would not be allowed with BBT testing alone *is* possible every other day. This combination relies on cervical mucus changes to identify infertile days during the follicular phase (dry days). At-risk days start when changes in cervical mucus are noted and end after both techniques agree intercourse is safe: 4 days after peak mucus and 3 days after the onset of temperature rise.

Cycle length methods can also be added to BBT shifts with or without cervical mucus determinations. The consistency of the cervix (hard vs. soft), its position (verted or more central), and external os characteristics (open or closed) can also be monitored as part of mixed FABMs. Mittelschmerz, breast tenderness, vulvar swelling, and other symptomatic indications of impending ovulation can also be added to the list of techniques that are used to identify at-risk days.[60]

Symptohormonal Methods

One version, the Marquette method (nfp.marquette.edu), combines urinary LH and estrone-3-glucuronide levels measured with the Clearblue Easy-Fertility Monitor and cervical mucus methods. In one study, this approach was associated with a first-year failure rate of 2%.[61,62] A multicenter U.S. study used those elements along with BBTs, which resulted in a perfect-use 12-month pregnancy rate of 0.6% and a total 12-month pregnancy rate of 6.6%.[62]

A handheld monitor (Persona) combining dynamic recording of menstrual cycles for the woman with periodic testing of urinary LH and estradiol metabolite (estrone-3-glucuronide) using test strips placed into the device after being dipped in urine. This device enjoyed some success in Europe although there was controversy about its effectiveness, which was estimated to range from 6% to 12%.[63–65] In a European clinical trial, the overall first-year pregnancy rate was 12%.[66] While Persona is approved for use in European countries, ironically, the only vestige of that product in the United States is the Clearblue Easy-Fertility Monitor, which is approved in the United States for couples seeking pregnancy.[63,64]

Smart Phone Apps and Online Tools Used in Combination with Other Techniques

A recent evaluation of over 100 apps for fertility revealed that the majority were not based on evidence-based FABMs and did not include a disclaimer discouraging use for pregnancy avoidance.[67] The most basic applications collect only information about menstrual length, but others collect more detailed information, including menstrual flow, symptoms (such as breast tenderness), intercourse events, LH kit results, and usage of fertility drugs. Alerts are then provided by the application for subsequent cycles, including upcoming start of menses, cycle length averages, and fertility. Not all applications have all features, and with the rapid maturation of technology, applications change frequently. BBT measurements can be paired with a menstrual cycle length app. Three such applications are Natural Cycles (https://www.naturalcycles.com/en-us), DaysyView (https://usa.daysy.me/technology/how-daysy-works/), and Kindara (found at https://www.kindara.com).[68,69]

Natural Cycles is a smart phone app approved by the Food and Drug Administration in the United States and CE-marketed in the European Union for contraception in combination with BBT measurements. Women enter information about menstrual days, daily temperature readings, as well as additional information about urinary LH levels, urine pregnancy tests, and intercourse events (protected vs. unprotected). An analysis including 4,054 users who contributed 2,053 woman-years of data reported a first-year Pearl Index with correct and consistent use of 1.0 pregnancy per 100 woman-years.[70] The total group Pearl Index was 6.9 pregnancies per 100 woman-years. Although the authors label the total group failure rates as "typical use," that characterization is technically not correct. Additional objections have been raised about the accuracy of the data collected and the calculations used.[71,72]

DaysyView is an application combined with the Daysy electronic BBT thermometer.[69] Similar to Natural Cycles, the BBT measurements are combined with menstrual cycle length to identify at-risk days. A retrospective study consisting of women registered with the method who were invited to share their data anonymously and complete a survey (19% response rate) reported a 1.3% first-year failure rate after adjustments. After excluding women with less than 1-year use, data from 125 women were used to calculate the first-year perfect use of 0.8%.[69]

Symptopro (https://www.symptopro.org/) and Lady Cycle (http://lady-cycle.com/en_app.php) also help women record their BBT information and provide assessment of the woman's fertility status on a daily basis.

In the future, smart phone ultrasound technology may improve detection of ovulation and enhance the efficacy of methods that currently permit unprotected intercourse only after ovulation is complete. Other potential applications could include image processing algorithms that could more accurately interpret ferning patterns or BBT charts.

Other Concerns About FABM

Over the years, several theoretical concerns have arisen about possible adverse effects of FABM on the health of a fetus that resulted from a failure of the method. Would older gametes (either sperm or ova) be associated with higher rates of spontaneous abortion, aneuploidy, other birth defects, or preterm delivery? In each case, detailed research has proven reassuring.[73-78] Research has also demonstrated no discernable impact on sex ratios.[79]

Withdrawal

This method is available to couples whenever they lack other contraceptives or whenever they want to supplement another method. It is often referred to as Onanism after the son of Judah (Gen. 39, 7-10), who it is said was commanded by his father to impregnate his brother's widow to carry on the line. As the story goes, Onan knew that this was not right, so he "spilled his seed" on the ground. Hence, the term Onanism originally referred to coitus interruptus. However, in more recent times, the meaning of Onanism has been applied to other "seed spilling" situations, such as masturbation. In the late-19th century, withdrawal was introduced in France and other European countries; it had a profound and immediate impact on birth rates.[80]

The majority of Americans have used withdrawal at some time during their lives,[6] most commonly as an ongoing method among the youngest couples.[8] Based on NSFG 2006 to 2010 data, 14% of women 15 to 24 years and 17% of young men report *any* use of withdrawal at last sex, and 7% and 6%, respectively, report using only withdrawal.[81] Withdrawal was 2 to 2.5 times more commonly used by women who said they would be pleased about a pregnancy or, at the other extreme, by women who tended to "eroticize safety" or "de-eroticize risk."[80] Withdrawal is also more popular among men who have difficulty using male condoms.[81] Despite the interruption of thrusting, many users report using it because it enhances sexual pleasure and intimacy, especially when compared to condom use.[82] Withdrawal was added as a second or backup method in 10% of surveyed women, either with other coitally dependent methods or with more modern methods for extra protection.[80] Withdrawal is also used as an episodic method, when other methods are not available.

Couples using withdrawal often deny that they are using contraception, perhaps because the method does not require a prescription or purchase.

Users may consider it a "practice" rather than a "method." Other studies find that women themselves view withdrawal as ineffective and even describe their use of it with shame and regret.[83] More specific questioning may be needed to identify couples who practice withdrawal. It may be helpful to ask women, "when you and your partner have vaginal intercourse, how often does he pull out or withdraw before ejaculation?" Listing withdrawal as an option on intake history questionnaires and including it on contraceptive method charts may encourage users to reveal their reliance on it.

Withdrawal requires that the man recognize impending ejaculation, remove his penis from his partner's vagina, and redirect the flow completely away from her genitals. It is not always easy for the man or woman to judge the appropriate timing or act on this information. In many species, it has been recognized that the period of the fast intravaginal thrusting is associated with ejaculation.[84] Positron emission tomography (PET) in humans has shown that during the time immediately preceding ejaculation, there is activation of mesodiencephalic transition zone areas involved in rewarding behaviors, similar to heroin rush, which might make interruption particularly challenging.[85]

If practiced correctly and consistently, the first-year failure rate of withdrawal is impressive; only 4% of couples will experience a pregnancy. However, in typical use, first-year failure is estimated to be 18% to 20%.[9,86]

Risk of pregnancy due to sperm in the pre-ejaculate has been controversial. Quantitative studies find that only 40% of pre-ejaculatory samples contain spermatozoa.[87] On evaluation, only 37% of samples with sperm had motile sperm, the sperm counts were always low, and the pre-ejaculatory specimens were more cellular than the ejaculated ones. In essence, some men are less likely to leak spermatozoa in their pre-ejaculatory fluid and are able to practice withdrawal more successfully than others. Remembering the low rate of failure with correct and consistent use, it is doubtful that the pre-ejaculatory sperm presents a large risk for pregnancy. Until more is learned about the possible presence of sperm in the pre-ejaculate and how much of a pregnancy risk those sperm pose, counseling about this aspect should be couched in hypothetical terms.

The following practical suggestions may help promote more successful use and satisfaction with the method:

- If there has been any recent sexual activity, suggest the man urinate and wipe the tip of his penis off to remove residual ejaculate before initiating the next act.
- Plan ahead—place a towel or other absorbent material in the area where the ejaculate will be directed to minimize mess or the need to change bedding.
- Restrict coital positioning to missionary or some lateral positions. Avoid female-superior positioning that limits the man's ability to withdraw.

■ Counsel about the "pinch technique" to reduce the man's erection should he approaches ejaculation prior to completely satisfying his partner's desires. If the man does feel early desire to thrust, he can remove his penis and the woman can gently compress the tip to reduce that urge. Occasionally, the erection may be lost, but more time for mutual pleasuring has been created. This may help reduce the frustrations the woman may experience if coitus is over before she is ready.

While withdrawal does not protect women against sexually transmitted diseases, the amount of ejaculate-borne pathogens left in the vagina postcoitally is significantly reduced with this method. In monogamous discordant couples where the man was HIV-infected, use of withdrawal reduced the woman's seroconversion by at least 50%.[83,88] In one survey, women who used LARC methods were as likely to report use of withdrawal (13%) as they did condoms (11%).[89] Perhaps, they assumed it decreased STD risk.

Variations in Withdrawal (Coitus Interruptus)

Various cultures have evolved different practices that start as withdrawal of the penis prior to ejaculation, but follow that action with precise maneuvers to achieve other goals. For example, with *coitus obstructus*, the ejaculate is purposefully redirected by pressing the urethra between the scrotum and the anus. Practitioners thought this drove the semen through the spine, through all the chakras into the brain; in reality, it forced the semen into the bladder from whence later flowed out during urination. *Coitus reservatus* involved controlling (reserving) ejaculation. Practiced in China and India, the man maintained the plateau phase of intercourse; it was believed that ejaculation caused great loss of male Yang and, in excess, diminished a man's vigor and reduced the chance the woman would produce male heirs. Also, by reserving ejaculation, the man could gain some of his partner's Yin. In the Oneida Community in the 19th-century America, coitus reservatus was called "male continence."

Other Behavioral Sexual Practices

Outercourse avoids penetrative intercourse but involves genital-to-genital contact. Oral-genital intercourse is an increasingly common practice to seek/provide sexual pleasuring without the risk of pregnancy. Heterosexual anal intercourse may be practiced to avoid pregnancy or to provide the man more stimulation. Self-stimulation is readily available to release sexual tension and provide pleasure. Mutual masturbation provides bonding and pleasure sharing with no risk of pregnancy and only minimal risk of sexually transmitted infections. Short-term abstinence may be selected until other methods become available. With many women, promotion of abstinence may not be enough; concrete guidance about how to negotiate for abstinence in a variety of situations may improve her ability to maintain her commitment to the method. Acceptance of these different practices (and others) varies from culture to culture. But as with all things sexual, public pronouncements may differ from private practice. The clinician must learn what methods patients are using/want to use and provide education to help them be as successful as possible with their method of choice.

Postabortion/Postpartum Use

Lactational Amenorrhea Method

Breastfeeding protects infants against infection, offers an inexpensive supply of nutrition, contributes to maternal-infant bonding, and provides contraception. Urbanization, education, and modernization all contributed to a decline in breastfeeding, which was furthered with the introduction of bottle-feeding. In the United States, modification of cow's milk for infant feeding was not established until 1900. But it was not until the 1930s that the preparation of infant "formulas" moved from the home kitchen to commercial production and promotion. Breast milk substitutes were initially developed to meet specific needs (allergies and intolerance with cow's milk), but eventually came to be viewed as a means to free women from the responsibility of breastfeeding. In 1922, about 90% of infants were still being breastfed at 1 year of age. By the 1950s, breastfeeding prevalence at hospital discharge fell to 30%, and the downward trend reached its nadir (22%) in 1972.[90] This trend was followed in Europe a decade or two later.

The revival of breastfeeding can be attributed to the growth of knowledge regarding the health of infants.[91] The following reasons emerged as motivations to encourage breastfeeding:

1. Breastfeeding has a child-spacing effect, which is very important in the developing world as a means of limiting family size and providing good nutrition for infants.
2. Human milk prevents infections and illnesses in infants, both by the transmission of immunoglobulins and by modifying the bacterial flora of the infant's gastrointestinal tract.
3. Breastfeeding enhances the bonding process between mother and child.
4. Breastfeeding for at least 1 to 2 years provides protection for the mother against breast cancer and ovarian cancer.[92-95]

Lactation

During pregnancy, prolactin levels rise beginning about 8 weeks from the normal range of 10 to 25 ng/mL to higher concentrations, reaching a peak of 200 to 400 ng/mL at term.[96,97] The increase in prolactin parallels the increase in estrogen beginning at 7 to 8 weeks' gestation, and the mechanism for increasing prolactin secretion is believed to be estrogen suppression of the hypothalamic prolactin-inhibiting factor (PIF), dopamine, and direct stimulation of prolactin gene transcription in the pituitary.[98,99] There is marked variability in maternal prolactin levels in pregnancy, with pulsatile secretion and a diurnal variation similar to that found in nonpregnant subjects. The peak level occurs 4 to 5 hours after the onset of sleep.[100]

Made by the placenta and actively secreted into the maternal circulation from the sixth week of pregnancy, human placental lactogen (hPL), also called human chorionic somatomammotropin, rises progressively, reaching a level of approximately 6,000 ng/mL at term. hPL, though displaying less activity than prolactin, is produced in such large amounts that it may exert a lactogenic effect.

Although prolactin stimulates significant breast growth and is available for lactation, only colostrum (composed of desquamated epithelial cells and transudate) is produced during gestation. Full lactation is inhibited by progesterone, which interferes with prolactin action at the alveolar cell prolactin receptor level. Both estrogen and progesterone are necessary for the expression of the lactogenic receptor, but progesterone antagonizes the positive action of prolactin on its own receptor, while progesterone and pharmacologic amounts of androgens reduce prolactin binding.[101–103]

Prolactin is the principal hormone involved in milk biosynthesis. Without prolactin, synthesis of the primary protein, casein, will not occur, and true milk secretion will be impossible. The rapid disappearance of estrogen and progesterone from the circulation after delivery triggers the initiation of milk production within the alveolar cell and its secretion into the lumen of the gland. Prolactin clearance is much slower, requiring 7 days to reach nonpregnant levels in a nonbreastfeeding woman. These discordant hormonal events result in removal of the estrogen and progesterone inhibition of prolactin action on the breast. Breast enlargement and milk secretion begin 3 to 4 days postpartum when steroids have been sufficiently cleared, initiating the change from colostrum to transitional milk to, by about 14 days postpartum, mature milk. Maintenance of steroidal inhibition or rapid reduction of prolactin secretion (with a dopamine agonist) is effective in preventing postpartum milk synthesis and secretion. Augmentation of prolactin (by thyrotropin-releasing hormone [TRH] or sulpiride, a dopamine receptor blocker) results in increased milk yield.

In the first postpartum week, prolactin levels in breastfeeding women decline approximately 50% (to about 100 ng/mL). Suckling elicits increases in prolactin, which are important in initiating milk production. Until 2 to 3 months postpartum, basal levels are approximately 40 to 50 ng/mL, and there are large (about 10- to 20-fold) increases after suckling. Throughout breastfeeding, baseline prolactin levels remain elevated, and suckling produces a twofold increase that is essential for continuing milk production.[104,105] The pattern or values of prolactin levels do not predict the postpartum duration of amenorrhea or infertility.[106]

Maintenance of milk production at high levels is dependent on the joint action of both anterior and posterior pituitary factors. By mechanisms to be described shortly, suckling causes the release of both prolactin and oxytocin as well as thyroid-stimulating hormone (TSH).[107,108] Prolactin sustains the secretion of casein, fatty acids, lactose, and the volume of secretion, while oxytocin contracts myoepithelial cells and empties the alveolar lumen, thus enhancing further milk secretion and alveolar refilling. The increase in TSH with suckling suggests that TRH may play a role in the prolactin response to suckling. The optimal quantity and the quality of milk are dependent upon the availability of thyroid, insulin, and the insulin-like growth factors, cortisol, and the dietary intake of nutrients and fluids.

Secretion of calcium into the milk of lactating women approximately doubles the daily loss of calcium.[109] In women who breastfeed for 6 months or more, breastfeeding results in significant bone loss even in the presence of a high calcium intake.[110] The bone loss is due to increased bone resorption, probably secondary to the relatively low estrogen levels associated with lactation. Calcium supplementation has no effect on the calcium content of breast milk or on bone loss in lactating women who have normal diets.[111] Furthermore, any loss of calcium and bone associated with lactation is rapidly restored, and bone density rapidly returns to baseline levels in the 6 months after weaning[112,113]; therefore, there is no impact on the risk of postmenopausal osteoporosis.[114–117]

Antibodies are present in breast milk and contribute to the health of an infant. Human milk prevents infections in infants both by transmission of immunoglobulins and by modifying the bacterial flora of the infant's gastrointestinal tract. Viruses are transmitted in breast milk, and although the actual risks are unknown, women infected with cytomegalovirus, hepatitis B, or human immunodeficiency virus are advised not to breastfeed. Vitamin A, vitamin B_{12}, and folic acid are significantly reduced in the breast milk of women with poor dietary intake. As a general rule, approximately 1% of any drug ingested by the mother appears in breast milk. In a study of Pima Indians, exclusive breastfeeding for at least 2 months was associated with a lower rate of adult-onset non–insulin-dependent diabetes mellitus, partly because overfeeding and excess weight gain are more common with bottle-feeding.[118]

Frequent emptying of the lumen is important for maintaining an adequate level of secretion. Indeed, after the fourth postpartum month, suckling appears to be the only stimulant required; however, environmental and emotional states also are important for continued alveolar activity. Vigorous aerobic exercise does not affect the volume or composition of breast milk, and therefore infant weight gain is normal.[119] Maternal diet and hydration have little impact on lactation; the primary control of milk output is under the control of the infant's suckling.[120]

Suckling studied with ultrasonography indicates that the infant's instinctive attachment to a nipple immediately establishes a vacuum seal.[121] The tongue moves up and down, increasing the vacuum and producing milk flow during the downward motion. However, the ejection of milk from the breast does not occur only as the result of a mechanically induced negative pressure produced by suckling. Tactile sensors concentrated in the areola activate, via thoracic sensory nerve roots 4, 5, and 6, an afferent sensory neural arc that stimulates the paraventricular and supraoptic nuclei of the hypothalamus to synthesize and transport oxytocin to the posterior pituitary. The efferent arc (oxytocin) is blood-borne to the breast alveolus-ductal systems to contract myoepithelial cells and empty the alveolar lumen. Milk contained in major ductal repositories is ejected from 15 to 20 openings in the nipple. This rapid release of milk is called "letdown." This important role for oxytocin is evident in knockout mice lacking oxytocin who undergo normal parturition, but fail to nurse their offspring.[122] The milk ejection reflex involving oxytocin is present in all species of mammals. Oxytocin-like peptides exist in fish, reptiles, and birds, and a role for oxytocin in maternal behavior may have existed before lactation evolved.[120]

In many instances, the activation of oxytocin release leading to letdown does not require initiation by tactile stimuli. The central nervous system can be conditioned to respond to the presence of the infant, or to the sound of the infant's cry, by inducing activation of the efferent arc. These messages are the result of many stimulating and inhibiting neurotransmitters. Suckling, therefore, acts to refill the breast by activating both portions of the pituitary (anterior and posterior) causing the breast to produce new milk and to eject milk. The release of oxytocin is also important for uterine contractions that contribute to involution of the uterus.

The oxytocin effect is a release phenomenon acting on secreted and stored milk. Prolactin must be available in sufficient quantities for continued secretory replacement of ejected milk. This requires the transient increase in prolactin associated with suckling. The amount of milk produced correlates with the amount removed by suckling. The breast can store milk for a maximum of 48 hours before production diminishes.

Cessation of Lactation

Lactation can be terminated by discontinuing suckling, which results primarily in loss of milk letdown via the neural evocation of oxytocin. Within a few days, the swollen alveoli depress milk formation probably via a local pressure effect (although milk itself may contain inhibitory factors). With resorption of fluid and solute, the swollen breast diminishes in size in a week or so. In addition to the loss of milk letdown, the absence of suckling reactivates dopamine (PIF) production so that there is less prolactin stimulation of milk secretion.

Contraceptive Effect of Lactation and Lactational Amenorrhea

The contraceptive effectiveness of lactation depends on the level of nutrition of the mother (if low, the longer the contraceptive interval), the intensity of suckling, and the extent to which supplemental food is added to the infant diet.[123] If suckling intensity or frequency is diminished, contraceptive effect is reduced. Although different organizations have set different standards when defining the practices required to qualify for "lactational amenorrhea," the CDC has adopted the following in the U.S. MEC:

1. Amenorrhea
2. Fully or nearly fully breastfeeding (no interval of >4 to 6 hours between breastfeeds)
3. Less than 6 months postpartum (U.S. MEC Lactational Amenorrhea Method. https://www.cdc.gov/reproductivehealth/contraception/mmwr/mec/appendixg.html)

With menstruation or after 6 months, the chance of ovulation increases.[124,125] With full or nearly full breastfeeding, approximately 70% of women remain amenorrheic through 6 months and only 37% through 1 year; nevertheless with exclusive breastfeeding, the contraceptive efficacy at 1 year is high, at 92%.[126] Fully breastfeeding women commonly have some vaginal bleeding or spotting in the first 8 postpartum weeks, but this bleeding is not due to ovulation.[127] It has been suggested that pumping or milk expression does not provide the same level of contraceptive protection as direct breastfeeding with infant suckling (https://www.hhs.gov/opa/pregnancy-prevention/birth-control-methods/lam/index.html). Women who are not good candidates for breastfeeding such as those with infectious diseases, certain medicine use, or anatomical problems or galactosemia in the infant should not rely on this method.[128]

Although high concentrations of prolactin can work at both central and ovarian sites to produce lactational amenorrhea and anovulation,[127] the central action predominates. Prolactin appears to affect granulosa cell function in vitro by inhibiting the synthesis of progesterone. It also may change the testosterone to dihydrotestosterone ratio, thereby reducing aromatizable substrate and increasing local antiestrogen concentrations. Elevated prolactin levels inhibit pulsatile GnRH secretion.[129,130] Prolactin excess has short loop positive feedback effects on dopamine, which reduces GnRH by suppressing arcuate nucleus function, perhaps in a mechanism mediated by endogenous opioid activity.[131,132] However, blockade of dopamine receptors with a dopamine antagonist or the administration of an opioid antagonist in breastfeeding women does not always affect gonadotropin secretion.[133] The exact mechanism for the suppression of GnRH secretion remains to be unraveled. The importance of GnRH suppression by prolactin is reinforced by the demonstration that treatment of amenorrheic, lactating women with pulsatile GnRH fully restores pituitary secretion and normal ovarian cyclic activity.[134]

At weaning, as prolactin blood concentrations fall to normal, gonadotropin levels increase, and estradiol secretion rises. This prompt resumption of ovarian function is followed by the occurrence of ovulation within 14 to 30 days of weaning.

Prolactin concentrations are increased in response to the repeated suckling stimulus of breastfeeding. Given sufficient intensity and frequency, prolactin levels will remain elevated. Under these conditions, follicle-stimulating hormone (FSH) concentrations are in the low normal range (having risen from extremely low concentrations at delivery to follicular range in the 3 weeks postpartum), and LH values are also in the low normal range. These low levels of gonadotropins do not allow the ovary during lactational hyperprolactinemia to display follicular development and secrete estrogen. Therefore, vaginal dryness and dyspareunia are commonly reported by breastfeeding women. *Vaginal lubricants should be offered to the couple until ovarian function and estrogen production return.*

Ovulation in Breastfeeding Women

The return of ovulation in breastfeeding women has been documented in women from all parts of the world. In Chile, 14% of women ovulated during full breastfeeding, although full nursing provided effective contraception up to 3 months postpartum,[135,136] It has been argued that the threshold for suppression of ovulation is at least five feedings for a total of at least 65 minutes per day suckling duration.[137] However, in the studies from Chile, the frequency of nursing was the same in breastfeeders who ovulated and those who did not.

In Mexico, a study of 29 breastfeeding mothers and 10 nonbreastfeeders observed that in the absence of bleeding and supplementary feedings, 100% of the breastfeeders remained anovulatory for 3 months postpartum and 96% up to 6 months.[138] The median time from delivery to first ovulation was 259 days for breastfeeders compared to 119 days for nonbreastfeeders. However, by the third postpartum month, 18% of the breastfeeders had ovulated.

In a well-nourished population in Australia, less than 20% of breastfeeding women ovulated by the 6th postpartum month, and less than 25% menstruated.[139] Neither the time of first supplement nor the amount of supplement predicted the return of ovulation or menstruation. In other words, even in women giving their infants supplemental feedings, there is effective inhibition of ovulation during the first 6 months of breastfeeding.

With the use of life-table analysis, the probability of resumption of menstruation was calculated in data from a group of Eskimo women who nursed their babies on demand for up to 3 years and was compared with that for mothers who did not nurse.[140] Of the nonnursing women, 84% had resumed their cycles by the end of the second postpartum month and all by the end of the third postpartum month. The nursing mothers, however, had only about a 50% chance of resuming menstruation by the end of the 10th postpartum month.

Pregnancy Risk

While no estimates of typical use failure rates with LAM are available, international reports demonstrate considerable variability in pregnancy rates with use of this method in clinical trials. Among Australian women who have unprotected intercourse during lactational amenorrhea and use contraception when menses resume, 1.7% become pregnant in the first 6 months of breastfeeding, 7% after 12 months, and 13% after 24 months.[141] In a study of 422 middle-class women in Santiago, Chile, there was only one pregnancy (in month 6) when lactational amenorrhea was consciously relied upon for contraception.[142] This was equal to a cumulative 6-month life-table pregnancy rate of 0.45%. However, this accomplishment required an extensive program of education and support. In this study, 9% of exclusively breastfeeding women had resumption of menses by the end of 3 months and 19% by the end of 6 months.

This increased suppression of fertility undoubtedly reflected the intensity of the breastfeeding program and the motivation of the participants. In Chile, the probability of pregnancy in breastfeeding women who are amenorrheic was reported as 0.9% at 6 months and 17% at 112 months and in menstruating women, 36% at 6 months and 55% at 12 months.[143] In Pakistan, women who deliberately chose lactational amenorrhea as a method of contraception experienced a pregnancy rate of only 1.1% at 12 months if they remained amenorrheic.[144]

An international group of researchers in the area of lactational infertility reached the following consensus in 1989, called the Bellagio Consensus (after the site of the conference at Bellagio, Italy).[145]

The maximum birth-spacing effect of breastfeeding is achieved when a mother "fully" or "nearly fully" breastfeeds and remains amenorrheic. When these two conditions are fulfilled, breastfeeding provides more than 98% protection from pregnancy in the first 6 months.

The Bellagio degree of protection in the first 6 months of full or nearly full breastfeeding has been confirmed in clinical studies.[125,146] The WHO conducted a large prospective study examining the relationship between infant feeding and amenorrhea, as well as the rate of pregnancy during lactational amenorrhea.[147-150] Women who were still breastfeeding and remained amenorrheic had pregnancy rates of 0.8% at 6 months and 4.4% at 12 months, again confirming the Bellagio Consensus.

Only amenorrheic women who exclusively or nearly exclusively breast-feed at intervals of no longer than 4 to 6 hours, during the first 6 months, have the low (2%) failure rates. With menstruation or after 6 months, the risk of ovulation increases; ovulation returns without warning, prior to the first bleeding episode.[124,125,151] Supplemental feeding increases the risk of ovulation (and pregnancy) even in amenorrheic women.[143] Total protection against pregnancy is achieved by the exclusively breastfeeding woman for a duration of only 10 weeks.[126]

FABM and Withdrawal

Some behavioral methods may be well suited after delivery or following abortion or pregnancy loss. For example, once bleeding has stopped, methods that rely on cervical mucus detection (such as the TwoDay method) may be very useful. However, most of the FABMs that rely on cycle length alone will not be appropriate. From a practical standpoint, BBT measurement will probably also not be feasible for a young mother who must get up during the night to attend to her baby, but BBTs may be used by postabortal women. A methodology (called a "Bridge") for the Standard Day (CycleBeads) method has been developed to help women who are transitioning from breast-feeding and have menstruated at least once postpartum, until their cycles reestablish with a 6-month failure rate of 11.2%.[152] All methods are appropriate following abortion as fertility resumes rapidly, although bleeding may interfere with mucus evaluation. Withdrawal is always available to couples.

Resources

For more advice and supporting supplies (charts and written instructions).

Bedsider Birth Control Support Network
https://www.bedsider.org/
The Couple to Couple League Foundation
http://www.ccli.org/
The National Fertility Awareness and Natural Family Planning Service for the United Kingdom
https://www.nhs.uk/conditions/contraception/natural-family-planning/
The Natural Family Site, BYG Publishing Inc.
http://www.bygpub.com/natural/
The Fertility Awareness Center
http://www.fertaware.com
American Family Physician. Natural Family Planning
https://www.aafp.org/afp/2012/1115/p924.html
Planned Parenthood
https://www.plannedparenthood.org/learn/birth-control/fertility-awareness

References

1. **Fehring RJ, Schneider M, Barron ML, Pruszynski J,** Influence of motivation on the efficacy of natural family planning, MCN: Am J Matern Child Nurs 38:352–358, 2013.

2. **Daniels K, Abma JC,** Current contraceptive status among women aged 15–49: United States, 2015–2017, NCHS Data Brief (327):1–8, 2018.

3. **Hubacher D, Trussell J,** A definition of modern contraceptive methods, Contraception 92:420–421, 2015.

4. **United Nations, Department of Economic and Social Affairs, Population Division, Fertility and Family Planning Section 2018,** http://www.un.org/en/development/desa/population/publications/dataset/contraception/wcu2018.shtml

5. **Polis CB, Jones RK,** Multiple contraceptive method use and prevalence of fertility awareness-based method use in the United States, 2013–2015, Contraception 98:188–192, 2018.

6. **Daniels K, Mosher WD,** Contraceptive methods women have ever used: United States, 1982–2010, Natl Health Stat Report (62):1–15, 2013.

7. **Brauner-Otto S, Yarger J, Abma J,** Does it matter how you ask? Question wording and males' reporting of contraceptive use at last sex, Soc Sci Res 41:1028–1036, 2012.

8. **Jones RK, Lindberg LD, Higgins JA,** Pull and pray or extra protection? Contraceptive strategies involving withdrawal among US adult women, Contraception 90:416–421, 2014.

9. **Trussell J,** Contraceptive Efficacy in Contraceptive Technology, 21st ed., Ardent Media, Inc., New York, 2018, p 100.

10. **Grimes DA, Gallo MF, Grigorieva V, Nanda K, Schulz KF,** Fertility awareness-based methods for contraception, Cochrane Database Syst Rev (4):CD004860, 2004.

11. **Peragallo Urrutia R, Polis CB, Jensen ET, Greene ME, Kennedy E, Stanford JB,** Effectiveness of fertility awareness-based methods for pregnancy prevention, Obstet Gynecol 132:591–604, 2018.

12. **Grimes DA, Gallo MF, Grigorieva V, Nanda K, Schulz KF,** Fertility awareness-based methods for contraception: systematic review of randomized

controlled trials, Contraception 72:85–90, 2005.

13. **United Nations Department of Economics and Social Affairs,** 2015 UN Women. http://www.unwomen.org/en/what-we-do/ending-violence-against-women/facts-and-figures

14. **Lawrence RE, Rasinski KA, Yoon JD, Curlin FA,** Obstetrician-gynecologists' views on contraception and natural family planning: a national survey, Am J Obstet Gynecol 204:124.e1–124.e7, 2011.

15. **Choi J, Chan S, Wiebe E,** Natural family planning: physicians' knowledge, attitudes, and practice, J Obstet Gynaecol Can 32:673–678, 2010.

16. **Kudesia R, Chernyak E, McAvey B,** Low fertility awareness in United States reproductive-aged women and medical trainees: creation and validation of the Fertility & Infertility Treatment Knowledge Score (FIT-KS), Fertil Steril 108:711–717, 2017.

17. **Kennedy KI, Kotelchuck M,** Policy considerations for the introduction and promotion of the lactational amenorrhea method: advantages and disadvantages of LAM, J Hum Lact 14:191–203, 1998.

18. **Pyper CM,** Fertility awareness and natural family planning, Eur J Contracept Reprod Health Care 2:131–146, 1997.

19. **Elaut E, Buysse A, De Sutter P, Gerris J, De Cuypere G, T'Sjoen G,** Cycle-related changes in mood, sexual desire, and sexual activity in oral contraception-using and nonhormonal-contraception-using couples, J Sex Res 53:125–136, 2016.

20. **Pillsworth EG, Haselton MG, Buss DM,** Ovulatory shifts in female sexual desire, J Sex Res 41:55–65, 2004.

21. **Bullivant SB, Sellergren SA, Stern K, Spencer NA, Jacob S, Mennella JA, McClintock MK,** Women's sexual experience during the menstrual cycle: identification of the sexual phase by noninvasive measurement of luteinizing hormone, J Sex Res 41:82–93, 2004.

22. **Stirnemann JJ, Samson A, Bernard JP, Thalabard JC,** Day-specific probabilities of conception in fertile cycles resulting in spontaneous pregnancies, Hum Reprod 28:1110–1116, 2013.

23. **Wilcox AJ, Weinberg CR, Baird DD,** Timing of sexual intercourse in relation to ovulation. Effects on the probability of conception, survival of the pregnancy, and sex of the baby, N Engl J Med 333:1517–1521, 1995.

24. **Creinin MD, Keverline S, Meyn LA,** How regular is regular? An analysis of menstrual cycle regularity, Contraception 70:289–292, 2004.

25. **Che Y, Cleland JG, Ali MM,** Periodic abstinence in developing countries: an assessment of failure rates and consequences, Contraception 69:15–21, 2004.

26. **Lundsberg LS, Pal L, Gariepy AM, Xu X, Chu MC, Illuzzi JL,** Knowledge, attitudes, and practices regarding conception and fertility: a population-based survey among reproductive-age United States women, Fertil Steril 101: 767–774, 2014.

27. **Frank-Herrmann P, Freundl G, Gnoth C, Godehardt E, Kunert J, Baur S, Sottong U,** Natural family planning with and without barrier method use in the fertile phase: efficacy in relation to sexual behavior: a German prospective long-term study, Adv Contracept 13:179–189, 1997.

28. **Kambic RT, Lamprecht V,** Calendar rhythm efficacy: a review, Adv Contracept 12:123–128, 1996.

29. **Polis CB, Bradley SE, Bankole A, Onda T, Croft T, Singh S,** Typical-use contraceptive failure rates in 43 countries with Demographic and Health Survey data: summary of a detailed report, Contraception 94:11–17, 2016.

30. **Wilcox AJ, Dunson D, Baird DD,** The timing of the "fertile window" in the menstrual cycle: day specific estimates from a prospective study, BMJ 321:1259–1262, 2000.

31. **Arévalo M, Sinai I, Jennings V,** A fixed formula to define the fertile window of the menstrual cycle as the basis of a simple method of natural family planning, Contraception 60:357–360, 1999.

32. **Arévalo M, Jennings V, Sinai I,** Efficacy of a new method of family planning: the Standard Days Method, Contraception 65:333–338, 2002.

33. **Gribble JN, Lundgren RI, Velasquez C, Anastasi EE,** Being strategic about

contraceptive introduction: the experience of the Standard Days Method,
Contraception 77:147–154, 2008.

34. **Sinai I, Lundgren R, Arévalo M,
Jennings V,** Fertility awareness-based
methods of family planning: predictors
of correct use, Int Fam Plan Perspect
32:94–100, 2006.

35. **WHO,** Family planning/contracep-
tion key facts, http://www.who.int/
en/news-room/fact-sheets/detail/
family-planning-contraception

36. **Marston CA, Church K,** Does the evidence support global promotion of the
calendar-based Standard Days Method®
of contraception?, Contraception
93:492–497, 2016.

37. **Moglia ML, Nguyen HV, Chyjek K,
Chen KT, Castaño PM,** Evaluation of
smartphone menstrual cycle track-
ing applications using an adapted
APPLICATIONS scoring system, Obstet
Gynecol 127:1153–1160, 2016.

38. **Sohda S, Suzuki K, Igari I,** Relationship
between the menstrual cycle and timing
of ovulation revealed by new protocols:
analysis of data from a self-tracking
health app, J Med Internet Res 19:e391,
2017.

39. **Li D, Heyer L, Jennings VH, Smith
CA, Dunson DB,** Personalised estimation of a woman's most fertile days,
Eur J Contracept Reprod Health Care
21:323–328, 2016.

40. **Simmons RG, Shattuck DC, Jennings
VH,** Assessing the efficacy of an app-
based method of family planning: the
DOT study protocol, JMIR Res Protoc
6:e5, 2017.

41. **Shattuck D, Haile LT, Simmons RG,**
Lessons from the DOT contraceptive
efficacy study: analysis of the use of agile
development to improve recruitment and
enrollment for mHealth research, JMIR
Mhealth Uhealth 6:e99, 2018.

42. **Jennings VH, Haile LT, Simmons RG,
Fultz HM, Shattuck D,** Estimating
six-cycle efficacy of the Dot app for
pregnancy prevention, Contraception
99:52–55, 2019.

43. **Setton R, Tierney C, Tsai T,** The
accuracy of web sites and cellular phone
applications in predicting the fertile window, Obstet Gynecol 128:58–63, 2016.

44. **Lupton D,** Quantified sex: a critical
analysis of sexual and reproductive
self-tracking using apps, Cult Health Sex
17:440–453, 2015.

45. **Jin B, Jiang G, Pan Z, Yan J, Peng S, Lu
R,** The application of Billings for fertility
regulation method during the period
of breastfeeding, Reprod Contracept
10:163–169, 1999.

46. **Billings EL,** The simplicity of the
Ovulation Method and its application in
various circumstances, Acta Eur Fertil
22:33–36, 1991.

47. **Su HW, Yi YC, Wei TY, Chang TC,
Cheng CM,** Detection of ovulation, a
review of currently available methods,
Bioeng Transl Med 2:238–246, 2017.

48. **Connell-Tatum EB,** Ovulation method
of natural family planning, Fertil Steril
36:551–552, 1981.

49. **Frank-Herrmann P, Heil J, Gnoth C,
Toledo E, Baur S, Pyper C, Jenetzky
E, Strowitzki T, Freundl G,** The effectiveness of a fertility awareness-based
method to avoid pregnancy in relation
to a couple's sexual behavior during the
fertile time: a prospective longitudinal
study, Hum Reprod 22:1310–1319,
2007.

50. **Owen M,** Physiological signs of ovulation and fertility readily observable by
women, Linacre Q 80:17–23, 2018.

51. **Gallagher J,** More about natural family
planning, Aust Fam Physician 12:
786–792, 1983.

52. **Bhargava H, Bhatia JC, Ramachandran
L, Rohatgi P, Sinha A,** Field trial of
Billings ovulation method of natural family planning, Contraception
53:69–74, 1996.

53. **Indian Council of Medical Research
Task Force on Natural Family Planning
(NFP),** http://archst l.org/files/field-file/
WhatCanNFPDoForYou_Brochure%20
FINAL%20PDF.pdf

54. **Jennings JH, Polis CB,** Fertility
Awareness-Based Methods in
Contraceptive Technology, 21st ed.,
Ardent Media, Inc., New York, 2018,
p 411.

55. A prospective multicentre trial of the
ovulation method of natural family planning. II. The effectiveness phase, Fertil
Steril 36:591–598, 1981.

56. **Pallone SR, Bergus GR,** Fertility aware-ness-based methods: another option for family planning, J Am Board Fam Med 22:147–157, 2009.

57. **Arévalo M, Jennings V, Nikula M, Sinai I,** Efficacy of the new TwoDay Method of family planning, Fertil Steril 82:885–892, 2004.

58. **Behre HM, Kuhlage J, Gassner C, Sonntag B, Schem C, Schneider HP, Nieschlag E,** Prediction of ovulation by urinary hormone measurements with the home use ClearPlan Fertility Monitor: comparison with transvaginal ultrasound scans and serum hormone measurements, Hum Reprod 15:2478–2482, 2000.

59. **Eichner SF, Timpe EM,** Urinary-based ovulation and pregnancy: point-of-care testing, Ann Pharmacother 38:325–331, 2004.

60. **Gross BA,** Natural family planning indi-cators of ovulation, Clin Reprod Fertil 5:91–117, 1987.

61. **Fehring RJ, Schneider M, Barron ML, Raviele K,** Cohort comparison of two fertility awareness methods of family planning, J Reprod Med 54:165–170, 2009.

62. **Fehring RJ, Schneider M, Barron ML,** Efficacy of the Marquette Method of natural family planning, MCN: Am J Matern Child Nurs 33:348–354, 2008.

63. **Bonnar J, Freundl G, Kirkman R,** Personal hormone monitoring for con-traception, Br J Fam Plann 26:178–179, 2000.

64. **Guida M, Bramante S, Acunzo G, Pellicano M, Cirillo D, Nappi C,** Diagnosis of fertility with a personal hor-monal evaluation test, Minerva Ginecol 55:167–173, 2003.

65. **Trussell J,** Contraceptive efficacy of the personal hormone monitoring system Persona, Br J Fam Plann 25:34–35, 1999.

66. **Bonnar J, Flynn A, Freundl G, Kirkman R, Royston R, Snowden R,** Personal hormone monitoring for con-traception, Br J Fam Plann 24:128–134, 1999.

67. **Duane M, Contreras A, Jensen ET, White A,** The performance of fertility awareness-based method apps marketed to avoid pregnancy, J Am Board Fam Med 29:508–511, 2016.

68. **Berglund Scherwitzl E, Lundberg O, Kopp Kallner H, Gemzell Danielsson K, Trussell J, Scherwitzl R,** Perfect-use and typical-use Pearl Index of a contraceptive mobile app, Contraception 96:420–425, 2017.

69. **Koch MC, Lermann J, van de Roemer N, Renner SK, Burghaus S, Hackl J, Dittrich R, Kehl S, Oppelt PG, Hildebrandt T, Hack CC, Pöhls UG, Renner SP, Thiel FC,** Improving usability and pregnancy rates of a fertility monitor by an additional mobile applica-tion: results of a retrospective efficacy study of Daysy and DaysyView app, Reprod Health 15:37, 2018.

70. **Berglund Scherwitzl E, Gemzell Danielsson K, Sellberg JA, Scherwitzl R,** Fertility awareness-based mobile application for contraception, Eur J Contracept Reprod Health Care 21:234–241, 2016.

71. **Schimmoeller N, Creinin MD,** More clarity needed for contraceptive mobile app Pearl Index calculations, Contraception 97:456, 2018.

72. **Lundberg O, Berglund Scherwitzl E, Kopp Kallner H, Gemzell Danielsson K, Trussell J, Scherwitzl R,** Clarifications concerning contracep-tive mobile app Pearl Index calculations, Contraception 97:456–457, 2018.

73. **Castilla EE, Lopez-Camelo JS, da Graça Dutra M, Queenan JT, Simpson JL,** The frequency and spectrum of congenital anomalies in natural fam-ily planning users in South America: no increase in a case-control study. NFP-ECLAMC Group. Natural Family Planning. Latin-American Collaborative Study of Congenital Malformations, Adv Contracept 13:395–404, 1997.

74. **Barbato M, Bitto A, Gray RH, Simpson JL, Queenan JT, Kambic RT, Perez A, Mena P, Pardo F, Stevenson W, Tagliabue G, Jennings V, Li C,** Effects of timing of conception on birth weight and preterm delivery of natural fam-ily planning users, Adv Contracept 13:215–228, 1997.

75. **Gray RH, Simpson JL, Kambic RT, Queenan JT, Mena P, Perez A, Barbato M,** Timing of conception and the risk of spontaneous abortion among pregnan-cies occurring during the use of natural

family planning, Am J Obstet Gynecol 172:1567–1572, 1995.

76. **Mena P, Bitto A, Barbato M, Perez A, Gray RH, Simpson JL, Queenan JT, Kambic RT, Pardo F, Stevenson W, Tagliabue G, Jennings V, Li C,** Pregnancy complications in natural family planning users, Adv Contracept 13:229–237, 1997.

77. **Simpson JL, Gray RH, Perez A, Mena P, Barbato M, Castilla EE, Kambic RT, Pardo F, Tagliabue G, Stephenson WS, Bitto A, Li C, Jennings VH, Spieler JM, Queenan JT,** Pregnancy outcome in natural family planning users: cohort and case-control studies evaluating safety, Adv Contracept 13:201–214, 1997.

78. **Bracken MB, Vita K,** Frequency of non-hormonal contraception around conception and association with congenital malformations in offspring, Am J Epidemiol 117:281–291, 1983.

79. **Gray RH, Simpson JL, Bitto AC, Queenan JT, Li C, Kambic RT, Perez A, Mena P, Barbato M, Stevenson W, Jennings V,** Sex ratio associated with timing of insemination and length of the follicular phase in planned and unplanned pregnancies during use of natural family planning, Hum Reprod 13:1397–1400, 1998.

80. **Jones RK, Fennell J, Higgins JA, Blanchard K,** Better than nothing or savvy risk-reduction practice? The importance of withdrawal, Contraception 79:407–410, 2009.

81. **Higgins JA, Wang Y,** Which young adults are most likely to use withdrawal? The importance of pregnancy attitudes and sexual pleasure, Contraception 91:320–327, 2015.

82. **de Vincenzi I,** A longitudinal study of human immunodeficiency virus transmission by heterosexual partners. European Study Group on Heterosexual Transmission of HIV, N Engl J Med 331:341–346, 1994.

83. **Arteaga S, Gomez AM,** Is that a method of birth control? A qualitative exploration of young women's use of withdrawal, J Sex Res 53:626–632, 2016.

84. **Moralí G, Asunción Pía Soto M, Luis Contreras J, Arteaga M, González-Vidal MD, Beyer C,** Detailed analysis of the male copulatory motor pattern in mammals: hormonal bases, Scand J Psychol 44:279–288, 2003.

85. **Holstege G, Georgiadis JR, Paans AM, Meiners LC, van der Graaf FH, Reinders AA,** Brain activation during human male ejaculation, J Neurosci 23:9185–9193, 2003.

86. **Sundaram A, Vaughan B, Kost K, Bankole A, Finer L, Singh S, Trussell J,** Contraceptive failure in the United States: estimates from the 2006–2010 National Survey of Family Growth, Perspect Sex Reprod Health 49:7–16, 2017.

87. **Killick SR, Leary C, Trussell J, Guthrie KA,** Sperm content of pre-ejaculatory fluid, Hum Fertil (Camb) 14:48–52, 2011.

88. **Musicco M, Lazzarin A, Nicolosi A, Gasparini M, Costigliola P, Arici C, Saracco A,** Antiretroviral treatment of men infected with human immunodeficiency virus type 1 reduces the incidence of heterosexual transmission. Italian Study Group on HIV Heterosexual Transmission, Arch Intern Med 154:1971–1976, 1994.

89. **Higgins JA, Gregor L, Mathur S, Nakyanjo N, Nalugoda F, Santelli JS,** Use of withdrawal (coitus interruptus) for both pregnancy and HIV prevention among young adults in Rakai, Uganda, J Sex Med 11:2421–2427, 2014.

90. **National Academy of Sciences,** Nutrition during Lactation, Academy Press, Washington, DC, 1991.

91. **American Academy of Pediatrics,** Breastfeeding and the use of human milk, Pediatrics 129:e827–41, 2012.

92. **Collaborative Group on Hormonal Factors in Breast Cancer,** Breast cancer and breastfeeding: collaborative reanalysis of individual data from 47 epidemiological studies in 30 countries, including 50,302 women with breast cancer and 96,973 women without disease, Lancet 360:187, 2002.

93. **Rosenblatt KA, Thomas DB,** Lactation and the risk of epithelial ovarian cancer. The WHO Collaborative Study of Neoplasia and Steroid Contraceptives, Int J Epidemiol 22:192, 1993.

94. **Sung HK, Ma SH, Choi JY, Hwang Y, Ahn C, Kim BG, Kim YM, Kim JW, Kang S, Kim J, Kim TJ, Yoo KY, Kang**

D, Park S, The effect of breastfeeding duration and parity on the risk of epithelial ovarian cancer: a systematic review and meta-analysis, J Prev Med Public Health 49:349–366, 2016.

95. Chowdhury R, Sinha B, Sankar MJ, Taneja S, Bhandari N, Rollins N, Bahl R, Martines J, Breastfeeding and maternal health outcomes: a systematic review and meta-analysis, Acta Paediatr 104:96–113, 2015. doi: 10.1111/apa.13102.

96. Tyson JE, Hwang P, Guyda H, Friesen HG, Studies of prolactin secretion in human pregnancy, Am J Obstet Gynecol 113:14, 1972.

97. Kletzky OA, Marrs RP, Howard WF, McCormick W, Mishell DR Jr, Prolactin synthesis and release during pregnancy and puerperium, Am J Obstet Gynecol 136:545, 1980.

98. Tyson JE, Friesen HG, Factors influencing the secretion of human prolactin and growth hormone in menstrual and gestational women, Am J Obstet Gynecol 116:377, 1973.

99. Barberia JM, Abu-Fadil S, Kletzky OA, Nakamura RM, Mishell DR Jr, Serum prolactin patterns in early human gestation, Am J Obstet Gynecol 121:1107, 1975.

100. Ehara Y, Siler TM, Yen SSC, Effects of large doses of estrogen on prolactin and growth hormone release, Am J Obstet Gynecol 125:455, 1976.

101. Murphy LJ, Murphy LC, Stead B, Sutherland RL, Lazarus L, Modulation of lactogenic receptors by progestins in cultured human breast cancer cells, J Clin Endocrinol Metab 62:280, 1986.

102. Simon WE, Pahnke VG, Holzel F, In vitro modulation of prolactin binding to human mammary carcinoma cells by steroid hormones and prolactin, J Clin Endocrinol Metab 60:1243, 1985.

103. Kelly PA, Kjiane J, Postel-Vinay M-C, Edery M, The prolactin/growth hormone receptor family, Endocr Rev 12:235, 1991.

104. Battin DA, Marrs RP, Fleiss PM, Mishell DR Jr, Effect of suckling on serum prolactin, luteinizing hormone, follicle-stimulating hormone, and estradiol during prolonged lactation, Obstet Gynecol 65:785, 1985.

105. Stern JM, Konner M, Herman TN, Reichlin S, Nursing behaviour, prolactin, and postpartum amenorrhoea during prolonged lactation in American and !Kung mothers, Clin Endocrinol 25:247, 1986.

106. Tay CCK, Glasier AF, McNeilly AS, Twenty-four hour patterns of prolactin secretion during lactation and the relationship to suckling and the resumption of fertility in breast-feeding women, Hum Reprod 11:950, 1996.

107. Dawood MY, Khan-Dawood FS, Wahl RS, Fuchs F, Oxytocin release and plasma anterior pituitary and gonadal hormones in women during lactation, J Clin Endocrinol Metab 52:678, 1981.

108. McNeilly AS, Robinson KA, Houston MJ, Howe PW, Release of oxytocin and prolactin in response to suckling, Br Med J 286:257, 1983.

109. Kumar R, Cohen WR, Epstein FH, Vitamin D and calcium hormones in pregnancy, N Engl J Med 302:1143, 1980.

110. Sowers M, Corton G, Shapiro B, Jannausch ML, Crutchfield M, Smith ML, Randolph JF, Hollis B, Changes in bone density with lactation, JAMA 269:3130, 1993.

111. Kalkwarf HJ, Specker BL, Bianchi DC, Ranz J, Ho M, The effect of calcium supplementation on bone density during lactation and after weaning, N Engl J Med 337:523, 1997.

112. Kalkwarf HJ, Specker BL, Bone mineral loss during lactation and recovery after weaning, Obstet Gynecol 86:26, 1995.

113. Kovacs CS, Calcium and bone metabolism in pregnancy and lactation, J Clin Endocrinol Metab 86:2344, 2001.

114. Laskey MA, Prentice A, Hanratty LA, Jarjou LM, Dibba B, Beavan SR, Cole TJ, Bone changes after 3 mo of lactation: influence of calcium intake, breast-milk output, and vitamin D-receptor genotype, Am J Clin Nutr 67:685, 1998.

115. Ritchie LD, Fung EB, Halloran BP, Turnlund JR, Van Loan MD, Cann CE, King JC, A longitudinal study of calcium homeostasis during human pregnancy and lactation and after resumption of menses, Am J Clin Nutr 67:693, 1998.

116. Polatti F, Capuzzo E, Viazzo F, Colleoni R, Klersy C, Bone mineral changes during and after lactation, Obstet Gynecol 94:52, 1999.

117. **Kojima N, Douchi T, Kosha S, Nagata Y,** Cross-sectional study of the effects of parturition and lactation on bone mineral density later in life, Maturitas 41:203, 2002.

118. **Pettitt DJ, Forman MR, Hanson RL, Knowler WC, Bennett PH,** Breastfeeding and incidence of non-insulin-dependent diabetes mellitus in Pima Indians, Lancet 350:166, 1997.

119. **Dewey KG, Lovelady CA, Nommsen-Rivers LA, McCrory MA, Lönnerdal B,** A randomized study of the effects of aerobic exercise by lactating women on breast-milk volume and composition, N Engl J Med 330:449, 1994.

120. **McClellan HL, Miller SJ, Hartmann PE,** Evolution of lactation: nutrition v. protection with special reference to five mammalian species, Nutr Res Rev 21:97, 2008.

121. **Geddes DT, Kent JC, Mitoulas LR, Hartmann PE,** Tongue movement and intra-oral vacuum in breastfeeding infants, Early Hum Dev 84:471, 2008.

122. **Nishimori K, Young LJ, Guo Q, Wang Z, Insel TR, Matzuk MM,** Oxytocin is required for nursing but is not essential for parturition or reproductive behavior, Proc Natl Acad Sci U S A 93:11699, 1996.

123. **Wasalathanthri S, Tennekoon KH,** Lactational amenorrhea/anovulation and some of their determinants: a comparison of well-nourished and undernourished women, Fertil Steril 76:317, 2001.

124. **Campbell OM, Gray RH,** Characteristics and determinants of postpartum ovarian function in women in the United States, Am J Obstet Gynecol 169:55, 1993.

125. **Labbok MH, Hight-Laukaran V, Peterson AE, Fletcher V, von Hertzen H, Van Look PFA,** Multicenter study of the lactational amenorrhea method (LAM): I. Efficacy, duration, and implications for clinical application, Contraception 55:327, 1997.

126. **Visness CM, Kennedy KI, Gross BA, Parenteau-Carreau S, Flynn AM, Brown JB,** Fertility of fully breast-feeding women in the early postpartum period, Obstet Gynecol 89:164, 1997.

127. **Tyson JE, Carter JN, Andreassen B, Huth J, Smith B,** Nursing mediated prolactin and luteinizing hormone secretion during puerperal lactation, Fertil Steril 30:154, 1978.

128. **Curtis KM, Tepper NK, Jatlaoui TC, Berry-Bibee E, Horton LG, Zapata LB, Simmons KB, Pagano HP, Jamieson DJ, Whiteman MK,** U.S. Medical Eligibility Criteria for Contraceptive Use, 2016, MMWR Recomm Rep 65:1–104, 2016.

129. **Sauder SE, Frager M, Case GD, Kelch RP, Marshall JC,** Abnormal patterns of pulsatile luteinizing hormone secretion in women with hyperprolactinemia and amenorrhea: responses to bromocriptine, J Clin Endocrinol Metab 59:941, 1984.

130. **Tay CCK, Glasier A, McNeilly AS,** Twenty-four hour secretory profiles of gonadotropins and prolactin in breastfeeding women, Hum Reprod 7: 951, 1992.

131. **Ishizuka B, Quigley ME, Yen SSC,** Postpartum hypogonadotrophinism: evidence for increased opioid inhibition, Clin Endocrinol 20:573, 1984.

132. **Petraglia F, De Leo V, Nappi C, Facchinetti F, Montemagno U, Brambilla F, Genazzani AR,** Differences in the opioid control of luteinizing hormone secretion between pathological and iatrogenic hyperprolactinemic states, J Clin Endocrinol Metab 64:508, 1987.

133. **Tay CCK, Glasier AF, McNeilly AS,** Effect of antagonists of dopamine and opiates on the basal and GnRH-induced secretion of luteinizing hormone, follicle stimulating hormone and prolactin during lactational amenorrhea in breastfeeding women, Hum Reprod 8:532, 1993.

134. **Zinaman MJ, Cartledge T, Tomai T, Tippett P, Merriam GR,** Pulsatile GnRH stimulates normal cyclic ovarian function in amenorrheic lactating postpartum women, J Clin Endocrinol Metab 80:2088, 1995.

135. **Perez A, Vela P, Masnick GS, Potter RG,** First ovulation after childbirth: the effect of breastfeeding, Am J Obstet Gynecol 114:1041, 1972.

136. **Diaz S, Peralta O, Juez G, Salvatierra AM, Casado ME, Duran E, Croxatto HB,** Fertility regulation in nursing women. I. The probability of conception in full nursing women living in an urban setting, J Biosoc Sci 14:329, 1982.

137. **McNeilly AS, Glasier A, Howie PW,** Endocrine control of lactational infertility, In: Dobbing J, ed. Maternal Nutrition and Lactational Infertility, Nevey/Raven Press, New York, 1985, p 177.

138. **Rivera R, Kennedy KI, Ortiz E, Barrera M, Bhiwandiwala PP,** Breast-feeding and the return to ovulation in Durango, Mexico, Fertil Steril 49:780, 1988.

139. **Lewis PR, Brown JB, Renfree MB, Short RV,** The resumption of ovulation and menstruation in a well-nourished population of women breastfeeding for an extended period of time, Fertil Steril 55:529, 1991.

140. **Berman ML, Hanson K, Hellman IL,** Effect of breastfeeding on postpartum menstruation, ovulation, and pregnancy in Alaskan Eskimos, Am J Obstet Gynecol 114:524, 1971.

141. **Short RV, Lewis PR, Renfree MB, Shaw G,** Contraceptive effects of extended lactational amenorrhoea: beyond the Bellagio Consensus, Lancet 337:715, 1991.

142. **Pérez A, Labbok MH, Queenan JT,** Clinical study of the lactational amenorrhoea method for family planning, Lancet 339:968, 1992.

143. **Diaz S, Aravena R, Cardenas H, Casado ME, Miranda P, Schiappacasse V, Croxatto HB,** Contraceptive efficacy of lactational amenorrhea in urban Chilean women, Contraception 43:335, 1991.

144. **Kazi A, Kennedy KI, Visness CM, Khan T,** Effectiveness of the lactational amenorrhea method in Pakistan, Fertil Steril 64:717, 1995.

145. **Kennedy KI, Rivera R, McNeilly AS,** Consensus statement on the use of breastfeeding as a family planning method, Bellagio, Italy, Contraception 39:477, 1989.

146. **Ramos R, Kennedy KI, Visness CM,** Effectiveness of lactational amenorrhoea in preventing pregnancy in Manila, The Philippines, Br Med J 313:909, 1996.

147. **World Health Organization Task Force on Methods for the Natural Regulation of Fertility,** The World Health Organization multinational study of breast-feeding and lactational amenorrhea. I. Description of infant feeding patterns and the return of menses, Fertil Steril 70:448, 1998.

148. **World Health Organization Task Force on Methods for the Natural Regulation of Fertility,** The World Health Organization multinational study of breast-feeding and lactational amenorrhea. II. Factors associated with the length of amenorrhea, Fertil Steril 70:461, 1998.

149. **World Health Organization Task Force on Methods for the Natural Regulation of Fertility,** The World Health Organization multinational study of breast-feeding and lactational amenorrhea. III. Pregnancy during breast-feeding, Fertil Steril 72:431, 1999.

150. **World Health Organization Task Force on Methods for the Natural Regulation of Fertility,** The World Health Organization multinational study of breast-feeding and lactational amenorrhea. IV. Postpartum bleeding and lochia in breast-feeding women, Fertil Steril 72:441, 1999.

151. **Gray RH, Campbell OM, Apelo R, Eslami SS, Zacur H, Ramos RM, Gehret JC, Labbok MH,** Risk of ovulation during lactation, Lancet 335:25, 1990.

152. **Sinai I, Cachan J,** A bridge for postpartum women to Standard Days Method®: II. Efficacy study, Contraception 86:16–21, 2012.

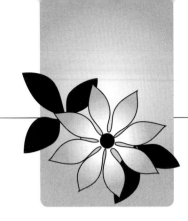

12

Emergency Contraception

Nora Doty, MD, MSCR and
Alison Edelman, MD, MPH

E mergency contraception (EC) is a method to prevent pregnancy after intercourse in which a primary contraceptive method was not used or failed.[1] Although this approach is commonly referred to as the "morning-after pill," this nomenclature fails to recognize that a copper intrauterine device (IUD) can also be used for EC, that methods are effective for many days after the "morning after," and that all EC methods should be initiated as soon as possible, not necessarily the "morning after." Numerous methods have been evaluated and vary in their ability to act as EC, but only three EC methods are primarily available worldwide: the copper IUD, ulipristal acetate (UPA), and levonorgestrel **(Table 12.1)**. EC is considered an essential treatment option for women wanting to avoid pregnancy following unplanned intercourse, barrier method failure, misuse of other contraceptive methods, or sexual assault. However, many women also report using EC simply due to fear of contraceptive method failure.[2]

The use of large doses of estrogen to provide EC was pioneered in the 1960s but was associated with significant gastrointestinal side effects.[3] Albert Yuzpe then developed a method utilizing a combination oral contraceptive or the "Yuzpe" method (ethinyl estradiol 100 mcg and norgestrel 1 mg given twice, 12 hours apart), resulting in a significant reduction in estrogen dose.[4,5] During the 1970s, a number of studies were undertaken, mostly in South America, to test the efficacy of various progestins given without estrogen for the potential use of progestins as on-demand contraceptives (i.e., after each act of intercourse). A WHO-sponsored multicenter trial found that levonorgestrel 0.75 mg had a failure rate of 0.8% per treated cycle without any serious side effects; however, this treatment regimen caused a high incidence of cycle disturbances.[6] These studies led to a large WHO-sponsored randomized trial comparing the Yuzpe and levonorgestrel regimens for EC.[7] The progestin-only EC containing levonorgestrel 0.75 mg given 12 hours apart not only had fewer side effects but was more effective than the Yuzpe method. Importantly, as a randomized comparative trial, this study was the first to prove that EC works, given the superiority of one regimen over the other; previously, studies only evaluated outcomes (pregnancy) compared to expected rates. This initially marketed two-dose progestin-only EC was replaced with a single-dose product based on studies demonstrating that taking both doses together

Table 12.1 Characteristics of Emergency Contraception Methods

EC Method	Dose	Effectiveness*	Timing	Approved	Accessibility	Notes
Intrauterine						
Copper IUD	380 mm^2	99%	Within 120 h	No	Requires office visit	
Oral antiprogestin						
Ulipristal acetate	30 mg	67%	Within 120 h	In most developed countries	Requires prescription in the United States, OTC in Europe	
Mifepristone	200 mg		Within 120 h	No	Limited access	
Oral progestin						
Levonorgestrel	1.5 mg	50%	Within 120 h	In most countries	OTC	FDA-approved in the United States for use within 72 h
Combined estrogen-progestin						
Ethinyl-estradiol/ norgestrel	100 mcg/1.0 mg†		Within 72 h for the first dose; repeat dose in 12 h	No	Requires prescription	Not recommended for routine use due to low efficacy

IUD, intrauterine device; OTC, over the counter.
*Calculated reduction in pregnancy risk.
†Norgestrel 1.0 mg is equivalent to levonorgestrel 0.5 mg.

provided similar effectiveness and no increase in side effects—leading us to the levonorgestrel regimen that is available today.[8,9] Subsequently, selective progesterone receptor modulators (like UPA) and the copper IUD were developed and implemented for EC.

Measuring Efficacy

EC pills are effective at delaying and/or inhibiting ovulation when taken during the correct window of time,[9-12] but determining EC effectiveness for a specific individual also depends on her actual risk of pregnancy. This risk is difficult to determine as it depends on an individual's inherent fecundability and on which cycle day unprotected intercourse occurred. The average woman's menstrual cycle has approximately 6 days when intercourse can result in pregnancy: the 5 days prior to ovulation and the day of ovulation itself.[13] This window is limited because sperm only have the capacity to fertilize an ovum for up to 5 days in the reproductive tract.[14] The risk of pregnancy is highest on the day prior to ovulation and negligible on the first few days of the cycle (**Figure 12.1**).[13] However, the day of ovulation is difficult to predict in each cycle due to lack of regularity even in women who report "regular" cycles; almost half of women will have a cycle range of 7 days or more over the course of four or more cycles.[15] Accordingly, 1% to 6% of women with reported regular cycles can be in their fertile window on the day that their next menses is expected to start.[13]

In EC trials, the number of pregnancies prevented by EC is typically obtained through subject recall as to the cycle day of unprotected intercourse. The likelihood of conception on that cycle day is based on

399

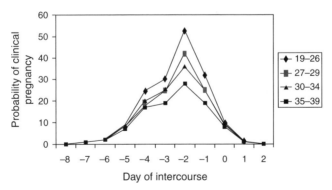

Figure 12.1 Probability of pregnancy relative to ovulation after intercourse on a given day of the cycle in women of different ages (years). (From **Dunson DB, Colombo B, Baird DD,** Changes with age in the level and duration of fertility in the menstrual cycle, Hum Reprod 17(5):1399–1403, 2002. Reproduced by permission of European Society of Human Reproduction and Embryology.)

pregnancy probability data from studies of women who were trying to conceive, which may not be same as the pregnancy probability in women who are not trying to conceive.[16] Thus, it is possible that the overall effectiveness of EC may be overestimated in trials.

At the individual level, EC effectiveness can be potentially influenced by factors like high BMI, weight over 75 to 80 kg, as well as further unprotected intercourse in the same cycle.[17,18] It can be difficult to determine the exact benefit an individual may get from EC, but because of its safety, it is recommended that women use EC at any point in the cycle even if it is outside the suspected fertile window because the benefits of use outweigh the risks.

In the United States, EC was initially touted as the answer to the high rate of unplanned pregnancies and projected to have the ability to reduce abortion rates by 40%.[19] Although many women report "ever having" used EC pills (3 in 10 women), population-level effects on unintended pregnancy rates have not been demonstrated.[19–21] This lack of a population-level effect is likely due to various factors including the incorrect and nonuse of EC, repeat acts of unprotected intercourse in the same month, and other patient-specific issues.[17,22,23] Advance prescription or provision does not appear to be a solution; a study of advanced provision of EC pills in Scotland did not demonstrate a change in abortion rates despite 45% of women using EC pills at least once.[24]

Types of EC

Copper IUD

The copper T380A IUD is the most effective form of EC and can prevent pregnancy for at least 120 hours after unprotected intercourse.[25] Some evidence exists that the copper IUD may be effective even if placed up to 14 days after unprotected intercourse as long as a urine pregnancy test is negative prior to placement.[26,27]

Copper ions impair sperm motility, viability, and the acrosomal reaction when used as a continuous contraceptive; these actions are unlikely to have any benefit when the IUD is inserted postcoitally.[28] The copper IUD is the only EC that may have a contragestive effect meaning that it may prevent implantation, but this action is entirely dependent on the timing of IUD placement in relationship to ovulation and intercourse.[29] Advantages of the copper IUD over oral EC methods include its cost-effectiveness,[30] its ability to be used as an ongoing contraceptive method for 10 or more years, and that weight or other patient characteristics are unlikely to impair its efficacy. In copper IUD EC studies, 1-year continuation rates range from 60% in a U.S. sample to 94% in a large Chinese sample.[25,31] Disadvantages of the copper IUD include initial upfront cost, discomfort with placement, and need for a time-sensitive office visit. Side effects of using the copper IUD as EC are the same as those associated with using the copper IUD for contraception and include an initial increase in menstrual bleeding and dysmenorrhea, which typically decrease with time.[25]

The copper IUD as EC is an excellent choice for women with access to an expedient office visit for placement and who desire to use it as their ongoing method of contraception. One project that investigated increasing copper IUD access found that 11% of women who were seeking EC but not necessarily IUD placement had same-day IUDs placed after a counseling intervention.[32] A copper IUD as EC has almost no contraindications for use. According to the U.S. Center for Disease Control's Medical Eligibility Criteria for Contraceptive Use (MEC), the copper IUD for EC is a category 4 for women who are currently pregnant and a category 3 for women who have undergone solid organ transplant and are having complications.[33] If placing a copper IUD for EC, patients should be counseled about the risk of failure and, if this occurs, the risk of having an IUD in place with an ongoing pregnancy. After insertion of copper IUD for EC, no additional or backup method of contraception is needed because the IUD is immediately effective.

Ulipristal Acetate

UPA is the most effective oral EC agent available. UPA is a selective progesterone receptor modulator that works by delaying ovulation.[34] Different from other oral EC methods, UPA appears to be able to delay ovulation even at the time of a rising LH surge. A pooled analysis from clinical trials demonstrated that rupture of follicles ≥18 mm in size is delayed by at least 5 days in 59% of cycles exposed to UPA compared to only 15% of levonorgestrel EC-exposed cycles.[34] The enhanced activity of UPA relative to levonorgestrel is due to its tissue-specific functions as a selective progesterone receptor modulator. When given prior to the luteinizing hormone (LH) surge, UPA acts at the hypothalamus as a progesterone receptor agonist (like levonorgestrel) and blocks or attenuates the LH surge. However, once the LH surge has initiated, many LH-triggered events in the follicle are mediated by progesterone receptor binding. As a result, UPA acts as an antagonist, blocking the pathways required for follicle rupture and extending the effective dosing window to the time of the LH peak. As a pure agonist, levonorgestrel cannot block these downstream progesterone receptor–mediated pathways (see Chapter 2).[35]

The efficacy of UPA compared to levonorgestrel has been established in clinical trials. UPA prevented more pregnancies than levonorgestrel both 0 to 72 hours and 72 to 120 hours after unprotected intercourse in a noninferiority trial; however, the 97- to 120-hour subgroup constituted only 3% of the study population, which limits this finding.[23] As sperm can be viable in the reproductive tract for up to 5 days,[16] UPA can effectively prevent ovulation during a woman's entire fertile window. UPA's consistency and duration of effect as well as its longer window of effectiveness are likely what make it a more effective method of EC compared to levonorgestrel.

Risk factors for failure of UPA include subsequent acts of unprotected intercourse during the same menstrual cycle without repeating the use of UPA. UPA delays follicle rupture for at least 5 days; thus, women are at risk for conception if they have unprotected intercourse again as ovulation just occurs later in that same cycle.[36] UPA efficacy *may* be impaired by obesity. A meta-analysis of two randomized controlled trials found an increased odds of pregnancy after taking UPA in women with a BMI $\geq$ 30 kg/m^2 compared to women with a BMI of less than 25 kg/m^2. However, this study was not sufficiently powered to definitively determine this outcome (OR 2.62, 95% CI 0.89 to 7.0).[17] Subsequent studies of UPA pharmacokinetics or drug levels demonstrate similar levels in normal and obese BMI subjects,[37] but as obesity can impact all aspects of drug function and transport, further pharmacodynamics and/ or sufficiently powered pregnancy trials are needed to ultimately answer this question.

Side effects of UPA are mild and include headaches (10%) and nausea (10%).[36] UPA is a good choice of EC for almost all patients; according to the MEC, UPA has no contraindications to use.[33] UPA EC users can expect onset of their next menses to occur slightly later than expected (average 2.1 days)[23] because UPA delays ovulation by 5 to 7 days, which in turn prolongs the follicular phase and lengthens the cycle.

Even in places where UPA is approved as EC, accessibility is limited as it is only available by prescription. In the United States, many pharmacies do not routinely stock it; a study of pharmacies in major U.S. cities in 2016 found that less than 10% had the ability to immediately fill a prescription for UPA EC.[38] Since 2015, UPA has been available without a prescription in all European Union members except Hungary.[39]

An important limitation of UPA use is that rapid initiation of a hormonal contraceptive method appears to interfere with UPA's efficacy. A blinded placebo crossover trial of UPA and a desogestrel progestin-only pill started on the next day found that only 1 ovulation event occurred in the 19 cycles when UPA was followed by placebo versus 13 ovulation events in 29 cycles when UPA was followed by desogestrel.[40] Another study of UPA, but with a combined oral contraceptive method, also demonstrated that early initiation of a hormonal contraceptive method interferes with UPA's efficacy.[41] Current clinical guidance recommends delaying hormonal contraceptive initiation following UPA EC for 5 days.[42,43] Although hormonal contraception can affect UPA's efficacy, it does not appear that UPA impacts the ability of subsequent hormonal contraception to suppress ovulation. A randomized controlled trial demonstrated that UPA does not impact the ability of a combined oral contraceptive pill started 1 day later to cause ovarian quiescence.[44] A woman could theoretically start a hormonal method earlier than 5 days after UPA if she is confident of the date of the last unprotected intercourse. Because sperm are only viable in the reproductive tract for 5 days, hormonal contraception could be initiated 5 days after the unprotected intercourse. A woman can have any IUD placed after oral EC use as long as it is reasonably certain she is not pregnant at the time of IUD placement.

Levonorgestrel

Levonorgestrel is less effective than UPA or a copper IUD[23,45] but more effective than the Yuzpe method.[7,8] Levonorgestrel prevents about 50% of expected pregnancies.[8,18] Although marketed for use within 72 hours of unprotected intercourse, some efficacy is present through 5 days. However, it is most effective when taken close to the time of unprotected intercourse and its effectiveness appears to wane over time. By waiting more than 12 hours from unprotected intercourse, the odds of pregnancy increase by 50%. Delaying the use of levonorgestrel for 5 days (120 hours) after unprotected intercourse has a five times increased risk of pregnancy compared to taking it within the first 24 hours.[46]

Levonorgestrel has a differential effect on the LH surge depending on when it is administered in the menstrual cycle.[38] If taken 2 days before the LH surge, the surge is usually suppressed completely, which means ovulation is prevented and pregnancy risk is decreased. If taken closer to the LH surge, the surge can be blunted or delayed but may not be suppressed completely resulting in ovulation that may be delayed and persistence of some pregnancy risk.

Levonorgestrel EC has significantly fewer side effects than the Yuzpe regimen but more than those reported with UPA EC. The most common side effects reported are nausea (23%) and emesis (19%).[7] Some women also report irregular bleeding in the week after use. Less common side effects include dizziness, fatigue, headache, breast tenderness, and abdominal pain.[8] These side effects tend to be mild and treatment is not typically needed for them. Levonorgestrel EC users can expect their next menstrual period slightly earlier (average 1.2 days), and in some women, the duration of bleeding was more than 8 days. Levonorgestrel EC taken earlier in the cycle is associated with a shorter menstrual cycle compared to taking it later in the cycle.[47]

Advantages of levonorgestrel EC include that it is available over the counter worldwide to anyone of any age, is well tolerated, and has no contraindications to use.[33] Another advantage of using levonorgestrel for EC is that any contraceptive method can be started immediately following its use without impacting the EC efficacy. **(Table 12.2).** Women should use abstinence or a backup method for 7 days following initiation

403

Table 12.2 Clinical Guidelines for Initiation of Contraception after Oral EC

	Implant	Levonor-gestrel IUS	Copper IUD	Depot Medroxy-progesterone	Combined Hormonal Methods	Condoms
Ulipristal acetate	Wait 5 d	Immediately	Immediately	Wait 5 d	Wait 5 d	Immediately
Levonorgestrel	Immediately	Immediately	Immediately	Immediately	Immediately	Immediately

of hormonal contraception after using any oral EC and should take a pregnancy test if no withdrawal bleed occurs in 3 weeks.[44]

The biggest risk factor for levonorgestrel EC failure is a subsequent act of unprotected intercourse in the same cycle. The most concerning issue regarding levonorgestrel EC is that obesity and weight may impact its effectiveness. Efficacy seems to wane at a weight of 75 kg, and for women 80 kg and over, levonorgestrel appears to not work at all.[17] A pooled analysis of 6,873 women from four studies found the pregnancy rates in obese women who used levonorgestrel EC are eight times that of normal-weight women.[48] Levonorgestrel EC pharmacokinetic studies have demonstrated that levonorgestrel drug levels are 50% lower in obese women compared to women with a normal BMI,[37,49,50] which is likely the reason for its impaired efficacy in women who are obese or weigh greater than 80 kg. Despite this concern, both the FDA and European Medicines Agency (EMA) have determined that not enough information exists to restrict use of levonorgestrel EC for women of higher weights or BMI.

Clinicians have hypothesized that increasing the dose of levonorgestrel may improve its effectiveness, but more research needs to be done in this area as only a small pharmacokinetic study exists. A study of five obese and five normal BMI women demonstrated that doubling the dose of levonorgestrel EC (levonorgestrel 3 mg) normalized the maximum serum concentration of levonorgestrel to that of a woman with a normal BMI.[50]

Other

Yuzpe Method

The Yuzpe method is no longer recommended for routine use given that other available methods are more effective and have fewer side effects.[18,51] Note that women are less likely to get pregnant even if they wait 24 hours to obtain levonorgestrel EC than if they were to take the Yuzpe method right away.[8]

Levonorgestrel 52 mg Intrauterine System

We have no data to support the use of levonorgestrel intrauterine system (IUS) alone for EC. However, a levonorgestrel 52 mg IUS may be quick-started following use of levonorgestrel EC in the setting of a negative pregnancy test. An observational study of 168 women who presented to an office for EC compared pregnancy rates with the copper IUS as compared to simultaneous use of levonorgestrel 1.5 mg orally with levonorgestrel 52 mg IUS placement.[52] Nearly two thirds of the women chose the levonorgestrel regimen and only one woman in that group became pregnant. A subsequent study demonstrated that among women who had a levonorgestrel 52 mg IUS placed simultaneously with oral levonorgestrel 1.5 mg, 70% were still using the levonorgestrel IUS at 1 year.[30] If an IUD is placed for EC or simultaneously with EC, patients should be counseled regarding the potential risk of EC failure resulting in an ongoing pregnancy and should undergo a follow-up pregnancy test several weeks after placement.

Mifepristone

Like UPA, mifepristone is a progesterone receptor modulator that acts by down-regulating progesterone receptors and delaying follicle maturation.[53] Doses as small as 10 mg are effective within 72 hours of unprotected intercourse,[54] and doses of 200 mg are effective in preventing 85% of pregnancies up to 120 hours after unprotected intercourse.[55] Mifepristone has different mechanisms of action depending on when it is taken during the menstrual cycle. In the follicular phase, it can inhibit ovulation, while in early luteal phase, mifepristone can alter endometrial receptivity.[55] While this regimen is available in many countries throughout the world, mifepristone is not FDA approved in the United States for this indication.

Other Clinical Considerations

What Is the Risk of Repeated Use of Oral EC?

Oral EC only covers a single act of unprotected intercourse. If a subsequent act of unprotected intercourse occurs in the same cycle, another dose of oral EC should be provided if a regular method of contraception has yet to be started and there is no contraindication to use.[51] Repeat EC use appears safe,[56,57] but results in a higher risk of pregnancy as compared to routine contraception.

Drug Interactions

Both levonorgestrel and UPA are metabolized in the liver by the cytochrome P450 CYP3A4 isoenzyme in addition to other isoenzymes.[58] Medications that induce CYP3A4 theoretically could decrease serum concentrations of UPA or levonorgestrel, possibly impacting efficacy. However, the U.S. MEC considers the concurrent use of CYP3A4 inducers with either UPA or levonorgestrel EC use a category 2 condition or safe to use.[32]

What to Do if Emesis Occurs After Taking Oral EC?

Unlike estrogen-containing EC regimens, levonorgestrel and UPA EC have a low risk of emesis; as such, routine pretreatment with antiemetics is not recommended.[7,42] However, if a patient vomits within 3 hours of taking either UPA or levonorgestrel, she can try using an antiemetic and repeating the dose.[45,59] Alternatively, the patient could be offered a copper IUD.

What Is the Risk of Ectopic Pregnancy Following EC Use?

Women who use EC are less likely to become pregnant than women who do not; therefore, the absolute risk of ectopic pregnancy is significantly lower after using EC. A systematic review of EC clinical trials found that of the pregnancies occurring post-EC use, ectopic pregnancy occurred in 0.6% with mifepristone EC and 1% with levonorgestrel EC use.[60] UPA clinical trial and postmarketing surveillance data report an ectopic pregnancy rate of 1.1%.[61] These rates are not higher than the ectopic pregnancy rate in the general population of 0.6% to 2.0%.[62,63]

What Are the Risks to a Pregnancy if Exposed to EC?

There are few data about intrauterine pregnancy outcomes after exposure to EC. An analysis of 376 pregnancies exposed to UPA from clinical trial and postmarketing surveillance data included 28 pregnancies which resulted in live-born infants with no pregnancy or neonatal complications. The miscarriage rate in exposed pregnancies was 14%.[61] A prospective cohort study of 332 women exposed to levonorgestrel EC in their conception cycle compared to unexposed pregnant women found no difference in rate of spontaneous abortion, congenital malformations, or adverse pregnancy outcomes.[64] Other studies have confirmed the safety of levonorgestrel exposure during pregnancy including normal neurologic and behavioral development of infants.[65,66]

Access Issues

The most effective EC methods still have barriers to access. The copper IUD requires an office visit within 5 days of unprotected intercourse. UPA currently requires a prescription and is not immediately available in pharmacies throughout the United States.[38] Theoretically, advanced provision of oral EC methods should increase effective use of this method, but studies have not demonstrated that advanced provision decreases pregnancy rates.[67-70] Advanced provision of EC however does increase its use without increasing the risk of using a less effective method of birth control.[68,70] Future options to increase access include expanding access to telemedicine, online prescribing,[71] and, ultimately, over-the-counter access to all oral methods.

EC Myths

- **EC is an abortifacient.** Pregnancy occurs after implantation of a fertilized embryo. Therefore, to be an abortifacient, EC would have to disrupt an implanted embryo. EC is not an abortifacient. Oral EC works primarily by preventing or delaying ovulation and by preventing fertilization.[72-75] Oral EC does not prevent implantation.[76-78] Even animal experiments using higher doses of levonorgestrel could detect no impact on the pregnancy once fertilization had occurred.[79,80] This evidence demonstrates that a postfertilization effect does not contribute to effectiveness of oral EC.[53,79-82] Health care providers and patients can be reassured oral EC is not an abortifacient. The copper IUD, when used for EC, has a contragestive effect meaning that it may prevent blastocyst implantation but will not impact an already implanted gestation.
- **Women use EC as routine contraception.** During the move to bring EC over-the-counter status, concerns were raised that women would rely on EC as a regular method of contraception. Studies have since refuted this and have demonstrated that EC access does not decrease the use of condoms or routine contraceptive use or increase the incidence of sexually transmitted infections.[83]

Postabortion and Postpartum EC Use

Women typically ovulate within 6 to 21 days after a first trimester surgical or medical abortion[84-88] and can therefore use EC at any time in the postabortion period based on clinical judgment. Women who are not breastfeeding ovulate on average 39 days postpartum. EC can be used at any time in the postpartum period. Women who are breastfeeding can use any method of EC. UPA is excreted in small amounts into breast milk. There is no evidence to recommend for or against using UPA while breastfeeding.[89] Remember that warnings related to hormonal contraceptive use within 5 days of UPA use are still relevant in both postabortion and postpartum women.[42,43]

Additional EC Resources

- The Office of Population Research at Princeton University maintains a website (ec.princeton.edu) that contains information for both patients and clinicians including information on how to obtain EC online and links to the Bedsider.org EC locator by zip code.
- The U.S. MEC and U.S. Centers for Disease Control's Selective Practice Guidelines provide evidence-based guidance on who can use and how to use EC (https://www.cdc.gov/reproductivehealth/contraception/mmwr/mec/summary.html).
- The American Society for Emergency Contraception (http://americansocietyforec.org/index.html) also provides evidence-based practical guidance for clinicians on EC and the issues impacting use.

References

1. **Croxatto HB, Devoto L, Durand M, et al.,** Mechanism of action of hormonal preparations used for emergency contraception: a review of the literature, Contraception 63:111–121, 2001.

2. **Daniels K, Jones J, Abma J,** Use of Emergency Contraception among Women aged 15–44: United States, 2006–2010. NCHS Data Brief, No. 112, National Center for Health Statistics, Hyattsville, 2013.

3. **Morris JM, Van Wagenen G,** Compounds interfering with ovum implantation and development, Am J Obstet Gynecol 96:804–815, 1966.

4. **Yuzpe AA, Percival Smith R, Rademaker AW,** A multicenter clinical investigation employing ethinyl estradiol combined with dl-norgestrel as a postcoital contraceptive agent, Fertil Steril 37:508–513, 1982.

5. **Ellerston C, Webb A, Blanchard K, et al.,** Modifying the Yuzpe regimen of emergency contraception: a multicenter randomized controlled trial, Obstet Gynecol 101:1160–1167, 2003.

6. **World Health Organization Task Force on Post-Ovulatory Methods for Fertility Regulation,** Post-coital contraception with levonorgestrel during the peri-ovulatory phase of the menstrual cycle, Contraception 36:257–286, 1987.

7. Randomised controlled trial of levonorgestrel versus the Yuzpe regimen of combined oral contraceptives for emergency contraception. Task Force on Postovulatory Methods of Fertility Regulation, Lancet 352:428–433, 1998.

8. **von Hertzen H, Piaggio G, Peregoudov A, et al.,** Low dose mifepristone and two regimens of levonorgestrel for emergency contraception: a WHO multicentre randomised trial, Lancet 360:1803–1810, 2002.

9. **Johansson E, Brache V, Alvarez F, et al.,** Pharmacokinetic study of different

dosing regimens of levonorgestrel for emergency contraception in healthy women, Hum Reprod 17:1472–1476, 2002.

10. **Hapangama D, Glasier AF, Baird DT,** The effects of peri-ovulatory administration of levonorgestrel on the menstrual cycle, Contraception 63:123–129, 2001.

11. **Noe G, Croxatto HB, Salvatierra AM, et al.,** Contraceptive efficacy of emergency contraception with levonorgestrel given before or after ovulation, Contraception 84:486–492, 2011.

12. **Brache V, Cohon L, Jesam C, et al.,** Immediate pre-ovulatory administration of 30 mg ulipristal acetate significantly delays follicular rupture, Hum Reprod 25:2256–2263, 2010.

13. **Dunson DB, Colombo B, Baird DD,** Changes with age in the level and duration of fertility in the menstrual cycle, Hum Reprod 17:1399–1403, 2002.

14. **Wilcox AJ, Weinberg CR, Baird D,** Timing of sexual intercourse in relation to ovulation, N Engl J Med 333:1517–1521, 1995.

15. **Creinin MD, Keverline S, Meyn LA,** How regular is Regular? An analysis of menstrual cycle regularity, Contraception 70:289–292, 2004.

16. **Raymond E, Taylor D, Trussell J, et al.,** Minimum effectiveness of the levonorgestrel regimen of emergency contraception, Contraception 69:79–81, 2004.

17. **Glasier AF, Cameron ST, Blithe D, et al.,** Can we identify women at risk of pregnancy despite using emergency contraception? Data from randomized trials of ulipristal acetate and levonorgestrel, Contraception 84:363–367, 2011.

18. **Shen J, Che Y, Showell E, et al.,** Interventions for emergency contraception, Cochrane Database Syst Rev (8):CD001324, 2017.

19. **Harper CC, Ellerston CE,** The emergency contraceptive pill: a survey of knowledge and attitudes among students at Princeton University, Am J Obstet Gynecol 173:1438–1445, 1995.

20. **The Kaiser Foundation,** Emergency Contraception fact sheet, September 2018. Accessed October 14, 2018. http://files.kff.org/attachment/emergency-contraception-fact-sheet.

21. **Trussell J, Ellerston C, con Hetzen H, et al.,** Estimating the effectiveness of emergency contraceptive pills, Contraception 67:259–265, 2003.

22. **Trussell J,** High hopes versus harsh realities: the population impact of ECPs, Eur J Contracept Reprod Health Care 18:S42–S46, 2013.

23. **Glasier AF, Cameron ST, Fine PM, et al.,** Ulipristal acetate versus levonorgestrel for emergency contraception: a randomised non-inferiority trial and meta-analysis, Lancet 375:555–562, 2010.

24. **Glasier A, Fairhurst K, Wyke S, et al.,** Advanced provision of emergency contraception does not reduce abortion rates, Contraception 69:361–366; 383, 2004.

25. **Wu S, Godfrey EM, Wojdyla D, et al.,** Copper T380A intrauterine device for emergency contraception: a prospective, multicentre, cohort clinical trial, BJOG 117:1205–1210, 2010.

26. **Turok DK, Godfrey EM, Wojdyla EM, et al.,** Copper T380 intrauterine device for emergency contraception: highly effective at any time in the menstrual cycle, Hum Reprod 28:2672–2676, 2013.

27. **Ivana Thompson, Jessica N Sanders, E Bimla Schwarz,** Christy Boraas, David K Turok. Copper intrauterine device placement 6–14 days after unprotected sex. Contraception 2019 (in press); DOI: https://doi.org/10.1016/j.contraception.2019.05.015.

28. **Gemzell-Danielsson K, Berger C, Lalitkumar PGL,** Emergency contraception—mechanisms of action, Contraception 87:300–308, 2013.

29. **Stanford JB, Mikolajczyk RT,** Mechanisms of action of intrauterine devices: update and estimation of post-fertilization effects, Am J Obstet Gynecol 187:1699–1708, 2002.

30. **Bellows BK, Tak CR, Sanders JN, et al.,** Cost-effectiveness of emergency contraception options over 1 year. Am J Obstet Gynecol 218:e1–e9, 2018.

31. **Schwarz EB, Papic M, Parisi SM, et al.,** Routine counseling about intrauterine contraception for women seeking emergency contraception, Contraception 90:66–71, 2014.

32. **Sanders JN, Turok DK, Royer PA, Thompson IS, Gawron LM, Storck KE,** One-year continuation of copper or levonorgestrel intrauterine devices initiated

at the time of emergency contraception, Contraception 96:99–105, 2017.

33. **Curtis KM, Tepper NK, Jatlaoui TC, et al.,** U.S. Medical Eligibility Criteria for Contraceptive Use, 2016, MMWR Recomm Rep 65:1–103, 2016.

34. **Brache V, Cochon L, Deniaud M, et al.,** Ulipristal acetate prevents ovulation more effectively than levonorgestrel: analysis of pooled data from three randomized trials of emergency contraception regimens, Contraception 88:611–618, 2013.

35. **Kim J, Bagchi IC, Bagchi MK,** Control of ovulation in mice by progesterone receptor-regulated gene networks, Mol Hum Reprod 15:821–828, 2009.

36. **Moreau C, Trussell J,** Results from pooled Phase III studies of ulipristal acetate for emergency contraception, Contraception 86:673–680, 2012.

37. **Praditpan P, Hamouie A, Basaraba CN, et al.,** Pharmacokinetics of levonorgestrel and ulipristal acetate emergency contraception in women with normal and obese body mass index, Contraception 95:464–469, 2017.

38. **Shigesato M, Elia J, Tschann M, et al.,** Pharmacy access to Ulipristal acetate in major cities throughout the United States, Contraception 97:264–269, 2018.

39. **The European Consortium for Emergency Contraception,** An update on access to emergency contraception in European union countries, April 2016, Accessed April 12, 2018. http://www.ec-ec.org/wp-content/uploads/2019/03/UPDATE-Access-to-EC-in-EU-countries-ECEC-April2016.pdf.

40. **Brache V, Cochon L, Duijkers IJM, et al.,** A prospective, randomized, pharmacodynamic study of quick-starting a desogestrel progestin-only pill following ulipristal acetate for emergency contraception, Hum Reprod 30:2785–2793, 2015.

41. **Edelman AB, Jensen JT, McCrimmon S, et al.,** Combined oral contraceptive interference with ability of ulipristal acetate to delay ovulation: a prospective cohort study, Contraception 98:463–466, 2018.

42. **Curtis KM, Tepper NK, Jatlaoui TC, et al.,** U.S. Selected Practice Recommendations for contraceptive use, 2016, MMWR Recomm Rep 65:1–66, 2016.

43. **Salcedo J, Rodriguez MI, Curtis KM, et al.,** When can a woman resume or initiate contraception after taking emergency contraceptive pills? A systematic review, Contraception 87:602–604, 2013.

44. **Cameron ST, Berger C, Michie L, et al.,** The effects on ovarian activity of ulipristal acetate when 'quickstarting' a combined oral contraceptive pill: a prospective, randomized, double-blind parallel-arm, placebo-controlled study, Hum Reprod 30:1566–1572, 2015.

45. **Creinin MD, Schlaff W, Archer DF, et al.,** Progesterone receptor modulator for emergency contraception: a randomized controlled trial, Obstet Gynecol 108:1089–1097, 2006.

46. **Piaggio G, Kapp N, von Hertzen H,** Effect on pregnancy rates of the delay in the administration of levonorgestrel for emergency contraception: a combined analysis of four WHO trials, Contraception 84:35–39, 2011.

47. **Raymond EG, Goldberg A, Trussell J, et al.,** Bleeding patterns after use of levonorgestrel emergency contraceptive pills, Contraception 73:376–381, 2006.

48. **Festin MPR, Peregoudov A, Seuc A, et al.,** Effect of BMI and body weight on pregnancy rates with LNG as emergency contraception: analysis of four WHO HRP studies, Contraception 95:50–54, 2017.

49. **Natavio M, Stanczyk FZ, Molins EAG, Nelson A, Jusko WJ,** Pharmacokinetics of the 1.5 mg levonorgestrel emergency contraceptive in women with normal, obese and extremely obese body mass index, Contraception 99:306–311, 2019.

50. **Edelman AB, Cherala G, Blue SW, et al.,** Impact of obesity on the pharmacokinetics of levonorgestrel-based emergency contraception: single and double dosing, Contraception 94:52–57, 2016.

51. **American Congress of Obstetricians and Gynecologists,** Practice bulletin no. 152: emergency contraception, Obstet Gynecol 126:e1–e11, 2015.

52. **Turok DK, Sanders JN, Thompson IS, et al.,** Preference for and efficacy of oral levonorgestrel for emergency contraception with concomitant placement of a levonorgestrel IUD: a prospective cohort study, Contraception 93:526–532, 2016.

53. **Marions L, Hultenby K, Lindell I, et al.,** Emergency contraception with mifepristone and levonorgestrel: mechanism of action, Obstet Gynecol 100:65–71, 2002.

54. Comparison of three single doses of mifepristone as emergency contraception: a randomised trial. Task force on postovulatory methods of fertility regulation, Lancet 353:697–702, 1999.

55. **Ashok PW, Wagaarachchi PT, Flett GM, et al.,** Mifepristone as a late post-coital contraceptive, Hum Reprod 16:72–75, 2001.

56. **Jesam C, Cochon L, Salvatierra AM, et al.,** A prospective, open-label, multicenter study to assess the pharmacodynamics and safety of repeated use of 30 mg ulipristal acetate, Contraception 93:310–316, 2016.

57. **Festin MP, Bahamondes L, Nguyen TMH, et al.,** A prospective, open-label, single arm, multicentre study to evaluate efficacy, safety and acceptability of pericoital oral contraception using levonorgestrel 1.5 mg, Hum Reprod 31:530–540, 2016.

58. **Pohl O, Osterloh I, Gotteland JP,** Effects of erythromycin at steady-state concentrations on the pharmacokinetics of ulipristal acetate, J Clin Pharm Ther 38:512–517, 2013.

59. **Rodriguez MI, Curtis KM, Gaffield ML, et al.,** Prevention and management of nausea and vomiting with emergency contraception: a systematic review, Contraception 87:583–589, 2013.

60. **Cleland K, Raymond E, Trussel J, et al.,** Ectopic pregnancy and emergency contraceptive pills: a systematic review, Obstet Gynecol 115: 1263–1266, 2010.

61. **Zhang L, Chen J, Wang Y, et al.,** Pregnancy outcome after levonorgestrel-only emergency contraception failure: a prospective cohort study, Hum Reprod 24:1605–1611, 2009.

62. **Levy DP, Jager M, Kapp N, et al.,** Ulipristal acetate for emergency contraception: postmarketing experience after use by more than 1 million women, Contraception 89:431–433, 2014.

63. **Stulberg DB, Cain LR, Dahlquist I, Lauderdale DS,** Ectopic pregnancy rates and racial disparities in the Medicaid population, 2004–2008, Fertil Steril 102:1671–1676, 2014.

64. **De Santis M, Cavaliere AF, Straface G, et al.,** Failure of the emergency contraceptive levonorgestrel and the risk of adverse effects in pregnancy and on fetal development: an observational cohort study, Fertil Steril 84:296–299, 2005.

65. **Zhang L, Ye W, Cheng L, et al.,** Physical and mental development of children after levonorgestrel emergency contraception exposure: a follow-up prospective cohort study, Biol Reprod 91:1–7, 2014.

66. **Hoover KW, Tao G, Kent CK,** Trends in the diagnosis and treatment of ectopic pregnancy in the United States, Obstet Gynecol 115:495–502, 2010.

67. **Meyer JL, Gold MA, Haggerty CL,** Advance provision of emergency contraception among adolescent and young adult women: a systematic review of literature, J Pediatr Adolesc Gynecol 24:2–9, 2011.

68. **Rodriguez MI, Curtis KM, Gaffield ML, et al.,** Advance supply of emergency contraception: a systematic review, Contraception 87:590–601, 2013.

69. **Polis CB, Schaffef K, Blanchard K, et al.,** Advance provision of emergency contraception for pregnancy prevention: a meta-analysis, Obstet Gynecol 110:1379–1388, 2007.

70. **Jackson RA, Schwarz EB, Freedman L, et al.,** Advance supply of emergency contraception effect on use and usual contraception—a randomized trial, Obstet Gynecol 102:8–16, 2003.

71. **Smith NK, Cleland K, Wagner B, et al.,** "I don't know what I would have done." Women's experiences acquiring ulipristal acetate emergency contraception online from 2011 to 2015, Contraception 95:414–418, 2017.

72. **Young DC, Wiehle RD, Joshi SG, et al.,** Emergency contraception alters progesterone-associated endometrial protein in serum and uterine luminal fluid, Obstet Gynecol 84:266–271, 1994.

73. **Swahn ML, Westlund P, Johannisson E, et al.,** Effect of post-coital contraceptive methods on the endometrium and the menstrual cycle, Acta Obstet Gynecol Scand 75:738–744, 1996.

74. **Trussell J, Raymond EG,** Statistical evidence about the mechanism of action of the Yuzpe regimen of emergency contraception, Obstet Gynecol 93:872, 1999.

75. **Croxatto HB, Fuentealba B, Brache V, et al.,** Effects of the Yuzpe regimen, given during the follicular phase, on ovarian function, Contraception 65:121–128, 2001.

76. **Novikova N, Weisberg E, Stanczyk S, et al.,** Effectiveness of levonorgestrel emergency contraception given before or after ovulation—a pilot study, Contraception 75:112–118, 2007.

77. **Lalitkumar PGL, Lalitkumar S, Meng CX, et al.,** Mifepristone, but not levonorgestrel, inhibits human blastocyst attachment to an in vitro endometrial three-dimensional cell culture model, Hum Reprod 22:3031–3037, 2007.

78. **Meng CX, Cheng LN, Lalitkumar PGL, et al.,** Expressions of steroid receptors and Ki67 in first-trimester decidua and chorionic villi exposed to levonorgestrel used for emergency contraception, Fertil Steril 91:1420–1423, 2009.

79. **Ortiz ME, Ortiz RE, Fuentes MA, et al.,** Post-coital administration of levonorgestrel does not interfere with post-fertilization events in the new-world monkey *Cebus apella*, Hum Reprod 19:1352–1356, 2004.

80. **Müller AL, Llados CM, Croxatto HB,** Postcoital treatment with levonorgestrel does not disrupt postfertilization events in the rat, Contraception 67:415–419, 2003.

81. **Trussell J, Ellertson C, Dorflinger L,** Effectiveness of the Yuzpe regimen of emergency contraception by cycle day of intercourse: implications for mechanism of action, Contraception 67:167–171, 2003.

82. **Okewole IA, Arowojolu AO, Odusoga OL, et al.,** Effect of single administration of levonorgestrel on the menstrual cycle, Contraception 75:372–377, 2007.

83. **Raine TR, Harper CC, Rocca CH, et al.,** Direct access to emergency contraception through pharmacies and effect on unintended pregnancy and STIs, JAMA 293:54–62, 2005.

84. **Marrs RP, Kletzky OA, Howard WF, Mishell DR,** Disappearance of human chorionic gonadotropin and resumption of ovulation following abortion, Am J Obstet Gynecol 135:731–736, 1979.

85. **Lahteenmaki P,** The disappearance of hCG and return of pituitary function after abortion, Clin Endocrinol (Oxf) 9:101–112, 1978.

86. **Lahteenmaki P, Luukkainen T,** Return of ovarian function after abortion, Clin Endocrinol (Oxf) 8:123–132, 1978.

87. **Cameron IT, Baird DT,** The return to ovulation following early abortion: a comparison between vacuum aspiration and prostaglandin, Acta Endocrinol (Copenh) 118:161–167, 1988.

88. **Schreiber CA, Sober S, Ratcliffe S, Creinin MD,** Ovulation resumption after medical abortion with mifepristone and misoprostol, Contraception 84:230–233, 2011.

89. **Ella Product Label.** Food and Drug Administration. Afaxys, May 2018.

411

INDEX

Page numbers followed by *f* indicate figures; those followed by *t* indicate tables; those followed by *b* indicate boxes.

A

Abortion
   induced in United States, 23
   medical, 56, 317–318
   with mifepristone and misoprostol, 55
   septic, 190–191
   spontaneous, 261, 406
Acne, 145–146
Actinomyces, 188–189
Adenomas
   liver, 267
   prolactin-secreting, 270–271
Adiana, 101, 104
Anemia, 262
Antibiotics, 9, 188, 266
Anticonvulsants, 334
Antimicrobials, 334
Antimüllerian hormone (AMH), 37
Antiprogestins, 56*f*
Apple®, 372
Arterial thrombosis
   myocardial infarction, 243–245, 244*t*
   stroke, 245–247, 245*t*
Atazanavir, 334

B

Backup method, 148
Bacterial vaginosis
   IUD, 187
   oral contraception, 269
Barrier contraception, 341
   cervical cap, 351, 351*f*
   clinicians counseling, 341
   condoms
      availability, 358
      benefits, 358–359
      breakage rates, 358
      female condoms (*see* Female condom)
      male (*see* Male condom)
      manufacturing quality, 358
      proper use of, 358
      risk for STIs and HIV infections, 358
      steps for maximal condom efficacy, 358–359
      withdrawal of, 358
   contraceptive sponge
      effectiveness, 352
      lower rates of infection, 352–353
      Protectaid®, 352
      side effects, 352–353
      Today®, 352
      vaginal, 352
   diaphragm, 343–350
      benefits, 344
      care of 350
      Chlamydia, 344
      choice and use of, 344–345
      distribution of, 343
      efficacy, 343–344
      fitting, 345, 346*f*–350*f*
      gonorrhea, 344
      Milex fitted silicone, 343
      Ortho All-Flex, 343
      pelvic inflammatory disease, 344
      reassessment, 345
      side effects, 344
      timing of, 345
      tubal infertility, 344
      urinary tract infections, 344
      vaginal irritation, 344
   modern history, 342
   physical, 341
   postpartum/postabortion period, 360
   protection against STIs and pelvic infection, 342
   risk of toxic shock syndrome, 342
   spermicides, 353–355
      acid-buffering gel, 353
      advantages, 354
      Amphora™, 353
      application instructions, 353
      BufferGel, 353
      commercial availability, 353
      Contragel®, 353
      efficacy, 354
      Gynol II®, 353
      modern, 353
      protection against STIs, 353–354
      RepHresh™ and Replens™, 353
      side effects, 354–355

Basal Body Temperature (BBT) Method, 369, 371
Behavioral methods
abstinence, 367
advantages, 369
classification, 367–368
coitus interruptus/withdrawal, 367
FABMs (*see* Fertility awareness–based methods (FABMs))
genital-to-genital contact, 380–381
lactational amenorrhea method (*see* Lactational amenorrhea method (LAM))
mutual masturbation, 380–381
oral-genital intercourse, 380–381
patient education and motivation, 367, 380–381
self-stimulation, 380–381
Benzalkonium chloride, 352
Bilateral total salpingectomy, 118–121
Billings ovulation method, 373–374
Bleeding profiles, 171
Breakthrough bleeding, management of, 40
Breast cancer, 251–254, 259–260
hormonal contraceptive, 82t
levonorgestrel system, 187
in LNG-IUS users, 185
Breast disease, 251–252
Breastfeeding. *See also* Lactational amenorrhea method (LAM)
inexpensive nutrition, 381
injectable progestin-only contraceptives, 317–318
motivation to, 381
ovulated women, 386
prevalence, 381
progestin-only pills, 336
revival of, 381

C
Cancer. *See specific types*
Cancer effects
breast cancer, 251–254, 259–260
cervical cancer, 256–260
colorectal cancer, 258
endometrial cancer, 255
liver cancer, 258–259
lymphatic/hematopoietic cancers, 259
melanoma, 259
ovarian cancer, 255–256
Candida, vaginal infection, 188–189
Carbohydrate metabolism, 232–233
Cardiovascular disease risks, 248–251

Cardiovascular effects
arterial thrombosis (myocardial infarction and stroke), 243–248
hypertension, 242–243
inherited thrombophilias, 241–242
thrombosis, 248–251
venous thromboembolism, 233–242, 250t
Case reports and case series, 74–75, 75t
Case-control studies, 73, 73t
Caya diaphragm, 342–343, 343f
Cervical cancer, 256–260
Cervical cap. *See* Barrier methods of contraception
Cervical mucus, 40–41
CHCs. *See* Combination hormonal contraceptives (CHCs)
Chemical barrier methods. *See* Spermicides
CHOICE project, 24, 170
Clauberg test, 62
Clinical practice guidelines
Centers for Disease Control and Prevention, 89
definition, 84–86
examples for family planning and reproductive health, 84–86, 85t
Medical Eligibility Criteria for Contraceptive Use, 84, 86t–90t
recommendations for clinical care, 84–86
Selected Practice Recommendations for Contraceptive Use, 84
sources of, 84–86
trustworthy, 84–86, 84t
updated guidance, 90
Clinical Practice Guidelines for Family Planning and Reproductive Health, 84–86, 85t
Clinical study designs
bias, distortions due to study design
confounding factors, 76–78, 76t, 77t
detection/surveillance/diagnostic bias, 75
information/observer bias, 76
publication bias, 75
reporting/recall bias, 75
selection bias, 75–76
sources of, 75
classification of, 67, 69f
hierarchy from USPSTF, 67, 68t
nonrandomized trials, 71, 71t
observational studies, 72
case reports and case series, 74–75, 75t
case-control studies, 73, 73t

cohort studies, 72, 72*t*
    cross-sectional studies, 74, 74*t*
    randomized trials, 69–70, 70*t*
Clinical trials database, 67
COCs. *See* Combined oral contraceptives (COCs)
Cohort studies, 72, 72*t*
Coitally related methods, 2*t*
Coitus interruptus. *See* Withdrawal
Colorado Family Planning initiative, 170
Colorectal cancer, 258
Combined hormonal contraceptives (CHCs)
    cancer effects
        breast cancer, 251–254, 259–260
        cervical cancer, 256–260
        colorectal cancer, 258
        endometrial cancer, 255
        liver cancer, 258–259
        lymphatic/hematopoietic cancers, 259
        melanoma, 259
        ovarian cancer, 255–256
    cardiovascular effects
        arterial thrombosis (myocardial infarction and stroke), 243–248
        hypertension, 242–243
        inherited thrombophilias, 241–242
        thrombosis, 248–251
        venous thromboembolism, 233–242, 250*t*
    contraceptive effects, 228–229
    ethinyl estradiol, 219–220
    eye/ear diseases, 271
    gastrointestinal
        gallbladder, 267
        general inflammatory bowel disease, 267–268
        liver adenomas, 267
        ulcerative colitis, 267–268
    hematologic effects, 270
    hepatic effects, 229
    infectious disease
        cervicitis, 269–270
        human immunodeficiency virus, 268
        pelvic inflammatory disease, 270
        vaginitis (BV/Trichomonas/ Candidiasis), 269
    initiation and management, 271–274
    libido, 265–266
    mestranol, 219–220
    metabolic effects, 230–233
        carbohydrate metabolism, 232–233
        lipoproteins and oral contraception, 231–232
        weight gain, 230

mood and PMS, 265
multiple sclerosis, 271
pharmacodynamics
    contraceptive effects, 228–229
    hepatic effects, 229
postpartum and postabortion use, 274–275
prolactin-secreting adenomas, 270–271
reproductive system
    during early pregnancy, 260–261
    fertility, 261
    gynecologic effects, 262–264
    polycystic ovary syndrome, 263–264
    pregnancy outcome, 262
    spontaneous abortion, 261
skin, 266–267
variations in oral formulations
    extended cycle, 223–224
    extended regimen, 221–223
    phasic regimens, 221
    unrelated to hormonal content, 224–225
Combined oral contraceptives (COCs). *See* Combined hormonal contraceptives (CHCs)
Condoms. *See also* Barrier methods of contraception
    declined to teens, 19
    female, 341–342, 359–360
        Cupid, 359–360
        FC1® condom, 359
        FC2® condom, 359
        multiple uses, 359
        prelubrication, 359
        protection from STIs, 342
        as single-use internal condom, 360
    male (*see* Male condom)
Confidence interval, 78–79
Contraception
    declination of teen pregnancy, 19
    education methods of effectiveness, 24, 25*f*
    efficacy, 12–16
    failures, 14–16, 15*t*
    Family Planning Health Encounter, 24, 25*f*
    historical background, 6–12
        birth control pill, 8–10
        hormonal contraception development, 8–10
        intrauterine device, 10–11
        LARC revolution, 11
        male contraception development, 11–12
        prior to modern era, 7–8

Contraception (*Continued*)
  life-table analysis, 14
  and litigation, 24, 26
  Pearl Index, 12–13
  perfect and typical failure rate for, 14–16,
    15*t*
  public funding of, 20–23
  in United States
    induced abortion, 23
    LARC methods and permanent
      methods, 17
    nonuse women, 16–17
    NSFG surveys, 16
    teen pregnancy, 19
    trends, 17–18, 18*f*
    unintended pregnancy, 17, 18*f*
Contraceptive effects, 228–229
Contraceptive gel, 343
Contraceptive sponge
  effectiveness, 352
  lower rates of infection, 352–353
  Protectaid®, 352
  side effects, 352–353
  Today®, 352
  vaginal, 352
Copper intrauterine device (Cu-IUD), 171,
    173–174, 315
  emergency contraception
    accessibility, 401
    advantages/disadvantages, 400
    complications, 401
    copper T380 IUD, 400
    effectiveness, 400
  intrauterine contraception
    Copper 7, 172*f*
    Cu-Fix, 173–174
    emergency contraception, 201–202
    FlexiGard, 173–174
    GyneFIX, 173–174
    magnetic resonance imaging, 187
    Multiload-375, 173
    Nova T, 171–173, 172*f*
    Saf-T-Coil, 172*f*
    TCu-380 Slimline, 172*f*, 173
    TCu-380A, 172*f*, 173
    TCu-200B, 172*f*
    TCu-220C, 173
Corticotropin-binding globulin (CBG), 229
Counseling, 12
Crossover randomized trials, 69
Cross-sectional studies, 74, 74*t*
Cu-IUD. *See* Copper intrauterine device
    (Cu-IUD)
Cupid female condom, 359–360
Cycle length–based methods

Apps based, 372–373
  algorithms, 372
  DaysyView, 377
  DOT model, 372
  features, 377
  on menstrual cycle data, 373
  Natural Cycles, 377
  ovulation timing, 372
  Symptopro and Lady Cycle, 378
calendar method and rhythm method,
    370–371
Standard Days Method (CycleBeads),
    371–372, 371*f*
CycleBeads, 371–372, 371*f*
Cytochrome P450 (CYP) enzymes, 57–58,
    334

D
Dalkon Shield, 170–173, 187–188
Darunavir, 334
DaysyView, 377
Depot medroxyprogesterone acetate
    (DMPA), 2*t*, 14–16, 301, 302*t*
  advantage, 316
  amenorrhea, 40
  availability, 301–303
  bleeding irregularities, 303–304
  comparative trial of NET-EN and, 303
  dosage level, 301–303
  duration of action, 309
  indications, 301–303
  by intramuscular/subcutaneous injec-
    tion, 301
  late reinjections, 309
  medical eligibility criteria, 316
  metabolic effects, 311–313
    bone, 311–312
    cardiovascular, 312
    general metabolism/weight gain,
      312–313
  with mifepristone, 317–318
  pharmacodynamic effects, 309
  pharmacokinetic studies, 304–306, 304*f*
  prevalence, 303
  protects against ectopic pregnancy, 308
  self-injection, 303
  unscheduled bleeding, 310–311
Desogestrel, 53, 53*f*, 329, 330*t*, 331–333
Diabetes mellitus, 232
  insulin-dependent, 233
  IUD insertion, 193
  non–insulin-dependent, 383
Diaphragm. *See* Barrier methods of
    contraception

Dienogest, 54, 55*f*, 61
DMPA. *See* Depot medroxyprogesterone acetate (DMPA)
D-norgestrel, 53
Doxycycline, 310–311
Drospirenone, 55, 55*f*, 61, 329, 330*t*, 331–334
Dynamic optimal timing (DOT) model, 372

E
EC. *See* Emergency contraception (EC)
Ectopic pregnancy, 141
    emergency contraception, 405
    lowest rates, 184–185, 185*t*
    women with previous ectopic, 184
EE. *See* Ethinyl estradiol (EE)
Efavirenz, 334
Ehrlich, Paul, 1, 5
Emergency contraception (EC)
    abortifacient, 406
    characteristics, 397, 398*t*
    copper IUD, 400–401
    drug interactions, 405
    levonorgestrel
        advantages, 403–404
        clinical guidelines, 403–404, 403*t*
        differential effect on LH, 403
        efficacy, 403
        side effects, 403
    levonorgestrel 52 mg intrauterine system, 404
    measuring efficacy, 399–400, 399*f*
    mifepristone, 405
    as "morning-after pill," 397
    in postabortion and postpartum period, 407
    progestin-only, 397–399
    randomized comparative trial, 397–399
    resources, 407
    risk of
        access issues, 406
        ectopic pregnancy, 405
        emesis, 405
        intrauterine pregnancy, 406
        repeated usage risk, 405
    as routine contraception, 406
    side effects, 397–399
    ulipristal acetate, 401–402
        accessibility in U.S., 402
        clinical guidance recommendation, 402
        clinical trials, 401
        delay ovulation, 401
        efficacy, 401
        IUD placement, 402
        limitation, 402
        oral agent, 401
        as progesterone receptor agonist, 401
        randomized controlled trial, 402
        risk factors, 401–402
        side effects, 402
    Yuzpe method, 404
Endometrial cancer, 255
    IUD, 181–182
    Norplant, 146–147
Endometriosis
    and dysmenorrhea, 262–263
    levonorgestrel IUS, 180–181
    progestin-only contraceptive methods, 146–147
    suppression of, 180
Enovid, 46
Epidemiology
    attributable risk, 79
    cause-and-effect relationship, 81, 84
    confidence interval, 78–79
    definition, 81
    examples, 82*t*
    number of individuals, 79
    odds ratio, 78, 81
    p value, 79
    rate of disease, 81
    relative risk, 78, 81
EQUATOR Network, 83
Essure, 101–104, 103*f*
Estetrol, 48
Estradiol, 47
Estriol, 48
Estrogens
    in combined hormonal contraception, 48–49, 49*f*
    estetrol, 48
    estradiol, 47
    estriol, 48
    estrone, 47
    production, 37
    SHBG induction by, 57–58
Estrone, 47
Ethinyl estradiol (EE), 48, 57–58, 219–220, 310–311
Ethynodiol diacetate, 329, 330*t*, 331
Etonogestrel, 61, 135
Etonogestrel single-rod implant, 133, 134*f*
EU Clinical Trials Register, 67
Evidence for Contraceptive Options and HIV Outcomes (ECHO) study, 315
Extended cycle, 223–224
Extended regimen
    "escape" follicular activity, 223
    hormone-free interval, 221–222

Extended regimen (*Continued*)
 hypothalamic-pituitary-ovarian (HPO)
  axis, 221
 withdrawal bleeding, 222

F
FABMs. *See* Fertility awareness–based
  methods (FABMs)
Factor V Leiden mutation, 241
Failure rates
 perfect, 14, 15*t*
 typical, 14, 15*t*
Fallopian tube
 anatomy, 97*f*
 laparoscopic methods, 94
 postpartum, 97–98
 removal, 114
Family Planning Health Encounter,
  24, 25*f*
Female condom, 341–342, 359–360
 Cupid, 359–360
 FC1® condom, 359
 FC2® condom, 359
 multiple uses, 359
 prelubrication, 359
 protection from STIs, 342
 as single-use internal condom, 360
Female permanent contraception
 complications, 95–96
 counseling for, 114–117
 disadvantages, 95
 ectopic pregnancy, 112–114
 hysteroscopic methods, 101–109
 interval procedures, 95–96
 menstrual function, 115–116
 ovarian cancer risk reduction, 113–114
 reversibility, 116–117
 sexuality, 115
 total salpingectomy, 100
 transcervical approaches, 100–101
 tubal occlusion or excision, 96–100, 97*f*
 vaginal approach, 109
Female sterilization. *See* Permanent
  contraception
FemBloc™, 101
FemCap, 342, 351, 351*f*
Fertility, 261
 awareness approaches, 369*b*
 Billings technique, 373
 effects, future, 144
 IUD removal, 199
 reproduction after discontinuing combined hormonal contraception,
  261–262

Fertility awareness–based methods
  (FABMs), 2*t*, 341
 clinical trials, 368
 cycle length–based methods (*see* Cycle
  length–based methods)
 to detect at-risk days, 367, 369, 369*b*
 estimation of, 367–368
 failure rates, 368–369
 mixed methods
  symptohormonal methods, 376–377
  symptothermal methods, 376
 natural family planning, 369–370
 ovulation cycles and fertilization, 370
 reproductive plan, 368
 sign/symptom-based ovulation detection,
  373–376
  Basal Body Temperature Method, 375
  Billings ovulation method, 373–374
  hormonal testing, 375–376
  mucin composition, 373
  time of ovulation, 373
  TwoDay Method, 374–375
 systematic review, 368
 theoretical concerns, 378
 and withdrawal, 387
Fibroplant, 176
Filshie clip, 97–98, 98*f*–99*f*
Flexible cycle, 224
Follicle-stimulating hormone (FSH), 32, 385
Fosamprenavir, 334

G
Galactorrhea, 144
Gastrointestinal
 gallbladder, 267
 general inflammatory bowel disease,
  267–268
 liver adenomas, 267
 ulcerative colitis, 267–268
Generic oral contraceptives, 62
Gestodene, 53, 53*f*
Gonadotropin-releasing hormone (GnRH),
  32
Google®, 372
Gynecologic effects, 262–264
 dysmenorrhea/endometriosis, 262–263
 heavy menstrual bleeding/anemia, 262

H
Healthy user effect, 238–239
Heart disease, 193, 316
 coronary, 110, 232
 rheumatic, 243–245

Heavy uterine bleeding, 171
Hematologic effects, 270
Hepatic effects, 229
Hirsutism, 37, 55, 57, 144, 187, 263–264
Human chorionic gonadotropin (hCG), 32
Human population
    contraception history, 6–12
        birth control pill, 8–10
        hormonal contraception development,
            8–10
        intrauterine device, 10–11
        LARC revolution, 11
        male contraception development,
            11–12
        prior to modern era, 7–8
    and environment, 5–6
    growth, 2–5, 2*t*
    hazards of unchecked, 1
    peak population, 2–5, 3*f*
    rate of, 1
    resources of Earth, 1
    technologic associated with, 2
    voluntary family planning, 1
Hypertension
    cardiovascular effects, 242–243
    during pregnancy, 237
    risk factor for stroke, 246, 249
    women with treated hypertension, 243
Hypothalamic gonadotropin-releasing
        hormone (GnRH), 32
Hypothalamic-pituitary-ovarian (HPO)
        axis, 35–36, 35*f*
Hysteroscopic methods, 94, 101–109
    Adiana, 101, 104
    advantage, 99–100
    disadvantage, 100
    Essure, 101–104, 103*f*
    vs. laparoscopic method, 104–109, 107*t*

I
Implanon, 133, 135, 151–153
Implantable contraception, 133
    acne and, 145–146
    advantages, 138–139
    body weight and, 137–138
    bone density, 144
    breastfeeding women and, 148
    counseling women, 157–158
    cross-sectional anatomy of upper arm,
        149, 149*f*
    disadvantages, 139–140
        complicated removals, 139
        cost, 139–140
        disruption of bleeding patterns, 139

        protection against sexually transmitted
            infections, 139
        visible under the skin, 140
    drug interactions, 136*f*, 137–138
    effects on future fertility, 144
    efficacy, 140–141
    etonogestrel single-rod implant, 133, 134*f*
    galactorrhea and, 144
    Implanon, 133, 135, 151–153
    implant discontinuation, 146
    implant systems
        etonogestrel, 135
        levonorgestrel, 134–135
    indications, 136–158
    insertion technique
        anesthesia, 150
        complications, 151–152
        expulsion, 152
        infection, 152
        local reactions, 152
        marking and location, 149, 149*f*
        patient positioning, 148–149
        placement, 150–151, 155*f*–156*f*
    Jadelle, 151
    levels of sex hormone-binding globulin
        (SHBG) and, 137–138
    mastalgia and, 144
    mechanism of action, 136–137, 136*f*
    modes of action, 138
    Norplant, 133–135, 140, 146, 152–153
    ovarian cysts, 146
    postpartum and postabortal use, 158
    progestin blood levels, 146–147
    protection against sexually transmitted
        infections, 139
    reinsertion, 156
    removal techniques
        modified vasectomy forceps, 155*f*,
            156*f*, 155
        nonpalpable implant, 155
        palpable implant, 153–154
    return of fertility, 138–139
    risk of breast and cervical cancer, 146–147
    risk of endometrial cancer, 146–147
    risk of ovarian cancer, 146–147
    side effects, 144–145
    treatment of bleeding with implants, 157
    user acceptance of contraceptive
        implants, 157
    weight change, 145
Implants. *See* Implantable contraception
Inert devices (historic), 172–173
Infectious disease
    cervicitis, 269–270
    human immunodeficiency virus, 268

Infectious disease (*Continued*)
  pelvic inflammatory disease, 270
  vaginitis (BV/Trichomonas/Candidiasis),
    269
Inherited thrombophilias, 241
Inhibin B, 32
Injectable contraception
  alternative delivery formulations, 317
  combined injectable methods, 302*t*,
    303–304
  depot-medroxyprogesterone acetate (*see*
    Depot medroxyprogesterone acetate
    (DMPA))
  efficacy, 308–310
  estradiol cypionate/estradiol valerte, 301,
    302*t*
  incidence, 301
  mechanism of action/pharmacodynam-
    ics, 306–308, 307*f*
  medical eligibility criteria, 316
  medroxyprogesterone acetate, 301, 302*t*
  pharmacokinetics, 304–306, 304*f*
  postpartum and postabortion use,
    317–318
  progestin norethindrone enanthate
    (NET-EN), 301, 302*t*
  risk factors
    cancer, 314
    sexually transmitted infection and
      HIV, 314–315
  single injection dose, 301
  in special populations, 315–316
  unique features, 313
Insulin
  fasting, 264
  sensitivity, 232
Insulin-dependent diabetes mellitus
  copper IUD, 193
  women with, 233
Intrauterine contraception
  actinomyces, 188–189
  adolescents, 192
  amenorrhea and, 185
  antiproliferative effect, 186–187
  bacterial vaginosis, 187
  bleeding and cramping, 186
  CHOICE study, 170
  chorioamnionitis, 191
  congenital anomalies, 191
  copper IUD
    Copper 7, 172*f*
    Cu-Fix, 173–174
    emergency contraception, 201–202
    FlexiGard, 173–174
    GyneFIX, 173–174

magnetic resonance imaging, 187
Multiload-375, 173
Nova T, 171–173, 172*f*
Saf-T-Coil, 172*f*
TCu-380 Slimline, 172*f*, 173
TCu-380A, 172*f*, 173
TCu-200B, 172*f*
TCu-220C, 173
efficacy of, 181
  ectopic pregnancy and, 184–185
  expulsion, 184
  intrauterine pregnancy, 175*t*,
    182–184
history, 170–174
hormone-releasing, 174–176, 175*t*
inert devices (historic), 172–173
infections
  bacterial infection, 187–188
  endometritis, 189
  protection against STIs, 187–188
  risk of human immunodeficiency
    virus (HIV) transmission, 189–190
  risk of pelvic inflammatory disease,
    188, 189*b*
  vaginal infection, 188–189
insertion of the IUD, 193–198
  in breast-feeding, 193
  CDC recommendations, 194, 194*b*
  Chlamydia and gonorrhea screening,
    194
  follow-up, 198
  Liletta® inserter, 196, 197*f*
  Mirena® inserter, 196, 197*f*
  Paragard® inserter, 196, 196*f*–197*f*
  suspected perforation management,
    197–198
  timing, 194–195
IUD evidence *vs.* myths
  emergency contraception, 179
  evidence-based statements, 176
  mechanism of action, 177–179, 178*f*
IUD removal, 199–201
  embedded IUDs, 199–201
  missing IUD, 201
Lippes loop, 172–173, 172*f*
lowest ectopic pregnancy rates, 184–185,
  185*t*
menstrual blood loss, 186
menstrual pain, 185
noncontraceptive benefits, 179–182, 180*b*
  LNG 52-mg IUS, 179, 180*b*
patient selection, 191–193
  abnormalities of uterine anatomy,
    192–193
  diabetes mellitus, 193

immunosuppressed patients, 193
in patient counseling, 191, 192*b*
Wilson's disease, 192–193
placental abruption, 191
post abortion, 202
postpartum use, 202–203
preterm labor and birth, 191
progestin-related side effects, 187
prophylactic antibiotics, 187–188
risk of invasive cervical cancer, 181–182
risks of endometrial cancer, 181–182
septic abortion, 190–191
spontaneous miscarriage, 190
treatment with a NSAID, 186
women with previous ectopic
lowest rates, 184–185, 185*t*
pregnancies, 184
worldwide use, 169–170, 169*t*
Intrauterine device (IUD), 10–11, 343
Intrauterine pregnancy
exposure to emergency contraception,
406
Irving method, 118, 121*f*
IUD-related bacterial infection, 187–188

J
Jadelle, 133

L
Lactational amenorrhea method (LAM), 367
bottle-feeding, 381
breastfeeding
inexpensive nutrition, 381
motivation to, 381
ovulated women, 386
prevalence, 381
revival of, 381
failure rates with, 386–387
lactation
antibodies, 383
calcium secretion, 383
cessation of, 384
contraceptive effect of, 384–385
maternal diet and hydration impact
on, 383
oxytocin effect, 383–384
prolactin secretion, 381–383
ovulation in breastfeeding women, 386
pregnancy risk, 386–387
Lady Cycle, 378
Laparoscopic methods, 94
LARC. *See* Long-acting reversible contraceptive (LARC) method

Latex condoms, 356
Levonorgestrel (LNG), 34, 38, 53, 61,
134–135, 310, 315, 329, 330*t*,
331–333, 336
emergency contraception, 397–399
advantages, 403–404
clinical guidelines, 403–404, 403*t*
differential effect on LH, 403
efficacy, 403
side effects, 403
LH. *See* Luteinizing hormone (LH)
Libido, 265–266, 369–370
Life-table analysis, 14
Liletta® inserter, 196, 197*f*
Lipoproteins, 231–232
Lippes loop, 10, 172–173, 172*f*
Liver cancer, 258–259
Long-acting progestin-releasing system, 171
Long-acting reversible contraceptive
(LARC) method, 2*t*, 11, 24, 341
Lowest-dose oral contraceptives, 62
Luteinizing hormone (LH), 32, 36, 401
Lymphatic/hematopoietic cancers, 259

M
Male condom, 341–342, 356–358
in clinical practice, 357
failure, 357–358
forms, 357
latex, 356
oil-based lubricants, 357–358
placements, 357–358, 357*f*
polyurethane, 356–357
prevents HPV and herpes simplex virus
transmission, 356
protection against STIs and HIV, 356
Male sterilization. *See* Permanent
contraception
Marker degradation, 43
Mastalgia, 144
Medical Eligibility Criteria for
Contraceptive Use (MEC), 84–86,
86*t*–90*t*
Medroxyprogesterone acetate (MPA), 301
Mefenamic acid, 310–311
Melanoma, 259
Men who have sex with men (MSM),
355–356
Menstrual bleeding effects, 141–143
Menstrual cycle length, Smart phone apps,
372–373
algorithms for fertility prediction, 372
Apple® and Google®, 372
DaysyView, 377

Menstrual cycle length, Smart phone apps (*Continued*)
DOT model, 372
features, 377
on menstrual cycle data, 373
Natural Cycles, 377
ovulation timing, 372
Symptopro and Lady Cycle, 378
ultrasound technology, 378
Menstruation, 39–40
Mesosalpinx bleeding, Silastic ring application, 100
Mestranol, 219–220
Metabolic effects, 230–233
carbohydrate metabolism, 232–233
lipoproteins and oral contraception, 231–232
weight gain, 230
Mifepristone, 56*f*, 317–318, 405
Migraine headaches, 246–247
Milex fitted silicone diaphragm, 343
Milex® Wide-Seal diaphragm, 344–345
Minilaparotomy
interval procedures, 95
tubal occlusion, 95
Minimally invasive vasectomy (MIV) technique, 110
Mirena® inserter, 196, 197*f*
Miscarriage, 190
Multiload-375, 173
Multiple sclerosis, 271
Multipurpose prevention technologies (MPT), 341
Myocardial infarction, 243–245, 244*t*, 247–248

N
National Survey of Family Growth (NSFG), 14, 367
Natural Cycles (smart phone app), 377
Nelfinavir, 334
Nestorone®, 317
NET-EN. *See* Norethindrone enanthate (NET-EN)
Nexplanon inserter, 133, 134*f*
Nomegestrol acetate, 61
Non-insulin-dependent diabetes mellitus, 193
Nonoxynol-9 (N-9) spermicide, 342, 352–355
Nonrandomized trials, 71, 71*t*
Nonsteroidal anti-inflammatory drugs (NSAIDs), 310–311
Norethindrone, 50*f*, 52, 329, 330*t*, 331–333

Norethindrone enanthate (NET-EN), 1, 301
availability, 303
combination injectables, 303
comparative trial of DMPA and, 303
Norethisterone, 329, 330*t*
Norgestimate, 53, 53*f*, 61
Norgestrel, 53, 329, 330*t*, 331, 333
Norplant, 133–135, 140, 146, 152–153
Nova T, 171–173, 172*f*

O
Obesity, 226, 232
Observational studies, 72
case reports and case series, 74–75, 75*t*
case-control studies, 73, 73*t*
cohort studies, 72, 72*t*
cross-sectional studies, 74, 74*t*
Odds ratio, 78, 81
Office-based removal procedures, 200
Oil-based lubricants, 357–358
Opportunistic salpingectomy, 100
Oral contraception. *See* Combined hormonal contraception
Oral emergency contraception (EC), 405–406
Oral formulations, variations in
extended cycle, 223–224
extended regimen, 221–223
phasic regimens, 221
unrelated to hormonal content, 224–225
Oral-genital intercourse, 380–381
Ortho All-Flex diaphragm, 343
Ovarian cancer, 255–256
Ovarian cysts, 146
Ovarian follicular cysts, 333

P
ParaGard, 171
Paragard® inserter, 196, 196*f*–197*f*
PATH (female condom), 359–360
Pearl Index (PI), 12–13, 377
Peptide hormones, 32–34
action, 32, 34*f*
binding nature, 32–33
effects of, 32–33
FSH and LH, 32
inhibin B, 32
receptor agonists and antagonists, 33–34
reproductive, 32
Periodic abstinence, 354, 367, 369, 371
Permanent contraception
barriers, 117–118
cumulative failure rate, 111–112, 111*t*

efficacy of, 111–112
in female
  complications, 95–96
  counseling for, 114–117
  disadvantages, 95
  ectopic pregnancy, 112–114
  hysteroscopic methods, 101–109
  interval procedures, 95–96
  menstrual function, 115–116
  ovarian cancer risk reduction, 113–114
  reversibility, 116–117
  sexuality, 115
  total salpingectomy, 100
  transcervical approaches, 100–101
  tubal occlusion or excision, 96–100, 97*f*
  vaginal approach, 109
history
  family planning, 93
  hysteroscopic methods, 94
  laparoscopic methods, 94
  risk of obstructed labor due to a contracted pelvis, 93
  Uchida method, 93
in male
  postvasectomy semen analysis, 109–110
  reversibility, 110–111
  vasectomy methods, 110
postabortion, 122–123
postpartum partial salpingectomy
  Irving method, 118, 121*f*
  Pomeroy method, 118, 119*f*–121*f*
  Uchida method, 118, 120*f*
in regions/countries, 93, 94*t*
in select regions/countries, 93, 94*t*
Permanent methods, 2*t*
Pharmacokinetics
  injectable contraception, 304–306, 304*f*
Physical barrier methods. *See* Barrier methods of contraception
Pinch technique, 380
Polycystic ovary syndrome (PCOS)
  androgenic symptoms, 263–264
  benign ovarian tumors and cysts, 264
  menstrual regulation, 263
  metabolic changes, 264
Polyurethane condoms, 356–357
Pomeroy method, 118, 119*f*–121*f*
POPs. *See* Progestin-only pills (POPs)
Postabortion, 274–275, 360
  considerations for, 335–336
  emergency contraception, 407
  injectable progestin-only contraceptives, 317–318
  vs. interval placement, 158
  lactational amenorrhea method, 381–386

period, emergency contraception in, 407
procedures, 122–123
progestin-only pills after, 335–336
use of IUDs, 202
Postpartum partial salpingectomy
  Irving method, 118, 121*f*
  Pomeroy method, 118, 119*f*–121*f*
  Uchida method, 118, 120*f*
Postpartum period
  emergency contraception in, 407
  injectable progestin-only contraceptives, 317–318
  progestin-only pills during, 335–336
Postvasectomy semen analysis (PVSA), 109–110
Power analysis, 81
Pregnancy
  mifepristone during, 56
  preventing method (*see* Emergency contraception (EC))
  probability of, 399, 399*f*
  teen, 19
  unintended, 17, 18*f*
Progestasert® IUD, 10
Progesterone
  actions of, 37, 38*f*
  albumin, binding globulin for, 56
  commercial manufacture, 44
  derivatives, 54, 54*f*, 55*f*
  levels of, 37–39
  marker degradation and, 43
  natural estrogens and, 47–48
  oral, 46
  ovulation inhibition by, 45
  production, 36, 38
  receptor, 34–36
  SPRMS (*see* Selective Progesterone Receptor Modulators)
  synthesis, 50
  withdrawal, 39
Progesterone vaginal ring (PVR), 335
Progestin-only pills (POPs)
  in adolescents, 332
  chlormadinone acetate, 329
  and combined oral contraceptives, 331
  desogestrel, 329
  drospirenone, 329
  drug interactions, 334
  efficacy, 331–332
  ethynodiol diacetate, 329
  levonorgestrel, 329
  mechanism of action, 331
  norethisterone, 329
  norgestrel, 329
  patient selection, 332

Progestin-only pills (POPs) (*Continued*)
  pill taking, 332–333
  for postpartum and postabortion use,
    335–336
  risks and benefits, 333–334
  side effects, 333
  transdermal and vaginal progestin-only
    contraceptives, 335
  U.S. availability, 329, 330*t*
Progestins/Progestogens, 51*t*, 60
  cardiovascular side effects, 50
  chemical structures, 57–58
  development, 50
  effect on liver, 57
  free form, 58
  history, 49–50, 43
  metabolism of, 57–58
  19-nortestosterone agents, 52–53,
    52*f*, 53*f*
  progesterone derivatives, 54, 54*f*, 55*f*
  spironolactones, 54–55, 55*f*
  synthetic, 48
Prolactin-secreting adenomas, 270–271
Protectaid® sponge, 352
Pulmonary embolism, 219–220

R
Randomized controlled trials (RCTs),
    69–70, 70*t*
Rapid reviews, 84
Relative risk, 78, 81
Reproduction and hormonal contraception
  development of, 31
  estrogen in combined hormonal contra-
    ceptives, 38*f*, 48–49
  historical background, 42–47
    hormonal oral contraceptive creation,
      44–47
    marker degradation and progesterone,
      43
    norethindrone and norethynodrel,
      43–44
    synthetic progestational drugs, 43–44
  mechanisms of action, 41–42
  oral contraceptive
    generation classification, 60
    high-dose and low-dose concept, 60
    history, 44–45
    progesterone, 45
  pharmacology *vs.* marketing
    dose *vs.* generation, 60
    generic products, 62
  potency, 62–63
  progestins (*see* Progestins)

reproductive endocrinology and physiol-
    ogy, 31
  cervix, 40–41
  corpus luteum, ovulation and develop-
    ment, 37–39, 38*f*
  dominant follicle development, 37
  hypothalamic-pituitary-ovarian axis,
    35–36, 35*f*
  menstruation, 39–40
  peptide hormones, 32–34, 34*f*
  steroid hormones (*see* Steroid hormones)
  selective progesterone receptor modula-
    tors, 55–56
Reproductive system
  during early pregnancy, 260–261
  fertility, 261
  gynecologic effects, 262–264
    dysmenorrhea/endometriosis,
      262–263
    heavy menstrual bleeding/anemia, 262
  polycystic ovary syndrome
    androgenic symptoms, 263–264
    benign ovarian tumors and cysts, 264
    menstrual regulation, 263
    metabolic changes, 264
  pregnancy outcome, 262
  spontaneous abortion, 261

S
Saquinavir, 334
Scoping reviews, 84
Selected Practice Recommendations for
    Contraceptive Use (SPR), 84–86
Selective estrogen receptor modulators
    (SERMs), 34
Selective progesterone receptor modulators
    (SPRMs), 34, 55–56
Self-stimulation, 380–381
Sex education
  and contraception counseling of teens, 19
Sex hormone–binding globulin (SHBG),
    229, 333
Sex steroids, 32, 48
Sexually transmitted infections (STIs)
  barrier methods, 342
  condoms, 115, 342
  and HIV risk, 314–315
  rate of, 188
  social impact, 341
  tubal infertility, 342
Short-acting hormonal methods, 14–16, 15*t*
Shorter-acting progestin-only methods. *See*
    Progestin-only pills (POPs)
Silastic, (Falope or Yoon) ring, 97, 99–100, 99*f*

Skin, 266–267
  acne, 266
  chloasma, 267
Smoking
  arterial thrombosis, 243
  effect in women, 247–248
  and estrogen, 249
  ischemic stroke, 245–246
  venous thromboembolism risk, 237, 248
Spermicides, 351, 353–355
  acid-buffering gel, 353
  advantages, 354
  Amphora™, 353
  application instructions, 353
  BufferGel, 353
  commercial availability, 353
  Contragel®, 353
  efficacy, 354
  Gynol II®, 353
  modern, 353
  nonoxynol-9, 342
  protection against STIs, 353–354
  RepHresh™ and Replens™, 353
  side effects, 354–355
17α-spirolactones, 54
Spironolactones, 54–55, 55f
Sponge. *See* Contraceptive sponge
Spontaneous abortion, 261
SPRMs. *See* Selective progesterone receptor
        modulators (SPRMs)
St. John's wort, 334
Standard Days Method, 371–372
Standard diaphragm
  fitting set, 345, 346f–350f
  placement, 345, 346f–350f
  self-insertion of, 345, 346f–350f
  self-removal technique, 345, 346f–350f
State-of-the-art reviews, 84
Statistical tests, 80–82
Sterilization
  failure, 106–108
  female, 97
  hormonal, 31
  hysteroscopic, 106, 107t, 112
  laparoscopic, 96, 112
  male, 94–95
  quinacrine, technique of, 100–101
  tubal, 115–117
Steroid hormones
  biologic response, 31–32
  blood transport, 56
  circulation, 32
  classical mechanism of, 32, 33f
  discovery, 42–43
  lipid-like nature of, 31

  metabolism, 56–59
  pharmacology of
    combined hormonal contraceptives,
        estrogen in, 48–49, 49f
    estrogens, 47–48
    progestins (*see* Progestins)
    progestogen, 48
  route of administration, metabolism, and
        excretion, 57–59
  practical aspect of, 58–59, 59f
STIs. *See* Sexually transmitted infections (STIs)
Stroke
  arterial thrombosis, 245–247
  in healthy, nonsmoking women, regard-
        less of age, 249
  incidence in reproductive age women,
        245–246, 245t
  risk in migraineurs, 247
Symptohormonal methods, 376–377
Symptopro, 378
Symptothermal methods, 376
Syntex, 8, 43–44, 46–47
Systematic reviews
  clinical practice guidelines
    Centers for Disease Control and
        Prevention, 89
    definition, 84–86
    examples for family planning and
        reproductive health, 84–86, 85t
    Medical Eligibility Criteria for
        Contraceptive Use, 84–86, 86t–90t
    recommendations for clinical care,
        84–86
    Selected Practice Recommendations
        for Contraceptive Use, 84
    sources of, 84–86
    trustworthy, 84–86, 84t
    updated guidance, 90
  Cochrane Database of Systematic
        Reviews, 84
  evidence
    clinical practice guidelines, 84–90,
        84t, 85t
    reporting, 83–84
    synthesizing, 83
  fertility awareness-based methods, 368
  and meta-analysis, 84
  sources, 83
  types of, 83

T
Tamoxifen, 40
Teen pregnancy, 19
TFR. *See* Total fertility rate (TFR)

Thrombosis
case-control study, 219–220
and combination hormonal
contraceptives, 248–251
arterial thrombosis, 243–248
epidemiological studies, 234–240
Thyroid-binding globulin (TBG), 229
Thyroid-stimulating hormone (TSH), 382–383
Thyrotropin-releasing hormone (TRH), 382
Tipranavir, 334
Today® sponge, 352
Total fertility rate (TFR), 1–4, 3*f*
Total salpingectomy, 100
Toxic shock syndrome, 342
Tranexamic acid, 310–311
Trichomonas, 344
Trustworthy clinical practice guidelines,
84–86, 84*t*
Tubal occlusion
with clips and rings
Filshie clip, 97–98, 98*f*–99*f*
silastic, (Falope or Yoon) ring, 97,
99–100, 99*f*
by electrosurgical methods, 96–97, 97*f*
TwoDay method, 374–375, 387
Typical failure rate, 14, 15*t*

U
Uchida method, 93, 118, 120*f*
Ulcerative colitis, 267–268
Ulipristal acetate (UPA), 34
emergency contraception, 401–402
accessibility in U.S., 402
clinical guidance recommendation, 402
clinical trials, 401
delay ovulation, 401
efficacy, 401
IUD placement, 402
limitation, 402
oral agent, 401
as progesterone receptor agonist, 401
randomized controlled trial, 402
risk factors, 401–402
side effects, 402
structure of, 56*f*
Unintended pregnancy, 78
U.S. Medical Eligibility Criteria for
Contraceptive Use, 84–86, 86*t*–90*t*

U.S. Preventive Services Task Force
Evidence Grading Scheme, 67, 68*t*

V
VA w.o.w.®, 359–360
VACTERL complex, 260
Vaginal approach, 109
Vaginal estrogen-progestin contraception,
251
Vasectomy. *See* Permanent contraception
Venous thromboembolism (VTE), 241
attributable risk, 79
cardiovascular effects, 233–240, 236*t*
EE administration risk, 57
incidence, 241–242, 242*t*
and inherited thrombophilias, 241–242
vs. oral contraceptives, 9
with POPs, 333–334
relative risk and incidence, 242*t*

W
Weight gain, 145, 230
Wilson's disease, 192–193
Withdrawal method
estimation, 367–368
and FABM, 387
first-year failure rate, 379
history, 378
impending ejaculation, 379
Onanism, 378
practice, 378–379
pregnancy rate, 368
prevalence, 378
reproductive plan, 368
risk of pregnancy, 379
use and satisfactory method, 379–380
variations in, 380
Women's Contraceptive and Reproductive
Experiences (CARE), 314
World Health Organization's Special
Programme of Research in Human
Reproduction, 303
World population, 2–3, 3*f*

Y
Yuzpe method, 397–399, 404